UNDERSTANDING YOUR HEALTH

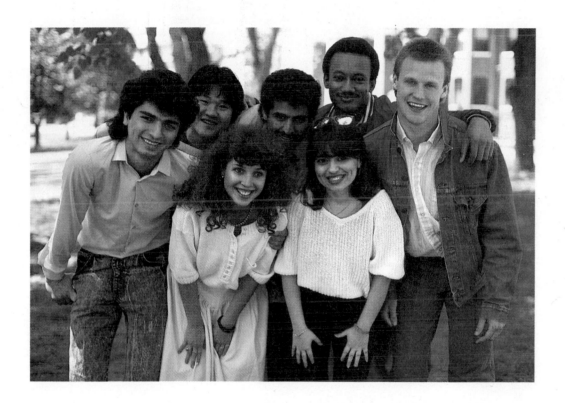

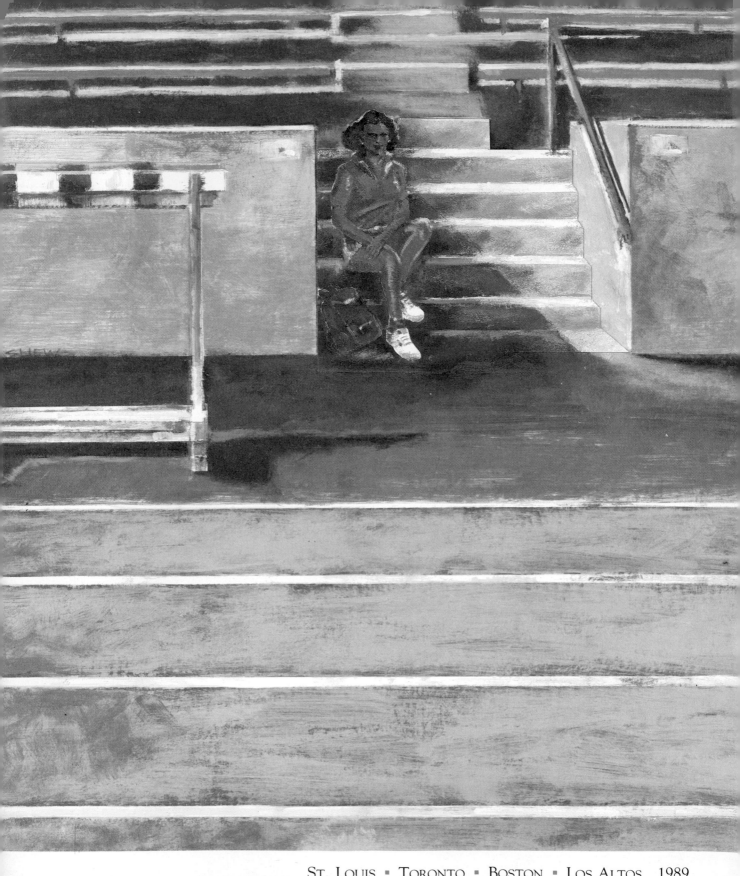

ST. LOUIS ▪ TORONTO ▪ BOSTON ▪ LOS ALTOS   1989

UNDERSTANDING YOUR HEALTH

WAYNE A. PAYNE, Ed.D.

DALE B. HAHN, Ph.D.

BALL STATE UNIVERSITY
MUNCIE, INDIANA

SECOND EDITION

Illustrated

TIMES MIRROR/MOSBY ▪ COLLEGE PUBLISHING

Publisher **Nancy K. Roberson**
Senior Developmental Editor **Michelle A. Turenne**
Project Manager **Suzanne Seeley**
Production Editor **Kathy Burmann**
Designer **Liz Fett**
Illustrator **Don O'Connor, Barbara Cousins**
Cover Illustration **John Shew**

Credits for all materials used by permission appear after the index.

SECOND EDITION

Copyright © 1989 by Times Mirror/Mosby College Publishing

A division of The C.V. Mosby Company
11830 Westline Industrial Drive
St. Louis, Missouri 63146

Previous edition copyrighted 1986

Printed in the United States of America

Library of Congress Cataloging in Publication Data

Payne, Wayne A.
    Understanding your health / Wayne A. Payne, Dale B. Hahn.—2nd
ed.
        p.   cm.
    Includes bibliographies and index.
    ISBN 0-8016-5164-6
    1. Health. 2. College students—Health and hygiene. I. Hahn,
Dale B. II. Title.
    RA777.3.P39   1989   88-13627
    613—dc19   CIP

C/VH/VH 9 8 7 6 5 4 3 2 1

To
Our Wives
Ruth and Ellen
and
Our Children
Andrew and Ellen
Leslie and Laura

Preface

When we wrote the first edition of *Understanding Your Health*, we realized that we were taking a risk by making a major departure from traditional college personal health textbooks. To make a health text really meaningful for college students, we were convinced that the book had to carry students *beyond* standard health information, healthful suggestions, and personal inventories. Our book had to make meaningful connections between health information and the lives of college students. The overwhelming success of the first edition indicates to us that our risk was worth taking.

The second edition of *Understanding Your Health* continues our approach of framing health content around two independent but related focuses: the *multiple dimensions of health* and the *developmental tasks of young adults*. Only when using our text will students be able to consistently consider health information from the physical, emotional, social, intellectual, and spiritual dimensions. *Understanding Your Health* also clearly and consistently reminds students that their health allows them to achieve personally satisfying lives by helping them master the important developmental tasks that confront them:

- Forming an initial adult self-identity
- Assuming increasing levels of responsibility
- Establishing a sense of relative independence
- Developing the skills for social interaction

This second edition of *Understanding Your Health* retains this academic approach with a carefully written, well-documented manuscript. *Understanding Your Health* is written by two health educators who teach the personal health course on a daily basis. None of our text has been written by journalists, contributors, graduate students, or ghost writers. It continues to acknowledge that students and professors seek sound, up-to-date material in an attractive, meaningful manner.

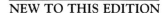

NEW TO THIS EDITION

The second edition of *Understanding Your Health* incorporates several new features to enhance student learning. The following summarizes these new features.

Presentation of Conceptual Theme Modified. Based on feedback from users and nonusers alike, application of the two conceptual threads (health dimensions and developmental tasks) helps this book stand alone. However, we have decided in this edition to alter the manner in which these threads are presented. Rather than being presented on a chapter-by-chapter basis, these threads are now presented at the start and completion of each of the text's seven units. By organizing the text in this fashion, we have been able to retain the significance

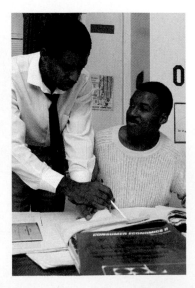

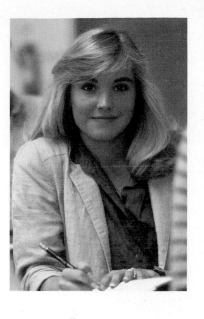

of the two conceptual threads and free up additional space for new health information.

Reorganization of Chapters. Users of the first edition of *Understanding Your Health* will immediately notice three changes in chapter organization. Our mental health chapter ("Achieving Emotional Maturity and Spiritual Growth: Keys to Your Mental Health"), Chapter 2, now comes *before* our stress management chapter ("Stress: Managing the Unexpected"), Chapter 3. The chapter on drug use ("Psychoactive Drugs: Use, Misuse, and Abuse"), Chapter 7, now precedes the chapter on alcohol use ("Alcohol: Responsible Choices"), Chapter 8.

The reorganization of some of the content in our sexuality unit (Chapters 13 through 16) should enhance student learning. We have now placed much of the anatomical and physiological information earlier in this unit. Also, our contraception chapter ("Fertility Control: An Exercise of Responsible Choice") has become Chapter 15 and now precedes the chapter on parenthood and birth.

New and Expanded Content Areas. In addition to updating information that appeared in the first edition (for example, we greatly expanded the section on AIDS), we have added many new topics that will be of interest to today's students. Approximately 40 new sections or subsections have been written for this edition. A sampling of some of the new topics is presented below:

Chapter 2 ▪ Factors that influence personality
▪ Characteristics of a mentally healthy person

Chapter 3 ▪ Life-centered stressors
▪ Type T personality

Chapter 4 ▪ Exercise for older adults
▪ Low impact aerobics
▪ Crosstraining

Chapter 5 ▪ Nutrient density
▪ Low-calorie fat substitutes

Chapter 7 ▪ Crack and freebase cocaine
▪ Drug testing
▪ Designer drugs

Chapter 8 ▪ Denial, enabling, and confrontation
▪ Inherited alcohol predisposition and personality traits related to alcoholism
▪ Alcoholism and the family

Chapter 10 ▪ Peripheral artery disease
▪ Heart transplants and artificial hearts

Chapter 12 ▪ Chronic Epstein-Barr virus syndrome

Chapter 14 ▪ Love
▪ Improving marriage
▪ Sexual victimization (rape and sexual assault, date rape, child sexual abuse, sexual harassment, commercialization of sex)
▪ Bisexuality

Chapter 15 ▪ Outercourse
▪ Morning-after pill
▪ Vaginal contraceptive film
▪ Infertility (artificial insemination, in vivo fertilization, GIFT procedure, surrogate parenting, how to reduce the chances of infertility)
▪ Birth technology

Chapter 19 ▪ The joys of midlife
▪ Sexuality and aging

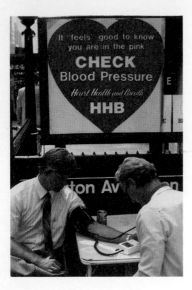

Full-color Throughout the Text. By no means has the emphasis on excellent content minimized *Understanding Your Health's* judicious use of illustrative support. As professors, we understand how important it is for students to be enthused about their assignments. Nearly all illustrations from the first edition have been replaced with full-color illustrations. We are certain that this full-color feature will make the second edition of *Understanding Your Health* especially exciting and inviting to today's college students in addition to enhancing comprehension of important concepts and applications.

Two New Appendixes. This edition features two new appendixes that depict the various systems of the body and mental disorders and therapies. These offer a quick reference to students and instructors seeking additional anatomical and mental health information.

Health Reference Guide. This guide lists the most commonly used resources that may have an impact on one's health. Perforated and laminated, this guide provides information students can keep for later use, such as national hotline phone numbers.

UNIQUE FEATURES

The second edition of *Understanding Your Health* continues to reflect our commitment to writing a text that provides a refreshingly different approach to the study of personal health. As hundreds of professors have indicated, this perspective is academically sound and personally meaningful to today's college students.

Conceptual Approach. This book's unique approach is consistently evident throughout the text. Each of the seven units in *Understanding Your Health* begins with a discussion of the upcoming content's relationship to the multiple dimensions of health. Each unit ends with a discussion of the relationship between the content and the four developmental tasks. Unlike other health books, we provide these two threads in a well-developed fashion throughout the book—not just in one or two isolated chapters or boxes.

Student Audience. This text is intended for traditional-age college students *and* older, nontraditional-age students. We have not ignored the increasing numbers of nontraditional students who have decided to pursue a college education. Frequent points within the discussion concern the lives of these nontraditional students. *Understanding Your Health* continues to encourage nontraditional students to achieve their goals in life.

Documentation. The second edition of *Understanding Your Health* continues its tradition of being the most comprehensively documented personal health text available. Numerous direct references to journals, scholarly books, and health agency materials help students and professors understand that they are reading the most current information concerning personal health issues.

Authorship. One continuing feature of this text is that it is written entirely by the authors. Both authors regularly teach the personal health course to nearly 1,000 students each year. By being colleagues at the same university, the authors have been able to maintain the highest level of content integration and consistency of writing style.

ADDITIONAL FEATURES

This book has been organized into seven major units that follow a sequence that seems appropriate for most personal health courses. However, instructors can easily rearrange the order in which they present the units or chapters to fit their personal needs. Each chapter can "stand alone" in terms of the order of presentation.

We encourage instructors and students to start with Chapter 1. "Health: Support for Your Future" introduces students to the two principal threads *Understanding Your Health* uses in all of its units—the multiple dimensions of health and the developmental tasks of young adulthood. Written clearly and concisely, Chapter 1 establishes the tone and framework for the remainder of the book.

As you read through the table of contents, you will see that all of the topics appropriate to a college personal health course are addressed. In addition, you will discover that Chapter 2 ("Achieving Emotional Maturity and Spiritual Growth: Keys to Your Mental Health") is unique. This is a mental health chapter that does not focus on pathology but rather on a process that students can use to enhance their emotional maturity, responsibility, independence, and happiness. One unique section in Chapter 2 expands on the concept of faith—not just in its religious application, but rather in the growth of beliefs that are important to the young adult.

The remaining chapter titles in *Understanding Your Health* will certainly seem familiar. However, within each chapter's content, the underlying strengths of this book emerge. Users of *Understanding Your Health* report that this book stands apart from other personal health books because it is skillfully written in a manner that conveys accuracy, sensitivity, and scholarship. It is challenging without being overwhelming to students. Technical, complex issues and concepts are presented in a clear, undistorted manner. We have made a concerted effort to elevate the consciousness of the students about the value of their health and how they must assume a personal responsibility for improving and maintaining it.

Here are some of the specific chapters where our coverage has been especially embraced by students and professors.

Chapter 4 "Physical Fitness: Enhancing Work, Study, and Play." This presents current findings in the field of exercise physiology to provide a basis for constructing your own cardiorespiratory fitness program. A special section concerning college students' attitudes toward fitness makes this chapter especially pertinent to today's students. One section entitled "Fitness: Questions and Answers" deals with such current topics as commercial fitness clubs and spas, fitness equipment, muscle fiber types, steroid use, bodybuilding, and sleep.

Chapter 8 "Alcohol: Responsible Choices." Although most health texts cover certain alcohol-related topics (especially the physical effects of alcohol and alcoholism), this chapter expands further to include sensitive, nonjudgmental coverage concerning responsible drinking patterns, responsible party hosting, first aid for acute alcohol intoxication, decisions concerning alcohol use or abstinence, alcoholism and the family, alcohol-related organizations, and fetal alcohol syndrome. Throughout this chapter we encourage students who use alcohol to do so in a judicious manner that best reflects both their independence and growing maturity.

Chapter 9 "Tobacco Use: A Losing Choice." In comparison to chapters on tobacco use found among other personal health textbooks, Chapter 9 is felt to be outstanding by reviewers. The chapter's central theme, that little of value can be derived through smoking, is supported by in-depth discussion and the most current documentation. Information pertaining to dependency formation,

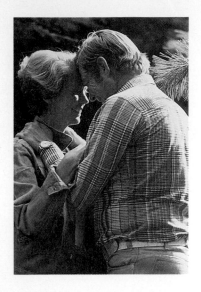

smokeless tobacco use, and constructive interchange between smokers and non-smokers highlights this chapter.

Chapter 13 "Sexuality: Biological and Psychosocial Origins." In this first of four chapters concerning sexuality, Chapter 13 effectively blends both the biological and psychosocial factors that contribute to the complex expression of our sexuality. The sensitive discussions of the concept of androgyny, and expanded definitions of sexuality, and the inclusion of basic anatomical and physiological information make this chapter unique when compared to other personal health texts on the market.

Chapter 19 "The Maturing Adult: Growing Older in America." Based on the most current theories of aging, this chapter treats the aging process with dignity and a great sense of optimism. From a variety of perspectives, we carefully examine two age groups: midlife adults and elderly adults. Perhaps for students the most intriguing and unique aspect of this chapter is the discussion of midlife adulthood. Students are asked to look closely at their own midlife parents or relatives to see how well they are mastering their own two key developmental tasks of midlife. This chapter helps prepare students for the probability of someday becoming "parents to their own parents."

PEDAGOGICAL AIDS

Understanding Your Health uses a variety of learning aids that will enhance student understanding.

Key Concepts. Each chapter opens with five to seven key concepts. The listing of these concepts will assist and direct the student's reading and comprehension of the chapter's most important topics.

Marginal Glossary. Key terms important to the student's understanding and application of the material are in boldface type and defined in the margin. Other significant terms in the text are in italics for added emphasis. Both approaches facilitate student vocabulary comprehension.

Comprehensive Glossary. At the end of the text, all terms defined in the margin, as well as pertinent italicized terms, are merged into a comprehensive glossary. This glossary improves the overall utility and study of the text. New for this edition is the added feature of page cross-references to the text; students will now be able to find a text location for any word in the glossary.

Personal Assessment Inventories. Each chapter contains a personal assessment inventory, starting with a comprehensive 64-question inventory ("Evaluating Your Health: A Personal Profile") in Chapter 1. These inventories serve two important functions: they capture the attention of the student and they serve as a basis for introspection and behavior change.

These assessments are presented in a variety of formats. We developed most of these assessments ourselves. Thus they apply directly to the chapter content and have stood the test of time in our own classes. Examples follow:

Chapter 2 (Mental Health) "How Creative Are You?"
Chapter 5 (Nutrition) "Seven-Day Diet Study"
Chapter 7 (Drug Use) "Nonchemical High Challenge"
Chapter 10 (Cardiovascular Disease) "RISKO"
Chapter 14 (Sexuality-Behaviors) "How Compatible Are You?"
Chapter 17 (Consumerism) "Health Consumer Skills"
Chapter 20 (Dying and Death) "Planning Your Funeral"

Boxed Material. In each chapter special material in boxes encourages the student to delve into a particular topic or to closely examine an important health issue.

Chapter Summaries. To help the student pull the chapter material together, each chapter concludes with a summary of the key ideas and their significance or application. The student can then return to any part of the chapter for repeated study or clarification as needed.

Review Questions. To help the student check for overall understanding, questions are given after each chapter for review and analysis of the material presented.

Questions for Personal Contemplation. To encourage students to apply a chapter's content to their own attitudes or life situation, questions with a philosophical orientation are given after each chapter. These questions promote student thinking to a degree beyond mere recall.

Documentation. We believe that it is critical for both instructors and students to be convinced that the material presented in a textbook is scientifically accurate, fully documented, and as current as possible. *Understanding Your Health* provides this kind of solid documentation with information fully referenced at the end of each chapter.

Annotated Readings. Since some students desire further reading in a particular area of interest or research, we provide an annotated reading list at the end of each chapter. This list comprises current books that can be readily obtained in bookstores or public libraries.

Appendixes. Understanding Your Health includes five appendixes that are valuable resources for the student.

Commonly Used Over-the-Counter Products. Popular categories of over-the-counter drugs are discussed in detail, with recommendations for the consumer of these products.

First Aid and Personal Safety. This appendix outlines practical safety recommendations in seven key areas: General first aid, personal safety, residential safety, recreational safety, firearm safety, motor vehicle safety, and home accident prevention.

A Look at Canadian Health. Statistical information pertinent to the health of Canadians is presented. These statistics, supplied by the Canadian government, include information about such topics as accidents, marriage and divorce rates, cardiovascular disease, and cancer rates.

Categories of Mental Disorders. New to the second edition, categories of mental disorders and therapeutic approaches have been added.

Body Systems. Also new with the second edition, the anatomical systems of the human body have been included.

ANCILLARIES

An extensive ancillary package is available to adopters to enhance the teaching-learning process. We, as well as the publisher, have made a conscious effort to produce supplements that are extraordinary in utility and quality. This package has been carefully planned and developed to assist instructors in deriving the greatest benefit from the text. To that end you will find several unique features within them, and a quality in their use that enhances use of this book. Each of these ancillaries has been thoroughly reviewed by personal health instructors,

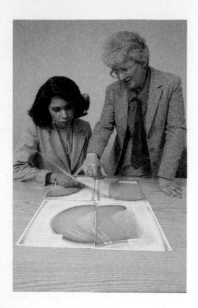

and we have subsequently refined them to ensure clarity, accuracy, and a strong correlation to the text. We encourage instructors to examine them carefully. Beyond the following brief descriptions, additional information on these helpful packages may be obtained from Times Mirror/Mosby College Publishing.

Instructor's Manual and Test Bank. One of the unique and most useful features of the supplementary materials for *Understanding Your Health* is the inclusion of conversion notes in the instructor's manual. At the beginning of each chapter, we describe how the content and focus in *Understanding Your Health* differs from similar chapters or coverage in other popular personal health textbooks. These conversion notes are intended to make the transition to *Understanding Your Health* as convenient and pedagogically sound as possible.

The instructional portion of the manual was prepared by Susan Cross Lipnickey, Ph.D., of Miami University, Ohio. This valuable tool features chapter overviews, learning objectives, suggested lecture outlines with recommended notes and activities for teaching each chapter, personal assessments, issues in the news, individual activities, community activities, suggestions for guest lectures, current media resources including software, and full-page transparency masters of helpful illustrations and charts. The manual is perforated and three-hole punched for convenience. The Test Bank has been revised by Kim Stassen, M.A., of Ball State University. It contains over 2,000 multiple choice, true/false, matching, and essay test questions. All test items have been thoroughly checked for accuracy, clarity, and range of difficulty by several instructors who also served as reviewers of the text.

Computerized Test Bank. Qualified adopters of this text may request a Computerized Test Bank package compatible with the IBM PC, Apple IIc, or Apple IIe microcomputers. This software is a unique combination of user-friendly computerized aids for the instructor. The following summarizes these software aids.

Testing. A test generator allows the user to select items from the test bank either manually or randomly; to add, edit, or delete test items through a preset format that includes multiple choice, true/false, short answer, or matching options; and to print exams with or without saving them for future use.

Grading. A computerized record keeper saves student names (up to 250), assignments (up to 50), and related grades in a format similar to that used in manual grade books. Statistics on individual or class performance, test weighting, and push-button grade curving are features of this software.

Tutoring. A tutorial package uses items from the Test Bank for student review. Student scores can be merged into the grading records.

Scheduling. A computerized datebook makes class planning and schedule management quick and convenient.

Student Study Guide. New with the second edition, the Student Study Guide was prepared by James F. McKenzie, Ph.D., M.P.H., of Mankato State University, Minnesota. The comprehensive manual offers invaluable help to students by reinforcing concepts presented in the text and integrating the concepts with innovative application activities. Reviewed for clarity and accuracy, the guide provides:

- A variety of questions to help students prepare for tests.
- Abundant activities and exercises to encourage students to apply what they've learned from the text to their daily routines.

Personal Health Self-Assessment Software. This interactive software allows students to assess their personal health status by helping them to better understand their individual behaviors and habits, and how these affect health. Students are asked a series of short questions about lifestyle and habits. Then they receive a personal health score that compares their health status with the optimal health score for a person of the same age, along with suggestions for gaining or maintaining high-level health. It is available to qualified adopters for use on IBM and Apple computers.

Overhead Transparency Acetates. Sixty of the text's most important illustrations, diagrams, tables, and charts are available as acetate transparencies. Attractively designed in full- and two-color, these useful tools facilitate learning and classroom discussion, and were chosen specifically to help explain difficult concepts. This package is also available to adopters of the text.

ACKNOWLEDGMENTS

The publisher's reviewers made excellent suggestions and criticisms that were carried out whenever possible. Their contributions are present in every chapter. We would like to express our sincere appreciation for both their critical and comparative readings of the early drafts. They were:

For the Second Edition:

DAN ADAME, Emory University

JUDITH BOONE ALEXANDER, Evergreen Valley College

JUDY B. BAKER, East Carolina University

ROBERT C. BARNES, East Carolina University

LOREN BENSLEY, Central Michigan University

ERNST BLEICHART, Vanier College

SHIRLEY F.B. CARTER, Springfield College

VIVIEN C. CARVER, Youngstown State University

CYNTHIA CHUBB, University of Oregon

JANINE COX, University of Kansas

DICK DALTON, Lincoln University

SHARRON K. DENY, East Los Angeles College

EMOGENE FOX, University of Central Arkansas

GEORGE GERRODETTE, San Diego Mesa College

RAY JOHNSON, Central Michigan University

JAMES W. LOCHNER, Weber State College

LINDA S. MYERS, Slippery Rock University

VIRGINIA PETERS, Central State University

JAMES ROBINSON III, Univesity of Northern Colorado

MERWIN S. ROEDER, Kearney State College

JAMES H. ROTHENBERGER, University of Minnesota

RONALD E. SEVIER, El Camino Community College

REZA SHAHROKH, Montclair State College

ALBERT SIMON, University of Southwestern Louisiana

DENNIS W. SMITH, University of North Carolina at Greensboro

LORETTA R. TAYLOR, Southwestern College

For the First Edition:

STEPHEN E. BOHNENBLUST,
Mankato State University

NEIL RICHARD BOYD, JR.,
University of Southern Mississippi

WILLIAM B. CISSELL,
East Tennessee State University

VICTOR A. CARROLL,
University of Manitoba

DONNA KASARI ELLISON,
University of Oregon,
Umpqua Community College

NEIL E. GALLAGHER,
Towson State University

SUSAN C. GIARRATANO,
California State University at Northridge

RAYMOND GOLDBERG,
State University of New York College
at Cortland

MARSHA HOAGLAND,
Modesto Junior College

CAROL ANN HOLCOMB,
Kansas State University

SHARON S. JONES, Orange Coast College

DANIEL KLEIN,
Northern Illinois University

SUSAN CROSS LIPNICKEY,
Miami University of Ohio

GERALD W. MATHESON,
University of Wisconsin at La Crosse

HOLLIS N. MATSON,
San Francisco State University

DAVID E. MILLS, University of Waterloo

PEGGY PEDERSON, Montana State University

VALERIE PINHAS,
Nassau Community College

JACY SHOWERS,
Formerly of Ohio State University

PARRIS WATTS,
University of Missouri at Columbia

WAYNE E. WYLIE, Texas A & M University

The second edition of this text could not have been written without the encouragement and support of numerous people. The challenge to pursue this project came 6 years ago from our now-deceased department chair, Warren E. Schaller, H.S.D. His belief that we could complete a project of this magnitude motivated us to persevere with the manuscript. As a personal and professional role model, Warren Schaller was one of the best. He is missed not only by us, but by all who knew him.

Our special thanks go to a number of physicians who provided us with current information and insights related to medicine and medical practice. These include Robert E. Hunter, M.D., Dennis F. Lawton, M.D., William B. Fisher, M.D., and Ralph F. Montgomery, M.D. We are further indebted to Meredith J. Sprunger, Ph.D., Larry Stewart, Ph.D., James F. Comes, Ed.D., Lilyan M. Goossens, M.S., and Jeffrey Bowman for technical assistance in their areas of expertise. We also thank secretaries Jane Lesh and Billie Kennedy for their cheerful, supportive inquiries about our work.

It is obvious to us that this book would not have been completed without the help of many dedicated people at Times Mirror/Mosby. We must give a special thanks to these people: our publisher, Nancy K. Roberson, whose dedicated interest and support remained constant; our developmental editor, Michelle Turenne, who devoted her professional energy to this project; and our manuscript and production editor, Kathy Burmann, who made certain that the manuscript was clear and the deadlines absolute. We also wish to thank numerous people in the production areas of this project. Their expertise has made this book both attractively organized and visually appealing.

Finally we wish to acknowledge the contributions of our parents, James and Blanche Payne, and Will and Marty Hahn. Through their life-long efforts as loving parents, we have been able to struggle successfully with many of our own developmental tasks. We hope to be able to supply the same support and encouragement to our own children.

WAYNE A. PAYNE ▪ DALE B. HAHN

Contents in Brief

Contents

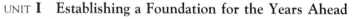
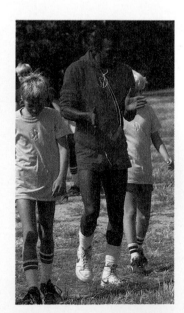

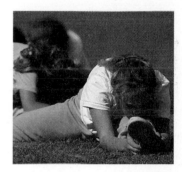

UNIT **III**   Products of Dependency: A Focus for Responsible Use

7   Psychoactive Drugs: Use, Misuse, and Abuse, 164

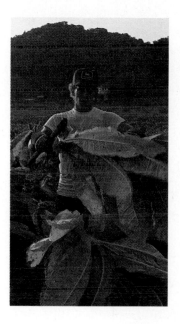

8   Alcohol: Responsible Choices, 196

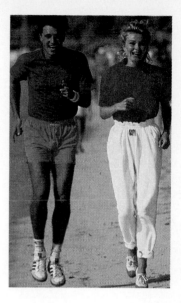

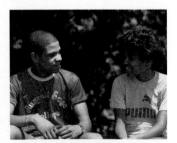

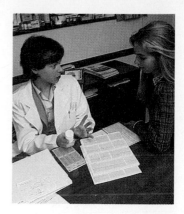

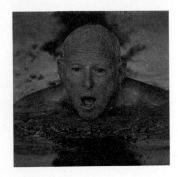

UNIT **VII**   **Growing Older: Balancing Your Future with Your Past**

19   The Maturing Adult: Growing Older in America, 552

20   Dying and Death: The Last Transitions, 580

CHAPTER
1

Health
Support for Your Future

Key Concepts

Health can be defined in several different ways.

Developmental tasks are central to the young adult years.

Health can be described in conjunction with developmental tasks.

Health is dynamic and can be modified to become a better tool for mastering developmental tasks throughout the life cycle.

We can all assess the composition of our health and the role it plays in our lives.

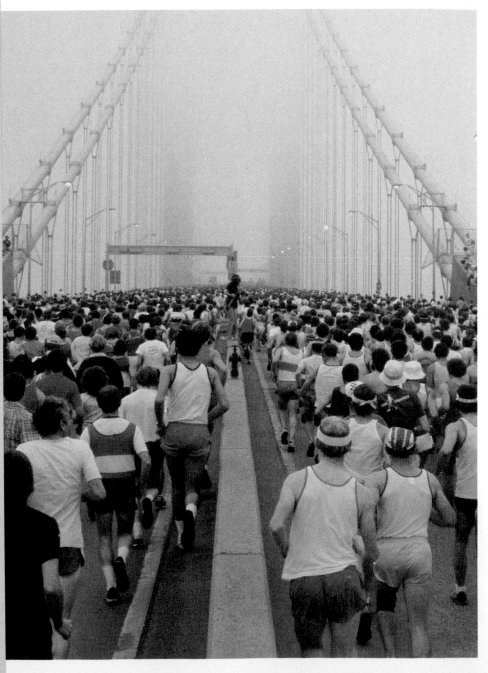

Have people ever warned you about your health by saying, "You'd better pay more attention to your health, because when it's gone, you'll be sorry"? If so, they were probably also telling you that without good health you cannot continue to be a productive and satisfied person.

For us to suggest that health can contribute to a productive and satisfying life is to invite the questions "What is health?" and "How does health contribute to the process of living a satisfying life?" Of course, ultimately only you can answer these two questions. We will help you to answer these questions by providing a framework around which to view health. We will encourage you to study your own health as it relates to your growth and development throughout the stages of the life cycle.

HEALTH CONCERNS OF THE 1990s

As we move closer to the turn of the century, it is evident that most of us are not too far removed from a number of health issues. Heart disease, cancer, accidents, drug use, and mental health are important concerns for us, even if we are not directly affected by them. The growing problems of environmental pollution, health care costs, and sexually transmitted diseases are becoming increasingly significant. World hunger, population control, and the threat of nuclear war represent major issues that will affect us, as well as the generations that follow.

These health concerns are not unmanageable. Indeed, by the turn of the century, we hope to see advancements in the way our society successfully tackles these problems. Fortunately, it appears that we as individuals can make choices in the way we decide to live our lives. At least on a personal level, we can decide to select a plan of healthful living. We can choose a healthy lifestyle that incorporates a sound diet, proper exercise, adequate rest, periodic medical checkups, and elimination (or moderation) of drug use, including tobacco and alcohol use. One goal of this textbook is to provide you with the information and motivation to help you select the lifestyle that will make you a happy and healthy person.

DEFINITIONS OF HEALTH

A Traditional Definition

One of the most widely recognized and most frequently quoted definitions of health is that given by the Geneva-based World Health Organization[1].

"Health is a state of complete physical, mental, and social well-being and not merely the absence of disease and infirmity."

This is a multifaceted view of health, with physical, mental, and social dimensions. This definition indicates that health extends beyond the structure and function of your body to include feelings, values, and reasoning. It also includes the nature of your interpersonal relationships. Furthermore, it can be implied that health can exist in the presence of disease and infirmity. You do not have to be a "picture of health" to be a productive and satisfied person. Nevertheless, for all the definition's value, one question remains unanswered: "How does health contribute to the process of living a satisfying life?"

1

Holistic Health

holistic health
encompassing view of the composition of health; views health in terms of its physical, emotional, social, intellectual, and spiritual makeup.

A currently popular description of health expands the definition supplied by the World Health Organization. **Holistic health** extends the physical, mental, and social aspects of the definition to include intellectual and spiritual dimensions. The holistically healthy person functions as a *total person*. Some experts say that holistically healthy people have reached a "high level of wellness."[2-4]

Holistic health may be the most encompassing explanation of the composition of health. Through a holistic concept of health, we are better able to understand how a person who has a serious physical illness can also claim to be quite healthy.

We think a holistic view of health would be even more appropriate if it further addressed itself to health's role in the events of daily living. Like other definitions of health, the holistic definition may not assist you to see the specific developmental targets toward which your health should be directed. As a consequence, you might not be certain how your health is to be used, and you might not discover the specific accomplishments that can generate a *sense of well-being*.

Health Promotion

health promotion
movement in which knowledge, practices, and value stances are transmitted to people for their use in lengthening their lives, reducing the incidence of illness, and feeling better.

If television talk shows were an accurate reflection of the times, then **health promotion** would reflect the state of the art. Health promoters believe that if you accept scientific opinion regarding health and adopt specific health-enhancing practices, you will become a healthy person. On the basis of this view of health, if you have enhanced your health, you should live longer than average, experience fewer health problems, and feel better than an unhealthy person.

As worthy as these outcomes are, we believe that this interpretation presents health as an end rather than as a means. Indeed, living a long time, not being sick, and doing only healthy things are important, but will they assure you of growing and developing your potential?

Wellness

wellness
a broadly based term used to describe a highly developed level of health.

While health promotion is a term that many in the health field are trying to define,[5,6] the terms **wellness** and "high level wellness" may represent the most popular health-related buzz words of the 1980s. Introduced by Dunn[7] in 1961, high level wellness reflects a new way of looking at a person's health. Wellness supports the concept that a person's health should not be judged primarily from a medical or disease standpoint, but from the standpoint of reaching or achieving human potential.

Some in the field of health promotion indicate that wellness is synonymous with the familiar terms "robust health," "excellent health," and simply "health."[8] Wellness is seen as a process for the continuous self-renewal that is needed for an exciting, creative, fulfilling life. In describing corporate employees engaged in a wellness program, Patton, et al., indicate that they[8]:

. . .continuously renew themselves, are highly energetic, live close to the potential for which they were hired, and whose lifestyle serves as an inoculation agent against many debilitating conditions such as mental depression, alcoholism, obesity, self-doubt and despair, myocardial infarction, and ulcers.

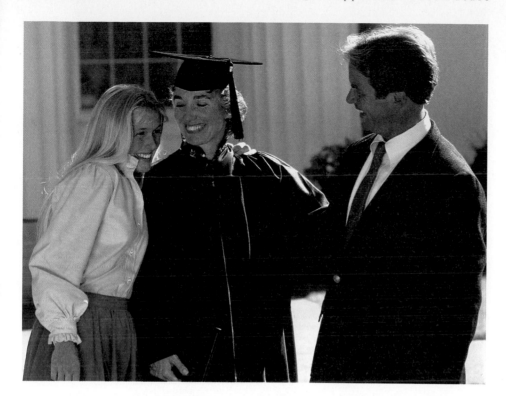

A nontraditional student achieves her goal of a college education.

TODAY'S COLLEGE STUDENTS

Although many terms have been used to identify the transitional years between adolescence and adulthood,[9-11] we will refer to these as the **young adult years.** The young adult period of the life cycle varies in length and in time of onset and completion. For our purposes it can be viewed as the traditional undergraduate years, from ages 18 to 22. Students of this age group are both chronologically and developmentally young adults.

For those of you who are **nontraditional students,** we offer two challenges: to review your own young adulthood and to examine your *current developmental stage* to see in what ways the decisions you made as a young adult are influencing the quality of your life now. All students, regardless of age, should be able to call themselves, at least in part, young adults, because they are working on the tasks that society has given to persons in this period of life.

Most of the students reading this text will be traditional-age college students. However, because the percentage of nontraditional students enrolled in colleges is growing rapidly, we will also identify throughout the text a variety of life experiences and developmental tasks appropriate to nontraditional students. Certainly, the nontraditional students in our classes help our traditional-age students appreciate the role that health plays throughout the life cycle.

young adult years
segment of the life cycle from ages 18 to 22; a transitional period between adolescence and adulthood.

nontraditional students
administrative term used by colleges and universities for students who, for whatever reason, are pursuing undergraduate work at an age other than that associated with traditional college years (18-22).

DEVELOPMENTAL TASKS OF THE YOUNG ADULT PERIOD

The four developmental tasks that we feel are critical for young adults to accomplish include (1) forming an initial adult self-identity, (2) establishing a sense of

Figure 1-1
This text will explore the multiple dimensions of health and how they relate to four tasks of young adulthood. Mastery of these tasks through a balanced involvement of the five dimensions will lead to your enjoying a more productive and satisfying life. The four tasks of young adulthood and the five dimensions of health will be indicated throughout this book by the symbols shown below:

- Physical
- Emotional
- Social
- Intellectual
- Spiritual
- Developmental tasks

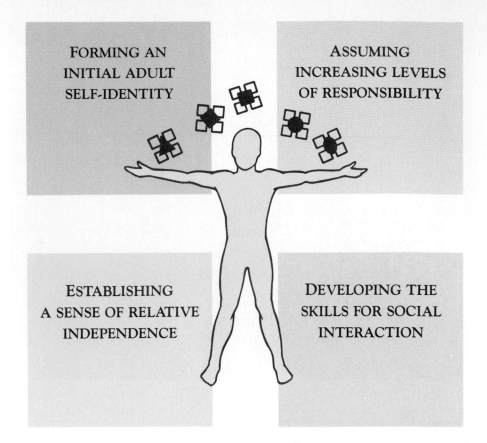

FORMING AN INITIAL ADULT SELF-IDENTITY

ASSUMING INCREASING LEVELS OF RESPONSIBILITY

ESTABLISHING A SENSE OF RELATIVE INDEPENDENCE

DEVELOPING THE SKILLS FOR SOCIAL INTERACTION

relative independence, (3) assuming increasing levels of responsibility, and (4) developing the skills for social interaction (see Figure 1-1). Through the gains you make on each of these tasks, you will find yourself moving further into adulthood.

 ## FORMING AN INITIAL ADULT SELF-IDENTITY

For most of childhood and adolescence, you were seen by adults within your neighborhood or community as someone's son or daughter. You were, and to some degree may still be, known as a unique person by only a few people. Except for your immediate family, teachers, and peers, most people have dealt with you as "so-and-so's child." That stage has now nearly passed; both you and society are beginning to look at each other in new ways.

Regardless of the nature of the push or pull supporting this process, it appears developmentally desirable for both parties to begin interacting on the basis of your growing *uniqueness and competencies*. As an emerging adult, you probably wish to present a unique identity to society. Internally you are constructing a perception of yourself as the adult you wish to be, while externally you are formulating the behavioral patterns that will project this identity to others.

We believe that the completion of this first developmental task is necessary so that you can experience a productive and satisfying life. Through your experiences in achieving self-identity, you will eventually be capable of answering the central question of young adulthood: "Who am I?"

ESTABLISHING A SENSE OF RELATIVE INDEPENDENCE

In contemporary society the primary responsibility for socialization during childhood and adolescence is assigned to the family. For nearly two decades your family was the primary contributor to your knowledge, values, and behaviors. By this time, however, you should be demonstrating an interest in moving away from the dependent relationship that has existed between you and your family.

Travel, peer relationships, marriage, military service, and, of course, college have been traditional avenues for disengagement from the family. Generally your ability and willingness to follow one or more of these paths will help you to establish your independence. Your success in these endeavors will be based on your willingness to use the resources you have. You will need to draw on physical, emotional, social, intellectual, and spiritual strengths to undertake the new experiences that will bring about your independence. In a sense your family laid the foundation for the resources and experiences you will use to draw yourself away from the family's midst.

ASSUMING INCREASING LEVELS OF RESPONSIBILITY

The assumption of increasing levels of responsibility is a third developmental task in which you are expected to progress. Paraphrasing a popular television commercial, we might ask you, "How do you spell RESPONSIBILITY?" You might respond, "TO TAKE CHARGE." Others would say, "TO PROVIDE LEADERSHIP," and others might respond, "TO CARRY YOUR FAIR SHARE." Regardless of how you spell it, responsibility is a significant part of adulthood.

For adults the opportunity to assume responsibility can come from a variety of sources. You may sometimes accept responsibility voluntarily, such as when

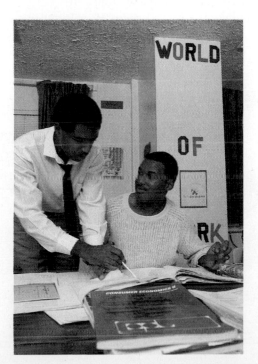

Are you assuming responsibility for your future?

you join a campus organization or establish a new friendship. Other responsibilities are placed on you when professors assign term papers, when dating partners exert pressure on you to conform to their expectations, or when employers require that you be a consistently productive employee. In other situations you may accept responsibility for doing a particular task not for yourself but for the benefit of someone else.

As important and demanding as these areas of responsibility are, a more basic responsibility awaits the adult: the responsibility of maintaining and improving your health and the health of others. You will be challenged to be responsible for recognizing, improving, and then using the strengths that constitute your physical, emotional, social, intellectual, and spiritual makeup. At the same time you will be equally responsible for recognizing, accepting, and working within your limitations. None of the specific areas of responsibility associated with school, employment, and parenting can be undertaken with maximum effectiveness unless you make a commitment to be responsible for your own health.

Because of your relationships with other people, the health of others will become an important component in the satisfying and productive life you seek. In its own right, the good health of your friends and family is rewarding. Healthy, productive friends, colleagues, and family members can also be valuable resources in your own quest for developmental task mastery. Thus their health becomes a matter for which you will want to share some measure of responsibility.

 ## DEVELOPING THE SKILLS FOR SOCIAL INTERACTION

The fourth developmental task that we believe is a part of the young adult years is that of developing appropriate and dependable social skills. Adulthood will probably require your "membership" in a variety of groups that range in size from a marital pair to a national political party or international corporation. These memberships will demand of you the ability to function in many different social settings and with a variety of people.

Social interaction takes place in many settings.

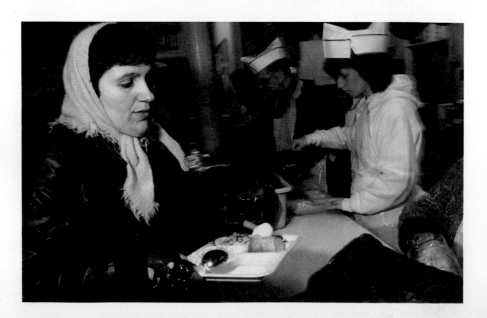

The college experience has traditionally prepared students very well in this regard, but the interactions in friendships, work relationships, or parenting may require that you make an effort to grow and develop beyond levels you might achieve as a result of being a college student. You will probably need to refine a variety of social skills, including communication, listening, and conflict management.

This need to interact socially will at times negatively influence your health. Examples might be the weekend party that prevents you from doing well on a Monday morning examination, or the recreational or intramural activities that sometimes result in serious injury.

Generally, however, social interaction contributes to your total health and serves as an important aid in helping you experience a productive and satisfying life. You can work now at becoming the skilled and comfortable social interactor that the rest of the life cycle will require you to be.

After becoming familiar with the four developmental tasks of the young adult period, you should readily see that there is considerable overlap in the accomplishment of each task; a mutually supportive relationship exists among all four tasks. For example, your development and refinement of social skills can enhance your independence from the family. Your willingness to accept increasing responsibility lets you see yourself as a unique emerging adult.

THE ROLE OF HEALTH

Having been introduced to the four developmental tasks of the young adult period, you can better answer the question, "What is the *role of health* in my life?" We believe that the role of health is to assist you in mastering the developmental tasks that will make your life more satisfying and productive.

If you wanted to know about another person's health, you would probably ask, "How's your health?" However, if you asked us that question, we would respond by saying, "Our health? In relationship to what?"

We suggest that health is something that can only be described meaningfully in conjunction with a developmental task. We all have, you see, a level of health for everything we need or want to do. No one has just one level of health for all of life's many demands.

For traditional-age students, the tasks we are identifying as those likely to be accomplished with high-level health are the four developmental tasks already presented. For nontraditional students, the refinement of these tasks and the mastery of additional developmental tasks will depend on your level of health.

The lack of task **mastery** because of a lowered level of health would reduce your opportunity to have a productive, satisfying life. Just as a broken leg might temporarily curtail your social activities or a catastrophic illness could alter your plans for your young adult years, so too a chronically low level of health could reduce your ability to develop within a particular segment of the life cycle.

mastery
when applied to growth within the young adult segment of the life cycle, mastery implies becoming more self-aware, independent, responsible, and socially interactive.

THE COMPOSITION OF HEALTH

Throughout this book we will contend that your health is composed of five interacting, *dynamic* dimensions. By becoming familiar with these dimensions of your health, you can more easily recognize what it is about your health that may or may not be helping you to master the developmental tasks. Fortunately, since your health is dynamic, you can modify aspects of its dimensions to make it a better tool to help you accomplish developmental tasks and live a productive, satisfying life.

Your health is not static; it cannot be stored on a shelf or given to others. The health you had yesterday no longer exists. The health you aspire to having next week or next year is not guaranteed. However, scientific evidence suggests that what you do today will help determine the quality of your future health.

We will now briefly consider each of the five dimensions of health so that you can more clearly see how they each form a part of your total health.

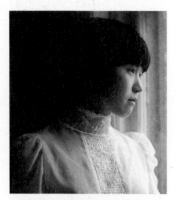

PHYSICAL DIMENSION OF HEALTH

You have a number of physiological and structural characteristics you can call on to aid you in accomplishing your developmental tasks. Among these physical characteristics are your level of susceptibility to disease, body weight, visual acuity, strength, coordination, level of endurance, and powers of recuperation. In certain situations the physical dimension of your health may be the most important dimension. Perhaps this is why many authorities have for so long equated health with the design and operation of the body.

EMOTIONAL DIMENSION OF HEALTH

You also possess certain emotional characteristics that can aid you as you grow and develop. The emotional dimension of health can include the degree to which you are able to cope with stress, remain flexible, and compromise to resolve conflict.

Your growth and development can have associated with it some vulnerability, which may lead to feelings of rejection and failure that could reduce your overall productivity and satisfaction. People who consistently try to improve their emotional health appear to lead lives of greater enjoyment than those who let feelings of vulnerability overwhelm them or block their creativity.

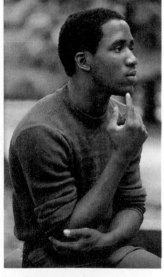

Exploring emotions.

SOCIAL DIMENSION OF HEALTH

A third dimension of total health is that of social abilities. Whether you label these as social graces, skills, or insights, you probably have many strengths in this area. Since most of your growing and developing has been undertaken in the presence of others, you can appreciate how this dimension of your health may be a critically important factor in your life.

INTELLECTUAL DIMENSION OF HEALTH

Your ability to process and act on information, clarify values and beliefs, and exercise your decision-making capacity ranks among the most important aspects of total health. Coping skills, flexibility, or the knack of saying the right thing at the right time may not serve you as well as does your ability to use information or understand a new idea. Certainly a refusal to grasp new information or to undertake an analysis of your beliefs could hinder the degree of growth and development your college experience can provide.

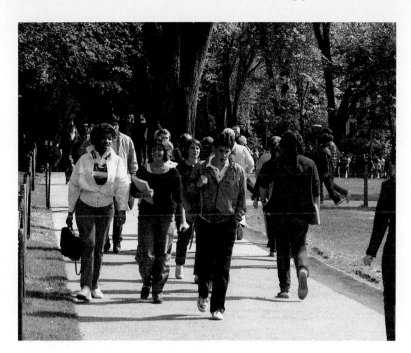

The college experience provides an arena for growth.

 ## SPIRITUAL DIMENSION OF HEALTH

The fifth dimension of health is the spiritual dimension.[12,13] Although you certainly could include your religious beliefs and practices in this category, we would extend it to include your relationship to other living things, the role of a spiritual direction in your life, the nature of human behavior, and your willingness to serve others. All are important components of spiritual health.

HEALTH: OUR DEFINITION

By combining the role of health with the composition of health, we offer a new definition of health that we believe is unique to this book:

Health is the blending of your physical, emotional, social, intellectual, and spiritual resources as they assist you in mastering the developmental tasks necessary for you to enjoy a satisfying and productive life.

FOCUS OF THIS TEXTBOOK

We feel confident that this health textbook can be an important aid in your study of health and its relationship to the demands of living. By detailing valid scientific information, discussing values, and describing behavior patterns that influence health, this text can help you explore your strengths and limitations. Armed with this information, you should then be able to recognize where changes in your lifestyle may be desirable and practical and where limitations may continue to hinder your development. Each of this book's topics, activities, and discussion questions should generate in you a recurring question:

How can I apply this new information about health to my daily life so that I can master the tasks necessary for having a productive, satisfying life?

Personal Assessment

A Personal Profile: Evaluating Your Health

Your health is influenced by behaviors in a number of aspects of living. This personal health profile will help you assess these behaviors. For each statement circle the number of the response that best describes your behavior, or how you think you will behave when confronted by a particular situation. At the end of each section, add the points received on the statements in that section and record your point total in the appropriate box. At the conclusion of the inventory you will be able to make a broad interpretation of the influence of your behaviors on your personal health status.

STRESS MANAGEMENT

	1	2	3	4
1 I seek out change and accept its presence with a sense of confidence and anticipation.	Rarely, if ever	Some of the time	Most of the time	Almost always
2 I participate regularly in a physical activity that allows me to expend nervous energy.	Rarely, if ever	Some of the time	Most of the time	Almost always
3 I turn to friends for counsel and assistance during periods of disruption in my life.	Rarely, if ever	Some of the time	Most of the time	Almost always
4 I periodically reevaluate my experiences with distressful events in anticipation of future events of the same type.	Rarely, if ever	Some of the time	Most of the time	Almost always
5 I seek the counsel of professional advisers when stress becomes too difficult to manage.	Rarely, if ever	Some of the time	Most of the time	Almost always
6 I seek comfort and support in my faith when faced with a difficult period of adjustment.	Rarely, if ever	Some of the time	Most of the time	Almost always

Points _____

PHYSICAL FITNESS

	1	2	3	4
1 I participate in rigorous activity for approximately 30 minutes four times per week.	Rarely, if ever	Some of the time	Most of the time	Almost always
2 I am active during the day and prefer a more vigorous approach to work and leisure activity.	Rarely, if ever	Some of the time	Most of the time	Almost always
3 I do exercises specifically designed to condition my muscles and joints.	Rarely, if ever	Some of the time	Most of the time	Almost always
4 I enter into vigorous activity only after I am warmed up, and I warm down following vigorous activity.	Rarely, if ever	Some of the time	Most of the time	Almost always

	1	2	3	4
5 I select properly designed and well-maintained equipment and clothing for each activity.	Rarely, if ever	Some of the time	Most of the time	Almost always
6 I listen to my body regarding injury and fatigue, and I seek appropriate care when injured.	Rarely, if ever	Some of the time	Most of the time	Almost always

Points _____

SOCIAL RELATIONSHIPS

	1	2	3	4
1 I feel comfortable and confident when meeting people for the first time.	Rarely, if ever	Some of the time	Most of the time	Almost always
2 I establish social relationships with both genders with equal ease and enjoyment.	Rarely, if ever	Some of the time	Most of the time	Almost always
3 I participate in a wide variety of groups, including educational, recreational, religious, and occupational groups.	Rarely, if ever	Some of the time	Most of the time	Almost always
4 I find the roles of leader and subordinate to be equally acceptable.	Rarely, if ever	Some of the time	Most of the time	Almost always
5 I seek out opportunities to become proficient at a variety of socially related skills.	Rarely, if ever	Some of the time	Most of the time	Almost always
6 I am open and accessible to others in the development of intimate relationships.	Rarely, if ever	Some of the time	Most of the time	Almost always

Points _____

NUTRITION

	1	2	3	4
1 I select a wide variety of foods in an attempt to eat a balanced diet.	Rarely, if ever	Some of the time	Most of the time	Almost always
2 I select breads, cereals, fresh fruits, and vegetables in preference to pastries, candies, sodas, and fruits canned in heavy syrup.	Rarely, if ever	Some of the time	Most of the time	Almost always
3 I select such foods as peas, beans, and peanut butter as my primary sources of protein while limiting my consumption of red meat and dairy products.	Rarely, if ever	Some of the time	Most of the time	Almost always

Continued.

Personal Assessment

A Personal Profile: Evaluating Your Health—cont'd

4 I select foods prepared with unsaturated vegetable oils while reducing my consumption of red meats, organ meats, dairy products, and foods prepared with lard or butter.

1 Rarely, if ever	2 Some of the time	3 Most of the time	4 Almost always

5 I limit snacking, and select nutritious foods when I do snack.

1 Rarely, if ever	2 Some of the time	3 Most of the time	4 Almost always

6 I attempt to balance my caloric intake with my activity level.

1 Rarely, if ever	2 Some of the time	3 Most of the time	4 Almost always

Points _____

ALCOHOL, TOBACCO, AND DRUG USE

1 I abstain from alcohol use, or I use alcohol infrequently and in very limited amounts.

1 Rarely, if ever	2 Some of the time	3 Most of the time	4 Almost always

2 I avoid riding with persons who are consuming alcohol, and I drive defensively, remaining aware that other drivers may be using alcohol.

1 Rarely, if ever	2 Some of the time	3 Most of the time	4 Almost always

3 I avoid the use of tobacco products in all forms, including cigarettes, cigars, pipes, and smokeless tobacco products.

1 Rarely, if ever	2 Some of the time	3 Most of the time	4 Almost always

4 I limit my contact with others who are using tobacco, particularly when in confined spaces or when exposure would be for an extended period.

1 Rarely, if ever	2 Some of the time	3 Most of the time	4 Almost always

5 I take prescription drugs only in the manner prescribed, and I use over-the-counter drugs in accordance with directions.

1 Rarely, if ever	2 Some of the time	3 Most of the time	4 Almost always

6 I refrain from using illegal drugs.

1 Rarely, if ever	2 Some of the time	3 Most of the time	4 Almost always

Points _____

SAFETY

1 I attempt to identify the sources of risk or potential danger in each new setting or activity.

1 Rarely, if ever	2 Some of the time	3 Most of the time	4 Almost always

2 I learn procedures and precautions before undertaking new recreational or occupational activities.

1 Rarely, if ever	2 Some of the time	3 Most of the time	4 Almost always

3 I select appropriate equipment for all activities and maintain equipment in good working order.	1 Rarely, if ever	2 Some of the time	3 Most of the time	4 Almost always
4 I curtail my participation in activities when I am not feeling well or am distracted by other demands.	1 Rarely, if ever	2 Some of the time	3 Most of the time	4 Almost always
5 I refrain from using alcohol or drugs when engaged in potentially dangerous recreational or occupational activities.	1 Rarely, if ever	2 Some of the time	3 Most of the time	4 Almost always
6 I repair or report dangerous conditions to individuals responsible for their maintenance.	1 Rarely, if ever	2 Some of the time	3 Most of the time	4 Almost always

Points _____

SELF-CARE

1 I maintain an accurate, updated personal health history.	1 Not at all	2 To a very limited degree	3 Almost completely	4 Completely
2 I routinely monitor my weight and blood pressure, as well as factors related to specific conditions applicable to my health.	1 Rarely, if ever	2 Some of the time	3 Most of the time	4 Almost always
3 I practice home dental health care, including brushing and flossing.	1 Rarely, if ever	2 Some of the time	3 Most of the time	4 Almost always
4 I maintain my immunization status and receive boosters when scheduled or required by specific conditions.	1 Not at all	2 To a very limited degree	3 Almost completely	4 Completely
5 I take prescription medication through the entire course of the prescribed period of use rather than stopping use when symptoms subside.	1 Rarely, if ever	2 Some of the time	3 Most of the time	4 Almost always
6 I consult a reliable home-medical reference book prior to beginning self-care.	1 Rarely, if ever	2 Some of the time	3 Most of the time	4 Almost always

Answer When Applicable

1 I routinely examine my testicles for the presence of small masses or other unusual signs.	1 Rarely, if ever	2 Some of the time	3 Most of the time	4 Almost always
2 I routinely examine my breasts for the presence of masses or other unusual signs.	1 Rarely, if ever	2 Some of the time	3 Most of the time	4 Almost always

Continued.

Personal Assessment

A Personal Profile: Evaluating Your Health—cont'd

3 I routinely receive a Pap smear test.

1	2	3	4
Rarely, if ever	Some of the time	Most of the time	Almost always

4 I use my birth control technique in the manner intended to maximize its effectiveness.

1	2	3	4
Rarely, if ever	Some of the time	Most of the time	Almost always

Points _____

HEREDITARY

1 I can identify members of my family tree for the previous three generations.

1	2	3	4
Not at all	To a limited degree	Almost completely	Completely

2 I can identify the age at death and the cause of death for all family members to whom I am genetically related for the previous three generations.

1	2	3	4
Not for any	For a few but not for most	For most but not for all	For all

3 I receive medical consultation for conditions for which I may have a genetic predisposition (diabetes, hypertension, etc.).

1	2	3	4
Not at all	To a very limited degree	Relatively continuous consultation	Continuous consultation

4 I limit my exposure to radiation and to toxic environmental pollutants.

1	2	3	4
Rarely, if ever	Some of the time	Most of the time	Almost always

5 I will openly share information concerning inheritance abnormalities with potential mates.

1	2	3	4
Not likely	Perhaps	Very likely	Certainly

6 I will seek genetic counseling for known inherited conditions before having children.

1	2	3	4
Not likely	Perhaps	Very likely	Certainly

Points _____

SLEEP, REST, AND RELAXATION

1 I plan my daily schedule to allow time for leisure activity.

1	2	3	4
Rarely, if ever	Some of the time	Most of the time	Almost always

2 I plan my daily schedule to allow time for contemplation, meditation, or prayer.

1	2	3	4
Rarely, if ever	Some of the time	Most of the time	Almost always

3 I receive between 7 and 8 hours of sleep daily.

1	2	3	4
Rarely, if ever	Some of the time	Most of the time	Almost always

	1	2	3	4
4 I refrain from using sleep-inducing over-the-counter drugs.	Rarely, if ever	Some of the time	Most of the time	Almost always
5 I curtail activities when I need to recover from illnesses and injuries.	Rarely, if ever	Some of the time	Most of the time	Almost always
6 I attempt to leave the demands of work, school, or parenting outside of my leisure or relaxation time of the day.	Rarely, if ever	Some of the time	Most of the time	Almost always

Points _____

HEALTH CONSUMERISM

	1	2	3	4
1 I am skeptical of practitioners and clinics who advertise or offer services at rates substantially below those charged by reputable providers.	Rarely, if ever	Some of the time	Most of the time	Almost always
2 I have the financial resources necessary to cover the costs associated with a major illness or hospitalization.	Not at all	To a limited degree	Almost completely	Completely
3 I am skeptical of claims that "guarantee" the effectiveness of a particular health care service or product.	Rarely, if ever	Some of the time	Most of the time	Almost always
4 I accept information that is deemed to be valid by the established scientific community.	Rarely, if ever	Some of the time	Most of the time	Almost always
5 I pursue my rights in matters of misrepresentation or consumer dissatisfaction.	Rarely, if ever	Some of the time	Most of the time	Almost always
6 I seek additional opinions regarding diagnoses indicating a need for surgery or other costly therapies.	Rarely, if ever	Some of the time	Most of the time	Almost always

Points _____

Your total points _____

Interpretation

196-240   Behaviors are very supportive of high-level health.
151-195   Behaviors are relatively supportive of high-level health.
106-150   Behaviors are relatively destructive to high-level health.
 60-105   Behaviors are very destructive to high-level health.

SUMMARY

Health is defined in a variety of ways; several were offered in this chapter. A widely recognized definition is one used by the World Health Organization. Other descriptions of health are drawn from movements in holistic health, health promotion, and wellness. In addition to these, this text offers you another view that extends these concepts to a more functional definition of health. This view reflects the needs of those persons in the transitional period between adolescence and adulthood but will also function for adults of all ages.

There are four developmental tasks that are central to the young adult years. These four tasks include forming an initial adult self-identity, establishing a sense of relative independence, assuming increasing levels of responsibility, and developing the skills for social interaction. This chapter suggested that health can be described in conjunction with developmental tasks. How you accomplish these tasks is based on your level of health.

REVIEW QUESTIONS

1 How does the World Health Organization's definition of health differ from the definition developed in this chapter?
2 Define holistic health, health promotion, and wellness.
3 Identify the four developmental tasks of the young adult years.
4 What is the difference between the *role* of health and the *composition* of health?
5 What is meant by "health is dynamic"?
6 What are the five dimensions of health?

QUESTIONS FOR PERSONAL CONTEMPLATION

1 If you had not read this chapter, how would you have defined health?
2 Can people who have a severe physical health problem still consider themselves healthy? In what ways?
3 Suppose that you had a severe physical health problem. Would you consider yourself healthy? In what ways?
4 In considering the four developmental tasks discussed in this chapter, how do you feel about how well you are mastering each task at this point in your life?
5 If you are a nontraditional student (not in the young adult years), how do you feel you can best apply the information in this chapter to your own life to gain the most from this textbook?

REFERENCES

1 World Health Organization: Constitution of the World Health Organization, Chronicle of the World Health Organization 1:29-43, 1947.
2 Ardell, DB, and Tager, MJ: Planning for wellness: a guidebook for achieving optimal health, ed 2, Dubuque, Iowa, 1983, Kendall-Hunt Publishing Co.
3 Ardell, DB: The history and future of wellness, Dubuque, Iowa, 1985, Kendall-Hunt Publishing Co.
4 Chester, SD: Wellness—what's it all about? Spiritus 8-13, 1985.
5 Duncan, D, and Gold, R: Reflections: health promotion—what is it? Health Values 10:47-48, 1986.
6 Nicholas, DR, Gobble, DC, and Schmottlach, RN: View point: health promotion: a discipline or a technology? American Journal of Health Promotion 1:75-77, 1987.
7 Dunn, H: High level wellness, ed 7, Arlington, Va, 1971, R.W. Beatty.
8 Patton, RW, et al: Implementing health/fitness programs, Champaign, Ill, 1986, Human Kinetics Publishers, Inc.
9 Erikson, E: Childhood and society, ed 3, New York, 1963, W.W. Norton & Co., Inc.
10 Levinson, D, et al: Seasons of a man's life, New York, 1979, Ballantine Books, Inc.
11 Sheehy, G: Passages, New York, 1974, Bantam Books, Inc.
12 Banks, RL, Poehler, DL, and Russell, RD: Spirit and human-spiritual interaction as a factor in health and in health education, Health Education 15:16-17, 1984.
13 Ardell, DB: Spirituality and wellness, ed 9, The Ardell Wellness Report, 2, 1986.

ANNOTATED READINGS

Chopra, D: Creating health: beyond prevention, toward perfection, Boston, 1987, Houghton Mifflin Co.
   Based on the tenets of Ayurveda, Chopra perceives health as inseparable from the integration of man and nature.
Pelletier, KR: Holistic medicine: from stress to optimum health, Magnolia, Mass, 1984, Peter Smith Publisher, Inc.
   Discusses theory that holistically oriented medical practice in combination with the individual's commitment to holistic lifestyle will signal the dawning of the optimal health.
Pelletier, KR: Mind as healer—mind as slayer: a holistic approach to preventing stress disorders, Magnolia, Mass, 1984, Peter Smith Publisher, Inc.
   An in-depth evaluation of stress and its relationship to major disease processes. A holistically based approach to the reduction and management of stress is detailed.
Smith, P, and Quillin, P: The LaCosta prescription for longer life, New York, 1985, Fawcett Crest.
   Using experiences gained at the famous spa, the authors discuss genetics, attitude, exercise, sexuality, and other personal health-related topics.

UNIT I

The first unit in this textbook covers two topics that are closely linked to how we handle change in our lives. Chapter 2 discusses emotional maturity and spiritual growth, and Chapter 3 deals with stress management. As we said in Chapter 1, we believe that your personal growth closely relates to the status of your health, as seen in each of the five dimensions of health. We will now make some connections between Unit I and the five dimensions of health.

■ **Physical Dimension of Health** Your physical dimension of health is concerned with the structure and physiological function of all body systems. Many of the profoundly important experiences that will shape your feelings about yourself and the value of life are made possible by a highly developed physical dimension. We experience life on the basis of our physical bodies and grow emotionally as the result. Our coping skills often involve responses that require a well-developed physical dimension of health.

■ **Emotional Dimension of Health** Unlike prehistoric humans, who primarily responded physically to confrontation, your responses to change will be largely emotional. Feelings of uneasiness arising from the demands of college, intimate relationships, parenting, or employment are the hallmarks of being "stressed." Fortunately, you can cope with threatening change by using the resources associated with the emotional dimension of your health. By employing your personal integrity, sense of humor, ability to be empathetic, and when necessary, your defense mechanisms, you can persist in the face of demanding change.

■ **Social Dimension of Health** Your growth and development rarely take place without influence from other people. At times, your growth and maturation can be bolstered by social relationships. When things go well with roommates, spouses, co-workers, or your own children, you begin to see how capable you are as a social person. Occasional failures in social relationships can be especially bothersome because of the stress they produce. Fortunately, these failures can remind you that emotional growth and stress management capabilities are critically important qualities that take time to develop.

■ **Intellectual Dimension of Health** Throughout your college experience and in the years to follow, your intellectual resources will be called upon with increasing frequency. Your ability to form creative ideas, integrate material, analyze situations, and think logically will help you function as an educated adult.

More importantly perhaps, these resources from your intellectual dimension of health will help you to enjoy life more fully. They may be able to help you understand and better control your expanding emotional and spiritual growth, regardless of when this growth takes place. It is quite possible that during difficult times, you may find your mind to be your most dependable coping source. A book, a lecture, a concert, or art may be a refuge from the stressful events of the classroom, family, or office.

■ **Spiritual Dimension of Health** A growing body of evidence suggests the presence of a spiritual focus in the lives of many college undergraduates. Although only a minority of students claim to have experienced a strong conversion, many more of today's students appear to be searching for a deeper understanding of the meaning of life. Although *you* may not feel personally pressured by the nature of your spiritual beliefs, many students do. The uncertainties arising from exploring what to believe and how to practice what you believe can create stress in the spiritual dimension of your health.

One explanation for the renewed interest in the spiritual dimension of health probably stems from its value as a resource during periods of personal stress. For some people, meditation, introspection, and prayer seem to effectively free them from the tribulations of living in a fast-paced, sometimes uncaring world. To believe deeply in something and to act on that belief through service to others leads to personal enrichment.

Establishing a Foundation for the Years Ahead

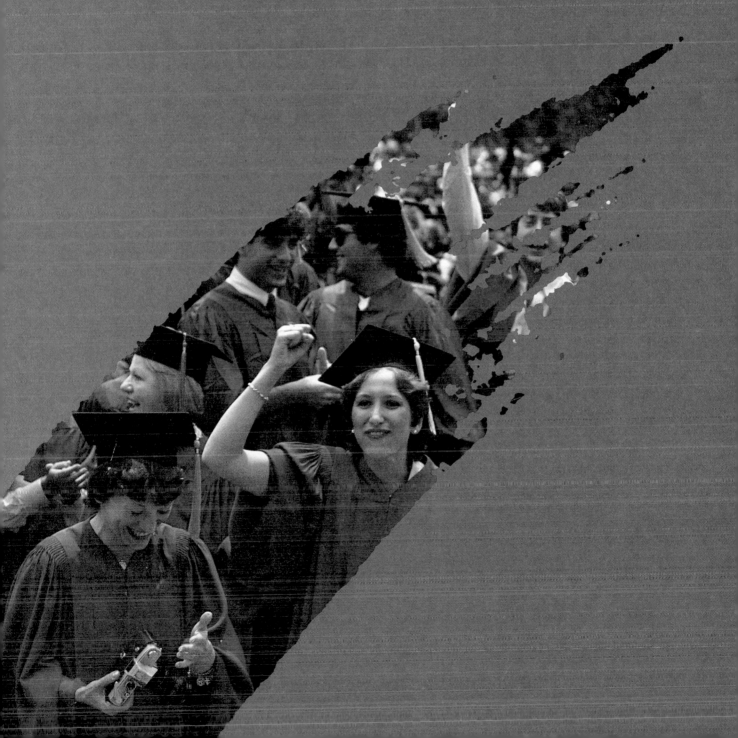

CHAPTER 2

Achieving Emotional Maturity and Spiritual Growth

Keys to Your Mental Health

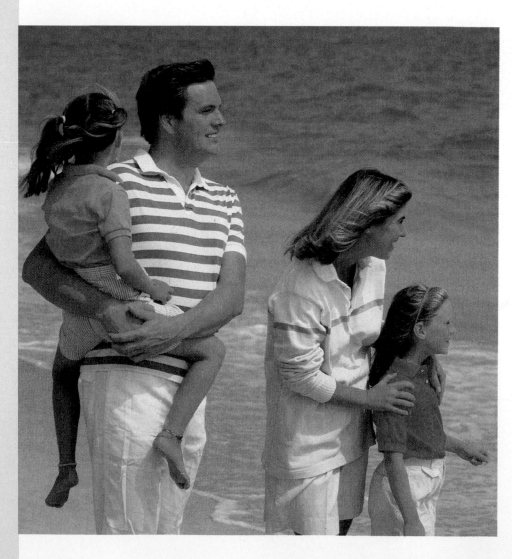

I n Chapter 2 we will explore your ability to grow dynamically to healthy emotional and spiritual maturity. In planning this chapter we decided to direct your attention to the development of emotional and spiritual maturity rather than describe emotional dysfunctions that can occur among young adults. By taking this approach we will be able to explore the experiences you can undertake that can help you achieve greater emotional maturity and spiritual development. Emotional dysfunctions and treatments are presented in Appendix 4.

CHARACTERISTICS OF A MENTALLY HEALTHY PERSON

When our students ask us to define a mentally healthy person, we often respond by asking them to consider our definition of health (see Chapter 1) and how health contributes to the quality of life. Thus a mentally healthy person is one who is capable of using significant resources from each of the five dimensions of health to achieve a satisfying and productive life. People who live satisfying and productive lives are, by our definition, mentally well.

A more specific yardstick for measuring mentally healthy people comes from the National Mental Health Association. This group describes mentally healthy people as those who[1]:

- *Feel comfortable about themselves.* They are not overwhelmed by their own emotions and they can accept many of life's disappointments in stride. They experience all of the human emotions (for example, fear, anger, love, jealousy, guilt, joy) but are not incapacitated by them.
- *Feel right about other people.* They feel comfortable with others and are able to give and receive love. They are concerned about the interests of other people and have relationships that are satisfying and lasting.
- *Are able to meet the demands of life.* Mentally healthy people respond to their problems, accept responsibility, plan ahead without fearing the future, and are able to establish realistic goals.

We do not wish to give a distorted view of mentally healthy people. At times, mentally healthy people experience stress, frustrations, feelings of self-doubt, failure, and rejection. What distinguishes the mentally healthy is their resilience—their ability to recapture their sense of mental wellness within a reasonable period of time.

TOWARD THE AUTHENTIC SELF

If you were privileged to receive a few minutes of time from the wisest person that you could imagine, what do you think that person would say to you about how you can lead a satisfying and productive life?

The suggestion we think this person would share with you would be, "Learn to live comfortably with yourself." The development of your adult self-identity is a reflection of this idea. Regardless of how the concept is transmitted to you, you must recognize that a productive and satisfying life is based on your ability to live comfortably with yourself. This ability requires that you first learn to know yourself.

Learning to know who you are is not as easy is it first seems. What you see in yourself is often determined by what you wish to see rather than what you should see. For either positive or negative reasons, the conscious or unconscious

We learn about ourselves through experiences with others.

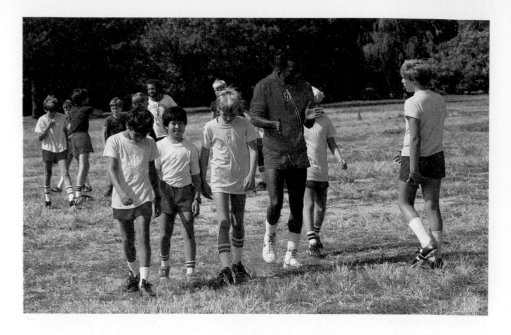

mind tends to color what you see. Since the last person you want to delude is yourself, you should look at yourself frequently and honestly. On pp. 31-35 you will find a plan for undertaking this process of self-evaluation.

Ultimately, to learn to live with yourself, you will have to extend the process of learning about yourself. You will need to make an honest commitment to learning to *accept yourself* on the basis of what you discover through self-examination. There are times when this acceptance will be difficult. Recognition of your limitations and imperfections can be depressing. You may find yourself concentrating too deeply on these temporary imperfections while failing to look closely enough at those positive aspects of yourself that seem consistent and predictable. Accepting yourself does not mean that you can never change; accepting yourself should include an acknowledgment of your desire to grow in a more positive direction.

To grow to real maturity, you must reach beyond mere acceptance of qualities you have discovered about yourself and begin *learning how to be yourself*. Being and becoming are the central challenges of life.

Your maturity will depend heavily on your ability and willingness to live as you are rather than as the person others might wish you to be. Your initial adult self-identity and your ability to assume increasing levels of responsibility will be enhanced when life is viewed through the eyes of your **authentic self**—the real you. The more mature you become, the more consistently your true nature will be reflected by your thoughts and behavior. By being authentic you will move closer to high-level emotional and spiritual health.

authentic self
positive self-identity that underlies the individual's more temporary mood identities; the most basic self-concept.

FACTORS THAT INFLUENCE PERSONALITY

For good or bad, a person's authenticity is judged on the basis of his or her personality. What factors shape one's personality? Although there are many viewpoints concerning personality development, there is general concensus that the following factors are influential in shaping a person's personality:

- *Genetic factors.* Genetic factors include those traits passed on from one or both parents. These are centered in the genes located on the 46 chromosomes found in the cell nucleus. Also related to the genetic factors are the changes to chromosomes that sometimes occur after conception.
- *Environmental factors.* These factors can influence a person's personality throughout a lifetime. They range from impacts in the intrauterine environment (nutrition, drug use, infection, maternal stress) to the daily environmental conditions that we face. Air quality, noise pollution, traffic congestion, weather, social relationships, family harmony, job concerns, academic rigors, and financial resources represent familiar environmental factors.

Of course, it must be pointed out that both genetic and environmental influences can shape a personality both positively and negatively. Genetic influences cannot be reversed (only responded to), whereas environmental influences may be altered to minimize disruptive influences to one's personality. For example, older students who have difficulty coping with the return to college may find their outlook on life much happier by seeking out other older students, perhaps through a campus organization for nontraditional students.

MODELS OF PERSONALITY AND GROWTH

Just as there is no single interpretation of the nature and role of health or of the exact nature of the developmental tasks that await you in each segment of the life cycle, there is also no universally agreed upon interpretation of how or why everyone's personality develops uniquely. Many schools of thought, most with widely recognized spokespersons, have advanced their interpretations of why you become the person you are. This text can do little more than present an overview of how these important schools of thought perceive the process of growth.

Piaget's view

Piaget emphasizes the importance of the intellectual-maturational aspects of growth. In the *sensorimotor period* (0 to 2 years of age), the infant distinguishes between himself or herself and exterior objects. During the *preoperational period* (2 to 7 years of age) the child tends to classify by single salient features and is able to think in terms of classes and numbers. He gradually develops conservation capacities. He is able to recognize that the amount of mass of something is not changed when it is formed into different shapes. At this stage the child is **egocentric.** Language, judgment, and thinking are influenced by the child's inabilty to see experiences through the eyes of others.

egocentric
unable to take into account the views of others; self-centered.

During the *concrete operations period* (7 to 11 years of age), the child is able to use logical operations, such as reversibility in working arithmetic problems, classification in organizing hierarchies of classes, and seriation in organizing objects in an ordered series of size. At the same time, the child's moral judgment is characterized by a literal interpretation of rules and **moral realism.**

The *formal operations period* (11 to 15 years of age) culminates intellectual development in enabling the individual to engage in abstract thinking, conceptualization, and hypothesis testing. Piaget describes growth primarily in terms of intellectual capacities. Egocentrism is now overcome. The differing points of view held by others can be recognized, as can the motives underlying the behavior of others. At this time the child is capable of making and actualizing moral decisions.[2]

moral realism
literal interpretation of rules; real values as opposed to idealistic assumptions.

Erikson's view

Erikson emphasizes the psychosocial aspects of growth. During the first year the child develops basic attitudes of trust or mistrust associated primarily with the mother. The second year establishes the beginning of autonomy or dependence in relation to both parents. From the third to the fifth year the child develops his or her own balance between initiative and hesitancy or guilt as it relates to the entire family. Social development from the sixth year to the onset of puberty is marked by characteristics associated with industry on the one hand and traits of inferiority on the other. The social range is extended to the neighborhood and school. During adolescence the individual establishes his identity and reputation. Difficulties arise when there is identity confusion and negative self-regard. Peer groups become very important and leadership role models may exert great influence.

The period of early adulthood establishes intimacy relationships or solitary social patterns. The more diffused peer group relationships narrow down into partner and small in-group interactions. Sex and the broader issue of competition and cooperation become an important part of life. Young and middle adulthood are times for the raising of children and establishing productive vocational relationships. For those who have established solitary patterns, self-absorption may become more pronounced. In later adulthood the individual culminates his or her life through an integration of purpose to achieve an integrity of being or disintegrates with failing physical capacities into a state of despair or helplessness.[3]

Erikson's eight stages of psychosocial development are outlined in the box on the opposite page.

Kohlberg's view

Kohlberg emphasizes the moral-ethical dimension of growth. At the *premoral stage* the individual obeys rules in order to avoid punishment or conforms to obtain rewards and favors. The morality of conventional role conformity is the "good boy" behavior pattern which acts in socially approved ways to get approval or avoid disapproval and dislike by others. This behavior generalizes to abide by laws and regulations to avoid punishment and guilt feelings.

The morality of **self-accepted moral principles** includes the morality of laws, contracts, and ethical principles. At this level of morality we conform out of respect for democratically established laws and personal integrity, or because we believe our behavior is in conformity with reality. Moral growth moves in the direction of harmonizing behavior with social values, personal integrity, and universal reality.[4]

Behavioralists' view

Pioneered by J.B. Watson in the early decades of this century and carried forward by a number of psychologists, child developmentalists, and therapists, *behavioralism* attempts to explain human behavior on the basis of *responses* to specific or generalized **stimuli.** Environmental events, mental images, and symbols serve as the stimuli to which responses are formulated. To the behavioralist, responses are purposeful in that they either stop the negative nature of certain stimuli or enhance the positive nature of others. Once established, however, the specific response pattern will continue to occur as long as the response is, by its own nature, rewarding, or is reinforced by an extraneous source. Responses can be elicited by **cueing** the individual through words or symbols to recall the particular stimulus that initially elicited the response. A *reinforcement schedule* can maintain the response for lengthy periods of time.[5]

Freud's view

Freud saw growth as a struggle between the unconscious-irrational forces and the conscious-rational forces of life. The two basic life forces, **eros** (urge toward life and love)

---

self-accepted moral principles
moral behavior selected by the individual as opposed to socially imposed ethical standards.

stimulus
changing condition within the environment to which the individual will respond.

cueing
providing clues to ensure that an individual responds to a stimulus.

eros
unconscious urge toward life and love; in Freudian tenets, the powerful life force.

Erikson's Eight Stages of Psychosocial Development

STAGE	AGES	FAVORABLE OUTCOMES
Trust versus mistrust	Birth to second year	Trust and optimism
Autonomy versus shame and doubt	Second to third year	Sense of self-control and adequacy
Initiative versus guilt	Third to sixth year	Direction and purpose; can initiate own activities
Industry versus inferiority	Sixth year to onset of puberty	Competence in intellectual, social, and physical skills
Identity versus role confusion	Adolescence to initial young adulthood	Integrated image of self; a sense of manliness or womanliness
Intimacy versus isolation	Young adulthood	Ability to form close and lasting relationships; ability to honor commitments and support causes
Generativity versus stagnation	Middle adulthood	A sense of paying back society; concern for the family, society, and future generations
Integrity versus despair	Late adulthood	A sense of fulfillment and satisfaction for having lived life fully; an acceptance of the reality of death and a willingness to face death

and **thanatos** (urge toward death and hate), are in competition. In life situations these two basic instincts are mixed; this conflict is called **ambivalence.** Ambivalence results in many polarities in human life; love-hate, activity-passivity, femininity-masculinity, pleasure principle–reality principle. He believed the *id* (unconscious pleasure drive) and the *superego* (higher social mores and values) were in a constant struggle for dominance.

Growth is the movement away from the domination of the irrational pleasure principle toward the control of the reality principle. Since we cannot cope with facing reality too quickly, we need to use defense mechanisms to guard our sensitive *ego* (see the box on p. 26).

Subconsciously, people use variations and combinations of these defense mechanisms daily. For example, some professors refuse to believe that they are weak lecturers (denial) and then place all of their professional energy into research projects (compensation). Students sometimes use rationalization or projection when they receive a low test score. They may feel that they had a bad test result because of a poor night's sleep (rationalization) or because the professor was at fault (projection). The use of defense mechanisms helps us feel better about our shortcomings. Freud would say that defense mechanisms help us keep our egos intact.

thanatos
unconscious urge toward death and hate; in Freudian tenets, the powerful and destructive death force.

ambivalence
simultaneous holding of two incongruent ideas or aspirations: love-hate, attraction-rejection.

Defense Mechanisms: Protecting the Ego

Stressors, particularly when they are dealt with poorly, can challenge our self-perception, or ego. In an attempt to protect the delicate nature of the ego we subconsciously use a variety of defense mechanisms. Many of the following will be familiar to you.

Compensation	Covering our weaknesses by emphasizing our more desirable traits; overachieving in one area to minimize our inadequacies in another
Denial	Refusing to accept the existence of something that should be obvious to us
Displacement	Redirecting our feelings about an original stressor to other persons, objects, or events
Fantasy	Escaping from reality through the use of our imagination
Intellectualization	Applying intellectual operations to resolve a stressor or to protect ourselves from dealing in a more personal or emotional manner; objectivity rather than subjectivity
Isolation	Detaching ourselves emotionally from the source and resolution of a stressor
Projection	Assigning our own unacceptable feelings to another person; often our own fear or uncertainty is said to be the fear or uncertainty held by another
Rationalization	Attributing a rational explanation to our own irrational behavior or feelings
Reaction formation	Responding in a manner that is generally directly opposite to the manner in which we feel or would like to respond
Regression	Escaping from stressors by returning to more childlike, less mature responses
Repression	Suppressing uncomfortable feelings from reaching a level of consciousness; frequently we forget that which we do not wish to remember

- Now that defense mechanisms have been reviewed, are they familiar in the sense that you have on occasion employed them?
- Are defense mechanisms innate, or are we subtlely taught what they are and how to employ them in particular situations?
- At what point is it possible that we are relying too heavily on the use of defense mechanisms?

Maturity is marked by the dominance of the reality principle in our lives. Freud thought that in most of the ordinary decisions of our lives we should rely primarily on rational thinking, but in great and fundamental decisions such as choosing our vocation or selecting our life partners, we should draw on the deep unconscious resources. Our imagination tends to win over our reason; our head is eventually dominated by our heart.[6]

Maslow's view

Maslow views growth in terms of inner needs and motivation. He lists motivational requirements in the following order: physiological needs, safety needs, belonging and love needs, esteem needs, and self-actualization needs (see Figure 2-1). Maslow distinguishes between the lower *deficiency needs* and the higher *being needs*. We do not seek the higher needs until the lower demands have been reasonably satisfied.

Maslow's theory of metaneeds and being values postulates that values are the distinctive and fundamental aspect of human motivation. *Metaneeds* are rooted in human biology; they are universal and not merely the product of culture. *Being values* are intrinsic, supracultural, transpersonal, universal, and are related to ultimate reality. When these values are not actualized in our lives, we become frustrated, maladjusted, and ill. Social pathology, such as crime, is the result of intrinsic value starvation—being value deficiency.

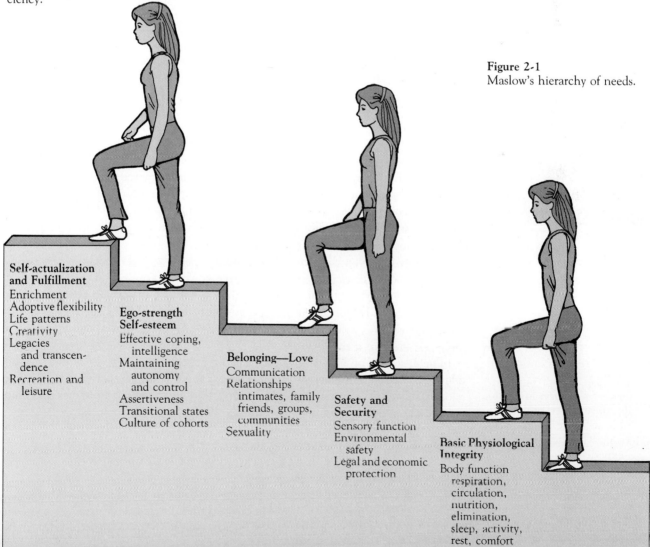

Figure 2-1
Maslow's hierarchy of needs.

Self-actualization and Fulfillment
Enrichment
Adoptive flexibility
Life patterns
Creativity
Legacies
    and transcen-
    dence
Recreation and
    leisure

Ego-strength Self-esteem
Effective coping,
    intelligence
Maintaining
    autonomy
    and control
Assertiveness
Transitional states
Culture of cohorts

Belonging—Love
Communication
Relationships
    intimates, family
    friends, groups,
    communities
Sexuality

Safety and Security
Sensory function
Environmental
    safety
Legal and economic
    protection

Basic Physiological Integrity
Body function
    respiration,
    circulation,
    nutrition,
    elimination,
    sleep, activity,
    rest, comfort

transcenders
self-actualized people who
have achieved a quality of
being ordinarily associated
with higher levels of spiritual growth.

self-actualization
highest level of personality
development; self-actualized
persons recognize their roles
in life and use personal
strengths to the fullest.

The healthiest and most effective people in human society are those whose lives em-
body being values such as truth, beauty, goodness, faith, wholeness, and love. Maslow
labels these as "Theory Z" people or **transcenders. Self-actualization,** the highest level
of self-development, is clearly evident in the personality of the transcender. Transcenders
as described as follows[7]:

Transcenders have more peak or creative experiences and naturally speak the language of being values.

- Transcenders are more responsive to beauty, more holistic in their perceptions of
  humanity and the cosmos, adjust well to conflict situations, and work more whole-
  heartedly toward goals and purposes.
- Transcenders are innovators who are attracted to mystery and the unknown and see
  themselves as instruments for the acutalization of the transpersonal being values.
- Transcenders tend to fuse work and play. They are less attracted by the rewards of
  money and objects and more motivated by the satisfaction of being and service
  values.
- Transcenders are more likely to accept others with an unconditional positive regard,
  and they tend to be more oriented toward spiritual reality.

CREATIVE EXPRESSION

Whichever school of thought about personal growth seems most plausible to you,
we think that a productive and satisfying life also requires that you find creative
ways of expressing yourself. You may have noticed that individuals you consider
to be emotionally healthy and mature seem to enjoy life and get a great deal
accomplished. These individuals are productive workers who seemingly find interesting approaches to whatever they are doing. They engage in useful work
that contributes not only to their own sense of accomplishment and well-being,
but also to society.

These same persons seem to have personalities that are capable of supporting
warm, loving interpersonal relationships. You are attracted to these individuals
because they are interested in you and in what you are doing. They are pleasant
and courteous. You feel relaxed in their presence because you sense that they
are understanding and willing to give and receive love naturally and gracefully.

Emotionally healthy individuals have a free and open approach to life. You
have surely observed that they think and act positively. They also assess people
and situations realistically and constructively. When you interact with emotionally healthy people you quickly notice their flexibility in solving problems. How
did these individuals become so secure, competent, and constructive? Is it possible that you too will mature in this direction? What resources will you need to
help you grow in a similar fashion?

The Institute of Personality Assessment at the University of California has
identified traits that characterize creative people. Assuming that **creativity** is
closely related to emotional health, these traits might adequately describe emotionally healthy persons[8]:

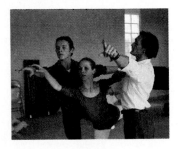

creativity
innovative ability; insightful
capacity to solve problems;
ability to move beyond ana-
lytical or logical approaches
to experience.

- Creative people are intuitive and have an openness to experience. They are
  spontaneous and expressive and have the courage to reveal themselves.
  They are relatively free from fear and are not disturbed by the unknown,
  the mysterious, or the puzzling.
- Creative people are not interested in detail but in meaning and implications. They tend to be more theoretical than pragmatic in their orientation.

Personal Assessment

How Creative Are You?

Do you possess tendencies toward high creativity? To determine this for yourself, circle the number that best reflects your relative position on each continuum.

More interested in the meaning and implications of things and ideas than in details and the practical value of things and ideas	1 2 3 4 5	More interested in details and the practical value of things and ideas than in their meaning and their implication
A combination of relatively equal measures of both reasonableness and passion	1 2 3 4 5	More reasonable than passionate or more passionate than reasonable
A combination of relatively equal measures of both rationality and irrationality	1 2 3 4 5	More rational than irrational or more irrational than rational
A combination of relatively equal measures of scientific interests and artistic interests	1 2 3 4 5	More interested in science than in art or more interested in art than in science
A combination of relatively equal measures of masculinity and femininity	1 2 3 4 5	More masculine than feminine or more feminine than masculine
More likely to concentrate on the possbility of finding the deeper meaning and possibilities inherent in something	1 2 3 4 5	More likely to be interested in becoming aware of or discovering something
More productive and contributive when working alone	1 2 3 4 5	More productive and contributive when engaged in group activities and brainstorming

Your total points _____

Interpretation

26-35   Relatively low creativity
17-25   Average creativity
 7-16   Relatively high creativity

These people have the ability to unify, synthesize, and integrate materials and experiences.

- Creative people are independent, self-accepting, and autonomous yet are not authoritarian in their attitudes. They tend to resist group work and function best when allowed to work independently in the field of their interest.
- Creative people are flexible. They do not use either-or nor black-white thinking but recognize that there are many ways to interpret the same situation.
- Creative people are governed by an internal set of values and are persistent in developing ideas and working toward goals.

You may recognize many of these characteristics as being already well developed in your personality. You may not have mastered some traits listed, and they may now appear beyond your reach. Nevertheless, you can increase your creativity if you let your high level of health help you face new challenges.

A search for spiritual understanding.

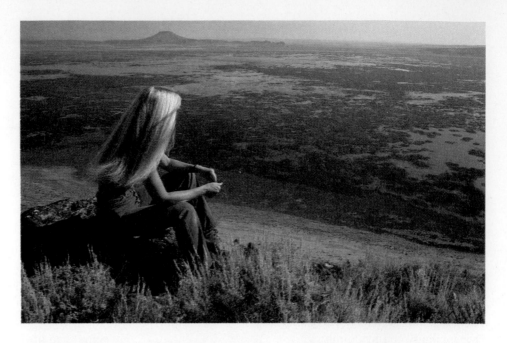

FAITH: A BASIS FOR THE SPIRITUAL DIMENSION OF HEALTH

You may have a growing recognition that a satisfying and productive life—with a resultant sense of well-being—may require a dimension of health beyond that generally associated with the emotional dimension of health. As important as it is to have an accurate perception of yourself and your role in life, many people are finding it increasingly important to discover what lies beyond the existence of a physical environment and a social structure.[9,10] These people are pondering the nature of an *ultimate environment* and are searching for a spiritual dimension to their lives that involves a concept we will refer to as **faith.**

faith
predisposition to apply one's concept of an ultimate environment to life's experiences; the purposes and meaning that underlie the individual's hopes and strivings.

James Fowler[11,12] describes the nature of faith as a fundamental, universal, but infinitely varied value response within the human experience. Faith is seen as being quite distinct from religious practice or belief. Faith is the most fundamental category in the human quest for a meaning to life. It is an orientation of the total person that gives purpose and meaning to thoughts and actions, hopes and strivings.

Synthetic-Conventional Stage

The stage of faith development seen among adolescents is frequently that of a value orientation, with a content and structure influenced heavily by forces from outside the individual. Fowler labels this a **synthetic-conventional stage** of faith. The family, congregation, and community provide values and information from which a young person draws an identity and outlook on life. The structure of faith during this stage of life is based on conformity and relies heavily on the expectations and judgments of authority figures and on social customs. Since the young person lives within this value ideology, the beliefs and needs of others are judged on the basis of their affiliations (religion, denominational affiliations, national or ethnic group membership) rather than on the basis of the needs common to all persons.

synthetic-conventional stage
stage of faith development generally associated with adolescence in which one lives within the constructs formulated for the individual by others.

The synthetic-conventional stage of faith may serve the individual reasonably well not only during adolescence but also into the adult years. For many, however, their experiences at college may stimulate exploration of a more personally defined structure for faith. When faith that has been largely structured by forces outside of the individual is gradually transformed into a faith that is based on personal interpretation and application, a **demythologization** is said to have occurred. When this happens, a person has reached an **individuative-reflective stage** of faith.

Individuative-Reflective Stage

An individuative-reflective stage of faith development is more likely to be seen in an adult who has begun to take seriously the burden of responsibility for his or her own commitments, lifestyle, beliefs, and attitudes. This stage of faith development involves tension and anxiety, since it may require the courage to make personal decisions. It demands objectivity and independence from family and social pressure; it requires finding a balance between wholly personal aspirations and a developing desire to serve others. At this stage of faith development, the person translates symbols, literal beliefs, and doctrines into conceptual meanings whereby the essence of spiritual truths can be seen. The person's faith has matured to become a unique value or orientation. Identity, independence, and relationships are viewed in a different light.

Dynamic faith is the foundation of effective living and creative service. Adult life will be enhanced by the satisfaction of serving others. As Erikson suggests, the major task awaiting you as an adult is that of "paying back" the collective society for the support that has been extended to you during your childhood, adolescence, and young adult years. Your sense of well-being grows as you recognize that you are a part of a community—a community you are obligated to serve. Good health supports this service.

demythologization
transfer of faith from an orientation based on teachings gained outside oneself to an orientation developed within oneself.

individuative-reflective stage
state of faith development generally associated with the young adult; stage in which one translates symbols into personally meaningful concepts; living within one's own structure of faith.

A PLAN FOR ENHANCING YOUR EMOTIONAL GROWTH

A greater understanding of your emotional nature, and consequently your emotional dimension of health, can be visualized as a four-component cyclic process that continues throughout life. Figure 2-2 shows the sequence of these components as they would occur during one revolution of the cycle. Although you may experience emotional growth and mental health without having a concrete plan of action, we support the use of this active four-component plan.

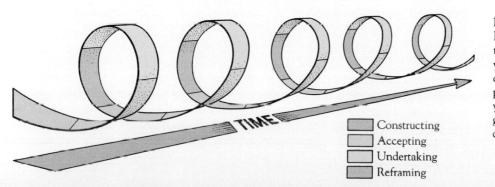

TIME

Constructing
Accepting
Undertaking
Reframing

Figure 2-2
If you visualize the growth of the emotional dimension of your health as a four-component process, you will perceive the *cyclic* nature of your continued emotional growth throughout the life cycle.

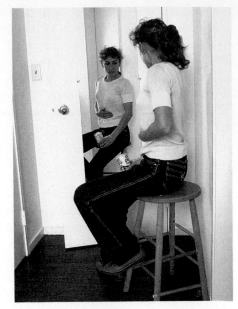

How do you see yourself?

Constructing Mental Pictures

Actively taking charge of your emotional development begins when you construct a mental picture of what you are like. This mental picture or perception should be composed of the most recent and accurate information you have about yourself. Information concerning **cognition, affect,** how you arrange priorities, and **performance** are the materials from which this picture will take shape.

To construct this mental picture of yourself, you will need to set aside a period of uninterrupted quiet time. Commitment to this period for reflection is essential. Even in the midst of a busy schedule, most of us can "free up" several moments if we feel the task is important. It will be helpful to write down your perceptions of yourself.

Before continuing to the second component in your plan for active emotional development, it is important that you formulate, in addition to a mental picture about *yourself,* similar mental pictures about yourself in relation to *other people* and *material objects,* including your college environment, residence, belongings, wardrobe, and so on. Since few of you will have the opportunity to live without thinking about yourself, other people, and material objects, it is important that you formulate your perceptions in a broad triangular fashion. Again, jot down some of the perceptions you have about yourself and how you relate to other people and material objects.

Accepting Mental Pictures

The second component of the plan involves an *acceptance* of your mental pictures. Acceptance implies a willingness on your part to honor the **validity** of the pictures you have formed about yourself and other people. The concept of acceptance also reflects your willingness to use material objects in support of your own development. Start believing that there is a way in which the components in your mental picture can help you grow emotionally.

cognition
information-processing skills; cognition influences *affect* and *performance.*

affect
priorities, predispositions, and values; affect influences *cognition* and *performance.*

performance
psychomotor skills or behaviors in which an individual is engaged; performance influences *cognition* and *affect.*

validity
the accuracy and soundness of one's perceptions.

As in the first component of the plan, the second stage requires time and commitment from you. Growth and development are rarely passive processes. You must be willing to be *introspective* about yourself and the world around you. It is impossible to think that you can ignore your need to grow.

Undertaking New Experiences

Of the 31 students who traveled to London, England, for one semester, 29 spent every free evening and weekend "exploring." No part of the United Kingdom was beyond their reach. Two students, however, spent nearly all of their free time in the hotel room that they shared—writing letters, doing each other's hair, or watching the small television they had rented.

This vignette is an experience that one of us had with a group of undergraduate students. The two students who preferred the unchanging nature of their small hotel room generated these questions in the minds of all who witnessed their inactivity: "Why did you bother coming to London?"; "What are you afraid of finding?"; and "Does it bother you that we do so much, while you stay behind all the time?"

To mature emotionally you must progress beyond the first two components of the prescription and test the newly established perceptions you have constructed. This *testing* is accomplished by *undertaking a new experience* or reexperiencing something in a modified way.

These new experiences do not require high levels of risk, nor do they necessitate foreign travel or the outlay of money for equipment or facilities. They may, in fact, be no more "new" than deciding to try an advanced course in a particular discipline, to move from the dorm into an apartment, to take a summer job that is different from your last, or to pursue a new friendship. The experience itself is not the end you are seeking; rather, it is a means of reaching a new "pool" of information about yourself, others, or the objects that form your material world.

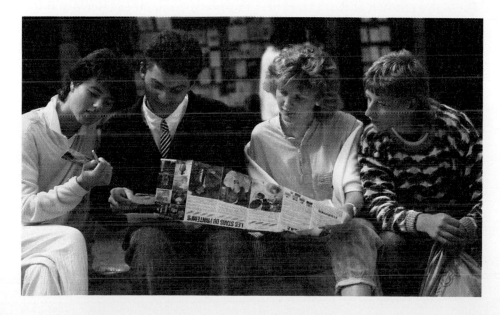

Foreign travel offers opportunities for new experiences.

Although your life is shaped by many factors, including heredity, biological characteristics, environment, and cultural conditioning, new experiences can have a profound influence over the course your life will take. The occasionally powerful impact of a single experience is no more vividly seen than it was in the life of Abraham H. Maslow[13]:

Abraham H. Maslow, former president of the American Psychological Association and one of the greatest creative thinkers in the history of psychology, had become a world authority on the psychology of sexuality because he saw this as the area which would be most helpful to mankind.

His entire career was changed by an experience which he had shortly after Pearl Harbor. While driving home, he was stopped by a war parade. As he watched, suddenly he saw the parade as a march of death with skeletons walking and corpses smiling. Tears began to run down his face. He had a vision of a peace table where men were talking about human nature. "It was at that moment," he says, "that I realized that the rest of my life must be devoted to discovering a psychology for the peace table. That moment changed my whole life and determined what I have done ever since. Since that moment in 1941 I've devoted myself to developing a theory of human nature that could be tested by experiment and research."

"I wanted to prove that human beings are capable of something grander than war and prejudice and hatred. I wanted to make science consider all of the problems that non-scientists have been handling—religion, poetry, values, philosophy, art."

A second example of a single profound experience that forever changed the life of a person is that of Candy Lightner, the mother of a 13-year-old child killed by a drunk driver in 1980. After seeing how leniently the judicial system treated the driver who killed her child, Lightner formed the now-famous organization MADD (Mothers Against Drunk Driving). Much of her time is now spent combating drunk driving.

Our unique experiences do shape our lives, but perhaps the most constructive interpretation of new experiences is to view them first as a means of achieving continued growth and enhanced health. You should never dismiss the possibility that a single experience may profoundly alter the direction your life will take. The active creation of new experiences to guide you toward emotional and spiritual maturation may be the very process that generates the single profound event that transforms your future. In some ways the current phrase "go for it!" expresses this thought.

Reframing Mental Pictures

If you have completed the first three steps in this plan for achieving emotional growth, the newly gleaned information about yourself, others, and objects now becomes the most current source of information available for your use. Regardless of the type of new experience you have undertaken and regardless of its outcome, you are now in a position to modify the initial perceptions you constructed during the first component of this plan. You have new insights, new knowledge, and a new perspective.

Your new experience may have altered the way you value and assign priorities to what you know and do. You have used, modified, and developed new behaviors.

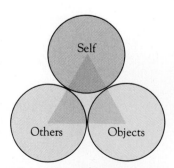

The individual interacts with the self, others, and material objects to grow.

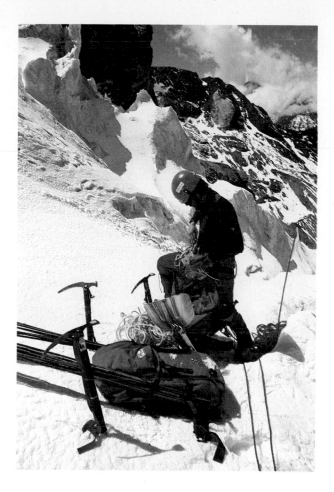

Challenges can lead to new pictures of yourself.

This *new picture* of yourself may not be too different from the perceptions it replaced. However, it will have resulted from a process that is itself growth-oriented. By continuing to engage in this four-step process, your growth will continue over your entire life cycle.

SUMMARY

This chapter challenged you to work toward emotional maturity and spiritual growth. You have learned that genetic and environmental factors can influence personality. Also, a mentally healthy person is one who feels comfortable about himself or herself, feels right about other people, and is able to meet the demands of life.

There is no universally agreed upon interpretation of how one's personality develops; this chapter presented an overview of the traditional views of emotional growth developed by six theorists.

Creative expression is another essential component of emotional maturity. Traits that characterize this component include independence, flexibility, self-acceptance, and openness.

Developing the spiritual dimension of health is a process that involves several stages, including Fowler's synthetic-conventional stage and the individuative-reflective stages. This process of spiritual development leads to a dynamic faith that is the foundation of effective living and creative service.

To develop emotional maturity you must learn to live comfortably with yourself. A periodic self-evaluation and a four-component plan was outlined to help you understand and learn about yourself.

REVIEW QUESTIONS

1 Identify and explain the four components of the cyclic process that will help you understand your emotional nature.
2 List the characteristics of a mentally healthy person.
3 Compare and contrast the six traditional views of growth presented in this chapter.
4 List five characteristics of creative people.
5 Identify the two stages of faith development mentioned in this chapter. Explain when each stage normally occurs and what happens at each stage.
6 What is meant by Erikson's suggestion that the major task awaiting you as an adult is that of "paying back" the collective society?
7 How are emotional maturity and spiritual growth related to overall health?
8 How can faith, as defined in this chapter, help you understand yourself better? How can faith help you serve others?

QUESTIONS FOR PERSONAL CONTEMPLATION

1 If you constructed the mental pictures this chapter suggested, were you able to accept them and plan a new experience that might enhance your future mental pictures?
2 How close do you come to meeting the characteristics of a mentally healthy person described in this chapter?
3 This chapter presents five characteristics of creative individuals. Which of these characteristics are already well-developed within your own makeup? Which of them would you like to start developing? How would you do this?
4 The authors identify two of Fowler's stages of faith development. Which stage do you feel you are in? Do you see this changing in the next few years? If so, why?

REFERENCES

1 National Mental Health Association: Characteristics of mentally healthy people, Alexandria, Va, The Association.
2 Piaget, J, and Inhelder, B: The psychology of the child, New York, 1969, Basic Books, Inc.
3 Erikson, E: The life cycle completed: a review, New York, 1982, WW Norton & Co.
4 Kohlberg, L: The psychology of moral development, San Francisco, 1983, Harper & Row, Publishers, Inc.
5 Lefton, LA: Psychology, Boston, 1985, Allyn & Bacon.
6 Freud, S: General psychological theory, New York, 1963, Macmillan Publishing Co.
7 Maslow, AH: The farthest reaches of human nature, Magnolia, Mass, 1983, Peter Smith Publisher, Inc.
8 Creativity, Carnegie Corporation of New York Quarterly 9:1-8, 1961.
9 Russell, RD: How goes the future, Hygeia? Health Education 16:90-91, 1985.
10 Young, EWD: Spiritual health—an essential element in optimum health, Journal of American College Health 32:273-276, 1984.
11 Fowler J: Stages of faith, San Francisco, 1981, Harper & Row Publishers, Inc.
12 Fowler, JW: Becoming adult, becoming Christian: adult development and Christian faith, San Francisco, 1984, Harper & Row Publishers, Inc.
13 Hall, M: A conversation with Abraham H. Maslow, president of the American Psychological Association, Psychology Today 2:35-37, 54-57, 1968.

ANNOTATED READINGS

Dauten, D: Taking chances: lessons in putting passion and creativity in your work life, New York, 1986, Newmarket Press.

The author describes ways in which people can take chances that will stimulate excitement in life through their work.

Gawryn, M: Reaching high: the psychology of spiritual living, Berkeley Calif, 1980, Spiritual Renaissance Press.

A synthesis of practical psychological insights with spiritual content; presents a comprehensive overview of the process of spiritual living.

Peale, NV: You can if you think you can, Englewood Cliffs, NJ, 1982, Prentice-Hall, Inc.

This book is designed to help you organize your personality forces into actions to help you to think, act, and live victoriously.

Pearsall, P: Superimmunity: master your emotions and improve your health, New York, 1986, McGraw-Hill.

This book encourages the reader to follow a plan of mastering your emotions so that you can improve your overall health.

Raschke, CA: The interruption of eternity: modern gnosticism and the origins of the new religious consciousness, Chicago, 1980, Nelson-Hall Publishers.

An investigation of the renewed interest in gnosticism, with its concomitant disillusionment with external values and its search for an inner spiritual reality.

Rusk, T, and Read, R: I want to change but I don't know how, Los Angeles, 1983, Price/Stern/Sloan Publishers, Inc.

A comprehensive handbook for mastering change, and a guide to personal growth for lay people who want to change.

Siegel, B: Love, medicine and miracles, San Francisco, 1986, Harper & Row Publishers, Inc.

Written by a physician, this best selling book focuses on the role of emotions in treating serious illnesses.

Wood, C, Britt, C, and Jackson, J: Spiritual life, Nashville, 1986, Graded Press.

A comprehensive discussion of three essential stages—hunger, transformation, and discipline—associated with a person's spiritual growth.

CHAPTER 3

Stress
Managing the Unexpected

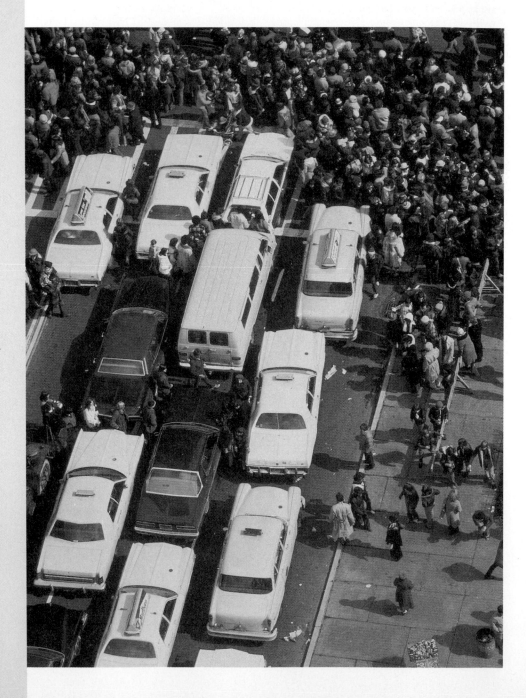

I n the midwestern states there is a familiar saying that suggests that if you do not like the weather, "just wait a few minutes and it will change." Rapid and often unanticipated change characterizes the weather of this region. People who choose to live in this part of the country need to be prepared for dealing with such rapid climatic fluctuations.

Inasmuch as the weather is characterized by change, growth and development are also influenced by change. Each person, program, and object in your immediate environment holds the potential for altering the predictable pattern of living. How you handle change can enrich your life, since change is often challenging, stimulating, and renewing. When you handle change poorly, however, your response precipitates a state of stress that is potentially disruptive to developmental task mastery.

STRESS AND STRESSORS

Almost every day on a college campus you can hear people comment about how much stress they are under. College administrators feel **stress** as they strive to maintain a positive image for their school. Department chairpersons feel pressures to maintain course enrollments. Professors may feel stress when they are assigned new courses to teach or when their journal articles are rejected. Coaches want to apply "positive stress" to their athletes to improve their performances. Even sitting next to a person you are attracted to can cause you to feel stressed.

Although people often use *stress* and *stressor* interchangeably, the words represent different concepts. Hans Selye,[1] world-famous biological scientist, described stress as "the nonspecific response of the body to any demand made on it." Stress can be viewed as a physiological response that results after one is exposed to some factor, agent, or event that forces the body to change or adapt. These factors or events that produce stress are called **stressors.** From a time standpoint, stressors always precede the development of stress in an individual. Stressors are the cause; stress is the effect.

The scientific study of stress has produced a number of general concepts; we will explore them next.

Variation in response to stressors Because individuals are unique, a stressor for one person might not be a stressor for another. While a blizzard could prove stressful for many persons, especially the elderly and the sick, others could find the shut-in days peaceful, relaxing, and utterly enjoyable. Standing in a long line or a crowded elevator can be a stressor for some people but not for others.

Generalized physiological response to stressors Once under the influence of a stressor, people's bodies respond in remarkably similar, predictable ways. When confronted with an uncomfortable situation (for example, being asked to stand up in front of a group and talk), your heart rate increases, your throat becomes dry, your palms sweat, and you feel a little dizzy, despite the fact that you are breathing faster. You may even feel sick to your stomach. It is clear that the stressor has produced these common bodily reactions.

Selye[1] described the typical response to a stressor in his **general adaptation syndrome** model. Selye stated that our bodies move through three stages when confronted by stressors.

stress
physiological and psychological state of imbalance caused by the body's response to an unanticipated, disruptive, or stimulating event.

stressors
factors or events, real or imagined, that elicit a state of stress.

general adaptation syndrome
sequenced physiological response to the presence of a stressor; the alarm, resistance, and exhaustion stages of the stress response.

39

College life presents many stressors.

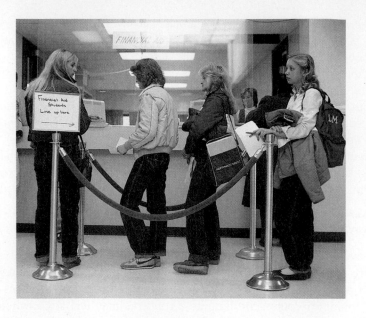

ALARM STAGE Once we are exposed to any stressor, our bodies immediately prepare for possible confrontation. The physiological changes just mentioned appear. These involuntary changes are controlled by hormonal and nervous system functions and in effect quickly prepare the body for Selye's classic **fight-or-flight response.** This response refers to the observation that when people are exposed to a stressor, they will do one of the following: (1) confront the stressor or (2) flee from the stressor. Fleeing eventually removes one from the stressor, whereas confrontation leads one to the next stage of the general adaptation syndrome.

RESISTANCE STAGE The second stage of response to a stressor, the resistance stage, reflects your body's attempt to reestablish internal equilibrium. The high level of energy seen in the initial alarm stage cannot be maintained for an extended period. Your body attempts to redirect the high level of generalized response to a more manageable level.

EXHAUSTION STAGE Body adaptations required through long-term exposure to a stressor often result in an overload. Specific organs and body systems that were called on during the resistance stage may not be able to resist a stressor indefinitely. Exhaustion results when resistance cannot be continued. In extreme or chronic cases, exhaustion can become so pronounced that physiological function deteriorates. Ultimately, prolonged stress can cause death.

Stressors categorized according to origin Stressors can originate from one of at least three different sources. Physical stressors are those whose initial impact is on the body's structural components. Heat, cold, pain, hunger, exercise, lack of sleep, disease organisms, and even sexual arousal can all be considered physical stressors. Psychosocial stressors are those whose initial impact is on the mental processes. Societal or family expectations, course examinations, loss of a friend, fears, and loneliness are all psychosocial stressors. Environmental stressors stem from changes in the natural environment that can affect your physical or mental well-being. Among environmental stressors are pollution, noise, floods, famine, and overcrowding. Some stressors may originate from more than one source.

fight-or-flight response the reaction to a stressor by confrontation or avoidance.

Life Stressors

Which of the following events have you experienced within the last year?

LIFE EVENTS	POINTS
1 Death of spouse	100
2 Death of a close family member	95
3 Divorce from spouse	90
4 Diagnosis of serious illness	85
5 Divorce of parents	80
6 Dismissal from university	75
7 Broken engagement	73
8 Difficulty in parenting	70
9 Getting married	70
10 Loss of job	60
11 Marital reconciliation	45
12 Change in health of a family member	44
13 Pregnancy	40
14 Beginning a new dating relationship	39
15 Lessened harmony in a marital relationship	39
16 Change in financial status	38
17 Death of a close friend	37
18 Lessened harmony in a dating relationship	35
19 Assumption of a large loan	30
20 Outstanding personal achievement	29
21 Relocation of family	28
22 Completion of degree	25
23 Change in living conditions	25
24 Change in personal habits	24
25 Conflict with a faculty member	23
26 Scheduling conflicts	20
27 Change in residence	20
28 Change in religious practices	19
29 Change in school (transfer)	19
30 Change in level of social involvement	18
31 Assumption of small loan	17
32 Change in sleeping patterns	16
33 Being at home for school holidays	15
34 Change in eating habits	13
35 Change in activity patterns	13
36 Minor violations of the law	11

Your total points _____

Interpretation

Life events can function as stressors that influence the body through activation of the stress response. It has been suggested that an accumulation of 150 or more points in a 1-year period may predispose a person to increased physical illness within the coming year. Of course you must remember that for a given person, certain events may be more or less stressful than the point values indicated.

Intensity of stressor Not everyone reacts similarly to a given stressor.[2] For increasing numbers of people, cigarette smoke is a stressor, yet two nonsmokers may have different reactions to being near someone else's cigarette smoke. One person might feel only mild stress or annoyance, while another person could feel severe stress. Thus we might expect different behavioral responses by people exposed to the same stressor.

Positive or negative stressors Stressors produce the same generalized physical response, whether an individual perceives the stressor as positive or negative. Poor academic performance, loss of a friend, or having a wisdom tooth extracted can result in stress, just as giving birth, receiving a promotion, or starting a passionate romance can be potential stressors. In each case the impact on body systems is relatively similar.

Selye[1] coined the word **eustress** for positive stress. Stressors that produce eustress can enhance longevity, productivity, and life satisfaction. Examples might be the mild stress that helps you stay alert during a midterm examination, the pain that causes you to seek medical attention, and the exhilarating stress you feel while exercising.

Selye calls harmful, unpleasant stress **distress.** Distress that goes uncontrolled can result in maladaptation, sickness, and even death.[3] Examples of distress are chronic pain, lack of meaningful relationships, and living in an unpleasant, demanding environment. For some, when distress becomes overwhelming, thoughts of suicide may occur (see Chapter 20).

Inevitability of stress Only in death can stress be avoided. We live our lives trying to accommodate a variety of stressors—many of which we are unaware. Stress motivates us and stimulates us into action. The key to lifelong satisfaction seems to lie in our ability to accommodate a myriad of positive and negative stressors. Selye, in his book *Stress Without Distress,* encourages us to identify the stress levels at which we can best function as productive, contributing, happy people.

Uncontrolled stress related to disease states According to the general adaptation syndrome theory, if the impact of the stressor is not minimized or resolved, the effect on the human body is exhaustion. This exhaustion produces psychological and physiological breakdown. Depending on the severity of the stressor and the resistance of the person, this breakdown may occur quickly or after many years. Exposure to a high-level stressor—intense cold or heat, for example—will result in death within a few moments. Constant exposure to a low-level stressor, such as an unpleasant co-worker or a polluted environment, might not cause disease symptoms to develop for years.

Clearly, the effects of unresolved stress are cumulative. The impact builds until the body begins to break down. This breakdown is manifested by the development of stress-related diseases and disorders.[4] Among the major diseases that have some origin in unresolved stress are hypertension, stroke, heart disease, kidney disease, depression, alcoholism, and gastrointestinal disorders (ulcers, irritable bowel syndrome, and diverticulitis). Other stress-related disorders are migraine headaches, allergies, asthma, hay fever, anxiety, insomnia, impo-

eustress
stress that adds a positive, enhancing dimension to the quality of life.

distress
stress that diminishes the quality of life; commonly associated with disease, illness, and maladaptation.

How Vulnerable Are You to Stress?

This self-assessment inventory can help you to determine how likely you are to be affected by stressors. Beside each item, indicate how much of the time each statement applies to you. Score each item based on the scale shown below. Calculate your total score at the end of the test.

 1 Always
 2 Almost always
 3 Most of the time
 4 Some of the time
 5 Never

 1 I eat at least one hot, balanced meal a day. _____

 2 I get 7 to 8 hours sleep at least four nights a week. _____

 3 I give and receive affection regularly. _____

 4 I have at least one relative within 50 miles on whom I can rely. _____

 5 I exercise to the point of perspiration at least twice a week. _____

 6 I do not smoke or smoke less than half a pack of cigarettes a day. _____

 7 I take fewer than five alcoholic drinks a week. _____

 8 I am the appropriate weight for my height. _____

 9 I have an income adequate to meet basic expenses. _____

10 I get strength from my spiritual beliefs. _____

11 I regularly attend club or social activities. _____

12 I have a network of friends and acquaintances. _____

13 I have one or more friends to confide in about personal matters. _____

14 I am in physical good health (including eyesight, hearing, teeth). _____

15 I am able to speak openly about my feelings when angry or worried. _____

16 I have regular conversations with the people I live with about
     domestic problems, (e.g., chores, money, and daily living issues). _____

17 I do something for fun at least once a week. _____

18 I am able to organize my time effectively. _____

19 I drink fewer than three cups of coffee (or tea or cola drinks) a day. _____

20 I take quiet time for myself during the day. _____

                              Your total points _____

Interpretation

To get your score, add up the figures and subtract 20. Any number over 30 indicates a vulnerability to stress. You are seriously vulnerable if your score is between 50 and 75, and extremely vulnerable if it is over 75. Please note that your score on this assessment may not relate closely to your score on the Life Stressors Assessment on p. 41. This instrument assesses behavior while the box on p. 41 assesses events that occur in your life. Also, keep in mind that such assessments are not intended to be substitutes for evaluations made by trained professionals.

Personal
Assessment

tence, and menstrual irregularities. The dependency-related behaviors of cigarette smoking, overeating or undereating, and underactivity relate in part to
unresolved stress. The role of stress in the development of cancer is not fully
understood. If a link should develop, it will likely involve cancers caused by an
immune system weakened by unresolved stress.

COLLEGE-CENTERED STRESSORS

For some people who have not attempted college coursework, the idea that college life could be stressful must seem too silly to consider. After all, isn't college
the "good life?" Four more years of high school? Parties, romances, and sunbath-
ing?

For those of us who study or teach on college campuses, these perceptions are
hard to understand. We know all too well that the undergraduate experience is
serious because of its role in preparation for life. For the part-time, nontraditional student who comes to campus for coursework (often at night) and then
returns to work, family, and community responsibility, college classes can be
especially stressful.

In college and university settings, we think stressors could arise from one or
more of the following areas.

Employment expectations For those students who believe that the major purpose of a college education is to prepare them for a job and a higher standard of
living than that enjoyed by their parents, the question of having chosen the
"right" course of study is at times extremely stressful. Uncertainty about job
opportunities, technical capabilities, starting salaries, and the need for a graduate degree become increasingly pressing when one begins to realize that college
will soon end and that the world of employment (or nonemployment) awaits.

Institutional expectations For entry into the "community of educated people,"
college places demands of various types on students. Concerns centered in course
selection, course withdrawal, maintaining a desired grade point average, and
admission to upper division or graduate school are all potential stressors. For
those who are only beginning the process of orchestrating a schedule of class
work that will encompass eight semesters or twelve quarters, the frustration arising from this responsibility can be quite stressful.

Financial support How much does a college education cost? Is it worth the
money, particularly at a time when loans are difficult to find and expensive to
repay? Should you consider ROTC as a source of assistance in light of the fact
that a military obligation awaits you after graduation? For some students these
questions are not stressful, but for many students these are among the most
pressing of all questions. Each registration period, each loan application, and
each statement of need introduces anew these feelings of frustration and uncertainty for college students.

Personal expectations While addressing the new freshmen during their orientation meeting, a college dean may tell you to shake the hands of the people

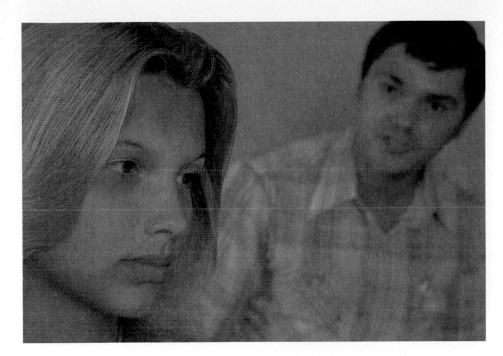

Interpersonal relationships can be a source of stress.

sitting next to you, since, on the basis of the school's attrition rate, one will not be in your class at the end of the year. As you extend your hand to the person next to you, the reality strikes you that a hand is being extended toward you. Will you be among the students who will fail to complete the freshman year? Will you be forced to return home or to your job and explain why you are no longer at school?

Beyond these are a variety of stressors that stem from personal decisions, including those related to part-time jobs, weight management, sexuality, and interpersonal relationships.

Family expectations For most students, college is an experiment in disengagement. For 9 months each year you are given a relatively free hand at structuring your own lifestyle—managing your own time, being responsible for completing course requirements, and establishing social relationships.

If these responsibilities seem difficult, then you may be stressed by the feeling that you are not capable of doing what others expect that you should be able to do. For many, this "disengagement shock" is the most pressing stressor that they will face. For some, the adjustment will be too great and they will return to their families before making further educational decisions.

For many students, the belief that college performance is being judged against the sacrifices being made by the family will be a draining source of stress. How should you feel when you learn that parents and siblings are "doing without" so that you can pursue your educational goals? If you are the first in your family to attempt higher education, will your success be an important determinant in your younger brother's or sister's chances of going to school? Could your failure be their failure too? In many ways, not only you, but also your family, has matriculated to the college campus.

For nontraditional students, family expectations may come from spouses, children, friends, and co-workers who are counting on you to do well in college.

Religious faith Consider this scenario: By the end of your first semester at college you no longer attend religious services. You become an agnostic by the middle of the second semester, and by the end of your first year in college you are a confirmed atheist.

As ridiculous as the above may sound, this scenario could be the anticipated "falling from grace" imagined by your parents as they see you leave the security of their home for life on the "radical" college campus. A current twist to this theme is that of your being captured by one of the religious cults that exist on every campus. Interfaith dating may represent an even more common religious-oriented stressor.

Questions about religion can become a part of your educational experience and be the source of uncertainty and stress.[5] Higher education is designed to challenge your knowledge, values, and practices so that they may serve you better in the future. Expect your religious beliefs to be challenged.

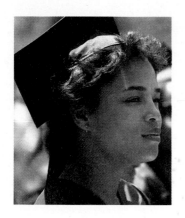

Faculty expectations Faculty members consider the college classroom a very real part of the world. It is an arena in which they experience success or failure. It is one of their major ways of achieving a sense of contribution. Most professors take their teaching seriously, and they expect you to pursue your studies with equal seriousness. Should you disregard this academic reality, stressors could occur in the form of poor grades or weak employment recommendations. Indeed, faculty expectations can be a major stressor for students.

Although we could have expanded our list of campus-centered stressors to include peer interactions, political activism, and other stressful activities, it is sufficient to say that each college or university holds the potential not only for enriching your life but also for making demands of you.

Growth is never passive; growth often necessitates conflict. It will nearly always demand active participation and effort and at times may demand more than you believe you are capable of giving.

LIFE-CENTERED STRESSORS

When we were college students during the 1960s, we had the notion that the traditional college years simply had to be the most stressful of times. We found out differently. Stressors remain, although they differ in their focus and intensity. In a study conducted for a major manufacturer,[6] adults were asked to identify the roots of their stress. Not surprisingly, many familiar factors surfaced.

Cost of living For most adults, the cost of living is a factor that can introduce distress into an otherwise tranquil life. From necessities (such as food and shelter) to luxury items (fancy cars and fashionable clothes), we can be routinely confronted by desires that exceed our financial resources. Unfortunately, not only can the inability to fulfill our needs be a source of stress, but frequently the activities necessary to secure financial resources prove to be stressful as well.

Being too busy An all too frequently voiced concern of today's active adults is that of being too busy. School, employment, parenting, and community service must all fit into a day that remains only 24 hours long. When we cannot effectively manage our time we can experience hours, days, weeks, and years that ask more of us than we have time to give. For most people, the remark "too busy" is never far removed from the feelings of stress.

Money concerns Contracts, estates, taxes, and investments are money concerns that are sources of stress to adults during the college years and beyond. Few of you will be able to escape these familiar sources of stressors.

Not only are we stressed by the cost of things that we need or want, but the events associated with being a wage earner are also stressful.

Trouble relaxing Interestingly, experiencing trouble relaxing is a concern to many. Perhaps at the base of this stressor is our inability to relax when we consciously know that relaxation is in our best interests. We are, at times, stressed by our inability to cope well with other stressors.

Family illness Family illness, particularly when serious, is an important component of life-centered stressors. As you may have noticed on the stress inventory on p. 41, family-related concerns are the most prevalent sources of stress for adults. Particularly, illness in children and elderly parents can be stressful for those attempting to balance the many demands of college, employment, and community involvement.

Personal illness Although not mentioned as often as other life stressors, personal illness is another obvious source of stress. When health-related limitations occur in our own lives, the relationships that we hold with others and the expectations that we hold for ourselves are challenged. We eventually become stressed by both the discomfort of the illness and by the inconvenience that it may cause our busy schedules.

THE STRESS RESPONSE

Why does something as familiar as a telephone ringing late at night cause you fear and near-panic? Why is it that your hands sweat, your muscles tense, and your appetite leaves as you wait in the hallway outside the classroom in which your final examination is to be held? Is the "cottonmouth" feeling described by athletes a valuable aid to performance?

The answers to these questions can be found in an understanding of the body's innate ability to be in a state of readiness to respond to situations associated with change. When the body must confront an aggressor, escape from a hostile situation, or respond sexually, it is being asked to perform primitively. From a functional perspective these survival demands are characterized by a common element—energy—rapid in its availability, generous in its amount, but costly in its potential danger to the body. Historically these demands were almost always short lived, thus allowing the energy to be expended quickly and the body to return to its preferred state of functional efficiency, **homeostasis.** Rarely are modern demands so easily resolved.

homeostasis
the body's preferred state of dynamic balance among body systems.

To understand and appreciate the energy production response, you must understand the functions of the nervous and endocrine pathways. Figure 3-1 shows the process of the body's response to a stressor as it stimulates energy production the body will require.

Stressors

For a state of stress to exist, you must first be confronted by an event, real or imagined, that you interpret as disruptive, frightening, exciting, or dangerous. On the basis of your interpretation, the event becomes the stressor.

Other people may not interpret a given event in the same way you do. Thus several persons may experience the same event as you, yet only you report that the event was stressful.

Factors Influencing the Perceptions of Stressors

A variety of factors influences how a particular person perceives stressors.

Genetic predispositions The manner in which persons perceive and respond to stressors may be influenced by genetic predispositions. In all likelihood, humans inherit different capacities for nerve conductivity and neurotransmitter function. Thus some people may be able to cope well with a stressor (cold weather, for example) because they may have inherited a greater physical capacity to confront that stressor. Some studies now suggest that certain people may be more likely to develop certain forms of mental illness or depression because they have inherited a genetic predisposition to those disorders.[7]

Past experiences Our responses to stressors are colored by our past experiences. As quickly as you are able to perceive a stressor, your brain searches its storehouse of past experiences. This past information then influences how you interpret the current stressor. Since past experiences differ from person to person, our interpretations of the same stressor can differ considerably. For example, children who have experienced a number of health problems might not feel as apprehensive about "getting a shot" as children who have rarely been sick.

Expectations As with past experiences, we also possess a storehouse of expectations about how we will react when confronted with a stressor. At times, we react according to how we think we might react. For example, if we have conditioned ourselves to expect a positive response to a stressor, we may be less easily stressed than people who have conditioned themselves to "expect the worst."

Setting and time Important factors that shape our individual reactions to stressors are setting and time. On occasion, normally routine events become stressors because of where we are and what we are doing. Noticing a police officer in your rear view mirror is enough to make a routine drive to the store a stressful experience.

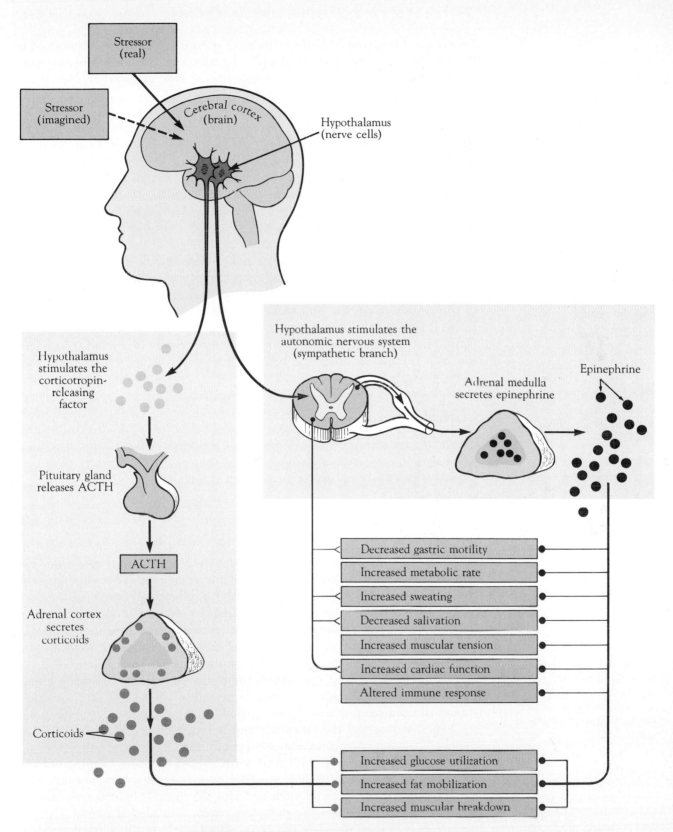

Figure 3-1
The stress response: physiological reactions to a stressor.

Number and frequency Our perceptions of stressors may also be conditioned by the number and frequency of stressors to which we are exposed. By being overwhelmed with stressors, we may be less able to manage many of our routine tasks.

Amount of support Finally, our response to stressors may differ according to the amount of support we have to confront the stressor. Thus how we handle a stressor might depend on our network of helpful and concerned friends, family, co-workers, and *mentors.* Perhaps this is what the Beatles had in mind when they sang "I'll get by with a little help from my friends."

Sensory Modalities

Before you can assess an event as stressful or nonstressful, it must be sensed by your *central nervous system.* With the exception of those stressors that are a product of your imagination, you become aware of most stressors through one or more of the *sensory modalities.* You must hear, smell, taste, feel, or see something before it becomes real to you, and thus potentially a stressor. Covering your eyes during the most bloody scenes of a horror movie reflects your attempt to reduce the stress of the event. Likewise, pinching your nostrils helps you avoid the stress of an unpleasant odor.

Cerebral Cortex

Events become stressors when, on entering the *cerebral cortex* of your brain, mental images of those events are assessed as stressors. The complexity of this interpretive process is far beyond the scope of this book.

Endocrine System Involvement

In a physiological sense, your body's response to the presence of a stressor involves not only the brain and nervous system but also your *endocrine system.* The endocrine system stimulates production of the energy needed for dealing with stressors.

The process of interconnecting your nervous system and endocrine system is the task of the **hypothalamus,** a structure located deep within the brain. The hypothalamus is located immediately above the gland that plays the major role in regulating the endocrine system—the **pituitary gland.**

The interplay between the hypothalamus and the pituitary gland is accomplished both by an exchange of nerve fibers and by the sharing of a small self-contained circulatory system. During periods of stress, communication between the hypothalamus and the pituitary gland is accomplished by the release from the hypothalamus of a chemical messenger into the blood flowing directly to the pituitary gland. This chemical, called **corticotropin-releasing factor,** stimulates the pituitary to produce its own powerful hormone, **adrenocorticotropic hormone (ACTH).** ACTH is then released into the general circulation, ultimately reaching a pair of glands of the endocrine system, the **adrenal glands.** The purpose of ACTH is to stimulate the outer layer (*cortex*) of the adrenal glands to

---

hypothalamus
portion of the midbrain that provides a connection between the cerebral cortex and the pituitary gland.

pituitary gland
"master gland" of the endocrine system; the wide variety of hormones produced by the pituitary are sent to structures throughout the body.

corticotropin-releasing factor
chemical messenger produced by the hypothalamus and released into the closed circulatory pathway shared with the pituitary gland; stimulates the pituitary's production of ACTH.

adrenocorticotropic hormone (ACTH)
hormone produced in the pituitary gland and transmitted to the cortex of the adrenal glands; stimulates production and release of corticoids.

adrenal glands
paired triangular endocrine glands situated above each kidney; site of epinephrine and corticoid production.

produce chemical substances called **corticoids.** Corticoids support the powerful hormone **epinephrine** (commonly known as **adrenaline**) in the production of energy.

The hypothalamus also activates the adrenal gland directly through a branch of the body's autonomic nervous system. This direct innervation of the adrenal gland is responsible for the production of epinephrine. Epinephrine causes most of the functional changes that occur in the body to produce the rapid, short-term high energy levels required in the presence of a stressor.

Many of the physiological responses that we will discuss in terms of the influence of epinephrine are also directly influenced by branches of the autonomic nervous system that connect directly to tissues or organs. Thus epinephrine's role in the general adaptation syndrome is supported by both corticoids and direct autonomic innervation.

Epinephrine-Influenced Responses

Once epinephrine is released by the adrenal gland, many of the following tissue responses can be expected in a normally healthy individual who is under the influence of a real or imagined stressor.

Decreased gastric motility Because the body needs energy when a stressor must be avoided or defeated, it cannot wait for the relatively slow process of digestion to change food into glucose in the stomach and small intestine. Rather, the body must turn to the *glucose* already circulating in the blood or in a storage form within tissue. Therefore the large volume of blood that is normally near the intestinal wall to absorb nutrients is now used to carry glucose to skeletal muscles. As a consequence, the entire digestive system slows down. It is not surprising that people who are under chronic stress may report gastric distress, constipation, hemorrhoids, or irritable bowel syndrome.

Increased metabolic rate Epinephrine will increase the **metabolic rate.** Glucose already within the system is rushed by blood circulation to the cells, where it will be combined with oxygen (oxidation) for the release of energy. In the presence of a stressor, the rate of this conversion of glucose to energy is increased. The body becomes a more efficient furnace, in the sense that it can "fire up" more quickly than usual.

Increased sweating To control the elevated temperatures generated by the accelerated energy production, the body sweats. The accumulated fluid forms on the skin surface, where it evaporates. As the water is converted to a vapor, heat is drawn from surrounding tissues, thus lowering the temperature. In those few persons who lack the ability to sweat, strenuous activity and stress can generate a state of **hyperthermia.**

Decreased salivation As a result of the overall shutdown of the digestive system, the production of saliva, a fluid that contains digestive enzymes, is also curtailed. Persons who are under the influence of any type of stressor may quickly report a "cottonmouth" sensation, which is caused by the absence of normal amounts of saliva.

---

corticoids
hormones generated by the adrenal cortex; corticoids influence the body's control of glucose, protein, and fat metabolism.

epinephrine
powerful adrenal hormone whose presence in the bloodstream prepares the body for maximal energy production and skeletal muscle response.

adrenaline
common name for epinephrine.

metabolic rate
rate or intensity at which the body produces energy.

hyperthermia
excess production of body heat; abnormally elevated core body temperature.

Increased muscular tension Twitching and tautness of the arms and legs during times of stress reflect how close to the fully contracted state the body has taken its skeletal muscles. By maintaining the muscles in this condition, the body is prepared for "fight or flight" in the shortest time.

Increased cardiac and pulmonary function The production of energy and the removal of waste products formed during that process require the presence of an efficient and dependable transport system. The circulatory system provides this transport. During periods of stress, the heart and lungs go into high gear. Epinephrine helps increase *cardiac* and *pulmonary* function, and thus assists the fight-or-flight response. An overall upsurge in heart output and blood pressure and the rate and depth of breathing ensure maximum oxygenation of tissue.

antigens
disease-producing microorganisms or foreign substances that, on entering the body, trigger an immune response.

antibodies
chemical compounds produced by the body's immune system to destroy antigens and their toxins.

T lymphocytes
small circulating white blood cells that, in the presence of specific antigens, form small sensitized lymphocytes—the basic components of the body's cellular immunity.

Altered immune system response In response to such **antigens** as invading microorganisms, foreign proteins (such as those found in bee venom), and, at times, the body's own cells, our immune system responds by producing **antibodies** and specific chemical substances (see Chapter 12). Cell-mediated immunity, a major component of the body's overall immune system, develops from **T lymphocytes** and helps counteract viruses, fungi, and foreign tissues. Cell-mediated immunity also helps to fight newly formed malignant cells and thus controls the development of cancers within the body.

During periods of prolonged stress, elevated levels of adrenal hormones appear to have a destructive effect on the T lymphocytes.[4] Illnesses contracted during or shortly after long periods of stress may be directly related to the suppression of this important component of the body's overall defensive system.

Influences of corticoids and epinephrine on energy release

Increased glucose utilization Because glucose is the body's most basic source of energy, an early feature of the stress response is the release of glycogen (the storage form of glucose) from its deposit sites, particularly the liver. Once glycogen is reconverted to glucose, the body will make increasing demands for glucose delivery to the tissues involved in resisting the stressor.

Increased fat utilization If a stressor is not eliminated promptly, the body's supply of glucose may become depleted. The body then turns to its two remaining energy reserves, fat deposits and muscle tissue. Of these two, fat breakdown will begin as the blood glucose level falls. Fat breakdown will result in the production of metabolic waste products, which will eventually cause the body to turn to its most protected energy deposits—muscle tissue.

Muscle tissue breakdown and utilization If the stressor is unusually powerful or the person's ability to deal constructively with that particular type of stressor is inadequate, energy demands will continue to the point that muscle tissue becomes involved. As seen in photographs of prisoners from World War II, when the body is forced to turn to its muscle mass as a source of energy, emaciation results. Fortunately, most college-related stressors (unlike nutritional deprivation) are resolved long before this drastic physiological response would be necessary.

Although in the short term all of the responses shown in Figure 3-1 are valuable when you confront a stressor, long-term exposure to these breakdown processes can only have a destructive effect on the integrity of the body and the physical component of health. Fortunately, most stressors are relatively short lived, but, as we pointed out in our discussion of the resistance stage of the general adaptation syndrome, the body will shift the efforts of a prolonged "fight" to specific body systems. When this shift occurs, the more specific disease processes associated with chronic stress begin to be seen.

COPING: REACTING TO STRESSORS

Perhaps because the effects of stress are cumulative, it is difficult for some people to realize that now is the time to examine their stress-related behaviors. We hear many undergraduate students say, "All right, I'm not that good at handling my stress now, but the moment I walk down the graduation aisle with my diploma in hand, I'll be ready to change my lifestyle. I'll finally be free to quit smoking [or to start an exercise program or to improve my eating habits]. I'll be able to cope well once my life gets easier."

For most persons, life won't get any easier once their college days are over. Just ask an older, nontraditional student in your class! The pressures of employment, finances, and family all seem to make life more difficult—more complicated. Obviously the best time to learn how to cope with your stress is now—before faulty habits have turned to dependencies, and the long-term effects of stress have started to damage your health.

The keys to coping with stressors are found in the ways we choose to live. Traditional methods of handling stress that have been both simple to accomplish and socially supported have included all of the *negative dependency behaviors* (smoking, excess drinking, overeating), withdrawal from the stressor, and at-

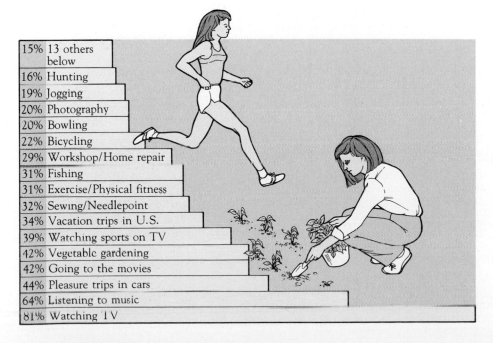

15%	13 others below
16%	Hunting
19%	Jogging
20%	Photography
20%	Bowling
22%	Bicycling
29%	Workshop/Home repair
31%	Fishing
31%	Exercise/Physical fitness
32%	Sewing/Needlepoint
34%	Vacation trips in U.S.
39%	Watching sports on TV
42%	Vegetable gardening
42%	Going to the movies
44%	Pleasure trips in cars
64%	Listening to music
81%	Watching TV

Figure 3-2
Based on a randomly selected national sample of 1,500 households, these data from the U.S. Bureau of the Census indicate that people spend their leisure time in a variety of ways. Which of these popular activities do you engage in? Which ones are most effective in helping you reduce stress?

tacking stress through direct confrontation. Although they may be effective in the short term, these coping methods may produce additional stress.

Perhaps as a consequence of the "Me decade" of the 1970s, efforts to develop coping skills have placed much more long-term responsibility directly on the stressed person. No longer is it socially acceptable to escape through negative dependency behaviors, withdrawal, or aggressiveness. The emphasis now is on lifestyle management, because the benefits appear to have immediate positive consequences and gradual long-term benefits.

Stress Management Techniques

Experts in stress management indicate that the most successful methods of coping with distress include relaxation training, physical exercise, dietary considerations, "hurry sickness" substitutions (including effective time management skills), and guided imagery.

Relaxation training

Although physicians can prescribe a wide variety of drugs to calm anxious patients, there is a growing interest today in the use of nonpharmacological relaxation techniques to reduce the effects of distress. Such efforts are relatively simple to learn, do not produce drug dependency or unusual side effects, and provide you with the necessary skills for dealing with future stressors.

For years physicians have encouraged patients to relax. Professors have told students to "relax and you'll do much better." What does it mean to relax? Is reading a book relaxing? Is sitting under a tree a way to relax? How about listening to music? Although enjoyable, these forms of relaxation are passive and may not permit you to cope effectively with some stressors.

Periods of reduced stress are vital for mental health.

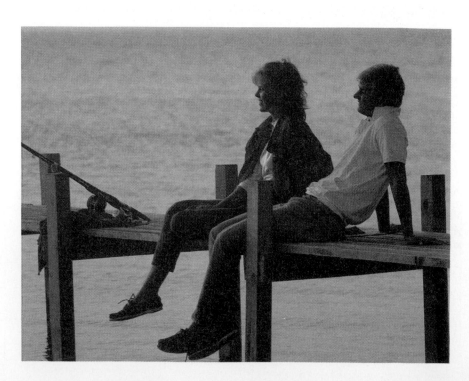

Through **relaxation training** people learn to control their own physiological reactions to stressors. Learning to relax is an active process. True relaxation is thought to occur only when an individual learns to control such functions as respiration, heart rate, and blood pressure—functions generally considered to be involuntary processes. Such self-control is indeed possible to master, even in a relatively short time.

relaxation training
the use of various techniques to produce a state of relaxation.

Various techniques appear useful in training persons to relax. Biofeedback, relaxation response, and muscle tension-relaxation exercise training all help to produce relaxation.

Biofeedback is the self-monitoring of physiological performance.[8] The subject is connected to various electronic instruments that measure heart rate, body temperature, respiration, brain waves, and muscle tension. These machines provide immediate objective information (feedback) about the degree of relaxation achieved by the user. Users of biofeedback equipment are amazed to see how quickly they can learn to relax muscle groups, slow breathing rates, reduce heart rates, and alter brain wave patterns. Biofeedback training familiarizes the user with the sensations associated with relaxation. Once the relaxation techniques are learned, a person should be able to relax without being attached to biofeedback equipment. Biofeedback training has been shown clinically to assist patients with hypertension and migraine headaches.

biofeedback
self-monitoring of physiological processes as they occur within the body.

The **relaxation response,** promoted by cardiologist Herbert Benson, is really a form of focused meditation. Benson believes that just as there is a "fight-or-flight response" in persons, there is also a "relaxation response."[9] The stimulation of this response, thought to originate in the hypothalamic region of the brain, will produce a lowering of blood pressure, oxygen consumption, and heart rate—all keys to deep relaxation. Achieving proper relaxation requires one to move through the following simple steps:

relaxation response
physiological state in opposition to the fight-or-flight response of the general adaptation syndrome.

- Sit quietly in a comfortable position.
- Close your eyes.
- Deeply relax all your muscles.
- Breathe in through your nose and mentally say the word "one" each time you exhale through your mouth.
- Do this for 10 minutes, maintaining a passive attitude.

Another means of coping with stressors involves the use of *muscle tension-relaxation exercises*. Also called progressive relaxation exercises, these exercises require a person to alternately contract and then relax the various muscle groups. Participants generally begin with one muscle group and then continue until all muscle groups have relaxed. These exercises allow the person to recognize and then control muscle tenseness. Some students report that these exercises help them fall asleep during episodes of insomnia. Edward Jacobson[10] developed these exercises in the 1930s, long before relaxation was considered a valuable component of overall health and stress management.

Physical exercise

One of the best ways to handle stress is to exercise. Health professionals are recognizing the value that exercise has on one's outlook and mental well-being. A good physical workout at the end of the workday appears to help minimize minor frustrations, replace mental fatigue with physical fatigue, and provide an excellent avenue for releasing excess muscle tension.[11,12]

Although most persons who exercise do so for only a relatively short time (30 to 45 minutes), the important stress-reducing benefits can extend for a number of hours. Respiration and heart rate lower. Muscle tension relaxes. People report feeling both relaxed and refueled at the same time. There is increasing evidence to suggest that during exercise, the body produces an influx of chemicals called **endorphins.**[12] Endorphins are opiate-like substances that produce a mild druglike euphoria in persons who exercise. Perhaps future research will indicate that it is the outpouring of endorphins that produces both the "chemical high" that some exercisers report and the repetitive behavior seen in exercisers who must exercise every day to maintain an internal equilibrium.

A word of caution: physical exercise can actually stimulate the stress response in people who become "addicted" to their exercise routine or become involved in competitive events. In the first case, people who become compulsively attached to their physical activity invite distress when their exercise routine is disrupted or when they are injured. In the second case, those persons who establish self-imposed levels of performance run the risk of distress whenever they fail to achieve their goals. From a stress management standpoint, the key seems to lie in your ability to put your fitness program in its proper perspective.

Dietary considerations

Dietary considerations apply to nearly every aspect of one's health status. With regard to stress management, it is important to consider the impact of consuming foods that tend to stimulate the body's central nervous system.

Caffeine, commonly found in coffee, tea, soft drinks, chocolate, and even some over-the-counter pain relievers, enhances the body's physiological response to stressors.[13] Caffeine stimulates heart rate, respiration, blood pressure, and overall alertness. People who use caffeine in heavy doses tend to think faster, talk faster, and walk faster. For this reason, you might consider caffeine to be a stressor by itself.

If you are a heavy consumer of caffeine products, you might consider curtailing your use of caffeine gradually, over a period of 2 or 3 weeks. Going "cold turkey" with caffeine products produces an unpleasant withdrawal symptom—headaches.

Books popular in the mid-1970s theorized the role of dietary sugar as a stressor. Foods containing high levels of sugar were thought to cause a rapid rise in blood glucose, followed by a release of high levels of insulin. When this insulin quickly depleted the blood glucose, a significant depression of physiological functioning ensued. Poor dietary practices involving excessive sugar consumption were thus thought to lead to a cyclic state of excitation-depression of the body. Sugar consumed in large amounts was seen as a powerful stressor because of the physiological changes it was thought to produce.

No carefully controlled research studies have substantiated the role of dietary sugar as a stressor of the magnitude once envisioned. Recent reports from physiologists on sugar's role as a stressor state that if double-blind studies were conducted, sugar consumption would not prove to be a major generator of stress.[14] In a related area, recently released results have shown little relationship between sugar consumption and childhood hyperactivity, as was also formerly theorized.[15,16]

---

endorphins
opiate-like substances within the central nervous system; endorphins are thought to create a euphoric effect 200 times greater than en equivalent dose of morphine.

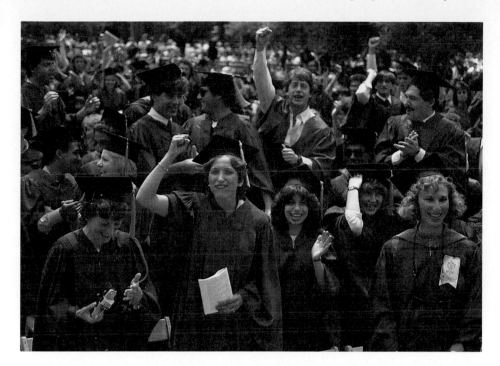

Graduation marks a transition from familiar stressors to new ones.

Hurry Sickness Substitutes

Since some scientific evidence suggests a correlation between a highly stressed personality type and cardiovascular disease, we should mention some recommendations offered by the noted cardiologists Friedman and Rosenman.[17,18] In their classic bestseller *Type A Behavior and Your Heart*, these physicians proposed ways of altering many of the typical behaviors that in effect keep some people chronically distressed—to a point that may cause premature death from cardiovascular degeneration.

To reduce the chances of developing stress-related *hurry sickness*, Friedman and Rosenman[17] suggest the following.

- *Reduce your sense of time urgency.* Constantly remind yourself that there will always be some unfinished business on your agenda. Few ventures ever failed because they were planned too well or too slowly.
- *Try to listen quietly when others are talking to you.* Do not try to finish the sentences of others or interrupt with such speed-up phrases as "Yes, yes" or "Uh huh, uh huh."
- *Reduce your polyphasic thinking.* Polyphasic thinking implies multiple simultaneous streams of thought. Try not to think of more than one thing at a time. Cluttering your mind produces unnecessary stress.
- *Take the time to offer sincere thanks to people that have performed services for you.* Do not merely grunt. Speak in full sentences while looking directly into the face of the person.
- *Smile at as many persons as often as you can.* This may be quite difficult at first, but this a great way of reducing your free-floating hostility.
- *Move more slowly.* Consciously attempt to walk at a slower pace. Drive your car more slowly. Be willing to give the other drivers a break.

Are You a Type A Personality?

Persons who display these behavioral traits have a Type A personality:

Overloads work schedule
Emphasizes speed over quality
Pays little attention to surroundings
Disregards the ideas of others
Competes with intensity
Moves rapidly (when walking, swimming, running)
Displays impatience with others
Checks the time frequently

- *Improve your speech by expanding your sentences.* Expand your vocabulary by learning the meaning of new words. Use longer sentences and speak more slowly while talking to people.
- *Hold your opinions more loosely.* Realize that you, indeed, may once be wrong or that others may sometimes be right. Stop saying "I told you so."
- *Seek time for yourself occasionally.* This means not just being alone, but searching your "inner self" for understanding and insight. Evaluate yourself and your behaviors during quiet times.
- *Become more satisfied with the understanding of overall concepts.* "Cramming facts" into your head should not be an end in itself. Life then tends to become a series of final examinations. Although at times knowledge of facts is essential, try to be more satisfied with understanding major concepts.

Whereas the Type A person would need to work to develop the healthful behaviors suggested above, the Type B person generally exhibits these on a regular basis. Type B people tend to be more relaxed, less aggressive, less time dependent, more readily satisfied, and less achievement oriented than Type A people. For years, Type B persons have been thought to be less likely to develop cardiovascular disease.

Recently, the link between personality, stress, and heart disease has been questioned.[19] Several recent studies suggest that the real culprits may be specific components of the Type A behavior—hostility and a cynical attitude. Regardless of the personality traits that may be most closely related to cardiovascular disease, many professionals continue to encourage Type A persons to evaluate their life-styles to seek a more balanced approach to living.

For certain people, a third personality type may be related to their ability to achieve eustress. In the opinion of Dr. Frank Farley at the University of Wisconsin, the *Type T personality* is one who intentionally pursues thrills through various risk-taking behaviors.[20] These risk-taking behaviors can include intellectual risks as well as physically demanding activities. As long as the activities chosen by the Type T person are not dangerous to others, thrill-seeking behaviors may lead to personal accomplishment and satisfaction.

Guided imagery

guided imagery
process of visualizing oneself responding in a positive and controlled fashion to a stressor.

Over 30 years ago Norman Vincent Peale referred to a process called *positive thinking.*[21] Today the term is more likely to be **guided imagery.** Regardless of its name, the active process of imagining yourself being successful in a particular endeavor is a technique for gaining a measure of personal control over events. Athletes use guided imagery to visualize their perfect performance before actual participation. Students prepare for final examinations by "seeing" the examination and "watching" themselves taking the imaginary examination with confidence and success. Cancer patients "visualize" their body's immune system attacking and subduing malignant cells. Guided imagery can also be used as a coping technique in resolving stress.

Although there is no one format to follow in using guided imagery as a coping technique, the following are frequently used by people who claim that guided imagery is a dependable tool for dealing with stressors:

- *Quiet time.* Identify a time and a place where you can find quietness.
- *Progressive relaxation.* As discussed on pp. 54-55, allow your body and mind to find the most relaxed state. Attempt to free yourself from cluttered, nagging thoughts.

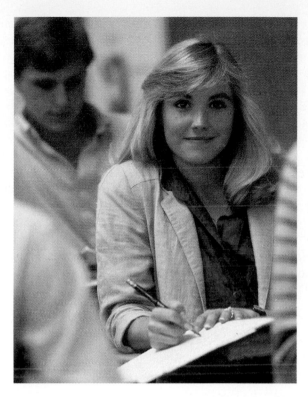

Envisioning success.

- *Support and security.* Create for yourself a visual image of relaxation, peace, and security. You should feel that you are in an environment of maximum support.
- *Participation and response.* Envision yourself participating, responding, and succeeding in exactly the manner you know is required to have total control over your stressor.
- *Recognize satisfaction.* Visualize yourself experiencing joy and personal satisfaction. Recognize that your satisfaction has come from your active involvement in stress management.

Guided imagery can be a successful coping technique for many of you. You may wish to experiment with your own version of the technique, perhaps doing so in combination with another coping technique with which you have already experienced success.

SUMMARY

Throughout an entire life one constantly reacts to changes (stressors) that can be unpredictable and potentially threatening—potentially enjoyable as well. These changes produce stress—the nonspecific response of the body to any demand made on it. Negative stress is called distress, whereas positive stress is called eustress. Selye characterized the body's general adaptation syndrome as a series of stages: the alarm stage, the resistance stage, and the exhaustion stage. Regardless of the stressor, our bodies respond in a similar, generalized manner.

Stressors can be classified according to origin: physical, psychosocial, or environmental. Through an intricate interplay involving the brain, nervous system, and endocrine system, the body undergoes a series of physiological changes that prepare the person to respond to stress. The stress response mobilizes the energy our bodies need to confront a stressor. Critical to the formation of this response are our sensory modalities, the cerebral cortex, the hypothalamus, the adrenal glands, and the hormones ACTH, the corticoids, and epinephrine.

It is evident that the effects of stress are cumulative. Unresolved stress frequently results in physiological breakdowns that predispose one to various disease states. Many major diseases and disorders are caused by or related to unresolved stress.

The college environment produces a number of stressors for students. Some clearly produce eustress, whereas others often produce distress. Studies, employment forecasts, personal and family expectations, and financial support are all potential sources of distress for students. Life-centered sources of stress influence all of us on a daily basis. Fortunately, a number of successful methods for coping with stress have been identified, including relaxation training (biofeedback, relaxation response, and muscle tension-relaxation exercise training), physical exercise, dietary changes, and hurry sickness substitutes.

REVIEW QUESTIONS

1 Can you specify the reactions that are thought to occur during each stage of Selye's general adaptation syndrome?
2 Differentiate between "stress" and "stressor."
3 Identify the endocrine hormones that influence the stress response. What is the source and function of each hormone?
4 Can you trace the pathways of the energy production response?
5 List three imagined stressors and three real stressors that produce the same physical responses in a person.
6 Why do people's metabolic rates increase when they are under the influence of a stressor? What causes a person to sweat when confronted with a stressor? Be specific.
7 Do you support the concept that people who are incapable of successfully coping with stress are also more likely to be incapable of fighting off relatively common illnesses? Can you support this concept with physiologically based findings concerning immune system changes that take place during stress the response?
8 How can stress be viewed as both positive and negative? Can you explain and provide examples of the concepts of eustress and distress?
9 Identify a specific physical stressor, a specific psychosocial stressor, and a specific environmental stressor.
10 Define Type A, Type B, and Type T personalities.

QUESTIONS FOR PERSONAL CONTEMPLATION

1 Which dimension of your own health (physical, emotional, social, intellectual, spiritual) do you most frequently rely on when you are confronted with a stressful situation? Can you explain why this one dimension is especially useful to you?

2 To what degree are you a Type A, Type B, or Type T personality? If you exhibit Type A behaviors, would you be interested in modifying them? How?

3 Can you remember a stressful experience you recently had in which your body responses clearly followed the pattern of Selye's general adaptation syndrome? How long did you remain in each of the specific stages?

4 If the body's responses to stressors are similar for both distress and eustress, how is it possible that we learn to distinguish between the responses from a passionate kiss and an electrical shock? Does a paradox exist?

5 If you believe that the future enhancement of your stress management skills will be important to you as a maturing person (regardless of your age), which of the suggested approaches to coping with stress could you most comfortably develop? Relaxation training? Physical exercise? Dietary change? Hurry sickness substitutes? When can you start to develop these skills?

REFERENCES

1 Selye, H: Stress without distress, New York, 1975, New American Library.

2 Selye, H: Selye's guide to stress research, vol 3, New York, 1983, Van Nostrand Reinhold Co, Inc.

3 Julius, M, et al: Anger-coping types, blood pressure, and all causes of mortality: a follow-up in Tecumseh, Michigan (1971-1983), American Journal of Epidemiology 124:220-233, 1986.

4 McGinnis, JM: Medicine for the layman: behavior patterns and health, U.S. Department of Health and Human Services, Public Health Service, National Institutes of Health, NIH Publication No. 85-2682, Washington, DC, 1986, US Government Printing Office.

5 Anderson, H, et al: God goes back to college, On Campus 10-16, 1986.

6 Mullins, ME: The roots of our stress, USA Today March 14, 1986, 1d.

7 Baron, M, et al: Genetic linkage between X-chromosome markers and bipolar affective illness, Nature 326:289-292, 1987.

8 Ross, CR: A guide to managing stress, Daly City, Calif, 1985, Krames Communications, Health Information Library.

9 Benson, H, and Proctor, W: Beyond the relaxation response: how to harness the healing power of your personal beliefs, New York, 1984, The New York Times Book Co, Inc.

10 Jacobson, E: You must relax, ed 5, New York, 1978, McGraw-Hill Book Co.

11 Getchell, B: Being fit: a personal guide, ed 2, Indianapolis, 1986, Benchmark Press.

12 Prentice, WE, Bucher, CA: Fitness for college and life, ed 2, St Louis, 1988, Times Mirror/Mosby College Publishing.

13 Caffeine: condensed report of the Institute of Food Technologists' Expert Panel on Food Safety and Nutrition, Contemporary Nutrition 9.1-2, 1984.

14 Nutrition update: sugar, Dairy Council Digest 55:21-24, 1984.

15 Williams, SR: Nutrition and diet therapy, ed 5, St. Louis, 1985, Times Mirror/Mosby College Publishing.

16 Guthrie, HA: Introductory nutrition, ed 7, St. Louis, 1989, Times Mirror/Mosby College Publishing.

17 Friedman, M, and Rosenman, R: Type A behavior and your heart, New York, 1981, Fawcett Group.

18 Friedman, M, and Ulmer, D: Treating Type A behavior: and your heart, New York, 1984, Alfred A Knopf.

19 Fischman, J: Type A on trial, Psychology Today 21:42-50, 1987.

20 Leo, J: Looking for a life of thrills, Time, April 15, 1985, p 125.

21 Peale, NV: Power of positive thinking, New York, 1978, Fawcett Group.

ANNOTATED READINGS

Eliot, R, and Breo, D: Is it worth dying for?: a self-assessment program to make stress work for you—not against you, New York, 1984, Bantam Books, Inc.

    The Type A personality pattern and its relationship to stress and premature death is examined. The authors provide an approach to self-improvement.

Peale, NV: Imaging, Carmel, NY, 1982, Guideposts.

    The application of imaging to a variety of personal problems is discussed; prayer is presented as an important component of imaging.

Quick, JC, and Quick, JD: Organizational stress and preventive management, New York, 1984, McGraw-Hill Book Co.

    Particularly appropriate for business majors, this book offers a complete discussion of the sources, consequences, and preventive management of stress.

Sheehy, G: Pathfinders, New York, 1982, Bantam Books, Inc.

    Overcoming the crises of adult life in a manner that is satisfying and productive is explored through profiles of people who have coped successfully with stressful life events.

Witkin-Lanoil, G: The male stress syndrome: how to recognize and live with it, New York, 1986, Newmarket Press.

    Males whose level of stress negatively influences their sex lives are given suggestions for managing stress and improving their love lives.

Mastering Tasks

The information you have mastered in Unit I will be helpful to you as you work on the four developmental tasks this book addresses. Also recall that the role of health is to assist you in completing the developmental tasks that will allow you to have a satisfying and productive life.

▪ **Forming an Initial Adult Self-Identity** You may have noticed that we have qualified the adult self-identity concept as "initial," or tentative. This suggests an identity that is temporary—one that can evolve over time. The idea that further changes in your identity are possible (even probable) can lead to feelings of uncertainty, confusion, and stress. However, we believe that as you increasingly come to grips with your evolving identity, you will find new opportunities for growth, creativity, and service. In many ways, this personal growth and development can be an exciting experience.

High-level emotional health encourages the formation of your emerging identity. Through healthy introspection and reflection, you learn a great deal about the person you are becoming. By exploring the ways you handle stressful situations, you learn even more about yourself. Indeed, interest in your emotional and spiritual makeup will serve you throughout your life as you repeatedly ask yourself "Who am I?"

▪ **Establishing a Sense of Relative Independence** This major developmental task is represented by your steady movement away from a dependent relationship with family and peers. For nontraditional students it may be represented by a similar pulling back from a spouse, limited employment opportunities, or parenting. Regardless, to progress toward independence you must be successful in dealing with people, institutions, programs, and yourself. It will without question be a process that exposes you to stressors, but it also will be a developmental progression in which your emotional health can play an extremely supportive role.

Your emotional maturity will be a major factor in determining the speed at which you progress toward independence. Stress will probably be produced in those who progress too slowly or too rapidly in their search toward independence. For those who move toward relative independence at a speed soundly based on their needs and health resources, this search will produce eustress. Enjoy the journey.

▪ **Assuming Increasing Levels of Responsibility** Although an adult of any age may lack an adequately developed sense of responsibility, it is in the young adult years that significant progress in that direction is expected. To whom is one most responsible? We take the position that your primary responsibility during the young adult years must be to yourself. For example, mastery of all four of the developmental tasks is your responsibility. Parents, faculty, and peers cannot force you to take charge of your own development; your growth in confidence, self-respect, and insight gained through new experiences rests in your own hands. Fortunately, this is the way most students want it.

▪ **Developing the Skills for Social Interaction** Since the costs of making friends and keeping friendships can sometimes be high, we would like to introduce someone who can be helpful in your search for improved social interaction—a mentor. For the purposes of this book, a mentor is a person slightly older than you (8 to 15 years older) who functions not as a peer nor as a parent substitute, but as an exemplar, counselor, and a person capable of sharing your aspirations.

The process of identifying potential mentors within an occupational, educational, or avocational setting cannot be prescribed. Potential mentors need not be of your own gender, nor do they necessarily need to hold a position significantly higher than yours.

It is through mentor relationships that some of you will find the most pleasurable social, occupational, and professional rewards. With your mentor you will sense a more deeply focused relationship against which to evaluate your initial successes and failures. Your mentor will listen, demand, share, critique, and counsel as you progress in this challenging period of your life.

UNIT II

The second unit is composed of three chapters whose topics are especially important to today's college students: physical fitness, nutrition, and weight management. We think these are interesting topics for students because most students tell us that they want to stay in good physical condition, eat well, and maintain a desirable weight. We will briefly discuss the upcoming content in terms with our philosophy that health is composed of five interacting dimensions.

Physical Dimension of Health Many health experts indicate that fitness, nutrition, and weight management are interrelated. How well our bodies work depends, in large measure, on what we eat and how we exercise. Since most of us need some degree of fitness just to complete our daily activities, we can appreciate the value of an appropriate exercise program. Bodies that are physically healthy can avoid costly repairs (figuratively and literally) and bounce back more quickly from illness and injury.

Emotional Dimension of Health When you start a fitness program or begin to monitor your food consumption behavior, you will learn a lot about your level of motivation and commitment. Undoubtedly, you will be challenged, but the mental and emotional rewards for your efforts can be monumental. Students who are conscientious about maintaining their fitness levels, food consumption habits, and body weight seem to bubble with an enthusiasm. There must exist some intrinsic, emotional rewards that go hand in hand with eating properly and being physically fit.

Social Dimension of Health The social dimension of our health is closely related to the content in Chapters 4, 5, and 6. Exercising with others offers opportunities for social interaction. Combined with most forms of group fitness activities are varying amounts of listening, sharing, and counseling by the participants. For college students of all ages, university facilities, commercial health clubs, local YMCAs and YWCAs, and competitive events provide social settings where we can improve social skills.

There is little question that food, like alcohol, can function as a "social lubricant." Food brings and holds people together. Kitchens and restaurants become meeting places, picnics and barbecues reunite scattered families and friends, and even supermarkets have served as contact points for "eligibles."

Food may also serve as a potentially dangerous agent that can hinder our social relationships with others. The overconsumption or underconsumption of food that results in a significant deviation from desirable weight can make our interactions with family members, friends, and employers more strained. Thus, we may become hindered in social developments regardless of our stage in the life cycle.

Intellectual Dimension of Health Whether being physically fit, eating well, and maintaining an appropriate weight level will have much effect on your intellectual functioning is a question that could be debated for years. Anecdotal evidence suggests that people do feel mentally sharper after exercise. Our students claim that they can study more efficiently after their workouts. As professors, we are able to teach with more enthusiasm, interest, and clear thinking when we are in good physical condition. People deprived of adequate exercise and nutrition may suffer intellectual impairment.

We believe that throughout your life, good fitness, a sound diet, and reasonable weight management will help you be able to experience the widest range of new experiences. These new experiences can lead to improved intellectual capacity. This thought is inherent in our "Plan for Enhancing Your Emotional Growth" in Chapter 2.

Spiritual Dimension of Health Throughout this text we emphasize that a major dimension of your spiritual growth will take the form of service to others. Physical fitness, good nutrition, and weight management can enhance your ability to serve others. You can better live your faith and assist others in bringing meaning into their lives when you feel the drive that results from a well-conditioned, adequately nourished body.

The Body
Your Vehicle for Health

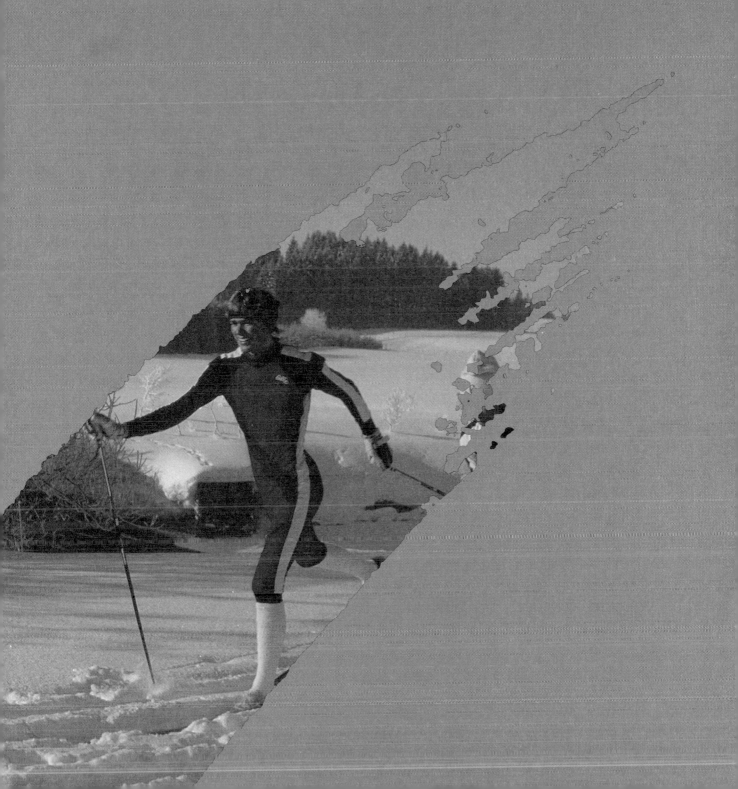

CHAPTER 4

Physical Fitness
Enhancing Work, Study, and Play

Key Concepts

A physically fit person is capable of responding to the demands of many activities.

▪

Physical fitness includes muscular strength and endurance, flexibility, agility, and cardiorespiratory endurance.

▪

Fitness influences other aspects of your life.

▪

The central components in an effective cardiorespiratory fitness program are type of activity, intensity, duration, and frequency.

▪

Controversies and questions abound concerning such topics as fluid replacement, fiber types, equipment, body building, and steroid use.

▪

Sleep is an important part of a well-planned exercise program.

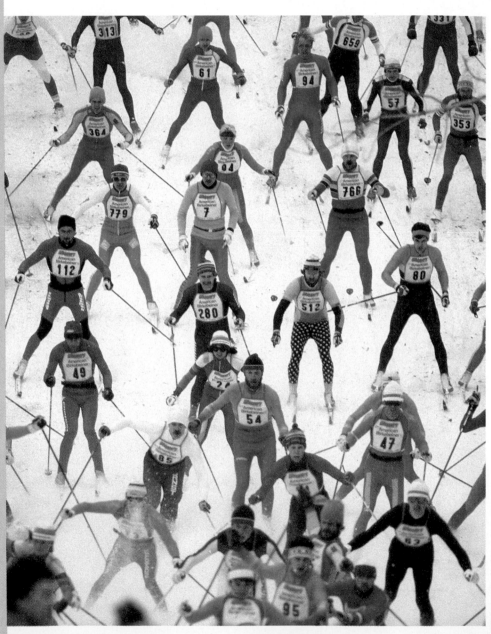

*W*hen your day begins early in the morning, then you go to class or work or immerse yourself in family activities, and your day does not end until after midnight, you must be physically fit. Even a highly motivated college student must have a conditioned, rested body to maintain such a schedule.

Fitness implies a concept similar to our earlier definition of health: To have your physical, emotional, social, intellectual, and spiritual dimensions functioning in a way that contributes to a satisfying and productive life. In a more familiar sense, fitness is often judged in terms of the physical dimension of your health. As a physically fit person, you have a body that is capable of responding to many demands—both in daily routine and in short-term activities.

When you have this level of conditioning, you will not only be capable of meeting the demands of your college schedule; more importantly, you will also master your developmental tasks with greater ease. Like many, you may find the psychological benefits are as rewarding as the physical benefits.

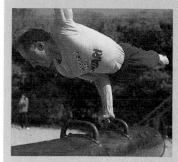

Muscular strength.

COMPONENTS OF PHYSICAL FITNESS

Physical fitness can be explored by examining several specific dimensions of the body's structure and function and how these dimensions influence the physical demands of work, study, and leisure. Although the number of components of physical fitness may vary, we will discuss muscular strength, muscular endurance, flexibility, agility, and cardiorespiratory endurance. Each dimension of your physical fitness will be defined, and its maintenance and further development will be discussed.

Muscular Strength

Muscular strength is essential for your body to accomplish any *work*. Your ability to maintain posture, walk, lift, push, and pull are familiar examples of the constant demands you make on your muscles to maintain or increase their level of *contraction*. The stronger you are, the greater will be your ability to contract muscles and maintain a level of contraction sufficient to complete tasks.

Many of the undertakings associated with being a college student require more than a minimal level of strength. Walking across campus, climbing stairs, and participating in physical education courses and intramural sports will maintain your strength. Occasionally your body's performance—or lack of performance—when you try to move furniture, lift weights, or sprint to catch a bus will remind you of the importance of developing more than minimal levels of muscle strength and tone.

Muscular strength can best be improved by training activities that use the **overload principle.** By overloading, or gradually increasing the resistance (load, object, or weight) your muscles must move, you can increase your muscular strength. The following three types of training exercises are based on the over-load principle.

In **isometric exercises** (meaning "same measure"), the resistance is so great that your contracting muscles cannot move the resistance object at all. Thus your muscles contract against immovable objects, usually in increasingly greater efforts (see Figure 4-1). Isometric exercises, because of the difficulty of precisely

muscular strength
the ability to contract skeletal muscles to engage in work; the force that a muscle can exert.

overload principle
principle (often used in training programs to increase muscular strength) whereby a person gradually increases the resistance load that must be moved or lifted.

isometric exercises
muscular strength training exercises that use a resistance so great that the resistance object cannot be moved.

67

Figure 4-1
Three types of training exercises to improve muscular strength. **A,** Isometric exercise. **B** and **C,** Progressive resistance exercises. **D,** Isokinetic exercise.

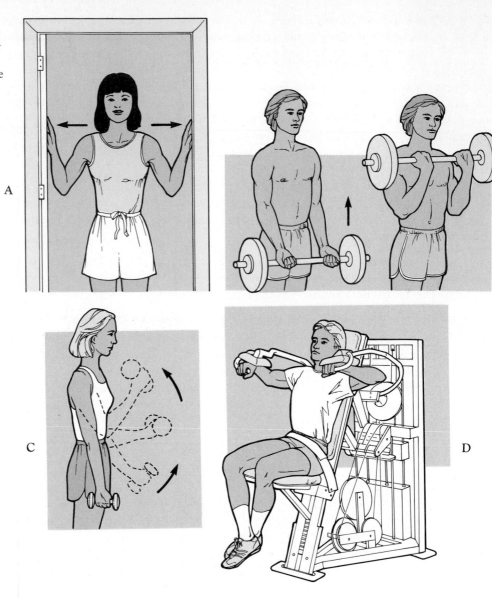

A

B

C

D

progressive resistance exercises
muscular strength training exercises that use traditional barbells and dumbbells with fixed resistances.

isokinetic exercises
muscular strength training exercises that use machines to provide variable resistances throughout the full range of motion.

evaluating the training effects, are not generally used as primary developers of muscular strength and can be dangerous for people with hypertension.

Progressive resistance exercises, once called *isotonic* or "same-tension" exercises, are currently the most popular type of strength-building exercises. Progressive resistance exercises are represented by the use of traditional weight training equipment, including dumbbells and barbells. Devotees of progressive resistance exercise use various muscle groups to move (or lift) specific fixed resistances or weights. Although during a given repetitive exercise the weight resistance remains the same, the muscular contraction effort required varies according to the joint angles in the *range of motion.*[1] The greatest effort is required at the start and finish of the movement.

Isokinetic exercises (meaning "same motion") employ mechanical devices that provide resistances that consistently overload muscles throughout the entire range of motion. Currently believed to be the most effective form of exercise to promote the strength of specific muscle groups, isokinetic training requires elaborate, expensive equipment. Thus the use of isokinetic equipment may be limited to certain athletic teams or to people who enroll at commercial fitness centers with this type of equipment.

The concept of *specificity* is of key importance. Specificity refers to the fact that by using carefully controlled exercises, muscular strength can be precisely increased for a particular task or series of skills. In most cases, specificity helps you accomplish particular goals. However, specificity can also create problems when muscle strength is highly developed in one part of the body and neglected in another part. In such a situation the risk of injury can be great. People should strive for appropriate, proportional balances of muscular strength throughout the body. Specificity applies to all components of fitness, not just muscular strength. Each fitness component responds to the specific demands made to it.

Muscular Endurance

Muscular endurance is a component of physical fitness associated with strength. When muscles contract and their individual muscle fibers shorten, energy is required. Energy production requires that oxygen and nutrients be delivered by the circulatory system to the muscles. Following the transformation of these products into energy by individual muscle cells, the body must remove the potentially toxic waste by-products. These coordinated efforts between the respiratory system, which delivers oxygen to the blood and removes carbon dioxide from the blood, and the circulatory system, which delivers oxygen and nutrients to the muscle cells and removes waste products from the cells, are the foundation of muscular endurance.

muscular endurance
the ability of a muscle or a muscle group to function over time; supported by the respiratory and circulatory systems.

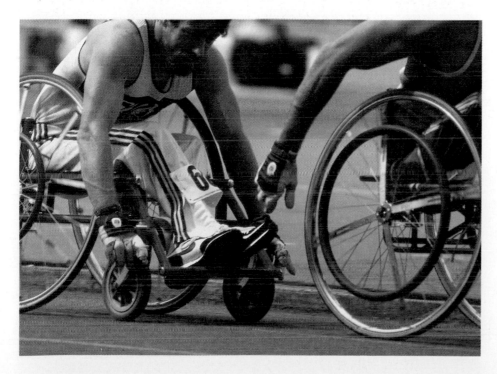

Muscular endurance.

Amateur and professional athletes often wish to increase the muscular endurance of specific muscle groups associated with their sports activities. They achieve such muscular endurance by using exercises that gradually increase the number of repetitions of a given movement. Interestingly, muscular endurance is not the physiological equivalent of cardiorespiratory endurance.[2] For example, a world-ranked distance runner with highly developed cardiorespiratory endurance and extensive muscular endurance of the legs may not have a corresponding level of muscular endurance of the abdominal muscles.

Flexibility

In the overall design of the human body, muscles must have an articulated (jointed) skeleton to function. To move an object, jump, run, swim, or just change position, your bones must be moved by the skeletal muscles that bridge their points of articulation, or joints. As joints move, so do you.

The ability of your joints to move through their natural range of motion is a measure of your **flexibility.** This fitness trait, like so many other aspects of structure and function, differs from point to point within your body or between different people. Not every joint in your body is equally flexible (by design), and over the course of time use or disuse will alter the flexibility of a given joint. Certainly sex, age, genetically determined body build, and current level of physical fitness will affect your flexibility. You may not be as flexible as a gymnast nor as inflexible as a person with arthritis, but certain inborn characteristics will influence your level of flexibility throughout life.

Your ability or inability to move easily during physical activity will be a constant reminder that aging and inactivity are the foes of flexibility. Failure to use joints regularly will quickly result in a loss of elasticity in the connective tissue and shortening of muscles associated with the joints. There is even the possibility that your body will neurologically "forget" how to use that particular joint effectively should you attempt to reactivate it in the future. Benefits of flexibility include improved balance, posture, athletic performance, and reduced risk of low back pain.

As seen in a young gymnast, flexibility can be highly developed and main-

flexibility
ability of joints to function through intended range of motion.

Flexibility.

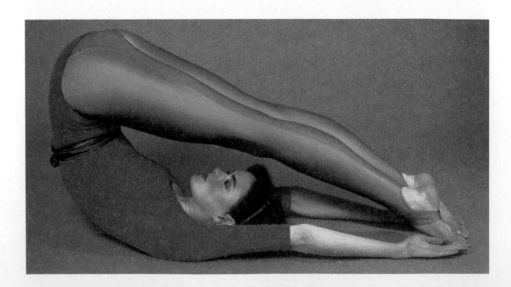

Guidelines for Stretching

The following precautions should serve as guidelines to reduce the possibility of injury during stretching:

- Warm up using a slow jog or fast walk before stretching vigorously.
- Stretch only to the point where you feel tightness or resistance to your stretching. Stretching should not be painful.
- Be sure to continue normal breathing during a stretch. Do not hold your breath.
- Exercise caution when stretching muscles that surround painful joints. Pain is an indication that something is wrong and should not be ignored.

tained by a program of activity that includes regularly exercising joints. Flexibility also helps reduce the risk of injury. Inactivity, far more quickly than aging, will be the factor that distinguishes adolescent levels of flexibility from adult levels. Guidelines for stretching are given in the box above and some valuable flexibility-stretching exercises are shown on pp. 72-73.

Agility

When muscular strength, muscular endurance, and flexibility are combined with speed and coordination, a fourth dimension of your physical fitness can be observed. **Agility,** or the ability to move quickly with frequent changes in direction or position, enhances your performance in a variety of activities. Dancing, walking on ice-covered sidewalks, balancing a cafeteria tray, and completing many aspects of employment are enhanced by an adequately developed level of agility. Although you probably do not need—or could not achieve—the level of agility of a professional basketball player, you need to be agile enough to function in the tasks of daily living.

agility
ability of the body to move quickly with frequent changes in direction

Like other dimensions of physical fitness, agility can be maintained when your lifestyle includes sufficient opportunity for vigorous activity. Dance, gymnastics, team sports, and many recreational pursuits (skiing, rock climbing, and backpacking) will provide opportunities for you to become more agile. If you require a more programmed and concise agility activity for your fitness program, you may wish to support the construction of a "parcourse" or fitness trail in your community.

Cardiorespiratory Endurance

If you were limited to improving only one area of physical fitness, which would you choose—muscular strength, muscular endurance, flexibility, or agility? Which would a dancer choose? Which would a marathon runner select? Which would an expert recommend?

We think the experts, exercise physiologists, would say that a fifth fitness dimension is of greatest importance. These research scientists regard enhancement of your heart, lung, and blood vessel function to be the most important focal point for a physical fitness program. **Cardiorespiratory endurance** forms the foundation for whole-body fitness.

cardiorespiratory endurance
ability of the heart, lungs, and blood vessels to process and transport oxygen required by muscle cells so that they contract over a period of time.

Ten Stretching Exercises

1 *Neck.* Start your stretching exercises with this one. Standing with your hands on your hips and your chin near your chest, slowly rotate your neck clockwise 5 times and then counterclockwise 5 times.

2 *Chest and shoulders.* With your elbows high, place your fists together at chest height. Gradually pull your elbows back and move your fists apart as far as possible. Hold for 10 seconds. Repeat 3 times.

3 *Back.* Lie on your back with your arms extended to the sides. Bring your knees toward your chin as far as possible without raising your arms off the floor. Hold the position for 5 seconds. Repeat 3 times.

4 *Hips and waist.* Stand with your feet comfortably apart. Extend your arms to each side. Keeping your arms outstretched, slowly bend from the waist as far as possible to the right. Hold this position for 5 seconds. Return slowly to your original position. Then bend to the left as far as possible. Repeat 3 times on each side.

5 *Lower back.* Stand and place your hands on your hips. Bend forward from the waist and lean forward as far as possible. Slowly return to the upright position and continue to extend your head and trunk back as far as possible. Repeat 5 times.

6 *Groin.* Sit on the floor with your knees bent and the soles of your feet touching. Slowly push down on your knees. When you feel a slight pulling in your groin area, hold your position for 5 seconds. As you continue this exercise over a period of weeks, attempt to push your knees closer to the floor.

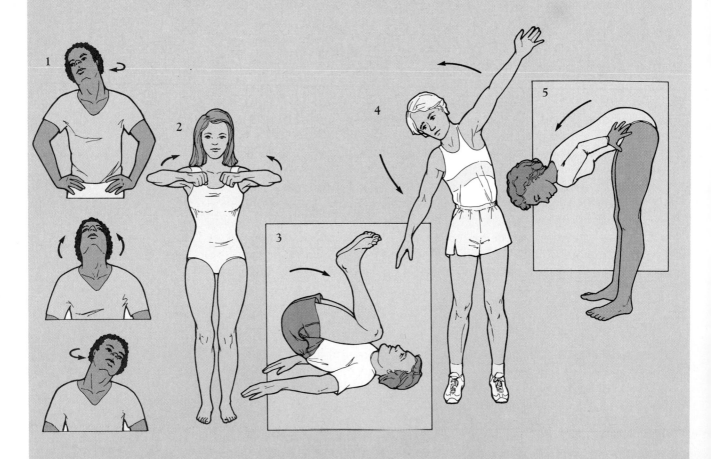

7 *Quadriceps.* In standing position, flex one leg behind you, grasp foot with hand, and pull the foot up toward buttocks until a good stretch is felt on the thigh. Repeat with opposite leg. Repeat 3 times with each leg, hold for 30 seconds.

8 *Hamstrings.* Sit on the floor with your legs comfortably spread. Slowly reach for your right foot with both hands. Gradually try to touch your forehead to your knee. (Don't force it.) Continue with your left leg. Repeat 5 times.

9 *Achilles tendon and calf muscles.* Stand and place your outstretched hands on a wall. Keeping your feet flat on the floor, slowly inch your feet backward. When you begin to feel a slight pulling in your calf muscles, hold your position for 10 seconds. As you continue this exercise over a period of weeks, gradually increase your distance from the wall.

10 *Feet and ankles.* Sit on the floor with your legs extended. With your hands on the floor by your hips, point your toes downward as far as you can. Return your toes to the upright position. Spread your toes apart and try to rotate each ankle outward until you feel some resistance. Repeat the sequence 5 times.

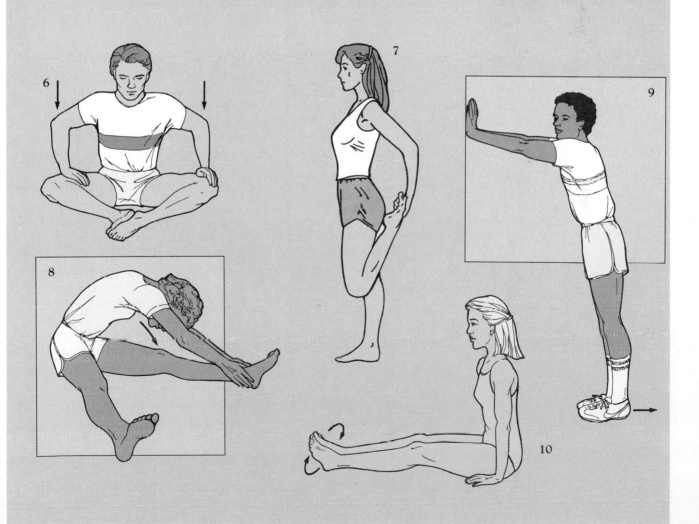

Cardiorespiratory endurance.

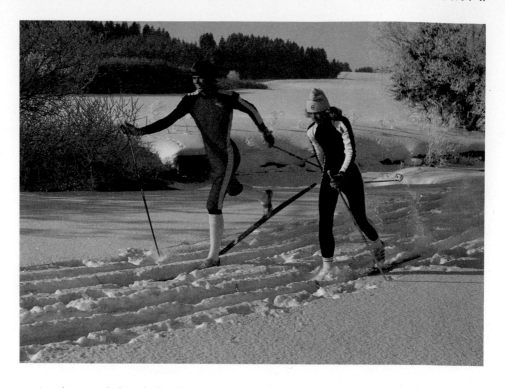

oxygen debt
physical state that occurs when the body can no longer process and transport sufficient amounts of oxygen for continued muscle contraction.

anaerobic energy production
body's production of energy when needed amounts of oxygen are not readily available.

lactic acid
chemical by-product of anaerobic energy production.

glycogen
storage form of the body's energy supplies; composed of a network of glucose molecules.

As discussed for skeletal muscle, an inability to supply muscle fibers with adequate oxygen, nutrients, and waste removal severely limits a muscle's ability to function. This is true for the rest of your body. When any tissue is deprived of an adequate supply of oxygen and nutrients, its capacity to function will be impaired. Cardiorespiratory endurance increases your capacity to sustain a given level of energy production for a prolonged period. Development of cardiorespiratory endurance helps your body to work longer and at greater levels of intensity.

Your body cannot always produce the energy needed for long-term activity. Certain activities require performance at a level of intensity that will outstrip your cardiorespiratory system's ability to transport oxygen efficiently to contracting muscle fibers. When the oxygen demands of the muscles cannot be met, a phenomenon called **oxygen debt** occurs. Any activity that must continue beyond the point at which oxygen debt begins will require a form of energy production that does not depend on oxygen.

This oxygen-deprived form of energy production is called **anaerobic** (without oxygen) **energy production,** the type of energy production regularly found in many intense, short-duration activities. Rope climbing, weight lifting for strength, and sprinting are short-duration activities that quickly cause muscle fatigue. These kinds of activities are generally considered anaerobic activities.

Muscle fatigue, or the inability of muscle tissue to maintain adequate exercise intensity, produces unpleasant sensations that force people to stop a particular exercise. For years it was thought that the buildup of a metabolic waste product called **lactic acid** was the culprit that produced muscle fatigue. This concept has largely been discounted. Currently muscle fatigue is thought to result from several factors, including depletion of **glycogen** stores in the affected muscles and a lowering of the pH level of the blood. When blood develops a more acid pH level than usual, the ability of muscle cells to formulate additional energy units is severely curtailed. The lowered pH levels may also stimulate pain receptors and cause exercisers to stop their activities.[3]

Activities that are not generally associated with anaerobic energy production (walking, distance jogging, and bicycle touring) become anaerobic activities when they are either increased in intensity or continued for an extended period.

If you usually work or play at lower intensity but for a longer duration, the ability to maintain **aerobic** (with oxygen) **energy production** is highly desirable. As long as your body can meet its energy demands in this oxygen-rich mode, you will not experience conversion to anaerobic energy production. Thus you will not find fatigue an important factor in determining whether you can continue to participate. Marathon runners, serious joggers, distance swimmers, bikers, and aerobic dancers can persist in their activities because of their highly developed aerobic fitness. These aerobically fit people take in, transport, and use oxygen in the most efficient manner possible.

Besides allowing you to participate in activities such as those mentioned above, aerobic conditioning (cardiorespiratory endurance conditioning) may also provide you with certain structural and functional benefits that may extend into other dimensions of your life. These recognized benefits (see the box below) have received considerable documented support. Some data even suggest that a conditioned cardiorespiratory system may increase your life expectancy.[4,5]

aerobic energy production body's production of energy when the respiratory and circulatory systems are able to process and transport sufficient amounts of oxygen to muscle cells.

Structural and Functional Benefits of Cardiorespiratory (Aerobic) Fitness

Aerobic fitness can help you:

    Complete your daily activities with enjoyment

    Strengthen your heart muscle and make it more efficient

    Increase your proportion of high-density lipoproteins

    Increase the capillary network in your body

    Improve collateral circulation

    Control your weight

    Cope with stressors

    Ward off infections

    Improve the efficiency of your other body systems

    Bolster your self-esteem

    Achieve self-directed fitness goals

    Reduce negative dependency behaviors

    Sleep better

    Recover more quickly from common illnesses

    Meet other people with similar interests

    Receive lowered insurance premiums

What is Your Level of Fitness?

You can determine your level of fitness in 30 minutes or less by completing this short group of tests based on the National Fitness Test developed by the President's Council on Physical Fitness and Sports. If you are over 40 or have chronic medical disorders such as diabetes or obesity, check with your physician before taking this or any other test. You will need another person to monitor your test and keep time.

Three-Minute Step Test

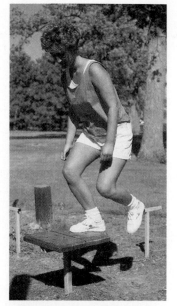

Aerobic capacity. Equipment: 12-inch bench, crate, block or step ladder, and stopwatch. Procedure: face bench. Complete 24 full steps (both feet on the bench, both feet on the ground) per minute for 3 minutes. After finishing, sit down, have your partner find your pulse within 5 seconds and take pulse for 1 minute. Your score is your pulse rate for one full minute.

Scoring Standards (heart rate for 1 minute)

Age	18-29		30-39		40-49		50-59		60 +	
Sex	F	M	F	M	F	M	F	M	F	M
Excellent	<80	<75	<84	<78	<88	<80	<92	<85	<95	<90
Good	80-110	75-100	85-115	78-109	88-118	80-112	92-123	85-115	95-127	90-118
Average	>110	>100	>115	>109	>118	>112	>123	>115	>127	>118

Sit and Reach

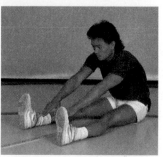

Hamstring flexibility. Equipment: yardstick and tape. Between your legs, tape yardstick to the floor. Sit with legs straight and heels about 5 inches apart, heels even with the 15-inch mark on the yardstick. While in a sitting position, slowly stretch forward as far as possible. Your score is the number of inches reached.

Scoring Standards (inches)

Age	18-29		30-39		40-49		50-59		60 +	
Sex	F	M	F	M	F	M	F	M	F	M
Excellent	>22	>21	>22	>21	>21	>20	>20	>19	>20	>19
Good	17-22	13-21	17-22	13-21	15-21	13-20	14-20	12-19	14-20	12-19
Average	<17	<13	<17	<13	<15	<13	<14	<12	<14	<12

Arm Hang

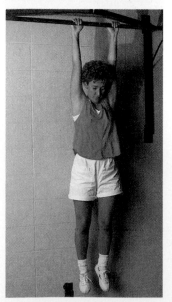

Upper body strength. Equipment: horizontal bar (high enough to prevent your feet from touching the floor), stop watch. Procedure: hang with straight arms, palms facing foward. Start watch when in position. Stop when subject lets go. Your score is the number of minutes and seconds spent hanging.

Scoring Standards (minutes and seconds)

Age	18-29		30-39		40-49		50-59		60 +	
Sex	F	M	F	M	F	M	F	M	F	M
Excellent	>1:30	>2:00	>1:20	>1:50	>1:10	>1:35	>1:00	>1:20	>:50	>1:10
Good	:46-1:30	1:00-2:00	:40-1:20	:50-1:50	:30-1:10	:45-1:35	:30-1:00	:75-1:20	:21-:50	:30-1:10
Average	<:46	<1:00	<:40	<:50	<:30	<:45	<:30	<:35	<:21	<30

Curl-ups

Abdominal and low back strength. Equipment: stopwatch. Procedure: Lie flat on upper back, knees bent, shoulders touching the floor, and your arms extended above your thighs or by your sides, palms down. Bend knees so that feet are flat and 12 inches from the buttocks. Curl up by lifting head and shoulders off the floor, sliding hands forward above your thighs or the floor. Curl down and repeat. Your score is the number of curl-ups in 1 minute.

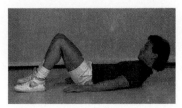

Scoring Standards (number in 1 minute)										
Age	18-29		30-39		40-49		50-59		60 +	
Sex	F	M	F	M	F	M	F	M	F	M
Excellent	>45	>50	>40	>45	>35	>40	>30	>35	>25	>30
Good	25-45	30-50	20-40	22-45	16-35	21-40	12-30	18-35	11-25	15-30
Average	<25	<30	<20	<22	<16	<21	<12	<18	<11	<15

Push-Ups (men)

Upper body strength. Equipment: stopwatch. Assume a front-leaning position. Lower your body until chest touches the floor. Raise and repeat for 1 minute. Your score is the number of push-ups completed in 1 minute.

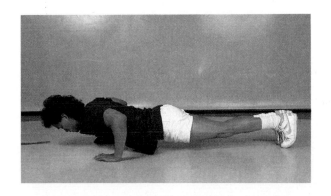

Scoring Standards (number in 1 minute)					
Age	18-29	30-39	40-49	50-59	60 +
Excellent	>50	>45	>40	>35	>30
Good	25-50	22-45	19-40	15-35	10-30
Average	<25	<22	<19	<15	<10

Push-Ups (women)

Upper body strength. Equipment: stopwatch. Assume a front-leaning position with knees bent up, hands under shoulders. Lower your chest to the floor, raise, and repeat. Your score is the number of push-ups completed in 1 minute.

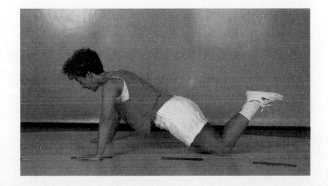

Scoring Standards (number in 1 minute)					
Age	18-29	30-39	40-49	50-59	60 +
Excellent	>45	>40	>35	>30	>25
Good	17-45	12-40	8-35	6-30	5-25
Average	<17	<12	<8	<6	<5

CURRENT ATTITUDES TOWARD PHYSICAL FITNESS

Recently we were told by a student that setting aside time for improving his physical fitness would be a total misuse of his working hours. He assured us that he would be no better served by a fitness program than by learning to play bridge. College and his preparation for a career were his only priorities.

This student has perceived being physically fit as an end rather than the means we know it to be. His opinion is one of the many feelings, pro or con, that people hold about their personal involvement in a physical fitness program.

Many people, including college students of all ages, spend little time in pursuit of physical fitness. Certainly some of these individuals may have physical limitations that make activity extremely difficult, and others are engaged in time-consuming activities that until finished do not permit opportunities for recreation. However, what about the majority who could do much more but do so little? Does one of the following statements sound like you?

- "I know it's important, but I just don't have time right now."
- "I'm already fit, and with my schedule, I'll have no difficulty staying that way."
- "I should do more than I do, but I just don't have facilities and I don't get much support from others."
- "Exercise makes me feel gross. Even when I shower, I get to my next class wet, sticky, and probably smelling like a locker room."

Unlike these people who have made no commitment to fitness, you may have made a commitment to a physical fitness program that might be rather narrow in scope. If one of the following comments fits you, perhaps you are failing to see the broader values of maintaining a high level of physical fitness.

- "Everyone in the dorm runs at night. That's why I run."
- "For every 3,500 Calories I can 'burn' during exercise, I'll lose a pound of fat. I have only 10 pounds more to drop before vacation."
- "This weekend will be cool and overcast. Saturday looks like a good day for a personal record."
- "Some would say I have a fear of death. Heck, I just want to live a long time."

If you see your own attitude represented by one of these comments, might you be shortsighted in your reason for valuing fitness? We would suggest that you reexamine your approach to fitness and its ability to positively influence other aspects of your life. Ask yourself, "What could I achieve if I were really in top physical condition?" Because fitness levels are easily observed and can be measured, you can quickly start to see the emerging person you are capable of becoming. Almost daily you can see progress and accomplishment. Keep in mind, however, that all people are different and some may progress faster than others. In the final analysis, we think that although fitness will not guarantee that you will live longer, it can help you enjoy the years you do live.

DEVELOPING A CARDIORESPIRATORY FITNESS PROGRAM

Although the pronounced benefits of exercise clearly exist, we expect that readers of this book fall into some rather distinct categories: (1) those who already exercise regularly, (2) those who exercise sporadically, (3) those who do not exercise, and (4) those who would like to start some kind of fitness program. A major limitation for readers in all groups is an uncertainty about how best to develop fitness. We ask ourselves, "Am I doing enough to develop my fitness?"; "How can I have fun and develop cardiorespiratory fitness at the same time?"; and "Could I be doing things that might be dangerous?"

For persons of all ages, cardiorespiratory conditioning can be achieved through many activities. As long as the activity you choose places sufficient demand on the heart and lungs, improved fitness is possible. In addition to the familiar activities of swimming, running, cycling, and aerobic dance, today many people are participating in brisk walking, cross country skiing, swimnastics, skating, rowing, and even weight training (when combined with some form of aerobic activity). Regardless of age or physical limitations, you can select from a variety of enjoyable activities that will condition the cardiorespiratory system.

This portion of the chapter may read like a fitness program "cookbook." Just as a master chef needs to rely on a recipe to produce a winning delicacy, so too must you rely on a proven strategy or master plan when you create your own fitness program. Experts have developed and refined effective cardiorespiratory fitness programs that are distinguished by four important components: (1) type of activity, (2) intensity, (3) duration, and (4) frequency.

Many people think any kind of physical activity is exercise. Golf, bowling, hunting, fishing, and archery are considered forms of exercise. However, these activities would generally fail to produce positive changes in your cardiorespiratory fitness; they may indeed by enjoyable and produce some fatigue after lengthy participation, but they do not meet standards recognized by exercise physiologists—including Bud Getchell, executive director of the National Institute for Fitness and Sport in Indianapolis, Indiana.[6]

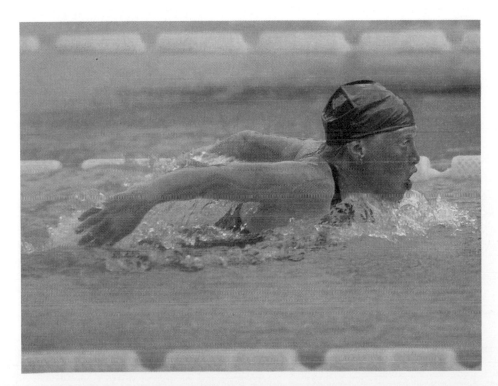

To produce cardiorespiratory fitness, physical activity must provide continuous, repetitive movements.

Type of Activity

Getchell believes the type of activity selected must be continuous and enjoyable. The activity should include repetitive movements (contractions) of large muscle groups. Among the activities that generally meet this requirement are continuous swimming, cycling, aerobic dancing, basketball, cross-country skiing, hiking, walking, and running. Tennis, racquetball, and handball are fine, as long as you and your partner are skilled enough to keep the ball in play; walking after the ball will do very little for you. Riding a bicycle is a fine activity, as long as you keep pedaling. Coasting through a residential neighborhood will do little to improve fitness. Softball and football are generally less than sufficient continuous activities—especially the way they are played by weekend athletes.

Regardless of the continuous activity you select, it should also be enjoyable. Running is not for everyone—despite what some accomplished runners will say! Find an activity you enjoy. If you need others around you to have a good time, corral a group of friends to join you. Vary your activities to keep from becoming bored. You might cycle in the summer, run in the fall, swim in the winter, and play racquetball in the spring. You should be aware that certain cardiorespiratory fitness activities may greatly enhance muscle strength and flexibility.

Intensity

intensity
level of effort one puts into an activity.

How much effort should you put into an activity? Should you run quickly, jog slowly, or swim at a comfortable pace? Must a person sweat profusely to achieve fitness? These questions all refer to **intensity** of effort.

target heart rate (THR)
number of times per minute that the heart must contract to produce a training effect.

You should sustain enough intensity to reach and maintain your **target heart rate (THR)** (see the box on p. 81). This rate refers to the minimum number of times your heart needs to contract (beat) each minute to have a positive effect on your heart, lungs, and blood vessels. This improvement is called the *training*

The pulse rate can be measured at the carotid artery *(left)* or at the radial artery *(right).*

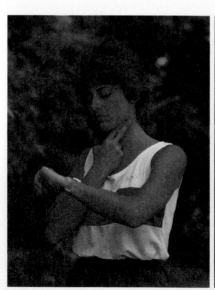
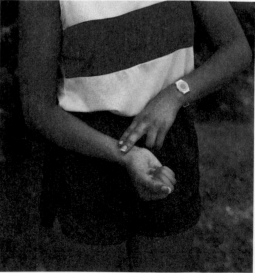

How to Calculate Your Target Heart Rate

The target heart rate (THR) is the optimal rate for increasing cardiovascular endurance. To maintain a training effect, you must sustain activity at your THR for 30 minutes. To find your THR, subtract your age from 220 (the maximum heart rate) and multiply by .75. Examples:

FOR A 20-YEAR-OLD PERSON

Maximum heart rate = 220 − 20 = 200

200 × .75 = 150

THR = 150 beats per minute

FOR A 52-YEAR-OLD PERSON

Maximum heart rate = 220 − 52 = 168

168 × .75 = 126

THR = 126 beats per minute

NOTE: The scientific literature presents various formulae which can calculate a THR. All calculate similar THRs for a given person.

effect. Intensity of activity below this level will be insufficient to make a significant improvement in your fitness. Intensity below the THR will still help you expend calories and thus lose weight, but it will probably do little to make you more aerobically fit. Intensity that is significantly above your THR will in all likelihood cause you to become so fatigued that you will be forced to stop the activity before the training effect can be achieved.

The younger person in the example in the box above would need to select a continuous and enjoyable activity and participate in this activity for an extended period while working at a THR of 150 beats per minute. The older person in the example would need to function at a THR of 126 beats per minute to achieve a positive training effect.

Determining your heart rate is not a complicated procedure. You need to find a location on your body where an artery passes near the surface of the skin. Pulse rates are quite difficult to determine by touching veins, which are more superficial than arteries. Two easily accessible sites for determining heart rate are the *carotid artery* (one is on either side of the Adam's apple at the front of your neck) and the *radial artery* (on the inside of your wrist, just above the base of the thumb).

You should practice placing the front surface of your index and middle fingertips at either of these locations and feeling for a pulse. Once you have found a regular pulse, look at the second hand of a watch. Count the number of beats you feel in a 6-second period and add a zero. This number will be your heart rate. With a little practice you can become very proficient at counting your heart rate.

Duration

How long should you exercise at your THR to achieve a training effect? The **duration** of exercise should be at least 30 minutes, not including your warm-up and cool-down activities.[6] While 30 minutes may sound like a long time for an out-of-shape person, remember that the THR is the key. Your jogging program

duration
length of time one needs to exercise at the THR to produce the training effect.

might start as a walking program; walking may be the only activity you can continue for 30 minutes while maintaining your THR. Once you become more fit, you probably will need to jog or run to be able to reach your THR. Obviously a person who is already conditioned and who plans to participate in a competitive endurance event will have a higher THR and require longer duration of exercise to improve significantly.

Frequency

frequency
number of times per week one should exercise to achieve a training effect.

Frequency refers to the number of days each week you need to exercise to receive a training effect. Early studies found that positive benefits could be reached with only two or three periods of exercise per week. More recent evidence indicates that you need to exercise four or five times each week.[6] Working out fewer than four times each week appears to be insufficient to develop a significant positive effect on your heart muscle, lungs, and blood vessels. Thus, although you may have a lot of fun cycling twice each week, do not expect to see a significant improvement in your cardiorespiratory fitness.

Exercise for Older Adults

An exercise program designed for younger adults may be inappropriate for older persons, particularly for persons over age 50. Special attention must be paid to matching the program to the interests and abilities of the participants. The goals of the program should include both social interaction and physical conditioning.

Older adults should take a physical examination before starting a fitness program. Included in this examination should be a stress cardiogram, blood pressure check, and an evaluation of joint functioning. It is a good idea for participants to learn how to monitor their own cardiorespiratory status during exercise.

Well-designed fitness programs for older adults will have activities that begin slowly, are monitored frequently, and are geared to the enjoyment of the participants. The professional staff coordinating the program should be familiar with the signs of distress (excessively elevated heart rate, nausea, *dyspnea*, pallor, and pain) and able to perform cardiopulmonary resuscitation (CPR). Periods of warm-up and cool-down should be included. (See stretching exercises on pp. 72-73.) Activities to increase flexibility are beneficial in the beginning and ending segments of the program. Participants should wear comfortable clothing, appropriate shoes, and be mentally prepared to enjoy the activities to the fullest.

A program designed for older adults will largely conform to the criteria (activity, intensity, duration, and frequency) specified earlier in this chapter. The principal exception is in the intensity component, where the THR should not exceed 120 beats per minute. This level of intensity is approximately 40% to 50% of the maximum heart rate. Also, because of possible joint or muscular/skeletal problems, certain activities may have to be done in a sitting position. Pain and discomfort should be reported immediately to the fitness instructor.

Fortunately, properly screened adults will rarely have health emergencies during a well-monitored fitness program. Like their youthful counterparts, many older adults find fitness programs socially enjoyable, physically beneficial, and occasionally addictive.

FITNESS QUESTIONS AND ANSWERS

Besides the four necessary elements to include in your fitness program, many additional issues should be considered when you start a fitness program.

Should I See My Doctor Before I Get Started?

This issue has probably kept thousands of people from ever beginning a fitness program. The hassle and expense of getting a comprehensive physical examination are excellent alibis for people who are not completely sold on the idea of exercise. A complete examination, including *blood analysis,* a *stress test,* a *cardiogram, serum lipid analysis,* and *body fat analysis,* is a valuable tool for developing some baseline physical data for your medical record.

Is this examination really necessary? Most exercise physiologists do not think so. The value of these measurements as safety predictors is questioned by many professionals. A good general rule of thumb to follow would be to undergo a physical examination if (1) you have an existing medical condition (diabetes, obesity, hypertension, heart abnormalities, or arthritis, for example), or (2) you are age 30 or over and have not pursued vigorous activity for at least 5 years.

What About the Value of Warming Up Before Exercise?

Stretching your muscles before participation should be an integral part of your activity. Take 5 to 10 minutes to stretch and lengthen all the major muscle groups of your body (see pp. 72-73). This preparation helps protect you from muscle strains and joint sprains.

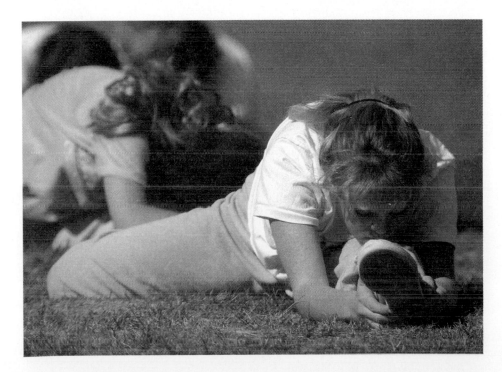

Warming up is an important part of a physical fitness program.

Warm-up is a fine time to socialize with others. Furthermore, you can mentally prepare yourself for your activity or think about the beauty of the morning sky, the changing colors of the leaves, or the friends you will meet later in the day. You may even enjoy contemplating the rigor of the activity you are about to undertake. Mental warm-ups can be as beneficial for you psychologically as physical warm-ups are physically.

Likewise, after finishing your activity take another 5 to 10 minutes to *cool down.*[7] Again, stretch the muscle groups and socialize with your friends. Think about your struggles and your accomplishments. Stretching helps to relax muscle fibers that have been under considerable stress and helps remove metabolic waste products.

What About Jumping Rope? I've Heard It Is a Great Conditioner

For most people jumping rope is a skill that takes a long time to develop well. Yet we hear claims that jumping rope only 10 minutes a day can make you fit. Jumping rope is not generally a good choice of activity unless you are already in good physical condition or are a member of an organized rope jumping program. The average person strains too hard to keep the jumping and rope maneuvering in synchronization. Thus the novice jumper quickly becomes fatigued and must stop.

Contrast this picture with that of a well-conditioned welterweight boxer. He is already in top cardiorespiratory condition and has developed excellent jump-rope skills. Thus he could (if he wanted to) keep the continuous activity going at his THR for the required 30 minutes. He does not become fatigued to the point of stopping. So comfortable is this athlete that he can even conduct an interview while he exercises.

Unless you too are already in good physical condition and have the requisite skills, you should hold off considering rope jumping as your only fitness activity.

How Beneficial Is Aerobic Exercise?

One of the most popular fitness approaches presently emerging is aerobic exercise, including aerobic dancing. Many organizations sponsor classes in this form of continuous dancing–movement. The rise in popularity of televised aerobic exercise programs reflects the enthusiasm for this form of exercise. While some extravagant claims are made for the value of these new programs, the wise consumer should observe at least one session of the activity before enrolling. Discover for yourself whether the program meets the four criteria outlined earlier in this chapter; type of activity, intensity, duration, and frequency.

Certainly this activity is enjoyable. Examine the program to see whether participants are in continuous motion for 30 minutes. Are heart rates periodically checked? Does the class meet at least four times each week? Many current classes meet only two times each week, but participants are encouraged to dance, jog, or swim on their own.

Research studies on aerobics are just beginning. Early data seem to suggest that aerobic exercise can produce a training effect for the participants—as long as the activity is carefully structured.

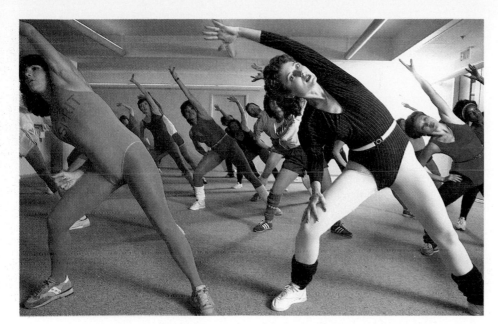

Low impact aerobics.

What Are Low Impact Aerobic Activities?

Because long term participation in some aerobic activities (for example, jogging, running, aerobic dance, and rope skipping) may cause damage to the hip, knee, and ankle joints, many fitness experts are promoting low impact aerobic activities. Low impact aerobic dance, swimnastics and brisk walking are examples of this kind of fitness activity. Participants still conform to the four principal components of a cardiorespiratory fitness program (activity, intensity, frequency, and duration). THR levels remain the same as in high impact activities.

The main difference between low and high impact aerobic activities is in the use of the legs. Low impact aerobics do not require having both feet off the ground at the same time. Thus, weight transfer does not occur with the forcefulness seen in traditional, high aerobic activities. Additionally, low impact activities may include exaggerated arm movements, the use of hand or wrist weights, and exaggerated lateral body movements. All of these variations are designed to increase the heart rate to the THR without damaging the joints of the lower extremities. Low impact aerobics may be especially beneficial to older adults.

What Is the Most Effective Fluid Replacement During Exercise?

Despite all the advertising hype associated with commercial fluid replacement products, for an average person involved in typical fitness activities, water is still the best fluid replacement available. It is more quickly absorbed by the body than any commercial products,[8] and the availability and cost are unbeatable. However, when activity is prolonged over an hour, commercial sport drinks may be preferable to water because they contain electrolytes (that replace lost sodium and potassium) and carbohydrates (that replace depleted energy stores).[9] Regardless of the drink you choose, it is recommended that you drink fluids at frequent intervals throughout your activity.

Choosing an Athletic Shoe

AEROBIC SHOES

When selecting shoes for aerobic dancing, J. Lynn Reese, president of J. Lynn & Co. Endurance Sports, Washington, DC, advises:

- Check the width of the shoe at the widest part of your foot. The bottom of the shoe should be as wide as the bottom of your foot; the uppers shouldn't go over the sides.
- Look for leather or nylon uppers. Leather is durable and gives good support, but it can stretch. Nylon won't stretch and gives support, but it's not as durable. Canvas generally doesn't offer much support.
- Look for rubber rather than polyurethane or black carbon rubber soles. Treads should be fairly flat in the forefoot. If you're dancing on carpet, you can go with less tread; if you're dancing on gym floors, you may need more grab.

COURT SHOES

What's important when choosing a tennis shoe? Jack Groppel, technical editor of *World Tennis* magazine and associate professor of bioengineering, University of Illinois, offers this list:

- Cushioning. Cushioning is especially important in the heel counter.
- Side support. Side support, also called lateral and medial support, is also important.
- Back-of-heel fit. Try on the shoe, and then put your little finger in behind the heel. It should fit snugly.
- Toe box (top front of shoe). Make sure the toe box isn't too tight or too loose.
- Traction. Keep in mind the surface you play on most often. Rubber gives better traction than synthetic materials such as polyurethane, but is less durable.

When buying shoes for racquetball, Doug Richie, podiatrist, Seal Beach, California, advises:

- Choose side-to-side over flexibility and cushioning.
- Choose a heavy shoe with lots of support.
- The tread should be relatively smooth—compatible with hardwood surfaces.
- Choose the brushed cotton jersey sock over terry liners.

RUNNING SHOES

Need new running shoes? Here's advice from Jeff Galloway, former Olympic runner, founder and president of Phidippides International aerobic sports stores, headquartered in Atlanta.

- Take time to shop, and get a knowledgeable salesman. Good advice is crucial.
- Check the wear pattern on your old shoes to see whether you have floppy or rigid feet. Floppy-footed runners wear out their soles on the outside and inside edges; rigid-footed runners wear out soles predominantly on the outside edges. Floppy-footed runners can sacrifice cushioning for support, while rigid-footed runners can sacrifice support for cushioning.
- Know your feet, whether they're curved or straight and whether you have high arches or are flat-footed. The shoe should fit the shape of your foot.

AEROBIC SHOES

Flexibility: More at ball of foot than running shoes, but less flexible than court shoes

Uppers: Most are leather or leather-reinforced nylon

Cushioning: More than court shoes, less than running shoes

Heel flare: Little or none

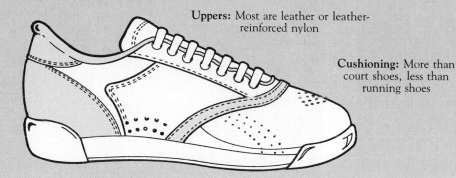

Tread: Should be fairly flat, especially on forefoot; may also have "dot" on the ball of the foot for pivoting

Soles: Rubber if you are dancing on wood floors; polyurethane for other surfaces

COURT SHOES

Flexibility: Less than running shoes; sole is firmer

Uppers: Usually leather or leather-reinforced nylon

Cushioning: Less than running shoes

Heel: Not flared (flared heels take away from side-to-side support)

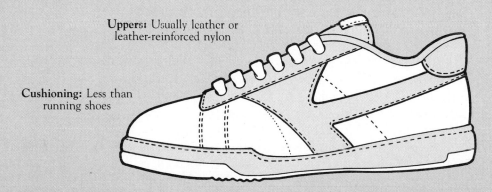

Soles: For tennis, flat; usually polyurethane is more durable for tennis courts; for racquetball, rounded (to allow quicker side-to-side movement); usually rubber less durable because wood courts are slicker and don't wear down shoes as fast

Tread: Much flatter than running shoes; may have tread pattern designed around ball of foot where the foot pivots

RUNNING SHOES

Flexibility: Shoe flexible at ball of foot

Uppers: Usually nylon mesh or nylon; a few leather; no canvas

Flared heel: Gives foot broader, more stable base

Cushioning: More than court shoes, especially at heel

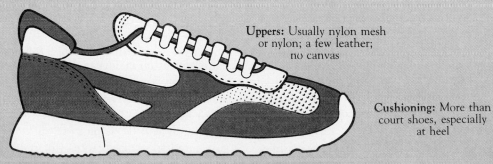

Tread: "Waffle" or other deep-cut tread for grip on many surfaces

Soles: Usually carbon-based for longer wear

Commercial fitness clubs should employ qualified instructors.

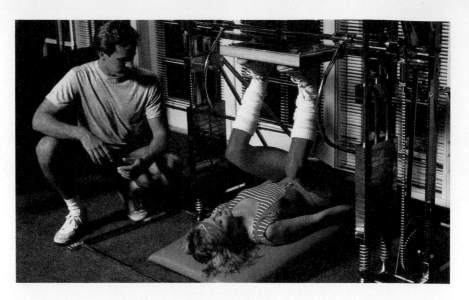

Why Has Bodybuilding Become So Popular?

It is true that *bodybuilding* has increased significantly in popularity in recent years. The reasons for this growth are many. Bodybuilders often start lifting weights to get into better shape—to improve muscle tone. They may just want to look healthier and feel stronger. Once they realize that they can alter the shape of their bodies, they find that bodybuilding offers challenges that—through hard work—are attainable. Bodybuilders also report enjoying the physical sensations (the "pump") that results from a good workout. The results of their efforts are clearly visible and measurable. Some bodybuilders become involved in competitive events to test their advancements.

Perhaps we should dispel a few myths about bodybuilding. Are bodybuilders strong? The answer is emphatically—yes! Will muscle cells turn into fat cells if weightlifting programs are discontinued? *No*, muscle cells are physiologically incapable of turning into fat cells. Will women develop bulky muscles through weight training? *No*, they can improve muscle strength and tone, but unless they take steroids, their muscle mass cannot increase like men's muscle mass. Is bodybuilding socially acceptable? *Yes*, for many people. Just observe all the new health clubs that cater to weightlifters and bodybuilders.

Where Can I Find Out About Proper Equipment?

College students are generally in an excellent setting to locate people and resources that can provide helpful information about equipment. Contacting physical education or health education faculty members who have an interest in your chosen activity might be a good start. Most colleges also have a number of clubs that specialize in fitness interests—cycling, hiking, and jogging clubs, for example. Attend one of their upcoming meetings. Since such clubs are often looking for new members, they surely will be helpful to you.

Sporting goods stores and specialized stores (for runners, tennis and racquetball players, and cyclists) are convenient places to obtain information. Employees of these stores are usually knowledgable about sports and equipment (see the box on pp. 86-87).

How Valuable Are Commercial Fitness Clubs and Spas?

These enterprises exist for one purpose—to make a substantial profit. To this end, spas and clubs provide a pleasant atmosphere in which members can socialize and feel pampered. After signing a contract, members often have use of hot baths, saunas, whirlpools, and devices that supposedly can make you fit with little effort on your part. Such passive machines that "roll your belly or pound your flab" cannot make you fit; neither will hot wraps or special mud packs.

Unless the spa provides the opportunity to sustain continuous movement at the proper intensity, little improvement in cardiorespiratory fitness could ever be accomplished even though some of the weight training machines that a few spas have can be helpful in increasing your muscle tone and development.

Before signing a contract at a health spa, do some careful questioning. Find out how long the business has been established, ask about the qualifications of the employees, contact some members for their observations, and request a thorough tour of the facilities. You might even consult your local Better Business Bureau for additional information. Finally, make certain you read every word typed on the contract. The Federal Trade Commission has reported that many of these businesses have abruptly declared bankruptcy. Unfortunately, few members of these defunct clubs were able to receive any reimbursements for their cancelled memberships. The message would seem to be: WATCH OUT.

What Is Crosstraining?

Crosstraining is the use of more than one aerobic activity to achieve cardiorespiratory fitness. For example, runners may use swimming, cycling, or rowing to periodically replace running in their training routines. Crosstraining allows certain muscle groups to rest and injuries to heal. Also, crosstraining provides a refreshing change of pace for the participant. You will likely find more enjoyment in your fitness program if you vary the activities.

What Are Steroids and Why Do Some Athletes Use Them?

Anabolic steroids are drugs that function like the male sex hormone *testosterone*. Steroids are used by athletes who hope to gain weight, power, strength, endurance, and aggressiveness (see the box on pp. 90-91). Numerous bodybuilders, weightlifters, and football players have found steroid use desirable. It is possible that steroids taken in clinically controlled dosages can accelerate the growth of muscle, bone, and red blood cells, and improve nerve conduction.[3] However, when taken in a medically unsupervised manner, as is done by most users, these effects are not as predictable.

Whether steroids actually are significant help in promoting these desired changes is debatable, but athletes who take steroids seem to believe that they provide them with a competitive edge. Certain athletes who are convinced that everyone else is taking steroids seem emotionally incapable of resisting steroid use. This perception is especially true in the case of some American athletes' perceptions of widespread steroid use by athletes from Eastern bloc countries.[10]

Aside from the fact that many organizations that control athletic competition have banned steroid use and are administering screening tests for illegal use by athletes, steroid use is associated with a variety of dangerous side effects, includ-

anabolic steroids
drugs that function like testosterone to produce increases in weight, strength, endurance, and aggressiveness.

What You Should Know About Steroids

WHAT THEY ARE

Anabolic steroids—anabolic referring to "building up"—are synthetic variants of the strongest male hormone, testosterone. Most common brand names are Anadrol, DecaDurabolin, and Anavar; nicknames include "roids" and "juice."

WHAT THEY DO

In conjunction with athletic training, they stimulate muscle growth by synthesizing protein and cause weight gain partly through increased water retention. They also increase aggression, which may make an athlete train harder.

HOW THEY ARE TAKEN

Mostly in tablet form, also by injection.

COST

Dosages vary widely. Users can spend $25 to $500 a month.

HOW THEY ARE OBTAINED

Legally, by prescription only; otherwise, several routes exist, including mail order.

WHY RESEARCH IS SKIMPY

It is considered unethical for testers to administer steroids in the high-dose levels athletes use.

HOW DANGEROUS THEY ARE

Experts agree the health risks outweigh any benefits—but whether steroids are as dangerous as, for example, cocaine, remains in dispute. "I think reaching out for steroids is bad but not as bad as reaching out for cocaine," says the Los Angeles Rams' Dr. Robert Kerlan, one of the United States' top sports medicine surgeons; "Steroids definitely are as dangerous as any prescription licensed drug that ever appeared on the market," says the New York Giants' Dr. Alan Levy.

MEDICAL APPLICATIONS

Doctors prescribe steroids as an aid to treatment for anemic and people who are growing inadequately and to aid recovery from surgery or chronic, debilitating diseases.

REDUCING AVAILABILITY

The Justice Department, Federal Bureau of Investigation (FBI), and the Food and Drug Administration (FDA) have been working together on a federal probe that has resulted in several arrests of the black market distributors they say may make $100 million a year.

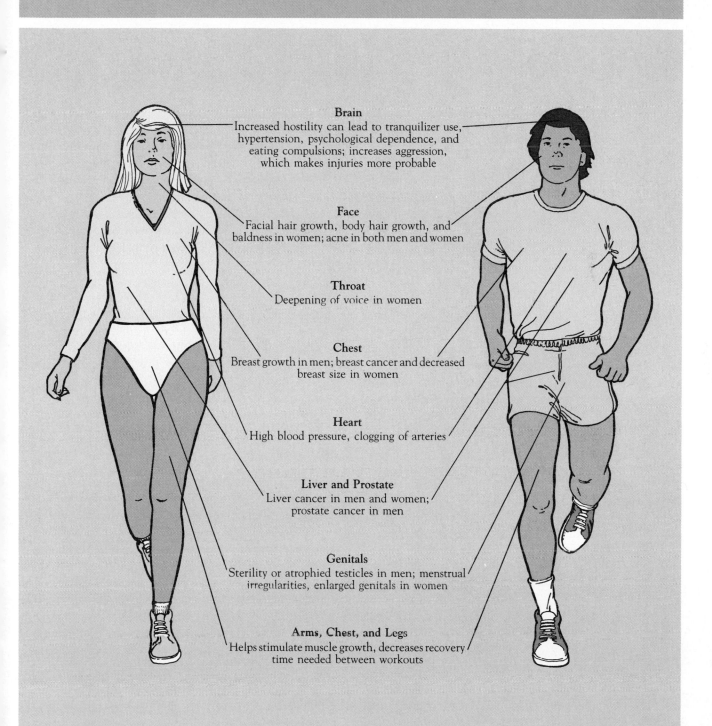

Brain
Increased hostility can lead to tranquilizer use, hypertension, psychological dependence, and eating compulsions; increases aggression, which makes injuries more probable

Face
Facial hair growth, body hair growth, and baldness in women; acne in both men and women

Throat
Deepening of voice in women

Chest
Breast growth in men; breast cancer and decreased breast size in women

Heart
High blood pressure, clogging of arteries

Liver and Prostate
Liver cancer in men and women; prostate cancer in men

Genitals
Sterility or atrophied testicles in men; menstrual irregularities, enlarged genitals in women

Arms, Chest, and Legs
Helps stimulate muscle growth, decreases recovery time needed between workouts

ing liver toxicity, hypertension, certain forms of cancer, heart disease, and decreased sperm production. Women who take steroids usually develop masculine characteristics, including lowered voice, increased facial and body hair, and increased baldness. Menstrual irregularity is a common side effect. A variety of more minor side effects have also been reported, such as muscle cramping, dizziness, sore nipples, and gastrointestinal distress.[1]

What Are the Two Types of Muscle Fibers and How Can They Affect Exercise Performance?

fast-twitch (FT) fibers
type of muscle cell especially suited for anaerobic activities.

slow-twitch (ST) fibers
type of muscle cell especially suited for aerobic activities.

Through a *needle biopsy procedure,* two basic types of fibers (muscle cells) can be seen in human muscle. These fibers are the **fast-twitch (FT)** and **slow-twitch (ST) fibers.** The high enzyme activity in FT fibers makes these fibers better suited for high-intensity activity, whereas the greater aerobic capacity of ST fibers makes them better suited for endurance-type activities."

People inherit varying proportions of these fiber types. People with greater percentages of FT fibers than ST fibers have a greater capacity for anaerobic activities. Those having a greater percentage of ST fibers than FT fibers seem more capable of endurance activities.

Although FT fibers cannot be converted to ST fibers, some research suggests that under proper exercise training, FT fibers are capable of developing some properties of ST fibers. One example of the application of this knowledge is in track and field, where increasing numbers of middle-distance runners are redirecting their training methods and finding great success at full-length marathons. Interestingly, ST fibers appear to be less able to develop the properties of FT fibers. Thus it is doubtful that marathon runners can be trained to be first-class sprinters. Indeed, it seems that we are born with predispositions to certain kinds of athletic activities. (For students interested in more in-depth analysis of fiber types and their subgroups, see the references at the end of the chapter.)

Are Today's Young Children Physically Fit?

The 1985 School Fitness Survey pointed out some alarming information about the fitness levels of today's youth. This study, which examined nearly 19,000 students age 6 to 17, found that levels of fitness were no better than those a decade earlier. The study concluded that many parents today are in better shape than their children. For measures of strength, flexibility, and cardiorespiratory endurance, children scored extremely poorly.

This information presents a challenge to educators and parents to emphasize the need for strenuous play activity. Television watching was implicated as a major culprit in this study. For students reading this text who are parents or grandparents of young chidlren, what can you do to encourage more physical activity and less sedentary activity?

How Can Sleep Contribute to Overall Fitness?

Although sleep may seem the opposite of exercise, sleep is an important adjunct to a well-planned exercise program (see the box on p. 93). In fact, sleep is so vital to health that people who are unable to sleep sufficiently (those with insomnia) or who are deprived of sleep experience deterioration in every dimen-

To Help You Sleep . . .

Can we work at being better sleepers? The answer is yes. There are many activities that when done at the appropriate time will aid you in your quest for sound sleep.

ACTIVITIES FOR THE DAY

Schedule. Maintain a consistent schedule of daily activities; a disrupted day makes sleeping difficult.

Physical activity. Regular vigorous activity promotes sleep; exercising too near bedtime, can, however, make you too energized to sleep soundly.

Eating. A large meal taken late in the evening interferes with sleeping; avoid large late-night snacks as well.

Alcohol use. A single drink in the evening may be relaxing, but too many drinks during the day make sleeping difficult.

CNS stimulants. Coffee, tea, soft drinks with caffeine, and some medications can disrupt normal sleeping patterns.

Worry. Problems and concerns should be put behind you by the time you retire; practice leaving your concerns at the office or in the classroom.

Rituals. A ritualistic "winding down" over the course of the evening promotes sleep; watching television, listening to records, and reading during the evening are excellent ways to prepare the body for sleep.

ACTIVITIES FOR THE END OF THE DAY

Bathing. For many people, a warm bath immediately before retiring promotes sleep.

Yoga. The quiet, relaxing exercises of yoga promote sleep by slowing the body's activity level.

Snack or nightcap. A light snack of foods high in L-tryptophan (eggs, tuna, and turkey) and a glass of milk will help you fall asleep.

Muscular relaxation. Alternating contraction and relaxation of the large muscles of the extremities aids the body in falling asleep.

Imaging. Quieting images can distract the mind, thus allowing sleep to occur more easily.

Fantasies. Escape into fantasies slows the mind and facilitates the onset of sleep.

Breathing. Slow, deep breaths set a restful rhythm the body can "ride" into sleep.

Thinking. By envisioning yourself as sleeping soundly, you may in fact fall asleep more quickly.

sion of their health. Fortunately exercise is frequently associated with improvements in sleeping.

Sleep is by no means a simple turning off of the body and mind, as some might imagine it to be. Rather, sleep reflects a progression of changes in the electrical activity of the brain. Through the course of the 6 to 8 hours of sleep per night that most adults achieve, the frequencies and intensities of electrical impulses being transmitted through the brain change in a cyclic and repetitive manner.[12] When recorded on an *electroencephalogram (EEG)*, activity patterns suggest two major states of sleep—**rapid eye movement (REM) sleep** and **slow wave (SW) sleep.** Slow wave sleep, a period producing primarily low-frequency, high-intensity delta waves, and REM sleep, in which dreaming predominates, completely recycle approximately every 90 minutes.

The value of sleep is expressed in a variety of positive changes in the body. Dreaming is thought to play a valuable role in supporting the emotional dimension of health. Problem-solving vignettes that occur during dreams seem to afford some carry-over value in actual coping experiences. A variety of changes in physiological functioning, particularly a deceleration of the cardiovascular system, occur while you sleep. The familiar feeling of being well rested is an expression of the mental and physiological rejuvenation you feel after a good night's sleep.

The amount of sleep needed varies among people. In fact, for any person, sleep needs vary according to one's activity level and overall state of health. As we become older, the need for sleep appears to decrease from the 6 to 8 hours young adults require. Elderly people routinely sleep less than they did when they were younger. This decrease may be offset by the short naps older people may take during the day. For all persons, however, periods of relaxation and day-dreaming generate electrical activity patterns that help regenerate the mind and body just as sleep does.

rapid eye movement (REM) sleep
dream stage of sleep characterized by twitching movements of the eyes beneath the eyelids.

slow wave (SW) sleep
stage of sleep characterized by minimal dream activity.

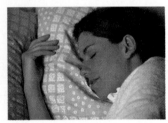

Adequate amounts of sleep are vital to every dimension of your health.

What Exercise Danger Signs Should I Watch For?

The human body is an amazing piece of equipment. It functions well whether or not you are conscious of its processes. It also delivers clear signals when something goes wrong.

You should monitor any sign that seems abnormal during or after your exercise. "Listen to your body" is a good rule for self-awareness. The following are some common signs to monitor:

- A delay of over 1 hour in your body's return to a fully relaxed, comfortable state after exercise.
- Difficulty in sleep patterns. Although it is not uncommon for a beginner to experience some sleep difficulties during the early stages of fitness development, continued problems may indicate overexertion. Reduce the intensity or frequency of your workouts for a while. Avoid exercising too close to bedtime.
- Any noticeable breathing difficulties or chest pains. Exercise at your THR should not initiate these problems. Recheck your level of intensity. Further problems should be referred to a physician.
- Persistent joint and muscle pains. Starting to exercise after years of inactivity will naturally bring on some muscle soreness and joint discomfort. How-

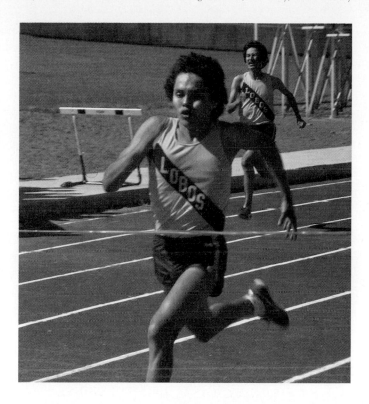

What do you hope to achieve with your fitness program?

ever, these should be temporary problems. Listen to your body. Any lingering joint or muscle pain might signal a problem. Seek the help of an athletic trainer, physical therapist, or your physician.

- Unusual changes in urine composition or output. Marked color change in your urine could signal possible kidney or bladder difficulties. Also, significant changes in volume of urine output might be a cause of concern. Remember, people who exercise need to consume much greater quantities of fluids than nonexercisers. Fluids lost through sweating need to be replaced. Drink plenty of water before, during, and after your activity.

- Anything of an unusual nature that you notice after starting your fitness program. Examples might be headaches, nosebleeds, fainting, numbness in an extremity, or hemorrhoids. However, such occurrences are extremely unusual. Fear of developing these difficulties should not deter you from starting a fitness program. The risks are minimal—and the benefits far outnumber the risks.

SUMMARY

A college student's life is busy and requires a high level of fitness. Physical fitness allows you to respond to routine demands on unexpected activities.

Physical fitness can be viewed in terms of several specific components related to body structure and function. The five components explored in this chapter include muscular strength, muscular endurance, flexibility, agility, and cardiorespiratory endurance. Some approaches to enhancing these fitness components were discussed. The well-documented benefits associated with cardiorespiratory endurance were also presented.

People hold many opinions about physical fitness programs. Many of the reasons given for being involved in a fitness program may be shortsighted. Chapter 4 recommended that your fitness be examined in relation to its ability to positively influence other aspects of your life.

The four important components of an effective cardiorespiratory fitness program were explained. These components are (1) type of activity, (2) intensity, (3) duration, and (4) frequency of the activity. Many other issues that you need to consider when you start a fitness program were also presented.

Finally, this chapter considered some of the current findings and trends related to fitness, including muscle fiber types (both fast-twitch and slow-twitch), bodybuilding, fluid replacement, steroid use, and sleep patterns.

REVIEW QUESTIONS

1 Identify the five components of fitness described in this chapter. Explain how each dimension relates to physical fitness.
2 What is the difference between anaerobic and aerobic energy production? What types of activities are associated with anaerobic energy production? With aerobic energy production?
3 Differentiate among the various methods used to promote muscular strength.
4 What do the principles of overload and specificity mean in regard to training programs used to develop fitness?
5 List some of the benefits of endurance conditioning.
6 Identify a few of the common reasons people give for not participating in a regular fitness program. Identify a few of the reasons people do particpate in a regular fitness program.
7 Identify the four important components of an effective cardiorespiratory fitness program. Explain the important aspects of each component.
8 Under what circumstances should you see a physician before starting a physical fitness program?
9 How do fast-twitch (FT) and slow-twitch (ST) muscle fibers differ?
10 Describe some of the negative consequences of anabolic steroid use.

QUESTIONS FOR PERSONAL CONTEMPLATION

1 Consider what your own schedule of daily activities is like. Do you feel that your present level of fitness allows you to effectively carry out the activities your schedule demands? Are there things that you would like to do but cannot because of your current level of fitness?
2 Describe your own level of fitness, taking into consideration the dimensions of strength, flexibility, agility, and cardiorespiratory endurance. Are there areas that you feel need improvement? How can you make these improvements?
3 What are your own attitudes toward physical fitness? If you do participate in a regular physical fitness program—why do you? If you do not participate in a regular program—why not? If you do participate in a regular program, do you feel you have made a commitment to physical fitness for the right reasons?
4 Examine your own physical fitness program in terms of the four important components: type of activity, intensity, duration, and frequency. What areas need improvement? How can you make these improvements?

5 Design a personal physical fitness plan for yourself, taking into consideration all of the dimensions of body structure and function and the four components of an effective fitness program described in this chapter. What are the chances that you will continue this program into your postcollege years?

6 After determining your own target heart rate (THR), calculate the THR for a parent or older friend. Talk to these people about starting their own fitness programs. Stand ready to help them with encouragement and accurate information. They may look to you as a role model for their own health.

REFERENCES

1 McArdle, WD, et al: Exercise physiology: energy, nutrition, and human performance, ed 2, Philadelphia, 1986, Lea & Febiger.

2 Hockey, RV: Physical fitness: the pathway to healthy living, ed 5, St. Louis, 1985, Times Mirror/Mosby College Publishing.

3 Brooks, GA, and Fahey, TD: Fundamentals of human performance, New York, 1987, Macmillan Publishing Co.

4 Gurin, J: Linking exercise with longevity, Runner's World 60:61, 1985.

5 Paffenbarger, R, et al: Physical activity, all-cause mortality, and longevity of college alumni, New England Journal of Medicine 314:605-613, 1986.

6 Getchell, B: The fitness book, Indianapolis, 1987, Benchmark Press, Inc.

7 Prentice, WE, and Bucher, CA: Fitness for college and life, ed 2, St. Louis, 1988, Times Mirror/Mosby College Publishing.

8 Foster, C, et al: Gastric emptying characteristics of glucose and glucose polymer solutions, Research Quarterly for Exercise and Sport 51:299-305, 1980.

9 Reynolds, G: Drink: don't dry, Runner's World 62:40-45, 1987.

10 Nightingale, D: Steroid wars: the crackdown on drug use intensifies as the 1984 summer games draw near, The Sporting News 197:2, 1984.

11 Noble, BJ: Physiology of exercise and sport, St. Louis, 1986, Times Mirror/Mosby College Publishing.

12 Thibodeau, GA: Anatomy and physiology, St. Louis, 1987, Times Mirror/Mosby College Publishing.

ANNOTATED READINGS

Coleman, R: Wide awake at 3AM: by choice or by chance, New York, 1986, WH Freeman & Co, Publishers.
    Explores the role of circadian rhythms in controlling sleep patterns. Adjustments are presented for persons whose lifestyles create sleep difficulties.

Cooper, KH: The aerobics program for total well-being, New York, 1982, M Evans & Co, Inc.
    Reevaluates more than three dozen kinds of exercises in terms of their aerobic benefits; analyzes various types of exercises in terms of toning and muscle building.

Edwards, S: Triathalon: a triple fitness sport, Chicago, 1983, Contemporary Books, Inc.
    For both the novice and the practitioner; how to rate yourself physically in swimming, bicycling, and running, and how to refine your skills for this ultimate competition.

Goldman, B: Death in the locker room: steroids and sports, South Bend, Ind, 1984, Icarus Press.
    Details the extent of steroid use among athletes. The tragic consequences of drug abuse among athletes are described in this landmark book.

McCullagh, JC: The complete bicycle fitness book, New York, 1984, Warner Books Inc.
    Complete guide to full body fitness through cycling; to trim you down, build you up, and provide life-enhancing pleasure at any age.

Prentice, WE, and Bucher, CA: Fitness for college and life, ed 2, St. Louis, 1988, Times Mirror/ Mosby College Publishing.
    Provides you with the basics of being physically fit; provides the necessary information to help you either begin or maintain a program of healthy and enjoyable exercise.

Sheehan, GA: Dr. Sheehan on fitness, New York, 1984, Simon & Schuster Inc.
    One of a number of bestselling books by the noted cardiologist who approaches running and fitness from a philosophical, psychological, and humanistic point of view.

CHAPTER 5

Nutrition
The Role of Diet in Your Health

Key Concepts

Six essential nutrients are required for growth, repair, and regulation of the body.

A nutritious diet contains selections from each of the four food groups.

The use of food additives should be viewed from a variety of perspectives.

There are risks associated with nontraditional dietary practices.

Older adults have special nutritional needs.

It is important to stay informed of nutritionally sound dietary recommendations.

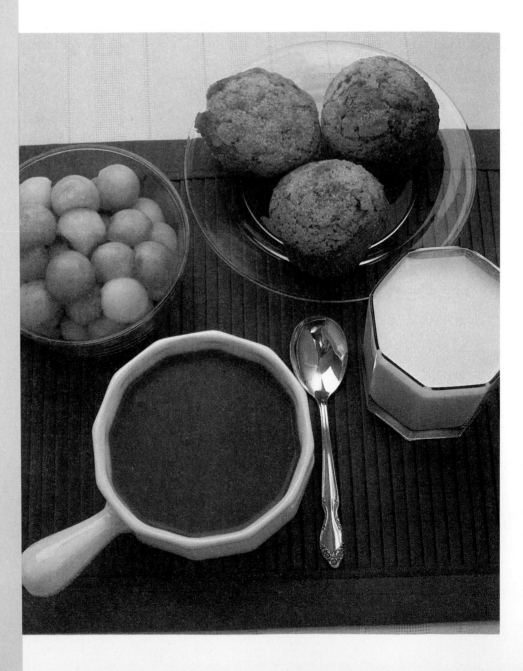

From the prenatal period throughout life, we must follow sound dietary practices to have a productive, satisfying life. Food provides the body with the raw materials for production of energy, repair of damaged tissue, growth of new tissues, and regulation of physiological processes.

Your mastery of developmental tasks can be compromised by inappropriate dietary practices. Failure to provide the body with nutrients essential for energy, repair, and regulation would eventually lead to a lowered level of health. Thus a careful and insightful structuring of your diet will be important throughout the course of your life cycle.

TYPES AND SOURCES OF NUTRIENTS

Nutrients are the elements in foods that are required for the growth, repair, and regulation of the body. Although nutritionists indicate that our bodies require six nutrients, our American culture is especially enamored of two of these: proteins and vitamins. It is difficult to watch television or listen to the radio for long without hearing someone describe how important these two nutrients are for your health. From peanut butter to high-powered dog food, we are sold on the value of protein. Breakfast cereals compete with each other in the battle to prove each contains more vitamins than any other cereal. Protein and vitamins are important nutrients but should be viewed in their proper perspective.

From the standpoint of the physical dimension of health, all six nutrient categories are essential. Serious nutritional deficiencies could occur should you neglect any nutrient. Despite Madison Avenue's preference for protein and vitamins, your body also requires fats, carbohydrates, minerals, and water, and nonnutritive fiber at levels adequate for sound maintenance and growth.

We will discuss the familiar carbohydrates, fats, and proteins first. These are the three nutrients that provide our bodies with **Calories.** * These Calories are either used by our bodies through energy metabolism or are stored in the form of glycogen or adipose tissue. Since the other nutrient groups are not sources of *energy* for the body, we will discuss them later.

Carbohydrates

Carbohydrates are various combinations of sugar units, or saccharides. The body uses carbohydrates primarily for the production of energy. Each gram of carbohydrate you consume provides your body with 4 Calories of energy. Carbohydrates that are composed of either one or two saccharides are generally called *sugars.* Carbohydrates that are composed of longer chains of saccharide units are known as polysaccharides, or starches. Nutritionists recommend that about 60% of our caloric intake be from carbohydrates.

Monosaccharides are the simplest sugar units. All carbohydrates, regardless of their original form, must be catabolized (broken down) by the body into this form before being utilized. Glucose is an important monosaccharide, since it makes up the blood sugar used for our body's fuel. Glucose, also known as dextrose, is found in vegetables, honey, molasses, fruits, and syrup. Fructose, also

nutrients
elements in foods that are required for the growth, repair, and regulation of body processes.

Calories
units of heat (energy); specifically, one Calorie equals the heat required to raise 1 kilogram of water 1° C.

carbohydrates
chemical compounds comprising sugar or saccharide units; the body's primary source of energy.

---

*Calorie with a capital C refers to kilocalorie (kcal), which is the accepted scientific expression of the energy value of a food.

Eating patterns established in childhood can continue throughout life.

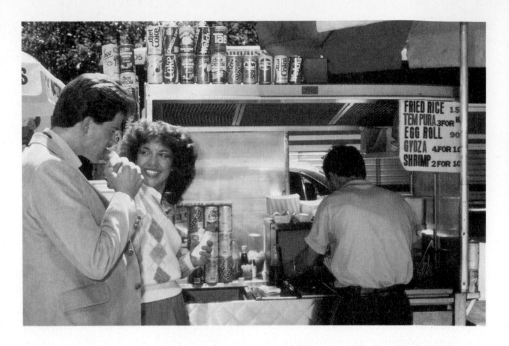

Eating on the Run

Select salads instead of french fries.

At a salad bar, choose the plain vegetables; avoid potato salad and cole slaw.

Opt for a plain hamburger without condiments; when you add your own, you control the amounts.

Add lettuce and tomato to hamburgers to add vitamins, not calories.

Plain chicken has fewer Calories than beef.

Avoid battered and fried foods.

Choose milk or juice, not sodas or shakes.

For dessert, bring a piece of fresh fruit with you.

Eat a small snack at 10 AM and then again at 2 PM. This kind of grazing can be healthier than gulping down one big, fat-filled meal at noon.

called levulose, is another monosaccharide that provides a source of simple sugar. This simple sugar is most often derived from fruits and berries.

Disaccharides are sugars composed of two monosaccharides. Sucrose is perhaps the most widely recognized disaccharide source, since it is better known as table sugar. Sucrose is a combination of glucose and fructose molecules. Other disaccharides include maltose, derived from germinating cereals, and lactose, the carbohydrate found in human and animal milk.

The average adult American now ingests approximately 100 pounds of sucrose each year—usually in colas, candies, and pastries, which offer few additional nutritional benefits.[1] For years excess sugar intake was implicated in a number of major health concerns, including obesity, micronutrient deficiencies, behavioral disorders, dental caries, diabetes mellitus, and cardiovascular disease. However, with the exception of dental caries, current scientific data fail to confirm that sugar per se directly causes any of these health problems.[2,3]

Much of the sugar we consume is hidden—that is, sugar is a principal product in a large number of food items we may overlook. Foods such as ketchup, salad dressings, cured meat products, and canned vegetables and fruit frequently contain much hidden sugar. After sugar and salt, corn syrup is the third most common food additive.[4] Corn syrup is a very concentrated sucrose solution.

Polysaccharides are carbohydrates that are composed of long chains of saccharide units. These long chains are better known as *starches*. However, these starches should not be confused with the adjective *starchy*. When people refer to starchy foods, they usually are referring to bland, bread-filled, or greasy foods. True starches are among the most important sources for dietary carbohydrates. Starches are found primarily in vegetables, fruit, and grains. Ingestion of these true starches helps us receive much overall nutritional benefit, since most starch sources also contain significant portions of vitamins, minerals, protein, water, and fiber. Starches are nutritional "good guys."

Polysaccharides, like disaccharides, must also be converted to separate glucose units before being used by the body.

Fats

Fats (lipids) are an important nutrient in our diets. Fats provide a concentrated form of energy (9 Calories per gram consumed) and help give our foods high *satiety value*. The fat in our foods helps to give our foods its pleasing taste, or *palatability*. Fats also serve as carriers of fat-soluble vitamins A, D, E, and K. Without fat, these vitamins would quickly pass through the body. Body tissues formed in part from fat help us retain heat.

The visible fats in our diet account for only about 40% of the fats we consume. Visible fats include margarine, butter, salad oil, and layers of fat in meat. The remaining 60% of our dietary intake of fat comes from the fat that is marbled throughout meat fibers, and from milk products, eggs, nuts, oil and grain cereals.[4] Nutritionists recommend that only 30% of our caloric intake come from fat.

Fats are composed of groupings of *glycerol* and *fatty acid* molecules. Biochem-

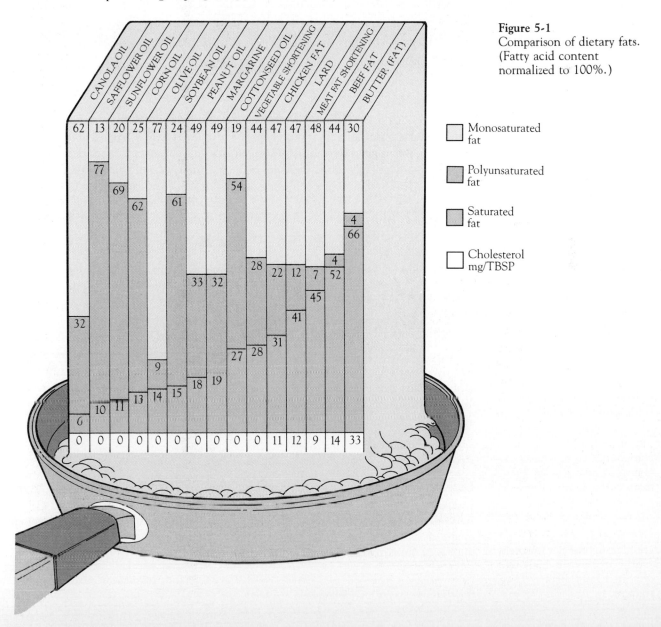

Figure 5-1
Comparison of dietary fats.
(Fatty acid content
normalized to 100%.)

Low-Calorie Fat Substitute

In early 1988, the Nutrasweet Company announced the development of a low-calorie fat substitute called Simplesse. By using high-protein sources such as egg whites and milk, food technologists were able to restructure the configurations of protein particles to resemble fat substances. This new product contains no cholesterol and has 80% fewer calories than fat. Because it becomes unstable in heat, Simplesse is expected to be used in foods such as ice cream, salad dressing, cheese spreads, and yogurt. At the time of this writing, Simplesse was awaiting possible approval by the Food and Drug Administration.

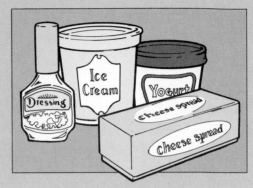

saturated fats
fats made up of compounds in which no further hydrogen bonding can occur; these are fats in solid form at room temperature; primarily animal fats.

triglycerides
fats made up of glycerol units each having three fatty acid molecules.

cholesterol
fat-related substance in alcohol form; lipid material manufactured within the body as well as derived through dietary sources.

proteins
compounds composed of chains of amino acids; primary components of muscle and connective tissue.

amino acids
chief components of protein; synthesized by the body or obtained from dietary sources.

ically fats are further classified according to their affinity for *hydrogen bonding*. **Saturated fats** are derived primarily from animal sources, *monounsaturated fats* are derived from peanuts and olive oils, and *polyunsaturated fats* are derived from vegetable sources—corn oil, safflower oil, and sunflower oil. Saturated fats, such as milk and meat fats, butter, and egg fats, have been critically accused of promoting a wide variety of cardiovascular diseases. Fortunately, the replacement of saturated fats with monounsaturated and polyunsaturated fats lowers blood cholesterol levels and the risk of cardiovascular disease. Figure 5-1 gives a comparison of dietary fats.

High blood levels of **triglycerides** and **cholesterol** (a fat-related substance in alcohol form) have also been reported to be risk factors in the development of cardiovascular disease (see Chapter 10). Cholesterol is a necessary constituent of all animal tissue and is synthesized by our own bodies from carbohydrate and fat sources. Some evidence suggests that increased intake of saturated fats may increase triglyceride and serum (blood) cholesterol levels. However, after extensive investigation, the relationship between the intake of dietary cholesterol and serum cholesterol levels remains unclear.[4,5] High-cholesterol foods include whole milk, shellfish, nuts, animal fat, and egg yolk. Acceptable fat substitutes may be available in the future (see the box above).

Proteins

Derived from a word meaning "first importance," **proteins** are found in every living cell. Proteins are composed of chains of **amino acids.** Of the 20 recognized naturally occurring amino acids, the body can synthesize all but nine *essential amino acids** from the foods we eat.[4] A food that contains all nine essential amino acids is called a *complete protein* food. Sources of complete protein are

*Eight additional compounds are sometimes classified as amino acids; thus some nutritionists consider that there are more than 20 amino acids.

animal products, including milk, meat, cheese, and eggs. A food source that does not contain all nine essential amino acids is called an *incomplete protein* food. Vegetables, grains, and *legumes* (peas or beans—including chickpeas, butter beans, soybean curd [tofu], and peanuts) are principal sources of incomplete protein.

Fortunately, one can combine various sources of incomplete protein to achieve appropriate complete protein intake. Many of us do this already when we combine peanut butter and bread, milk and cereal, and macaroni and cheese.

Protein serves primarily to promote growth and maintenance of body tissue. However, protein is also a primary component of enzyme and hormone structure, helps in maintaining the *acid-base balance* of our bodies, and serves as a source of energy (4 Calories per gram consumed). Nutritionists recommend that 12% of our caloric intake be from protein. Malnutrition in the world's under-developed countries is often seen in the protein deficiency disease called *kwashiorkor*. This disease is rarely seen in countries that have is an abundant supply of protein.

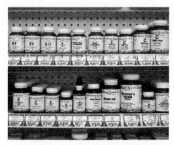

The vitamin industry thrives.

Vitamins

Vitamins are organic compounds that are required in small amounts for normal growth, reproduction, and maintenance of health. Vitamins differ from carbohydrates, fats, and proteins because they do not provide Calories or serve as structural elements for our bodies. Vitamins serve as *coenzymes*. By facilitating the action of *enzymes*, vitamins help initiate a wide variety of bodily responses, including energy production, utilization of minerals, and growth of healthy tissue. (See Table 5-1 for a listing of vitamin functions.)

Discovered just after the turn of the twentieth century, vitamins can be classified as *water soluble* (capable of being dissolved in water) or *fat soluble* (capable of being dissolved in fat or lipid tissue). Water-soluble vitamins include the B-complex vitamins and vitamin C. Most of the excess intake of these water-soluble vitamins will be eliminated from the body during urination. The fat-soluble vitamins are A, D, E, and K. Excessive intake of these vitamins is stored in the body in the adipose tissue or fat. It is therefore possible to consume and retain too many of these vitamins, particularly A and D. The resultant toxic condition is called **hypervitaminosis.**[4] Interestingly, hypervitaminosis seems to initiate body responses similar to those seen in people who consume too little of a fat soluble vitamin category. (See Table 5-1 for general properties of fat-soluble and water-soluble vitamins.)

Since water soluble vitamins dissolve rather quickly in water, you should be cautious in the preparation of fresh fruits and vegetables. One precaution is not to overcook fresh vegetables. The longer fresh vegetables are steamed or boiled, the more water-soluble vitamins will be lost. Even soaking sliced fresh fruit or vegetables can result in the loss of vitamin C and B-complex. You may wish to drink (or use in baking) any water in which fresh vegetables were boiled or steamed.

To ensure an adequate vitamin intake, do not rely on bottled vitamins sold in grocery stores or health food stores. The best way is really the simplest and least expensive way: just eat a variety of foods. Unless there are special circumstances, such as pregnancy, infancy, or an existing health problem, virtually everyone in our society who eats a reasonably well-rounded diet consumes appropriate levels of all vitamins.

vitamins
organic compounds that facilitate the action of enzymes.

hypervitaminosis
excessive accumulation of vitamins within the body, associated with the fat-soluble vitamins.

Table 5-1　The Major Vitamins

Vitamins	Physiological Benefits	Food Sources
Fat-soluble		
A	Night vision; growth of epithelial cells; mucus gland secretion; bone growth; sperm production; estrogen synthesis	Liver, eggs, cheese, milk; yellow, orange, and dark-green vegetables; carrots, broccoli, spinach, cantaloupe
D	Calcium and phosphorus absorption; bone growth; neuromuscular activity; kidney resorption of calcium and phosphorus	Fortified milk; egg yolk; fish-liver oil, tuna; sunlight stimulates the body's production of the vitamin
E	Antioxidation of unsaturated fatty acids and tissue lipids; vitamin A absorption; heme synthesis for red blood cell function	Vegetable oils; wheat germ, whole-grain cereal; liver; leafy green vegetables
K	Synthesis of blood clotting factors in the liver	Dark-green leafy vegetables, cabbage, cauliflower, tomatoes; liver; eggs; produced by intestinal flora
Water-soluble		
Thiamin (B_1)	Glucose metabolism; nervous system synaptic functioning	Enriched bread, enriched cereals; pork products, kidney; peas; pecans
Riboflavin (B_2)	Energy release from glucose and fatty acids; growth through cell proliferation; adrenal cortical activity; red blood cell formation; synthesis of glycogen	Liver, beef heart; yogurt, milk, cheese; broccoli, asparagus; almonds; produced by intestinal flora
Niacin (B_3)	Energy release from all nutrient forms; protein and fat synthesis	Liver, meat, poultry; peanut butter
Pyridoxine (B_6)	Protein metabolism; synthesis and breakdown of amino acids; neurotransmitter synthesis; hemoglobin synthesis; antibody production; lipid metabolism; carbohydrate metabolism; fetal nervous system function	Chicken, fish; whole-grain cereal; egg yolk; bananas, avocados
Cobalamin (B_{12})	Growth and function of the nervous system; red blood cell formation; metabolism of folic acid	Liver, kidneys, meats; eggs; dairy products
Folacin (folic acid)	DNA synthesis required in rapid cell division; red blood cell formation; fetal development	Oranges and orange juice; bread; asparagus, broccoli, lima beans, spinach; meat, fish, poultry, eggs
Ascorbic acid (C)	Collagen formation and formation of ground substance; maintenance of scar tissue; tooth development; neurotransmitter synthesis; absorption of iron and calcium; folic acid formation; additional functions have been suggested	Liver; peppers, broccoli, cauliflower, kale, lemons, strawberries, papayas, asparagus, spinach

*International Units.

Deficiency	Recommended Daily Allowance	Megadose Toxicity (10 × RDA)
Night blindness, corneal deterioration; respiratory infections; skin changes; diarrhea; enamel alteration	5000 IU*	Headache, drowsiness; nausea; loss of hair, dry skin, scaly dermititis; anorexia; amenorrhea; bone resorption, skeletal pain (children)
Rickets, osteomalacia, osteoporosis; tooth malformation	400 IU	Retarded linear growth; failure-to-thrive syndrome; anorexia, nausea, weight loss
Deficiency rarely seen in humans; destruction of cell membrane of red blood cells	30 IU	Reduced vitamin A storage; gastrointestinal disturbances; the use of high levels of vitamin E is not encouraged
Prolonged coagulation time, hemorrhage, bruising	Not established	Seen in infants only in conjunction with an overadministration of vitamin K at the time of birth
Anorexia; nausea; constipation; depression, mood swings, fatigue, irritability; gait changes, nystagmus (rapid eye movement); decreased work output; loss of hand-eye coordination; beriberi	1.5 mg	Not thought to be harmful to humans; excreted because of its water-soluble nature
Personality shifts, hypochondriasis, depression; cracks in corner of mouth and on lips, purplish-red color to tongue; dry skin; possible adverse effects on fetal development	1.7 mg	No evidence in humans
Pellagra-dermititis; diarrhea; depression, irritability, headaches, sleeplessness, personality disorientation; death	20 mg	Flushed skin, gastrointestinal distress, glucose intolerance when taken in extremely high dosage
No known deficiency in adults; decreased niacin production; poor growth; convulsions; anemia; decreased antibody formation; skin lesions	2 mg	Not observed in humans
Pernicious anemia; not caused however, by inadequate dietary B_{12}, but by a lack of an intrinsic factor influencing absorption	0.6 μg	Although often used in large amounts as a supplement, toxicity is rarely reported
Chronic alcohol use leads to inadequate absorption; toxemia of pregnancy; infections; rheumatoid arthritis; megaloblastic anemia	0.4 mg	No toxic effect noted
Scurvy; listlessness, fatigue, shortness of breath, muscle cramps, skeletal pain; anorexia; dry skin; hemorrhage of gums, pinpoint skin hemorrhage; depressed glucose tolerance; personality disorders	60 mg	Kidney stones; neonatal dependency when mother had taken megadose during pregnancy; destruction of vitamin B_{12}; increased plasma cholesterol; red blood cell destruction; gastrointestinal upset

Claims and Questions About Food Supplements

Some people choose to use one or more of the food supplements shown in conjunction with their regular diet to obtain additional benefits. However, current research questions the need for supplements and indicates there may be potential for harm in over-supplementation. Before using a food supplement, consider these questions: How valid are the claims made? Will use of these supplements really balance inadequate food intake?

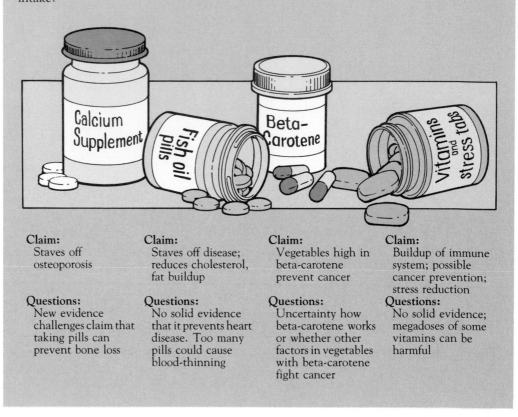

Claim:
Staves off
osteoporosis

Questions:
New evidence
challenges claim that
taking pills can
prevent bone loss

Claim:
Staves off disease;
reduces cholesterol,
fat buildup

Questions:
No solid evidence
that it prevents heart
disease. Too many
pills could cause
blood-thinning

Claim:
Vegetables high in
beta-carotene
prevent cancer

Questions:
Uncertainty how
beta-carotene works
or whether other
factors in vegetables
with beta-carotene
fight cancer

Claim:
Buildup of immune
system; possible
cancer prevention;
stress reduction

Questions:
No solid evidence;
megadoses of some
vitamins can be
harmful

Unfortunately many consumers are duped into believing that this is not possible; thus the over-the-counter vitamin industry has made millions of dollars on the gullibility of the average citizen. One recent source reported that 37% of all adult Americans take vitamin supplements in inappropriately large doses. The extravagant claims made for vitamins C and E as cures for the common cold and sexual lethargy have not been supported by scientific consensus. Furthermore, the claim that natural vitamins are superior to synthetic (laboratory produced) vitamins cannot be scientifically supported.

Minerals

Nearly 5% of our body is composed of inorganic ash materials, or *minerals.* Minerals function primarily as structural elements (seen in teeth, muscles, hemoglobin, and hormones.) They are also critical in the regulation of a number of body processes, including cell membrane permeability, muscle contraction, blood clotting, protein synthesis, and red blood cell synthesis. Approximately 21 mineral

Table 5-2   Minerals and Their Roles—Micronutrients

Micronutrient	Physiological Benefits	Food Sources	Recommended Daily Allowance
Iron	Oxygen and carbon dioxide transport; red blood cell formation; vitamin A synthesis; removal of lipids from blood; collagen synthesis; antibody production	Liver, spinach, asparagus, clams, beans, peas, greens, enriched bread and cereal	18 mg
Zinc	Enzyme formation; DNA/RNA synthesis; acid-base balance; hydrochloric acid production; collagen production; fetal development; wound healing; enhanced appetite and taste	Seafood, meats, whole-grain bread, whole wheat, cashew nuts	15 mg
Selenium	Antioxidation; energy release; heart muscle function	Organ meats, meats, cereal, milk, dairy products, fruits; plant sources depend on soil concentrations	Not established
Manganese	Skeletal development; connective tissue formation; cholesterol synthesis; urea formation; energy release	Whole-grain cereal, greens, vegetables, tea	Not established
Copper	Enzyme formation; hemoglobin synthesis; myelin sheath development; energy release; protein synthesis; cholesterol synthesis	Liver, oysters, nuts, cocoa, cherries, mushrooms, whole-grain cereal	2 mg
Iodine	Cell metabolism; synthesis of vitamin A, protein, thyroxine, and cholesterol	Drinking water (dependent on location), spinach, lobster, shrimp, oysters, dairy products, iodized salt	150 μg
Molybdenum	Enzyme formation, prevention of dental caries	Peas, beans, meats	Not established
Cobalt	Component of vitamin B_{12}; prevention of pernicious anemia; enzyme formation	Liver, kidney, oysters, beef, poultry, milk	Not established
Chromium	Utilization of glucose; lipid metabolism	Vegetables (dependent on soil type), whole-grain cereals, meat products, cheese	Not established
Fluoride	Prevention of dental caries and periodontal disease; skeletal stability; prevention of osteoporosis	Water supply, tea, mackerel, salmon, rice, spinach, soybeans	Not established
Silicon	Growth, calcification of bone, formation of connective tissue	Unrefined cereals, beer	Not established
Vanadium	Prevention of dental caries; potential role in iron and lipid metabolism, bone development	No specific source	Not established
Nickel	DNA/RNA synthesis	Cereal grains, fruits, vegetables	Not established

Table 5-3   Minerals and Their Roles—Macronutrients

Macronutrient	Physiological Benefits	Food Sources
Calcium	Bone ossification; tooth formation; general body growth; cell membrane maintenance; neuromuscular function; regulation of strontium uptake	Milk, milk products, cheddar cheese; turnip greens, collards, broccoli; soy products; shellfish; molasses
Phosphorus	Bone and tooth development; energy release (ADP/ATP); fat transport (phospholipids); synthesis of enzymes and proteins; DNA/RNA synthesis; acid-base balance	Meat, fish, poultry; eggs; cereal products; cheddar cheese; peanuts; carbonated soft drinks
Potassium	Energy release; protein synthesis; fluid balance; acid-base balance; nerve transmission	Avocados, apricots, cantaloupe; lima beans; potatoes; bananas; liver; milk; peanut butter
Sulfur	Metabolism; blood clotting; detoxification of body fluids; collagen synthesis	Protein foods
Sodium	Formation of digestive secretions; nerve transmission; acid-base balance	Olives; bacon; sauerkraut; processed cheese; table salt
Chloride	Acid-base balance; acidity of stomach content; carbon dioxide transport	Table salt
Magnesium	Energy production; carbohydrate, lipid, protein metabolism; protein synthesis; nerve transmission; tooth enamel stability	Green leafy vegetables; cocoa; nuts; soybeans; whole grain; molasses; clams; spinach

elements have been recognized as being essential minerals for human health.[6]

Macronutrient elements are those that are seen in relatively high amounts in our body tissues. Examples of macronutrients are calcium, phosphorus, sulfur, sodium, potassium, and magnesium. Examples of *micronutrient elements,* those seen in relatively small amounts in body tissues, include zinc, iron, copper, selenium, and iodine. Although micronutrient elements **(trace elements)** are required only in small quantities, they are still essential for good health. (See Tables 5-2 and 5-3 for listings of minerals and their functions.) As with vitamins, the safest, most appropriate way in which to receive a sufficient amount of all necessary minerals is to eat a balanced diet.

trace elements
minerals whose presence in the body occurs in very small amounts; micronutrient elements.

Water

Water may well be our most essential nutrient element, since without water most of us would die from **dehydration** effects in less than a week. We could survive for weeks and even years without some of the essential minerals and vitamins. Over half our body weight comes from water. Water provides the medium for nutrient and waste transport and plays a key role in nearly all of our body's biochemical reactions.

dehydration
abnormal depletion of fluids from the body; severe dehydration can lead to death.

Deficiency	Recommended Daily Allowance	Megadose Toxicity (10 × RDA)
Although not the result of a deficiency, osteoporosis is caused by calcium resorption; osteomalacia; tetany	1 g	No toxic effect established
Fatigue, anorexia; demineralization of bone seen in persons taking high levels of antacids	1 g	No toxic effect established
Muscle weakness; abdominal bloating; heart abnormalities; respiratory distress; deficiency most often seen in infants with vomiting and diarrhea	Not established	Hyperkalemia seen in some elderly with impaired kidney function
Sulfur deficiency is not clearly established	Not established	No toxic effect established
Very unlikely to occur; vomiting in children or profuse sweating could reduce sodium	Not established	Unlikely to occur; large dietary intake would enhance hypertension; megadose could be lethal
Unlikely dietary deficiency; loss as a result of vomiting	Not established	No toxic effect established
Difficult to determine; irritability, nervousness, convulsions; vasodilation; skin changes; deficiency related to vomiting rather than dietary inadequacy	400 mg	Coma; heart failure at extremely high levels

Most people seldom think about the importance of an adequate daily intake of water. Adults require about 6 glasses a day, depending on their exercise levels and environment. People who drink beverages that tend to dehydrate the body (tea, coffee, and alcohol) should increase their water consumption. Borderline dehydration can be seen in persons who fail to drink water in adequate amounts. Strained, uncomfortable bowel movements may be caused by this inadequate daily intake of water.

Interestingly, the average American drinks more soft drinks in a year than water. In 1986, each American drank an average of 42.1 gallons of soft drinks compared to 41.2 gallons of water. One syndicated columnist has speculated that the mesmerizing advertising campaigns have encouraged this movement toward soft drink consumption and away from water consumption.[7]

Fiber

Although not considered a nutrient by definition, *fiber* is an important nonnutritive food element. Fiber consists of plant materials that are not digested and thus move through the large intestine unchanged. Most of our dietary fiber comes from *cellulose*, the indigestible portion of vegetables, fruits, and cereals.

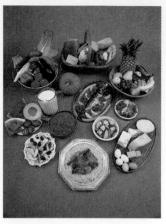

A variety of foods make up the four food groups.

Fiber has the ability to attract water and swell within the large intestine—thus producing larger, softer stools. Transit time through the large intestine is reduced in those persons who increase their fiber consumption. Because of this, fiber consumption has been linked to a reduction of colon cancer.

Aside from more comfortable bowel movements, fiber has recently been thought to play a role in reduction of the occurrence of many diseases. Can fiber really prevent such diseases as atherosclerosis, diabetes, cancer of the colon, or hemorrhoids? Probably not directly. However, a fiber-enriched diet might reduce the risk of colon cancer in some people.[8] Fiber can help those suffering from diverticular disease (an inflammation of the outpouchings of the colon) and chronic constipation.[9] Fiber consumption can be increased by eating more fresh fruits and vegetables, whole-grain cereals, and bran products.

THE FOUR FOOD GROUPS

As we mentioned, the best way to achieve adequate amounts of nutrients is to eat a *balanced diet;* that is, to eat a diet that includes selections from several food groups (see Table 5-4). Until the early 1950s nutritionists recommended selections from seven food groups. Now the recommendations designate only four food groups: milk, protein-rich foods, fruits and vegetables, and breads and cereals. Our discussion will highlight the nutritional benefit of each group and will identify the recommended daily adult serving minimums.

Milk and Milk Products

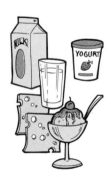

The milk group contributes two primary nutritional benefits—high-quality protein and calcium (required for bone and teeth development). Foods included in this group are whole milk, low-fat milk, skim milk, dried milk, yogurt, cheeses, and ice cream. The adult recommendation is 2 cups of milk or two equivalent servings from this group each day. For teenagers the recommendation is 4 cups of milk each day.

Because of the general concern over saturated fat, cholesterol, and additional calories, low-fat milk products are recommended in place of high-fat milk products. Both low-fat and high-fat dairy products provide similar nutritional benefits (see Table 5-5).

Protein-Rich Foods

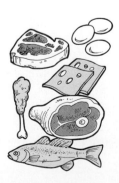

Our need for daily selections from the protein rich group is based on our daily need for protein, iron, and the B vitamins. Meats include all red meats (beef, pork, and game), fish, and poultry. Meat substitutes include eggs, cheese, dried peas and beans (legumes), and peanut butter. The current recommendation for adults is 4 ounces total per day, preferably in two or more servings. If you select a food that fits into both the meat and the milk categories, be careful not to include that food in both of your categories for that particular day.

The fat content of meat varies considerably. Some forms of meat yield only 1% fat, whereas others may be as high as 40% fat. Poultry and fish are generally significantly lower in overall fat than are red meats. Interestingly, the higher the grade of red meats, the more fat will be marbled throughout the muscle fiber and the higher will be its caloric value. Most of us prefer high-grade steaks because they appear to be more lean, yet just the opposite is true. Indeed, the higher grade steak usually tastes better, but that is because of the presence of a higher fat content.

Meats are generally excellent sources of iron. Iron is present in much greater amounts in red meats and organ meats (liver, kidney, and heart) than in poultry and fish.

Fruits and Vegetables

Four daily servings from the fruit and vegetable group are recommended for an adult. The important function of this group is providing vitamin A, vitamin C, and fiber in our diets. The American Cancer Society indicates that this food group may play an important role in the prevention of certain forms of cancer. Included foods are citrus fruits, dark green vegetables, yellow and orange vegetables, fruit juices, canned or cooked vegetables, and tossed salads. At least one serving high in vitamin C should be eaten daily, and at least one serving of a dark green, yellow, or orange vegetable containing fat-soluble vitamin A should be consumed every other day.

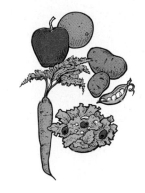

Breads and Cereals

The nutritional benefit from this group lies in its contribution of B-complex vitamins and energy (in the form of calories) to our diet. Some nutritionists believe that the use of foods from this group promotes protein intake, since many foods in this group are prepared with complete-protein foods: macaroni and cheese, cereal and milk, and bread and meat sandwiches.

enriched
the result of the process of returning to foods some of the nutritional elements (B vitamins and iron) removed during processing.

Four daily servings of any **enriched** or whole-grain bread or cereal are recommended. Milling of cereal grains into flour tends to deplete the flour of important nutrients, including fiber, vitamin B_6, vitamin E, magnesium, and various trace elements. The process of enrichment returns only four of these nutrients: thiamin, niacin, riboflavin (all B vitamins), and the mineral iron.

Fortunately, *whole-grain flour* is a healthy alternative for most consumers, since few, if any, nutrients are lost in the milling process. The *cereal germ*, the fiber, and additional nutrients are not destroyed.

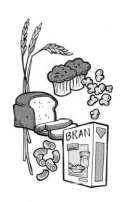

Foods in the breads and cereals group include noodles, rice, spaghetti, pancakes, tortillas, muffins, popcorn, cooked cereal, and boxed breakfast cereals.

Without *garnishes*, if a person selects the minimum adult recommendations from the four food groups, the total number of Calories equals only about 1,200. This low caloric total would not be enough for most of us to survive for very long. Of course, we add much more to our diets. We add gravies, margarine, drinks, salad dressings, desserts, and many other items to our daily intake. The 1,200-Calorie estimate refers to the "no-frill, no-garnish" daily minimum recommendations.

Junk Foods: A Fifth Category?

Where do such items as colas, cookies, corn chips, and pastries fit in? Most do not fit into any food group. Most just provide additional calories (generally from sucrose) and significant amounts of salt and fats. It is not surprising that these foods are collectively called *junk foods*. Of course, if the cookies are made from

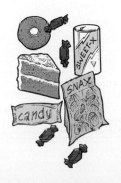

Table 5-4　Recommended Dietary Allowances

Nutrient	Men				Women					
	15-18	19-22	23-50	50+	15-18	19-22	23-50	50+	Pregnant	Lactating
Recommended dietary allowances, 1980										
Energy (kcal)*	2800	2900	2700	2400	2100	2100	2000	1800	+300	+500
Protein (g)	56	56	56	56	46	44	44	44	+30	+20
Vitamin A (RE)	1000	1000	1000	1000	800	800	800	800	+200	+400
(IU)†	(5000)	(5000)	(5000)	(5000)	(4000)	(4000)	(4000)	(4000)	(+1000)	(+2000)
Vitamin D (μg)	10	7.5	5	5	10	7.5	5	5	+5	+5
Vitamin E (mg)	10	10	10	10	8	8	8	8	+2	+3
Vitamin C (mg)	60	60	60	60	60	60	60	60	+20	+40
Thiamine (mg)	1.4	1.5	1.4	1.2	1.1	1.1	1.0	1.0	+0.4	+0.5
Riboflavin (mg)	1.7	1.7	1.6	1.4	1.3	1.3	1.2	1.2	+0.3	+0.5
Niacin (mg)	18	19	18	16	14	14	13	13	+2	+5
Vitamin B_6 (mg)	2.0	2.2	2.2	2.2	2	2	2	2	+0.6	+0.5
Folacin (μg)	400	400	400	400	400	400	400	400	+400	+100
Vitamin B_{12} (μg)	3	3	3	3	3	3	3	3	+1	+1
Calcium (mg)	1200	800	800	800	1200	800	800	800	+400	+400
Phosphorus (mg)	1200	800	800	800	1200	800	800	800	+400	+400
Magnesium (mg)	400	350	350	350	300	300	300	300	+150	+150
Iron (mg)‡	18	10	10	10	18	18	18	10	‡	‡
Zinc (mg)	15	15	15	15	15	15	15	15	+5	+10
Iodine (μg)	150	150	150	150	150	150	150	150	+25	+50

Estimated safe and adequate daily dietary intakes, Food and Nutrition Board

Vitamin K (μg)	50-100
Biotin (μg)	100-200
Pantothenic acid (mg)	4-7
Copper (mg)	2-3
Manganese (mg)	2.5-5
Fluoride (mg)	1.5-2.5
Chromium (mg)	0.05-0.2
Selenium (mg)	0.05-0.2
Molybdenum (mg)	0.15-0.5
Sodium (mg)	900-2700
Potassium (mg)	1525-4575
Chloride (mg)	1400-4200

*Energy recommendations represent average approximate needs; actual energy needs will vary depending on degree of physical activity.
†RE, retinol equivalent; until recently, vitamin A content in foods has been expressed as international units (IU), 1 IU being equivalent to 0.3 μg of retinol or 0.6 μg β-carotene. For the purposes of this discussion the conversion factor of 1 RE = 5 IU will be used.
‡The increased requirement during pregnancy cannot be met by the iron content of habitual American diets nor by the existing iron stores of many women; therefore the use of 30 to 60 mg of supplement iron is recommended. Iron needs during lactation are not substantially different from those of nonpregnant women, but continued supplementation of the mother for 2 to 3 months after parturition is advisable to replenish stores depleted by pregnancy.

high-quality flour and contain raisins and nuts, you can receive nutritional benefit from consuming such goodies. (See Nutrient Density on p. 126.)

Understandably the processed-food industry encourages this sweet-tooth approach to eating. Many vending machines are filled with relatively expensive junk foods. Indeed, advertising for nonnutritious food overwhelmingly exceeds advertising for nutritious foods. Although it is difficult to recall a television commercial for lettuce, broccoli, or green beans, we can all recall advertisements for

Table 5-5   A Nutritional Comparison of Familiar Dairy Products

Product	Calories	Carbohydrate (g)	Fat (g)	Saturated Fat (g)	Cholesterol (mg)	Protein (g)	Calcium (mg)
Milk							
Whole (3.3%) 1 cup	150	11	8	5.1	33	8	291
Lowfat (2%) 1 cup	120	12	5	2.9	18	8	297
Lowfat (1%) 1 cup	100	12	3	1.6	10	8	300
Nonfat (skim) 1 cup	85	12	Trace	0.3	4	8	302
Buttermilk 1 cup	100	12	2	1.3	9	8	285
Dried 1 cup	245	35	Trace	0.3	12	24	837
Milk beverages							
Chocolate milk (3.3%) 1 cup	210	26	8	5.3	31	8	280
Chocolate flavored 6 oz water + 1 oz powdered milk	100	22	1	0.6	1	3	90
Milk desserts							
Ice cream (11%) 1 cup	270	32	14	8.9	59	5	176
Ice milk (4%) 1 cup	185	29	6	3.5	18	5	176
Sherbet (2%) 1 cup	270	59	4	2.4	14	2	103
Yogurt							
Whole milk, plain 8 oz container	140	11	7	4.8	29	8	274
No fat plain 8 oz container	125	16	Trace	0.3	4	13	452
Lowfat fruit flavored 8 oz container	230	43	2	1.6	10	10	345
Cream							
Half and half							
1 cup	315	10	28	17.3	89	7	254
1 TBSP	20	1	2	1.1	6	Trace	16
Sour cream							
1 cup	495	10	48	30	102	7	268
1 TBSP	25	1	3	1.6	5	Trace	14

our favorite soft drink, breakfast snack, or candy bar. It takes a lot of willpower to say no to junk foods.

Fast Foods

Fast foods are convenience foods usually prepared in walk-in or drive-through restaurants. In contrast to junk foods, the nutritional value of fast foods can vary considerably (see the box below). Once billed as "hamburger joints," fast food restaurants have broadened their menus to include whole-wheat breads, salad bars, low-fat meat and milk products, and low-calorie foods. Many of the large fast food restaurants provide nutritional information for consumers. Unlike junk foods, fast foods may be reasonably nutritious, but to rely on these foods as one's primary source of nutrition would be both unwise and expensive.

Facts About Fast Foods

Are you stopping at a fast food restaurant today? Consider these points before you do: (1) Will this be an extra meal, or have I planned for it as a part of my food intake for the day? (2) Can fast foods be part of a balanced diet? (3) Do I realize how calorie-dense this meal will be? If you answer yes to these questions, then you are practicing responsible, healthful nutrition planning.

Food	Calories	Protein (g)	Carbohydrate (g)	Fat (g)	Cholesterol (mg)	Sodium (mg)
HAMBURGERS						
McDonald's hamburger	263	12.4	28.3	11.3	29.1	506
Dairy Queen single hamburger w/cheese	410	24	33	20	50	790
Hardee's 1/4 pound cheeseburger	506	28	41	26	61	1950
Wendy's double hamburger, white bun	560	41	24	34	125	575
McDonald's Big Mac	570	24.6	39.2	35	83	979
Burger King Whopper sandwich	640	27	42	41	94	842
Jack in the Box Jumbo Jack	485	26	38	26	64	905
CHICKEN						
Arby's chicken breast sandwich	592	28	56	27	57	1340
Burger King chicken sandwich	688	26	56	40	82	1423
Dairy Queen chicken sandwich	670	29	46	41	75	870
Church's Crispy Nuggets (one; regular)	55	3	4	3	—	125
Kentucky Fried Chicken Nuggets (one)	46	2.82	2.2	2.88	11.9	140
FISH						
Church's Southern fried catfish	67	4	4	4	—	151
Long John Silver's Fish & More	978	34	82	58	88	2124
McDonald's Filet-O-Fish	435	14.7	35.9	25.7	45.2	799
OTHERS						
Hardee's hot dog	346	11	26	22	42	744
Jack in the Box taco	191	8	16	11	21	406

FOOD EXCHANGE CATEGORIES

The American Dietetic Association has recently developed a food classification system designed to aid persons who wish to control the caloric and fat content of their diets. This food exchange list is available from the ADA.* By selecting the appropriate types and amounts of foods from each of the following six categories of food, people will achieve nutritional balance and better control of fat and Calorie intake. Sample menus for eating out or at home can be found in the box on p. 116-117.

*To receive a food exchange list, send $2.00 to The American Dietetic Association, 430 N. Michigan Ave., Chicago, IL 60611.

Food	Calories	Protein (g)	Carbohydrate (g)	Fat (g)	Cholesterol (mg)	Sodium (mg)
OTHERS—cont'd						
Zantigo taco	198	10.4	12.8	11.7	30.5	318
Arby's roast beef (regular)	350	22	32	15	39	590
Hardee's roast beef sandwich	377	21	36	17	57	1030
FRENCH FRIES						
Arby's french fries	211	2	33	8	6	30
McDonald's french fries (regular)	220	3	26.1	11.5	8.6	109
Wendy's french fries (regular)	280	40	35	14	15	95
SHAKES						
Dairy Queen	710	14	120	19	50	260
McDonald's						
Vanilla	352	9.3	59.6	8.4	30.6	201
Chocolate	383	9.9	65.5	9	29.7	300
Strawberry	362	9	62.1	8.7	32.2	207
SOFT DRINKS						
Coca-Cola Classic	144	—	38	—	—	14
Coca-Cola	154	—	40	—	—	6
Diet Coke	0.9	—	0.3	—	—	16
Sprite	142	—	36	—	—	45
Tab	1	—	1	—	—	30
Diet Sprite	3	—	0	—	—	9

Fast foods can be a part of a balanced diet. However, you should remember that they do have limitations, including their low calcium content, low vitamin A and C levels, and high Calorie content. Plan carefully for your fast food intake, remembering to eat a wide variety of all foods from each of the basic four food groups.

Create Your Own Diet

Starches/bread	**Minimum four choices a day, 80 Calories each**
	Examples: ½ cup cooked cereal
	½ cup pasta
	⅓ cup rice
	1 small potato
	½ bagel
Lean meats and substitutes	**Minimum two to three choices a day, 150 to 225 Calories each**
	Examples: ½ cup cottage cheese
	1 small pork chop
	1 small hamburger
	3 oz lean roast beef
Vegetables	**Minimum two choices a day, 25 calories each**
	Examples: ½ cup almost any cooked or raw vegetable
Fruit	**Minimum two choices a day, 60 Calories each**
	Examples: ½ banana
	15 grapes
	½ cup fruit juice
	¼ cup dried fruit
Milk	**Minimum two skim milk choices a day, 90 Calories each**
	Examples: 1 cup of skim milk, 90 Calories
	8 oz plain low-fat yogurt, 120 Calories
Fat	**Minimum three choices a day, 45 Calories each**
	Examples: 1 tsp margarine
	2 tsp diet margarine
	1 TBSP salad dressing
	2 TBSP reduced-calorie dressing

The exact number of choices from each of the six categories is determined by the maximum number of Calories each day that a person wishes to consume. However, should the total Calorie intake be limited to only 1,200 to 1,300 Calories, weight loss could occur at a rate exceeding that considered desirable.

SAMPLE MENUS (1,500 CALORIES)

DINING OUT		AT HOME		
Food Exchange	**Menu**	**Food Exchange**	**Menu 1**	**Menu 2**
Breakfast		*Breakfast*		
2 starch/bread	1 bagel or English muffin	2 bread/starch	1 bagel	1 English muffin
1 fat	1 tsp margarine	½ meat	1 oz part– skim milk cheese	¼ cup cottage cheese
1 fruit	½ grapefruit			
1 milk	1 cup (8 oz) skim milk	1 fruit	15 grapes	1 orange

DINING OUT		AT HOME		
Food Exchange	**Menu**	**Food Exchange**	**Menu 1**	**Menu 2**
Lunch		*Lunch*		
2 starch/bread	Burger King regular cheeseburger	2 starch/bread	Sandwich: 2 slices rye bread	Pasta salad: 1 cup cooked pasta with 2 oz diced chicken,
1 meat		1 meat	½ cup tuna fish and	1 TSBP salad dressing, ¾ cup mixed
1 fat		1 fat	1 tsp mayonnaise	peas, chopped
1 vegetable	Salad (avoid olives, seeds, bacon bits), low-cal Italian dressing	1 vegetable	1 large carrot	green pepper and scallions
1 fruit	Small apple (from home)	1 fruit	1 apple	2 TBSP raisins (in salad or alone)
		1 milk	1 cup skim milk	1 cup skim milk
Dinner		*Dinner*		
3 starch/bread	Large baked potato Small dinner roll 3 oz Broiled salmon or other fish	2 starch/bread	1 large baked potato	1 small roll ½ cup mashed potatoes
		1 fat	2 TBSP sour cream	1 tsp margarine
2 vegetables	Steamed broccoli (no butter), or sliced tomato Small mixed green salad	1 meat	3 oz London broil	3 oz baked fish
2 fat	1 tsp margarine or 2 TBSP sour cream 1 TSBP reduced-calorie salad dressing	2 vegetables	½ cup broccoli ½ cup tomato juice	½ cup stewed tomatoes ½ cup green beans
1 fruit	⅓ cantaloupe or ⅛ honeydew melon	1 fruit	1 cup strawberries	¾ cup sliced peaches
1 milk	1 cup skim milk	*Snack*		
		1 milk	1 cup skim milk	1 cup low-fat yogurt
		1 fruit	½ banana (blend above two ingredients with an ice cube or two for low-cal shake)	¾ cup blueberries

To cut down to a 1,200 Calorie diet: From Menu 1, omit 1 slice of rye bread, small baked potato, one fruit, and sour cream. From Menu 2, leave out ½ cup pasta, roll (or mashed potatoes), 1 fruit and margarine.

TOTAL: 1,500 Calories: 189 g carbohydrate (51% of diet); 78 g protein (21%); 45 g fat (28%); 135 mg cholesterol; 2,000 mg sodium.

TOTAL: 1,500 Calories: 190 g carbohydrates (51% of diet); 80 g protein (21%); 45 g fat (28%). Menu 1: 140 mg cholesterol, 2,000 mg sodium. Menu 2: 125 mg cholesterol; 1,500 mg sodium.

FOOD ADDITIVES

food additives
chemical compounds that
are intentionally or unintentionally added to our food
supply.

The lament about the "good old days" is certainly applicable to our current food supply. Today many people believe that the food they consume is dangerously compromised by intentionally and unintentionally introduced **food additives.**

The presence of additives in the food supply is not a totally modern occurrence. Salt, spices, and the chemicals imparted during the smoke-curing of meats have altered our food supply since the dawn of recorded history. Additionally, naturally occurring *biological toxins* and the foreign materials once added to food by processors made yesterday's food far less than pure and natural. Because of extensive federal regulation, it is doubtful whether many of today's approximately 2,800 food additives pose a significant health threat.[5,10] What is clear, however, is that if we wish to live in an urban setting, work outside the home, insist on convenience, and escape the limitations imposed by the seasonal nature of many foods, we will likely have to accept the presence of a considerable number of food additives.

Today's food processors add chemical compounds to the food supply for several reasons that they believe that we, as consumers, support. Compounds are added to food that (1) maintain the nutritional value of the food, (2) maintain the food's freshness by preventing changes in its color, flavor, and texture, (3) contribute to the processing of the food by controlling its texture, acidity, and thickness, and (4) make the food more appealing to the consumer by enhancing its flavor and standardizing its color.[11] Market research apparently indicates that we consumers will continue to accept these alterations regardless of what we might say about our desire that they not occur.

The Food Additives Amendment (1958) and the Color Additive Amendments (1960) to the federal Food, Drug and Cosmetic Act (1938) require that new additives to the food supply must be safe for human consumption. The process through which the manufacturer must go to gain approval is lengthy and expensive. Even compounds that have long been considered to be "generally recognized as safe" by experts are now undergoing reevaluation through modern laboratory technology. It is to be hoped that all truly harmful additives will soon be identified and removed from the food supply.

CURRENT DIETARY PRACTICES

For nearly 10 years the Senate Select Committee on Nutrition and Human Needs, under the direction of Senator George McGovern, gathered data and expert testimony from nutritionists, physicians, and educators about the current dietary practices of the American public. Based on evidence presented to them in 1977, the McGovern Committee summarized the current dietary practices, established dietary goals, and suggested appropriate changes for our consumption of certain foods (see Figure 5-2). The Committee made the following recommendations[12]:

- Consume only the Calories you expend. Maintain an *ideal weight*. (See Chapter 6 for an expansion of this concept.)
- Increase overall carbohydrate intake from 46% to nearly 60% of our current caloric intake. Within the carbohydrate group, increase complex carbohydrates (starches) from 22% to 48% of our caloric intake. Reduce simple sugar consumption from 24% to 15% of our overall caloric intake.

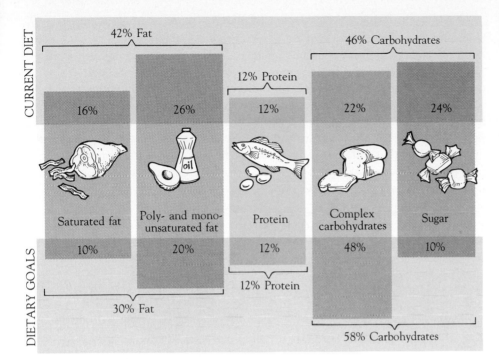

Figure 5-2
Where do your calories come from? The figure compares our present source of calories with the sources that were recommended by the U.S. Senate Select Committee on Nutrition and Human Needs. Can you identify the areas of recommended change?

- Reduce overall caloric fat intake from 42% of our diet to 30%. Reduce saturated fat from 16% to 10% of our caloric intake. Reduce polyunsaturated and monounsaturated fats from 26% to 20% of our caloric intake.
- Reduce cholesterol consumption to about 300 milligrams per day.
- Reduce sodium (salt) intake by about 85% to about 5 grams per day.

Since the McGovern Committee report was distributed in 1977, much controversy has risen about the recommendations. Some of the recommendations have received general approval, such as the suggestions to maintain an ideal weight and to reduce salt and sugar intake. However, criticism has been leveled at the recommendations concerning the reduction of saturated fat and dietary cholesterol. Some nutritionists and biochemists have also lamented the fact that the McGovern report neglected specific recommendations about obesity and alcohol use—two key factors affecting our nation's overall health.

Based on current knowledge, the American Dietetic Association published, through the U.S. Department of Health and Human Services and the U.S. Department of Agriculture, a slightly revised set of dietary recommendations— *Nutrition and Your Health: Dietary Guidelines for Americans*, second edition. The following recommendations are from these guidelines[13]:

- Eat a variety of foods.
- Maintain desirable weight.
- Avoid too much fat, saturated fat, and cholesterol.
- Eat foods with adequate starch and fiber.
- Avoid too much sugar.
- Avoid too much sodium.
- If you drink alcoholic beverages, do so in moderation.

These guidelines, although expressed in a rather simple form, represent our current understanding about the nutritional impact of our diet on the development of major health threats. These guidelines differ slightly from the McGovern Committee's recommendations by (1) tempering any irrational focus on saturated fats and cholesterol, (2) encouraging a varied diet that includes fiber, and (3) encouraging *moderate consumption* of alcohol in those who already drink alcoholic beverages. See Chapter 8 for a discussion on responsible alcohol use.

As a lifetime advocate for your own health, you must stay informed of any future changes in dietary recommendations generated by reputable institutions, professional associations, or government study committees. Although the ultimate influence that different foods have on the human body may never be completely understood, you owe it to yourself to examine your eating behaviors in light of generally accepted professional conclusions.

COLLEGIATE DIETARY PRACTICES

I figured that I had only $65 for the month's food so I decided to buy ground beef, bread, and KoolAid. I bought $50 worth of hamburger and froze it as patties, bought lots of day-old buns, and six large packages of KoolAid mix. Every day I fried a hamburger and drank a glass of KoolAid. After a week, I couldn't even look at a hamburger.

The above account was given to us by a student. We hope it represents an extremely atypical approach to collegiate dietary practices. Being a student, living in a residence hall, or attempting to balance college coursework with a job or family can compromise sound nutritional practices. Nutritionists have shared with us their concerns about some of the dietary practices observed among college students because they realize that dietary practices established during the college years may continue throughout life. Their recommendations are made with full knowledge that campus life does and will continue to force some compromises in the adoption of dietary patterns.

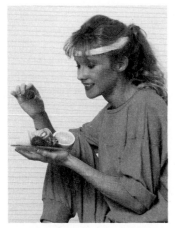

Fruit plays an important role in sound nutrition.

It is not uncommon for college students to pursue some form of nontraditional diet. Vegetarian diets, weight reduction diets, and over-reliance on *fast foods* represent some of these nontraditional diet approaches. Most nutritionists believe that these diets need not be discontinued or avoided, but they should be undertaken with care and with insight because of their nutritional limitations.

A *vegetarian diet* relies on plant sources for all or the vast majority of the nutrients needed by the body. Vegetarian diets encompass a continuum from diets that allow some animal sources of nutrients to those that not only exclude animal sources but are restrictive even in terms of the plant sources of nutrients permitted. We will briefly describe three vegetarian diets, beginning with the least restrictive in terms of food sources.

Ovolactovegetarian Diet

ovolactovegetarian diet
diet that excludes the use of all meat but does allow the consumption of eggs and dairy products.

Depending on the particular pattern of consuming eggs (*ova*) and milk (*lacto*) or using one but not the other, **ovolactovegetarianism** is an extremely sound approach to healthful eating during the entire course of the adult years. Ovolactovegetarian diets provide the body with the essential amino acids and limit the high intake of fats seen in more conventional diets. The exclusion of meat as a protein source lowers the total fat intake while the consumption of milk or eggs allows for an adequate amount of saturated fat to remain in the diet. The consistent use of vegetable products as the primary source of nutrients supports the current dietary recommendations for an increase in overall carbohydrates, an increase in complex carbohydrates, and an increase in fiber.

Meatlike products composed of *textured vegetable protein* are available in supermarkets. Nonmeat bacon strips, hamburger patties, and link sausage can be used by people who want to restrict their meat intake yet wish to plan menus with simulated meat to avoid a sense of deprivation. Soybeans are a primary source of this textured vegetable protein.

Two relatively minor concerns associated with some ovolactovegetarian diets are those of zinc deficiency and the overuse of a wide variety of **food supplements** (see the box on p. 106). Because of zinc's role in iron utilization, ovolactovegetarians may need to take this mineral in supplement form. The general use of large quantities of food supplements may be harmful or at best unnecessary.

food supplements
nutrients taken in addition to those obtained through the diet; powdered protein, vitamins, mineral extracts, etc.

Vegan Vegetarian Diet

A **vegan vegetarian diet** is one in which not only meat but also other animal products such as milk, cheese, and eggs are removed from the diet. When compared to the ovolactovegetarian diet, the vegan diet requires a higher level of nutritional understanding to avoid malnourishment.

vegan vegetarian diet
vegetarian diet that excludes the use of all animal products, including eggs and dairy products.

When plants represent the body's only source of nutrients, several possible difficulties can occur. The novice vegan will need to be particularly alert for these difficulties. One potential difficulty is that of obtaining all of the essential amino acids. Since a single plant source does not contain all the essential amino acids, the vegan dieter must learn to consistently employ a complementary diet. By carefully combining various grains, seeds, and legumes, amino acid deficiency can be prevented. This diet is not recommended for children, pregnant women, and **lactating** mothers.

lactating
breastfeeding, nursing.

In addition to the potential difficulty with amino acid deficiency, the vegan dieter could experience some difficulty in maintaining the necessary intake of vitamin B_{12}. Possible ramifications of inadequate B_{12} intake include depression, anemia, back pain, and menstrual irregularity. Vegan dieters often have difficulty maintaining adequate intakes of iron, zinc, and calcium.[4] Calcium intake must be monitored closely by the vegan dieter.

A final area of potential difficulty for the vegan dieter is that of an insufficient caloric intake because of the *satiation* resulting from the *voluminous* nature of the diet. Early satiation caused by a large amount of fiber may lower carbohydrate intake to the point that protein stores (muscle mass) are used for energy. The effects of this misuse of protein upon growth in children who follow a vegan diet should be given careful consideration by vegan parents.

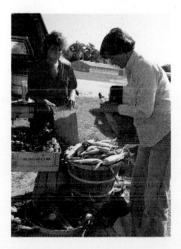

Because of its nutritional limitations, many nutritionists do not recommend the vegan vegetarian diet. Unless undertaken for reasons closely related to emotional, spiritual, or philosophical beliefs, the total exclusion of animal products seems to accomplish little from a nutritional-health point of view. Clearly, the ovolactovegetarian diet is much less likely to lead to malnutrition than is the vegan diet.

Personal Assessment

Seven-Day Diet Study

A primary requirement for good nutrition is a balanced diet. A variety of food selections from each food group forms the basis of this diet.

For a 7-day period, assign yourself the points indicated when each dietary requirement is met. Record your points in the appropriate column for each day. Total your daily and weekly points. Negative points for junk food consumption should be subtracted from your daily and weekly totals.

Food	Points	Maximum Score	Daily Score						
			M	T	W	T	F	S	S
Milk and Milk Products		30							
One cup of milk or equivalent	10								
Second cup of milk	10								
Third cup of milk	10								
Protein-Rich Foods		25							
One serving of egg, meat, fish, poultry, cheese, dried beans, or peas	15								
One or two additional servings of egg, meat, fish, poultry, or cheese	10 each								
Fruits and Vegetables		30							
One serving of green or yellow vegetables	10								
One serving of citrus fruit, tomato, or cabbage	10								
Two or more servings of other fruits and vegetables, including potatoes	5 each								
Breads and Cereals		15							
Four or more servings of whole-grain or enriched cereals or breads	5 each								
Junk Foods (or Negative Point Value Foods)									
Sweet rolls	−5								
Fruit pies	−5								
Potato chips, corn chips, or cheese twists	−5								
Candy	−5								
Nondiet sodas	−5								
		100							

Point Record

Weekly point total _____

Negative point total _____

Adjusted weekly _____
    point total

Interpretation

600-700   Excellent dietary practices

450-599   Adequate dietary practices

300-449   Marginal dietary practices

Below 300   Poor dietary practices

Assessing Your Dietary Practices

1 On which day of the week was it most difficult for you to eat a balanced diet? Why? _____

_____

2 Approximately what percent of your total points was from foods purchased in a restaurant? _____

3 Approximately how much money did you spend on food during this 7-day period? _____

_____

4 How much time do you estimate that you spent eating during this 7-day period? ____

_____

5 Was this a typical 7-day period in terms of the types of food eaten? If not, describe how a more typical 7-day period would appear. _____

_____

6 Your instructor may prepare a dietary profile of the class against which you can evaluate your personal 7-day diet assessment.

Macrobiotic Diet

At the extreme end of the vegetarian continuum is the *macrobiotic diet*. One form of this diet is the zen macrobiotic diet. Characterized by an almost total dependence on brown rice as the source of nutrients, this diet moves the individual through progressive stages—each of which gradually removes undesirable foods until little remains other than brown rice. So potentially harmful is this limited approach to nutrition (with deficiencies in vitamin C, calcium, and high-quality protein) that it is not recommended.[4] Regardless of the spiritual benefits or curative properties often claimed for the diet by its practitioners, any diet that prevents the body from meeting its nutritional needs is an unhealthy approach to eating.

Unbalanced and Fad Diets

After vegetarian diets, a second area of concern about collegiate dietary practices is that associated with an **unbalanced diet** to achieve or maintain weight loss. An unbalanced diet might consist of a *single food* (like pizza) or food selections from just one or two of the four food groups. Whether grapefruit, bananas, avocados, or any other "special foods" are used, the point remains the same: a diet lacking variety and balance generally cannot provide you with all of the needed nutrients.

unbalanced diet
diet lacking adequate representation from each of the four food groups.

Nutritionists at our university continue to inform us that college students, for some reason, tend to adopt these very unbalanced diets more frequently than nonstudents. Noticing the poor dietary practices of a friend or roommate should prompt you to look carefully at your own dietary practices (see the box on p. 125). Make certain that your own dietary pattern is not more unbalanced than you might otherwise have suspected.

RECOMMENDED DIETARY ADJUSTMENTS

In addition to the dietary patterns just discussed, nutritionists also recommend certain modifications in the diets of young adults.[14] These modifications include the following six considerations.

Additional milk consumption

Because of the tendency for aging women to develop a loss in bone mass density, a condition called *osteoporosis*, it is recommended that adult women increase their dairy product intake to achieve the equivalent of four servings. This additional intake provides needed calcium, which may prevent the incidence of hip, wrist, and vertebral fractures when they become older adults. Osteoporosis is statistically most likely to affect women who are thin, small boned, Oriental or Caucasian, have a family history of osteoporosis, who have reached menopause before age 50, smoke, and drink large amounts of alcohol or caffeine.[15] Excessive caloric and fat intake can be controlled by using skimmed milk or low-fat yogurt and by decreasing the daily intake of all fats. For students who do not like dairy products or who are allergic to milk, calcium supplements are an alternative. Of course, the other nutritional benefits from the milk group cannot be obtained through calcium supplements.[16] (Osteoporosis is discussed further in Chapter 11.)

Additional protein-rich sources

Nutritionists recommend that to maintain iron stores within the body to replace any iron lost during menstruation, college-age women who menstruate should include 3 ounces of red meat in their diets 3 or 4 times per week. Iron obtained from red meat (called *heme iron*) is iron in its most *biologically available* form. A general lowering of fat intake will allow this small inclusion of red meat to be undertaken without increasing overall fat intake or adding Calories.

Vegetarians can obtain adequate amounts of iron only if they carefully structure their diets to include appropriate vegetables, fruits, and grain products. Some excellent vegetable sources are lettuce, endive, beets, tomatoes, spinach, green peas, green beans, legumes, and broccoli. Good fruit sources of iron are apricots, cantaloupe, dates, prunes, and raisins. Enriched or whole-grain breads and cereals are good iron sources. Products prepared in iron cookware will often contain higher amounts of iron than those prepared in other forms of cookware. Interestingly, milk products contain little iron.

Iron supplements may be helpful in providing needed iron if they contain iron in the form of ferrous sulfate or ferrous gluconate. However, you might wish to consult a physician before taking iron supplements. Supplements alone do not provide the additional benefits from the protein-rich food group, and they may cause severe digestive complications.

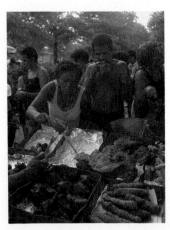

Food preferences vary widely.

Additional vitamins C and A

Within the fruit and vegetable food group, it is important to remember to include regular sources of vitamins C and A. The inclusion of the additional vitamin C will assist in the absorption of iron from bread, cereal, and eggs. For the female of reproductive age, iron stores are an important consideration, since iron is a component of the hemoglobin found in red blood cells that are lost during menstruation.

In addition to the recommendation concerning vitamin C, larger servings of fruits and vegetables, particularly the dark green vegetables, are recommended. By increasing intake in this food group, desirable increases in **folacin** and vitamin A can be achieved. Folacin's role in cellular development and in preventing **macrocytic anemia** makes its increased presence in the diet of critical importance. High levels of carotenes found in dark green vegetables aid in the production of vitamin A, a necessary fat-soluble vitamin.

folacin
folic acid; a vitamin of the B-complex group; used in the treatment of nutritional anemia.

macrocytic anemia
form of anemia in which large red blood cells predominate, but in which total red blood cell count is depressed.

Making Healthy Food Choices

EAT MORE HIGH-FIBER FOODS
- Choose dried beans, peas, and lentils more often.
- Eat whole grain breads, cereals, and crackers.
- Eat more vegetables—raw and cooked.
- Eat whole fruit in place of fruit juice.
- Try other high-fiber foods, such as oat bran, barley, brown rice, or wild rice.

EAT LESS SUGAR
- Avoid regular soft drinks. One 12-ounce can has nine teaspoons of sugar!
- Avoid eating table sugar, honey, syrup, jam, jelly, candy, sweet rolls, fruit canned in syrup, regular gelatin desserts, cake with icing, pie, or other sweets.
- Choose fresh fruit or fruit canned in natural juice or water.
- If desired, use sweeteners that don't have any calories, such as saccharin or aspartame, instead of sugar.

USE LESS SALT
- Reduce the amount of salt you use in cooking.
- Try not to put salt on food at the table.
- Eat fewer high-salt foods, such as canned soups, ham, sauerkraut, hot dogs, pickles, and foods that taste salty.
- Eat fewer convenience and fast foods.

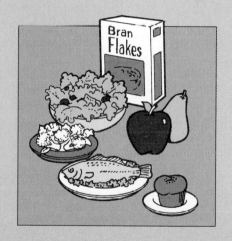

EAT LESS FAT
- Eat smaller servings of meat. Eat fish and poultry more often. Choose lean cuts of red meat.
- Prepare all meats by roasting, baking, or broiling. Trim off all fat. Be careful of added sauces or gravy. Remove skin from poultry.
- Avoid fried foods. Avoid adding fat in cooking.
- Eat fewer high-fat foods such as cold cuts, bacon, sausage, hot dogs, butter, margarine, nuts, salad dressing, lard, and solid shortening.
- Drink skim or low-fat milk.
- Eat less ice cream, cheese, sour cream, cream, whole milk, and other high-fat dairy products.

Additional grain product consumption

The grain products food group will play an important role in helping you achieve the recommended 60% of your total Calories from carbohydrates. By increasing the quantity of whole-grain breads and cereals in the diet, this 60% recommendation can be met.

Do you believe that breads and cereals are "bad" because of the Calories they provide? Remember that the current dietary recommendations presented earlier in this chapter encouraged you to reduce the intake of fats and *simple carbohydrates* and to increase consumption of *complex carbohydrate* foods. If you follow this recommendation your overall caloric intake will probably decrease. Whole-grain products are important because of the nutritional value of the complex carbohydrates and the nonnutritive fiber.

Moderation of alcohol consumption

The risks and benefits of alcohol use will be discussed at length in Chapter 8. However, because so many college students consume alcohol (90% in most surveys), we should indicate here that heavy use of alcoholic beverages can have a major impact on one's nutritional status.

Alcohol provides a significant amount of empty Calories. This can be a major concern for alcohol users who wish to control weight. Also, the overuse of alcohol can rob your body of its ability to absorb other nutrients successfully, may prevent you from consuming a sound diet, and is associated with a wide variety of diseases, including cancer and liver complications. From a health standpoint, moderation in the use of alcohol makes a lot of sense.

Nutrient density

For numerous college students, the consideration of nutrient density may prompt certain dietary adjustments. *Nutrient density* refers to the quantity of selected nutrients (mostly vitamins and minerals) in 1,000 Calories of food. Foods with a high nutrient density are better choices than those that supply only "empty" Calories. For example, a bag of potato chips or a bottle of beer has a much lower nutrient density than either a taco or a slice of pizza. Choosing to eat foods with high nutrient density is especially important for persons who are trying to limit caloric intake.

Nutrition and the Older Adult

Nutritional needs change as adults age. Age-related alterations to the structure and function of the body are primarily responsible for this. Included among the changes that alter nutritional requirements and practices are changes to the teeth, salivary glands, taste buds, oral muscles, gastric acid production, and peristaltic action. Older adults can find food less tasteful and harder to chew. Chronic constipation resulting from changes in gastrointestinal tract function can also decrease one's interest in eating.

The progressive lowering of the body's basal metabolism is also a factor that will eventually influence dietary patterns of older adults. As energy requirements fall, the body gradually senses the need for less food. This gradual recognition of lower energy needs results in a lessened food intake and "loss of appetite" seen in many elderly. Because of this decreased food consumption, nutrient density—

Remember That It Is Important To:

- Reach and stay at a reasonable weight
- Increase daily activity
- Be careful of serving sizes
- Avoid skipping meals

the nutritional value of food per Calories supplied—is an important factor for the elderly.

Besides the physiological factors that influence dietary patterns among the elderly, there are psychosocial factors that alter the role of food in the lives of many older adults. Social isolation, depression, chronic alcohol consumption, loss of income, transportation limitations, and housing are lifestyle patterns that can alter the ease and enjoyment associated with the preparation and consumption of food.[17]

SUMMARY

As you move into the independence of the adult years, your dietary practices may be the first of your health resources that are tested. Knowledge of dietary recommendations is essential for satisfactory completion of this developmental task.

From the standpoint of the physical dimension of health, the body requires six essential nutrients, including protein, vitamins, fats, carbohydrates, minerals, and water. Fiber is an important nonnutritive element in food. The best way to obtain adequate amounts of these nutrients is to plan a diet that includes selections from each of the four food groups: milk and milk products, protein-rich foods, fruits and vegetables, and breads and cereals.

The dietary practices of the American public have been studied, and several recommendations for our consumption of certain foods have been made. However, as more research is done and our knowledge of nutrition changes, these recommendations change. Therefore it is important to stay informed of the most recent dietary recommendations and to reexamine your eating behaviors.

Dietary practices often present special nutritional concerns. Many college students pursue forms of nontraditional diets, such as vegetarian diets, weight reduction diets, or diets that include a preponderance of fast foods.

Since campus life tends to force some compromises in the adoption of sound dietary patterns, certain modifications in the diets of college students are presented in this chapter. Additionally, modifications in the dietary practices of older adults are described.

REVIEW QUESTIONS

1 Define the term *nutrient*.
2 Identify the six essential nutrients and explain their contribution to the growth, repair, and regulation of the body.
3 Identify each of the four food groups.
4 Explain the nutritional benefit of each food group and the recommended daily adult serving minimums.
5 What are the dietary recommendations made by the McGovern Committee in 1977? Which of these recommendations have aroused controversy?
6 How do the guidelines published by the American Dietetic Association differ from those of the McGovern Committee?
7 Define a vegetarian diet. Explain the difference between an ovolactovegetarian diet and a vegan vegetarian diet. Which one poses more potential nutritional problems? In what ways?

8 What is nutrient density? How does this concept relate to the elderly?

9 Identify some general modifications recommended in the diets of college students and the reasoning behind each.

QUESTIONS FOR PERSONAL CONTEMPLATION

1 Consider the role that food plays in your life. Would you say that you live to eat or eat to live? If you lean toward the less-than-ideal situation of living to eat, what changes can you make in your dietary practices that will help you to eat to live?

2 We stated that protein and vitamins are the two major nutrients that we hear about from the mass media. Think about the impact this has had on your own diet. What nutrients are missing from your diet? Do you think that advertising for the other nutrients would affect your choice of foods?

3 Do your possible roles in parenting, employment, and home management compromise your ability to eat healthfully? If so, will this change in the future?

4 Analyze your diet in terms of the seven recommendations made by the American Dietetic Association. What changes do you need to make?

5 We stated that many college students eat nontraditional diets. Consider your own dietary practices as well as those of your friends. Are sound nutritional guidelines being followed?

6 Review the modifications recommended for college student diets. Take some time to examine your own diet and recognize your limitations (such as dorm living, lack of time, limited budget). See if you can make the necessary changes in your diet so that you obtain the nutrients that you need.

REFERENCES

1 Whitney, E, and Nunnelley, E: Understanding nutrition, ed 4, St. Paul, Minn, 1987, West Publishing Co.

2 Sugar: a balanced view? Child Health Alert, October, 1986, p. 6.

3 National Dairy Council: Nutrition update: sugar, Dairy Council Digest 55:21–24, 1984.

4 Guthrie, H: Introductory nutrition, ed 6, St. Louis, 1986, Times Mirror/Mosby College Publishing.

5 McNamara, DJ: The diet-heart question: how good is the evidence? Contemporary Nutrition 12:4, 1-2, 1987.

6 Christian, J, and Greger, J: Nutrition for living, Menlo Park, Calif, 1985, Benjamin/Cummings Publishing Co.

7 Greene, B: Water, water everywhere—but it's soda pop we drink, The Muncie Evening Press May 26, 1987, p. 4.

8 Greenwald, P, and Lanza, E: Dietary fiber and colon cancer, Contemporary Nutrition 11:1, 1-2, 1986.

9 Trowell, H, and Burkitt, D: Physiological role of dietary fiber: a ten-year review, Contemporary Nutrition 11:7, 1-2, 1986.

10 McBean, LD: A perspective on food safety concerns, Dairy Council Digest 58:1, 1-6, 1987.

11 Stare, F, and McWilliams, M: Living nutrition, ed 4, New York 1984, John Wiley & Sons, Inc.

12 Senate Select Committee on Nutrition and Human Needs: Dietary goals for the United States, ed 2, Washington, DC, 1977, US Government Printing Office.

13 Department of Agriculture/U.S. Department of Health and Human Services: Nutrition and your health: dietary guidelines for Americans, ed 2, Washington DC, 1985, US Government Printing Office.

14 Roepke, JB: Home Economics and Office of the Assistant Provost, personal interview, June 8, 1987, Ball State University, Muncie, Ind.

15 Osteoporosis fact sheet: He-xtra Newsletter 12:3, 5, 1987.

16 McBean, LD: Food versus pills versus fortified foods, Dairy Council Digest 58:2, 7-11, 1987.

17 Burdman, GM: Healthful aging, Englewood Cliffs, NJ, 1986, Prentice-Hall Inc, Prentice Hall Press.

ANNOTATED READINGS

Bailey, C: The fit-or-fat target diet, Boston, 1984, Houghton Mifflin Co.
  Helps you tailor a diet to your own tastes and needs and evaluate the wisdom or folly of any dietary scheme.
Brody, J: Jane Brody's nutrition book, New York, 1987, Bantam Books, Inc.
  Bestselling, comprehensive book answers lots of important questions: Is fast food junk food? Do we really need vitamin supplements? What is the truth about cholesterol? How to devise a diet without resorting to gimmicks.
Diamond, H, and Diamond, M: Fit for life, New York, 1985, Warner Books, Inc.
  A popular but scientifically controversial book that supports the concept that fruits and vegetables should constitute 70% of the diet.
Jacobsen, MF: Eater's digest: the consumer's factbook of food additives, Washington, DC, 1982, Center for Science in the Public Interest.
  Describes in detail over 100 additives commonly used by food manufactuers; tells you how to read a food label, which additives are harmful, which have not been adequately tested, and which are used to deceive the consumer.
Kirschmann, JD, and Durne, LJ: Nutrition almanac, ed 2, New York, 1984, McGraw-Hill Book Co.
  Assists you in working out a plan for personal nutrition and answers simple questions about food, nutrition, and health.
Wurtman, J: Managing your mind and mood through food, New York, 1986, Rawson Associates.
  The author contends that some foods initiate the production of stimulating neurotransmitters. Wurtman believes that alertness is heightened by foods high in protein.

CHAPTER 6

Weight Management
A Question of Calories

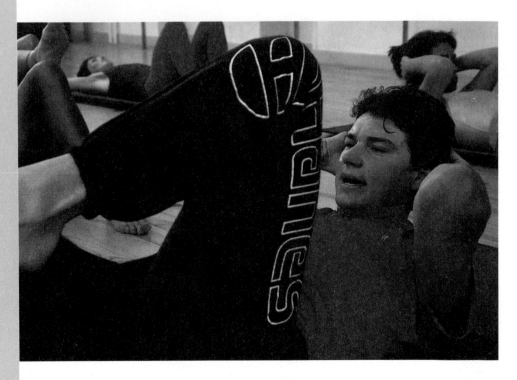

Y ou are probably aware that many people in our society think obesity is a serious health concern. Physicians counsel their patients about the need to maintain a desirable weight. People from virtually all backgrounds diet, participate in weight control programs, or engage in physical activity to lose weight, gain weight, or maintain their present weight. Yet most people are above their desirable weight, and a significant number of adults (25% to 50%) are classified as **obese.**[11] In a society that has an abundance of high-quality food and a vast array of labor-saving devices, **overweight** is almost the rule rather than the exception.

CONCERN OVER BODY IMAGE

When the body is supplied with more energy than it can expend, a predictable response is seen—the storage of excess energy in the form of body fat. This progressive accumulation of adipose tissue can eventually result in obesity. Some professionals claim that being even moderately overweight can pose serious health problems. The current consensus is that being mildly overweight may not be as dangerous as was once thought.[2] Few experts, however, question the potential dangers of extreme obesity.

For our image-conscious population, however, there is little debate about overweight being undesirable. All too often, advertisements tell us that being overweight can make our lives unpleasant, particularly when it interferes with our ability to conform to certain stereotypical body image perceptions. Interestingly, there has traditionally been little media attention to being **underweight,** yet the **body image** problems experienced by some markedly thin people are equally stressful.

OVERWEIGHT AND OBESITY DEFINED

The most prevalent forms of malnutrition in the more affluent countries of the world are overweight and obesity. Most of us think of malnourishment as a deprivation of certain types of essential nutrients. In developing countries this deprivation forms the basis of malnutrition. However, malnutrition can also be a disease of plenty. Since our food supply exceeds the needs of our population, we are able to eat more than is required for healthy living. We consume more Calories than we expend. We become overweight and may become obese.

How can we differentiate between overweight and obesity? Most nutritionists agree that obesity is apparent when one's fat accumulation produces a body weight that is more than 20% above an ideal or **desirable weight.** People are said to be overweight if their weight is between 1% and 19% above their desirable weight. The higher people move above their desirable weights, the more likely they are to become obese.

How prevalent is obesity? Some estimates indicate that up to 50% of the adult population is moderately overweight or obese. This high percentage may astound you, because among college students, certainly most are not this heavy. You must consider the fact that most obesity is seen in the older age groups. Obesity, although perhaps genetically and behaviorally determined early in life, often takes many years to develop fully. Consider the fact that a daily caloric surplus of only 10 Calories yields 10 unwanted pounds of fat in 10 years; 20 or 30 years of consistent food excess can easily result in obesity.

obesity
condition in which a person's excess fat accumulation results in a body weight that exceeds desirable weight by 20% or more.

overweight
condition in which a person's excess fat accumulation results in a body weight that exceeds desirable weight by 1% to 19%.

underweight
condition in which body weight is below desirable weight.

body image
our subjective perception of how our body appears.

desirable weight
weight range deemed appropriate for persons of a specific sex, age, and frame size.

A daily surplus of 10 calories yields 10 unwanted pounds in 10 years.

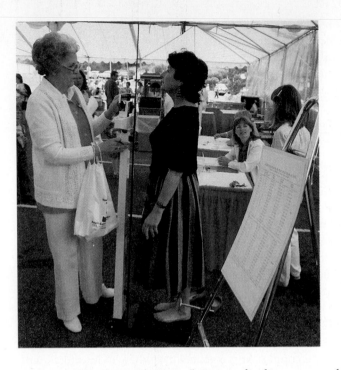

positive caloric balance greater caloric intake than caloric expenditure

As you read in Chapter 5, some foods are considered very healthy—lean meats, fresh fruits and vegetables, and low-fat dairy products, for example. However, the overconsumption of even high-quality foods will contribute to a **positive caloric balance.** The key to sustaining a specific weight (as you will soon read) is to maintain a balance between energy intake and energy expenditure. The key to taking weight off and keeping it off is exercise and dietary control.

Determining Obesity

How is obesity determined? The most widely used (and perhaps the least clinically accurate) method of determining obesity is to compare your body weight to tables of desirable weights. The Metropolitan Life Insurance Company provides a set of established standards for comparative purposes (see the box on p. 135).

Interestingly, the Metropolitan Life Insurance Company recently revised its *height-weight tables* for the first time since 1959.[3] Much criticism has been directed at these 1983 tables for their upward scaling of acceptable weights.[4,5] Health-conscious people must remember that these tables of desirable weights take into account only the relationship between longevity and weight. Of course, you may "desire" to weigh more or less than these tables indicate. Additionally, the data used for the tables are based only on those people who have purchased life insurance policies and perhaps have excluded a number of smokers, who tend to be thinner and who die at significantly younger ages.

One major factor that may further make most weight table comparisons inaccurate is that people must categorize themselves as small, medium, or large-framed before comparing weights. Since people prefer not to appear overweight or obese, they tend to place themselves in columns that make them appear to be of normal weight. To help determine your category, see the discussion of somatotypes on p. 136.

Height-weight tables may also be somewhat inaccurate because they take into account only a person's scale weight. Since muscle tissue is much more dense (and thus much heavier) than fat tissue, a muscular person with a low body fat percentage could easily be measured as overweight—even obese. Remember, the key to accurate obesity determination is the percentage of body fat—not merely overall weight.

Skinfold measurements and *hydrostatic weighing* (underwater weighing) provide relatively precise indicators of body fat percentages. Skinfold measurements rely on constant pressure calipers to measure the thickness of the layer of fat beneath the skin's surface. This layer of fat is called *subcutaneous fat*. Skinfold measurements of this fat layer are taken at several key places on the body (see Figure 6-1). Measurements of skinfold thickness are then compared to established standards. Obviously, the skill of the technician is critical to the accuracy of the measurements.

Hydrostatic or underwater weighing is a precise method that determines the relative amounts of fat and lean body mass that comprise body weight. A person's percentage of body fat is determined by comparing the underwater body weight with the body weight in air. Expensive equipment and trained technicians make this method impractical for the average person.

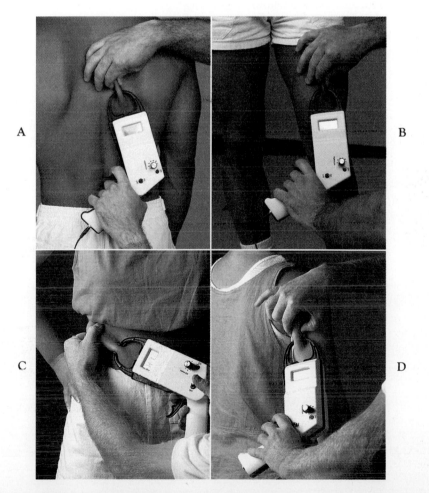

Figure 6-1
Body fat determination using skinfold calipers. Skinfold measurements can be taken at various points on the body. These measurements (in millimeters) are then used in equations that calculate body density and the percentage of body fat. Commonly measured skinfolds are the following: **A,** Subscapular. **B,** Thigh. **C,** Suprailiac. **D,** Triceps.

Young adult men normally have a body fat percentage of between 10% and 15%. The normal range for young adult women is 20% to 25%.[6] When a man's body fat percentage exceeds 20% and a woman's body fat percentage exceeds 30%, they are classified as obese. Why the discrepancy between men's and women's values? The answer is really quite simple. Because of the effects of female hormones, women naturally develop body forms that contain a higher percentage of fat. This phenomenon is probably related to the female biological role of childbearer and **lactator.**

Men and women also differ in terms of the areas of the body in which fat accumulates. Men have a tendency to develop a "spare tire" pattern of adipose storage. Women, however, are inclined to become "pear shaped" as weight is gained. It is now believed that the presence of an excessive roll of abdominal fat seen in men is associated with an increased risk of heart disease.

lactator
female who is producing breast milk.

Personal Assessment

Calculating Your Body Fat

Once the percent of body fat has been calculated, it becomes relatively simple to determine desired body weight. To calculate your percentage of body fat from skinfold measurements, use the following worksheet.

<u>Example: 20-year-old man</u>

Triceps skinfold = 14 mm

Subscapular skinfold = 15 mm

Percent body fat = $(0.43 \times 14) + (0.58 \times 15) + 1.47$

Percent body fat = $6.02 + 8.7 + 1.47$

Percent body fat = 16.19%

Worksheet For Calculating Percent Body Fat From Skinfold Measurements

1 Triceps skinfold thickness _____ mm

2 Subscapular skinfold thickness _____ mm

CALCULATION OF PERCENT BODY FAT

Men

___ % Body fat = $(0.43) \times$ _____ + $(0.58) \times$ _____ + 1.47
                                     Triceps skinfold   Subscapular skinfold

Women

___ % Body fat = $(0.55) \times$ _____ + $(0.31) \times$ _____ + 6.13
                                       Triceps skinfold   Subscapular skinfold

Some Common Sources of Error in Taking Skinfold Measurements

1 Midpoint incorrectly marked or measured

2 Arm not loose at side during measurement

3 Caliper placement too deep (muscle is involved)

4 Caliper placement too shallow (only skin grasped)

5 Caliper reading taken without marks in proper alignment

6 Skinfold grasp not maintained at time of caliper reading

BODY IMAGE

Despite the number of sophisticated ways in which obesity can be determined, the simplest method may be to look at yourself in the mirror. The old saying, "Mirrors don't lie," speaks for itself. For many large people, this method is relatively accurate, reasonably valid, and certainly inexpensive. Unless a person is especially muscular or has retained an excessive amount of water, the reflection in the mirror should be a good indicator of obesity. Although this simple method does not allow a person to pinpoint a body fat percentage, the person should be able to visually determine whether he or she is obese.

However, for many heavy people, it can be difficult to be objective. Just as many who have eating disorders (see pp. 154-155) may not judge their bodies, some heavy people do not perceive themselves as obese. Their perceived *body image* and their actual image are markedly different.

Some heavy people may rationalize their body size by saying that they are not different from others in their family. While this may be true, it is also probably

Metropolitan Life Insurance Company Weight Chart

Does your weight fall within the range established by this table? Weight tables published in 1983 reflect the fact that today's adults are on the average somewhat heavier than in recent decades. Figures include 5 pounds of clothing for men, 3 pounds for women, and shoes with 1-inch heels for both.

	Men				Women		
Height	Small Frame	Medium Frame	Large Frame	Height	Small Frame	Medium Frame	Large Frame
5 ft 2 in	128-134	131-141	138-150	4 ft 10 in	102-111	109-121	118-131
5 ft 3 in	130-136	133-143	140-153	4 ft 11 in	103-113	111-123	120-134
5 ft 4 in	132-138	135-145	142-156	5 ft 0 in	104-115	113-126	122-137
5 ft 5 in	134-140	137-148	144-160	5 ft 1 in	106-118	115-129	125-140
5 ft 6 in	136-142	139-151	146-164	5 ft 2 in	108-121	118-132	128-143
5 ft 7 in	138-145	142-154	149-168	5 ft 3 in	111-124	121-135	131-147
5 ft 8 in	140-148	145-157	152-172	5 ft 4 in	114-127	124-138	134-151
5 ft 9 in	142-151	148-160	155-176	5 ft 5 in	117-130	127-141	137-155
5 ft 10 in	144-154	151-163	158-180	5 ft 6 in	120-133	130-144	140-159
5 ft 11 in	146-157	154-166	161-184	5 ft 7 in	123-136	133-147	143-163
6 ft 0 in	149-160	157-170	164-188	5 ft 8 in	126-139	136-150	146-167
6 ft 1 in	152-164	160-174	168-192	5 ft 9 in	129-142	139-153	149-170
6 ft 2 in	155-168	164-178	172-197	5 ft 10 in	132-145	142-156	152-173
6 ft 3 in	158-172	167-182	176-202	5 ft 11 in	135-148	145-159	155-176
6 ft 4 in	162-176	171-187	181-207	6 ft 0 in	138-151	148-162	158-179

cellulite
term used by some clinicians to describe localized areas of fat with accompanying connective tissue strands that cause dimpling.

true that the entire family is obese. Others claim that their fat really isn't true fat. To these persons, fat has become **cellulite,** "baby fat," "love handles," or even "beer bellies." With so many euphemisms for body fat, it is not surprising that many people really do not consider themselves overweight. Their body images may remain distorted for an entire lifetime.

ORIGINS OF OBESITY

Experts continue to question the origins of obesity. As might well be expected, theories are numerous and focus on factors from within the individual as well as from the environment. If a definitive cause is ever identified, it will probably have a strong genetic and **neurophysiological** basis. However, until such a discovery, it is safe to assume that obesity is a complex condition whose cause involves a variety of factors. No two obese persons will have gained their excessive weight in exactly the same manner (or for the same reasons).

neurophysiological
nervous system functioning; processes through which the body senses and responds to its internal and external environments.

Genetic Basis for Obesity

A genetic basis for obesity would involve the interplay of *somatotype* (body type) and metabolic processes passed on from parents to their offspring.

The classic work of Sheldon[7] is credited with establishing the now familiar body types: **ectomorph, mesomorph,** and **endomorph.** In the case of the ectomorphic body type, a tall, slender body seems to virtually protect the individual from difficulty with excessive weight. Ectomorphs, more often than not, have difficulty maintaining normal weight for their height.

ectomorph
somatotype represented by the tall, thin individual; an individual who experiences little difficulty with excess weight.

The somewhat shorter, more heavily muscled, athletic body of the mesomorph represents a genetic middle ground in inherited body types. During childhood and adolescence, and during adulthood, as long as activity levels can be maintained, the mesomorphic individual will appear to be "solid" without appearing to be obese. For the well-conditioned mesomorph, scale weight may suggest obesity, but more than likely the excessive weight is the result of heavy muscular development. Mesomorphs experience their greatest difficulty with obesity during adulthood when their eating patterns fail to adjust to a decline in physical activity. Thus mesomorphs who do not change their eating patterns are likely to become heavy in middle age.

mesomorph
somatotype represented by the broad-shouldered, well-muscled individual.

Endomorphs have body types that tend to be round and soft. Many endomorphs have disproportionately large abdomens and report having had weight problems since childhood.

endomorph
somatotype represented by the short, round, obese individual.

Appetite Center

Building on the neurophysiological basis for obesity proposed by Mayer,[8] a theory has been developed that an appetite center is responsible for controlling food intake and caloric expenditure. Within the brain's hypothalamus, this genetically programmed center for hunger and satiety constantly monitors the blood for indications of the body's food needs. Precisely how the appetite center functions is not understood by scientists, but it is extremely likely that monitoring of blood levels of glucose and free fatty acids occurs.

According to this theory, the appetite center could account for the fact that some thin people can consume relatively large amounts of food without weight problems. The appetite center simply increases the **basal metabolism rate (BMR)** so that little food energy remains that needs to be stored as fat. (For further discussion of BMR, see pp. 143-144.) This protective mechanism, called **adaptive thermogenesis,** is thought to be highly functional within persons with genetic predispositions to thinness.[7]

Basing their conclusions on animal studies, some researchers believe that the control mechanism for thermogenesis resides in specialized adipose cells called **brown fat cells.** These cells are not like the common subcutaneous white or yellow fat cells that store lipid material. Through a process not fully understood, messages that activate the thermogenesis response are sent by the brown fat cells to the appetite control center of the hypothalamus. When brown fat cells are defective or the hypothalamus is insensitive to the instructions sent from the brown fat cells, obesity may result. It is possible that in obese persons the adaptive thermogenesis response may be entirely missing, or its effectiveness may be significantly reduced.

An additional dimension of the genetically controlled differences that could exist between the appetite centers of obese and nonobese persons is related to the sensitivity of the hunger and satiety areas of the appetite center. It is currently believed that in an obese person these areas are less sensitive than in a nonobese person. Thus in an obese person the desire to eat and the ability to sense when food needs have been satisfied are not as easily controlled as they are in a thin person. As a consequence obese people may consume more food than is required for their energy needs, and adipose tissue stores are increased.

Set Point Theory

Current theories suggest that the appetite center possesses a **set point.**[9] This set point is a genetically programmed range of body weights beyond which an individual will find it difficult either to gain or lose additional weight. The set point theory suggests that the body knows when it is near its "best" weight. Attempts to lower weight below that point are met with physiological resistance. In fact, heavy people trying to lose weight often report that their efforts are virtually fruitless below a certain weight. Perhaps it is impossible to achieve a weight level that is physiologically below the level your body was designed to carry, regardless of how much you desire to do so.

Infant and Adult Feeding Patterns

Many **bariatricians** categorize obesity according to the way in which feeding patterns seem to produce it. Two general feeding patterns are related to two forms of obesity: hypercellular and hypertrophic obesity.

The first of these patterns involves infant feeding. It is believed by many that the number of fat cells that a person has will be determined during the first 2 years of life. Through the process of *lipogenesis,* babies who are overfed during their early years will develop a greater number of adipose cells than babies who receive a balanced diet of appropriate, infant-sized portions. Overfed babies, especially those with a family history of obesity, will tend to develop **hypercellular obesity.**

---

basal metabolism rate (BMR)
amount of energy (in Calories) your body requires to maintain basic functions.

adaptive thermogenesis
physiological response of the body to adjust its metabolic rate to the presence of food.

brown fat cells
thought to be specialized fat cells responsible for regulating adaptive thermogenesis; not clearly identified in humans.

set point
genetically programmed range of body weights beyond which a person finds it difficult to gain or lose additional weight.

bariatrician
physician who specializes in the study and treatment of obesity.

hypercellular obesity
form of obesity seen in individuals who possess an abnormally large number of fat cells.

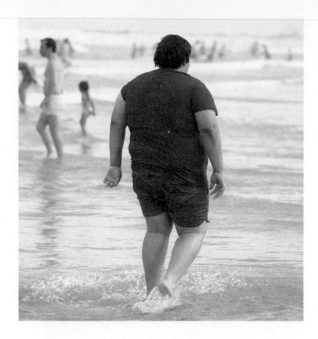

When these children grow into adulthood, they will have more adipose cells, which potentially can be filled with excess energy in the form of fat. Many researchers now believe that these fat cells drive the body's metabolic processes in the direction of a positive caloric balance (more than is needed for immediate energy requirements) and a filling of these cells. Indeed, adults who were overfed as babies often have a difficult time controlling their body weight. However, hypercellular obesity can develop at any stage of life, not just during infancy. If caloric intake is excessive, new adipose cell formation will occur.

Armed with the knowledge that overfeeding can contribute to future obesity, parents of newborns and small children are faced with a potentially troubling decision: how to "fat-proof" a child without crossing the fine line into undernourishment. Physicians consistently recommend a balanced diet, appropriate-sized servings, low-fat milk after the age of 1 year, use of cereals low in sugar, and regular physical activity. The use of these approaches is a good prescription for sound growth and development and the prevention of hypercellular obesity.

hypertrophic obesity
form of obesity in which fat cells are enlarged.

A second type of obesity that has its origins in a different eating pattern is called **hypertrophic obesity.** This form of obesity is related to a long-term, positive caloric balance that often starts shortly after the traditional undergraduate college years. Over a period of years, one's established fat cells increase in size to accommodate excess food intake. In our society, hypertrophic obesity becomes evident during middle age—a time when our physical activity declines but our food intake remains constant.

Externality

Studies have demonstrated what appears to be a more highly developed level of sensitivity to the outside world on the part of the obese.[1] In a study in which recently fed obese and nonobese subjects were "fooled" by a trick clock into believing it was time to eat, the power of this *externality* was demonstrated. When the obese subjects learned that it was meal time, they promptly ordered food, even though they had recently eaten and should not have felt hungry. The nonobese subjects, however, disregarded the message of the clock, contending that it couldn't be meal time because they did not feel hungry.

Other studies have reported that the obese are more attuned to food-oriented mass media messages and that they can more acutely smell food as it is being prepared. Further studies demonstrated that the obese dream more about food than do the nonobese.

Regardless of the mechanism accounting for this externality, it is clear that if an increased sensitivity to food does exist within an obese person, then the difficulty of adjusting to a controlled diet and disregarding temptation to eat more than is necessary is indeed a major obstacle.

Endocrine Influence

For a number of years, people believed that obesity was the result of "glandular" problems. Often the thyroid gland was said to be underactive, thus preventing the person from "burning up" food. Obesity supposedly resulted from a condition over which the individual had no control.

Today it is known that only a few obese people have an endocrine dysfunction of the type that would result in obesity. Clinicians report that no more than 3% to 5% of the obesity they observe is the result of **hypothyroidism.**

Pregnancy

During a normal pregnancy, approximately 75,000 additional Calories are required to support the development of the fetus and the formation of *maternal supportive tissues* and to fuel the elevated maternal metabolism rate. In addition, the woman will develop approximately 9 extra pounds of adipose tissue. This will be used as an energy source during lactation. In total, the typical woman enters childbirth having gained approximately 28 pounds over her prepregnancy weight.

Ideally, after the birth of the baby, the mother will display a weight gain of only 2 to 3 pounds over her prepregnancy weight. This small amount of additional weight will normally be lost by the end of the sixth to eighth month after the birth of the baby.[10] Some women experience an overall decrease in weight following pregnancy because of their concerted efforts to improve on their prepregnancy weight status.

In those women who do experience a significant weight gain as the result of having been pregnant, it is more than likely that their weight gain during pregnancy was excessive. For the majority of women, however, pregnancy and resultant obesity do not have to go hand in hand.

Decreasing Basal Metabolism Rate

The human body's requirement for energy to maintain basic physiological processes decreases progressively with age. Although on a short-term basis little adjustment needs to be made to maintain weight, weight gain can be significant over the course of time if adjustments are not made. A gradual decrease in caloric intake or a conscious effort to expend more Calories can be effective in preventing the gradual onset of obesity.

hypothyroidism
condition in which the thyroid gland produces an insufficient amount of its hormone, thyroxin.

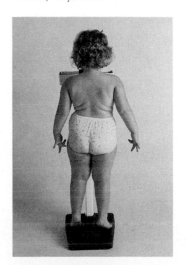

An overfed child may become an obese adult.

Family Dietary Practices

Subtly but effectively the family instructs its children on many topics; information, value stances, and diverse skills are passed from one generation to the next. Food preferences and dietary practices are among the many areas of instruction for which the family assumes responsibility. In some families the lessons are taught as though they were outlined from a nutrition textbook, while for others the patterns taught are destined to lead to a life of malnourishment, including obesity. Between-meal snacking, large serving sizes, multiple servings, and high-Calorie meals can lead to obesity.

Inactivity

When experts in the field of weight management are asked to identify the single most encompassing reason to explain the prevalence of obesity in today's society, they are almost certain to respond, "Inactivity." People of all ages tend to do less and therefore expend fewer Calories than did their ancestors only a few generations ago. Automation in the workplace, labor-saving devices in the home, the inactivity associated with watching television, and general disdain for sweating are but a few of the changes that account for this inactivity. As a society we do less than we once did. However, we have not adjusted our food intake to counterbalance this change.

In her overview of research studies related to this decreased activity, Guthrie identified a number of factors that account for our general inactivity. Some of these factors are ones many of us may take for granted[10]:

A decrease in the amount and intensity of physical activity tends to occur with increasing age. For homemakers often the activity associated with housework decreases. Not only do they exercise less in looking after the needs of their children and home but also expect the children to take over some of the household tasks they formerly did themselves. The increased availability of labor-saving devices and more readily available transportation has resulted in low energy expenditures among succeeding generations. For instance, power steering in a tractor reduces the operator's energy expenditure by 20% compared to regular steering. Secretaries working 6 hours a day on electric typewriters expend 450 kcal less per week than their counterparts using standard typewriters. Similarly, it has been estimated that the average man expends 210 kcal in walking 1.6 km (1 mile), 171 kcal in cycling the same distance, and 17 kcal in driving an automobile. The telephone company claims that the installation of an extension in the home will save 112 km of walking a year. This could account for 0.65 kg of weight a year.

The widespread use of school buses in transporting children to and from school further deprives young people of a mild but consistent form of exercise. To compensate for such things, these students must make a conscious effort to increase their activity, since prescribed periods of physical activity in schools are much too short to substitute for this. It has been shown similarly that obese women walked only half as much as control subjects, or 32 km less during a week. Frequently they sought ways of reducing activity, such as using elevators, efficient schedule planning to reduce activity, or choosing a mode of living that called for a minimum energy expenditure.

Today's renewed interest in physical activity may well indicate a reversal in this pattern of inactivity. Unfortunately, however, the observations we have made suggest that the obese college student is rarely among the physically active students seen on today's campus. For you who have not yet experienced weight problems, attention to physical fitness today will reduce the likelihood that you will have significant weight problems tomorrow.

CALORIC BALANCE

As previously mentioned, any surplus of Calories consumed beyond those that are used by the body is converted to fat stores. We gain weight when our energy input exceeds our energy output. Conversely, we lose weight when our energy output exceeds our energy input (see Figure 6-2). The basic formula is quite simple and can be analogous to a seesaw or lever with a fulcrum at the center-point. Weight remains constant when caloric input and caloric output are identical. In such a situation, our bodies are said to be in *caloric balance*.

Weight Loss

When we are in periods of reasonable physical activity (often in the spring and summer months), we tend to have greater energy expenditures than energy inputs; thus we lose weight. Obviously, when we are dieting or not eating because of illness, weight loss can occur.

Weight Gain

Some people wish to gain weight: the need to weigh more to fill out the frame, look better in particular types of clothing, or "bulk-up" for athletic events stimulates some persons to gain weight. Weight gain, of course, reflects a positive caloric balance and should be possible by increasing food intake. When combined with an exercise program designed to develop muscular strength, a moderate weight gain can be safely accomplished. We can also unintentionally gain weight when we are less active than normal.

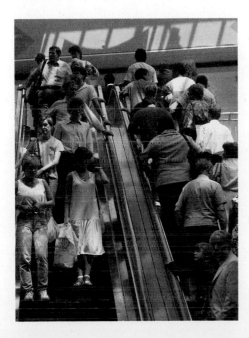

We search for ways to remain inactive.

Figure 6-2
Caloric balance: caloric input equals caloric output, some of which comes from physical activity.

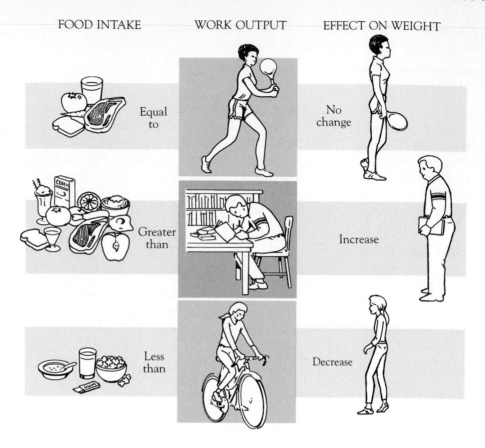

For those whose thinness is more pronounced and for whom weight gain has been very difficult, a genetic predisposition to thinness is probably the principal limiting factor. When an ectomorphic body type and an extremely sensitive thermogenesis mechanism exist, weight gain is difficult (see p. 154 for weight gain tips).

ENERGY NEEDS OF THE BODY

What are our energy needs? How many Calories should we consume (or expend) to achieve our ideal weight? There is no one answer for everyone. Although there are some ballpark estimates for college-age men (2,500 to 3,300 Calories) and women (1,700 to 2,500 Calories), we all vary in our specific energy needs.[11] These needs are based on three factors: (1) the person's activity requirements, (2) the person's basal metabolism, and (3) the dietary thermogenesis of food.

Activity Requirements

The caloric *activity requirements* of each individual vary in direct proportion to the amount of daily physical work one completes. Sedentary office workers will require a smaller daily caloric intake than will construction workers, lumberjacks, or farm workers. Even within a given general job type, the amount of caloric expenditure will vary according to the physical effort required. A police officer who walks a neighborhood beat will usually expend many more Calories than the typical police dispatcher or equestrian or motorcycle officer.

Physical activity that occurs beyond the occupational setting also adds to caloric needs. Sedentary office workers may be quite active in their recreational pursuits. Active employees may spend their off-hours lounging in front of the television. You must closely examine the total amount of work or activity expended by an individual to accurately estimate that person's caloric requirements. Physical activity uses between 20% and 40% of ones caloric intake.

Obviously recreational pursuits differ in the energy requirements needed for participation. Bowlers, golfers, and adult softball players expend far fewer Calories than do distance runners, swimmers, or backpackers. See Table 6-1 for a breakdown of caloric expenditures for various recreational pursuits.

Basal Metabolism

Of the three factors that determine caloric need, the basal metabolism uses the highest proportion (50% to 70%) of the overall Calories required by each person. Expressed as a basal metabolism rate (BMR), the basal metabolism reflects the minimum amount of energy the body requires to carry on all vital functions. We seldom consciously think of our blood circulation, respiration, glandular and brain activity, cellular metabolism, muscle tone, and body temperature as activities that require large amounts of fuel in the form of Calories. Obviously these functions do require energy. Even when you are totally relaxed or sleeping, these vital body functions continue to expend Calories.

Your basal metabolism is variable. Clearly your BMR changes with age. For both males and females BMR is relatively high at birth and continues to increase

Your Body at Rest: Basal Metabolism Rate

The basal metabolism rate (BMR) reflects the amount of energy in Calories (C) that your body requires to maintain basic functions. The formula below will help you calculate your approximate basal metabolism rate.

$$\text{BMR per day} = 1C \times \frac{\text{Body weight (pounds)}}{2.2} \times 24$$

Example: 150 pound person

$$\begin{aligned}
\text{BMR per day} &= 1C \times \frac{150}{2.2} \times 24 \\
&= 1C \times 68.2 \times 24 \\
&= 1{,}636.8\ C
\end{aligned}$$

You will need approximatley 1,637 Calories to maintain your body at rest, should you remain in that state for an entire day. Activity of any kind, of course, elevates your requirement for Calories.

NOTE: A woman's BMR will be approximately 5% lower than that of a man of the same age.

Table 6-1 Calories Expended During Physical Activity

To determine the Calories you have expended in an hour of activity, simply multiply the Calories per hour per pound column by your weight (in pounds). For example, after an hour of archery, a 120 pound person will have expended 209 Calories; a 160 pound person, 278 Calories; and a 220 pound person, 383 Calories.

Activity	Calories Per Hour Per Pound	Activity	Calories Per Hour Per Pound
Archery	1.74	Marching (rapid)	3.84
Basketball	3.78	Painting (outside)	2.10
Baseball	1.86	Playing music (sitting)	1.08
Boxing (sparring)	3.78	Racquetball	3.90
Canoeing (leisure)	1.20	Running (cross-country)	4.44
Climbing hills (no load)	3.30	Running	
Cleaning	1.62	11 min 30 sec per mile	3.66
Cooking	1.20	9 min per mile	5.28
Cycling		8 min per mile	5.64
5.5 mph	1.74	7 min per mile	6.24
9.4 mph	2.70	6 min per mile	6.84
Racing	4.62	5 min 30 sec per mile	7.86
Dance (modern)	2.28	Scrubbing floors	3.00
Eating (sitting)	0.60	Sailing	1.20
Field hockey	3.66	Skiing	
Fishing	1.68	Cross-country	4.43
Football	3.60	Snow, downhill	3.84
Gardening		Water	3.12
Digging	3.42	Skating (moderate)	2.28
Mowing	3.06	Soccer	3.54
Raking	1.44	Squash	5.76
Golf	2.34	Swimming	
Gymnastics	1.80	Backstroke	4.62
Handball	3.78	Breaststroke	4.44
Hiking	2.52	Crawl, fast	4.26
Horseback riding		Crawl, slow	3.48
Galloping	3.72	Butterfly	4.68
Trotting	3.00	Table tennis	1.86
Walking	1.14	Tennis	3.00
Ice hockey	5.70	Volleyball	1.32
Jogging	4.15	Walking (normal pace)	2.16
Judo	5.34	Weight training	1.90
Knitting (sewing)	0.60	Wrestling	5.10
Lacrosse	5.70	Writing (sitting)	0.78

until the age of 2. Except for a slight rise at puberty, your BMR will gradually decline throughout your lifetime. A variety of other variables also affect BMR, including body composition (muscular bodies are associated with higher BMRs), physical condition (fit people have higher BMRs), sex (males have 5% higher BMRs), hormone secretions (people with excessively active thyroid and adrenal glands have higher BMRs), sleep (BMRs are about 10% lower during sleep), pregnancy (a 20% increase in BMR is typical, especially in the last trimester), body temperature (a 1° rise in body temperature increases BMR about 7%), and environmental temperature (deviations above and below 78° F result in increased BMRs).[10]

For most of us the critical variable related to BMR is age. If you fail to recognize that your BMR declines significantly as you grow older, you might also fail to adjust your food intake accordingly.[12] Thus you will in all likelihood gradually put on unwanted pounds as you move through the life cycle.

Dietary Thermogenesis

Formerly called the specific dynamic effect of food, *dietary thermogenesis* represents the energy our bodies require for the digestion, absorption, and transportation of food; this energy need is in addition to activity needs and basal metabolism needs. Estimates are that the dietary thermogenesis of food represents about 10% of our total energy needs.[10] Some nutritionists now consider dietary thermogenesis of food merely a component of overall basal metabolism. This lack of distinction is understandable, since the digestive process does represent a vital body function. Thus some professionals categorize total energy needs into just two components—activity needs and basal metabolism needs.

WEIGHT MANAGEMENT TECHNIQUES

Dietary Alterations

Weight loss occurs when energy taken into the body is less than that demanded by the body for physiological maintenance and voluntary activity. Maintenance of body weight involves the establishment of an equilibrium between energy intake and energy expenditure. A number of approaches to weight management have been suggested.

A diet that reduces the Calories entering the body is the most common approach in what seems to be a national obsession with weight loss. The selection of foods included in the diet and the amount of food that can be consumed are the two factors that distinguish the wide range of diets currently available.

Balanced diets supported by portion control

For nutritional health, the most logical approach to weight loss and subsequent management of that loss is to establish a nutritionally sound balanced diet that controls portions. This approach is best undertaken with nutritionists and physicians who are knowledgeable in diet management. After a study of your day-to-day energy needs, they can establish a diet designed to produce a gradual loss. A working understanding of portion size can be achieved using diet scales or through a nutrition education program in which realistic models of food servings are used.

A balanced diet-portion control approach to weight loss reflects a nutritionally sound program which has some probability for success without the negative feature of forcing you to adapt to a restrictive approach to eating. People have extreme difficulty adjusting to a diet that presents them with uncommon foods. To these people dieting is often bad enough without feeling that they must be deprived of foods that satisfy their emotional needs.

Fad diets

People use a variety of fad diets in an attempt to achieve weight loss within a short period of time.[13] Almost without exception, these approaches are both ineffective and potentially unhealthy. Additionally, some require far greater expense than would be associated with weight loss or management techniques using portion control and regular physical activity. Important categories of fad diets are discussed below.

Diet drinks These powder or liquid products invariably contain too few Calories for safe, long-term weight loss. As a consequence of this caloric inadequacy, the body begins to use its muscle tissue as a source of energy. Blood chemistry is altered. Potassium levels are frequently lowered to unacceptable levels. Reliance on diet drinks also deprives dieters of the emotionally pleasing variety of foods associated with a balanced diet and prevents them from learning eating patterns that foster maintenance of weight loss.

Restrictive diets Many of the more familiar diet plans (for example, Atkins, Scarsdale, and Stillman) are too restrictive to be considered healthful for long-term use. In many cases, the low levels of nutrients found in these diets require the use of supplements to prevent malnourishment. As with diet drinks, restrictive diets are too frequently limited in variety and appeal of food choices and as a consequence prove difficult for persons to enjoy.

Quick weight loss diets When promises of weight loss much greater than 2 pounds per week are made, the diet being advocated will be low in carbohydrates. As a result of inadequate carbohydrate intake, the dieter will experience significant fluid loss, dehydration, and growing feelings of lethargy.

Rapid weight loss followed by an even more rapid regaining of lost weight is a characteristic too often associated with fad diets. When repeated frequently, weight loss followed by regaining weight forms the basis of the *yo-yo syndrome.*[14] Each failure enhances the chance of a future failure should weight loss be attempted again.

Franchised weight loss programs Programs that supply their clients with direction, counseling, and prepackaged foods are relatively new in the weight reduction field. Membership in these programs is generally expensive and often requires a contractual relationship with the company. Further, the foods included in the diet are often too high in protein and low in carbohydrates. Reliance on the program staff members for direction, encouragement, and reinforcement creates a level of dependency that can make eventual unsupervised weight loss difficult to sustain.

Should You Consider a Weight Loss Program?

Before you actually begin a weight loss program make a personal assessment of the reasons underlying your decision. Check all statements that you believe are applicable to your decision.

1　I feel that virtually everyone else I know is thinner than I am.　　　＿＿＿＿＿
2　The clothes I would like to wear are designed for people who are thinner than I am.　　　＿＿＿＿＿
3　I would be more active and outgoing if I could lose weight.　　　＿＿＿＿＿
4　My wardrobe is very limited because I can no longer fit into my clothing—pants can't be closed and shirts can't be buttoned.　　　＿＿＿＿＿
5　There are many activities that I can no longer take part in because my weight and size make active participation impossible.　　　＿＿＿＿＿
6　My physician has already told me that my life is seriously threatened by my obesity. Surgery could not even be safely performed on me because of my weight and size.

Many persons who undertake weight loss (and generally fail to reach their goal) do not need to do so. However, if you have checked numbers 4, 5, or 6, you should give consideration to a weight reduction program.

Personal Assessment

Low-calorie foods and controlled serving sizes

Recently a variety of familiar foods in a reduced-calorie form have been developed. By lowering the carbohydrate content with the use of nonnutritive sweeteners or reducing the fat content of the original formulations, manufacturers have given us "lite" versions of a wide variety of food products.

An even more recent addition to the diet arsenal has been the portion-controlled serving of food. Initially marketed as "single-serving" sizes, many familiar brands are now available in premeasured lunch or dinner servings. It is possible to find a fairly wide selection of attractively prepared frozen entrees with fewer than 300 Calories.

Low-calorie foods and portion-controlled servings of familiar foods can serve as valuable aids to the dieter who wants a moderate, comfortable approach to weight loss.

Controlled fasting

In cases of extreme obesity, some patients are placed on a *complete fast* in a hospital setting. The patient is maintained on only water, electrolytes, and vitamins. Weight loss is profound, because the body is quickly forced to begin **catabolizing** its fat and muscle tissues.

Complete fasting is such an extreme approach to weight loss that it must be done in an institutional setting so that the patient can be closely monitored. Sodium loss, a negative nitrogen balance, and potassium loss are particular concerns.

Today some people regularly practice short periods of modified fasting. Solid foods are removed from the diet for up to 12 days. Fruit juices, water, supple-

catabolism
metabolic process of breaking down tissue for the purpose of converting it into energy.

ments, and vitamins are used to minimize the risks described in association with total fasting. However, unsupervised short-term fasting can be dangerous and is not generally recommended.

Self-help weight reduction programs

In virtually every area of the country a person can find at least one version of popular, reputable weight reduction programs that are often operated commercially. Popularized by Weight Watchers, these programs currently feature a format consisting of (1) a well-balanced diet emphasizing portion control and low-calorie foods, (2) realistic weight loss goals over a realistic time period, (3) encouragement from supportive leaders and fellow group members, and (4) a weight management program (follow-up program).

These programs offer a reasonable, effective, noninstitutional approach to weight loss for people who cannot or will not participate in an activity program. As we will soon discuss, this program format, in combination with aerobic exercise, would be the most effective approach for most people.

Physical Intervention

A second approach to weight loss involves techniques and products designed to alter the basic patterns of eating. These techniques range from those that are self-selected and self-applied to those that must be administered within an institutional setting by highly trained professionals.

Appetite suppressants

One of the fondest wishes of overweight people is to not really want to eat—to actually have the feeling that food is not interesting or attractive. Today a variety of appetite suppressants are marketed in an attempt to achieve this for the dieter.

Pills, capsules, and candies containing sugar can be purchased that generate a short-term elevation in the body's blood glucose level. When the hypothalamus senses this elevated glucose level, the satiety center is triggered, causing the appetite to decrease. Since the active ingredient is usually some form of sugar, a piece of candy would probably accomplish the same result. These over-the-counter products are relatively harmless.

At the time of this writing, a large number of nonprescription appetite suppressants containing **phenylpropanolamine (PPA)** are being sold in supermarkets. Controversy concerning the safety of this active ingredient may alter its future availability.[15] Like its prescription counterparts, the amphetamines, this drug has only short-term value in weight reduction programs.

Stimulants (amphetamines) and depressants (tranquilizers) are prescription drugs that also have only short-term roles in weight reduction. The amphetamine's ability to influence the sensitivity of the hunger center results in a decreased desire to consume food. As a consequence, some weight loss can be experienced. In addition, the stimulating effect of the drug can elevate one's mood and thus reduce the tendency to snack.

In contrast to amphetamines, tranquilizers used for weight reduction exert their influence on the satiety area of the appetite center. By increasing the sensitivity of these centers, dieters feel more quickly satisfied by the food they con-

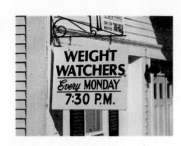

phenylpropanolamine (PPA)
active chemical compound found in most over-the-counter diet products.

Picking a Diet Book

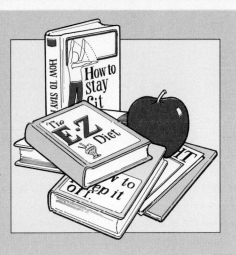

- Make sure the program incorporates a balanced diet, exercise program, and behavior modification.
- Beware of inflexible plans, such as those that require you to eat certain foods on certain days.
- Avoid plans that are lower than 1,200 Calories a day, the minimum needed to get essential nutrients.
- Make sure the recommended rate of weight loss doesn't exceed 2 pounds a week.
- Steer clear of books that promote vitamins, pills, shots, gimmicks, gadgets or brand-name diet foods.
- Read reviews to see if the book got a nod of approval from a reputable nutrition expert, institution, or journal.
- Check the authors' credentials. They should be trained in nutrition from an accredited university, or they should use reliable sources for their information?
- Make sure the book is based on up-to-date scientific research.
- Beware of diets that promise fast, easy or effortless weight loss, or "a new secret formula."
- Choose a plan that teaches how to keep the weight off once you've lost it.

sume. They stop eating sooner and consume fewer Calories. Additionally, tranquilizers may indirectly reduce the tendency to nibble and thus aid in the weight loss effort.

The use of amphetamines and tranquilizers is only a short-term approach to weight loss. The first limitation associated with their use is their relatively short period of effectiveness because the body develops a **tolerance.** Since physicians recognize this probable development of tolerance, they hesitate to prescribe larger dosages because of **dependency** problems associated with continuous use (see Chapter 7).

tolerance
increasing loss of sensitivity to the effects of a particular quantity of a given drug.

dependency
development of a psychological and/or a physical need for a particular drug.

Surgical measures

When weight loss is imperative and the initial level of obesity is great, surgical intervention may be considered. A *gastric resection* is a major operation in which a portion of the small intestine is bypassed in an attempt to decrease the body's ability to absorb nutrients. Although the procedure can produce major loss of body weight, it is associated with many unpleasant side effects (diarrhea and liver damage) and various nutritional deficiencies. Not only will surgery be re-

Figure 6-3
A new method for reducing weight; a balloon is placed in the stomach. There are some medical dangers.

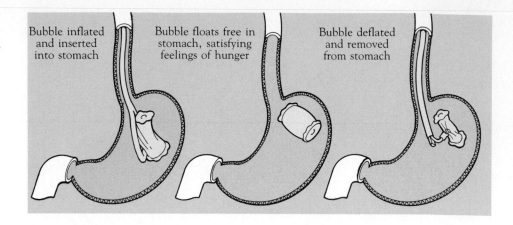

Bubble inflated and inserted into stomach

Bubble floats free in stomach, satisfying feelings of hunger

Bubble deflated and removed from stomach

quired for this approach, but lifetime medical management will also be necessary.

Gastroplasty (stomach stapling) is a surgical procedure that appears to be less dangerous than the intestinal bypass operation. During this operation about half of the stomach is sealed with surgical staples. Once the procedure is completed, the reduced capacity of the stomach decreases the amount of food that can be processed at any one time. As a result patients feel full more quickly after eating a small meal. This procedure is reversible but carries the risks associated with surgery and the costs of a major surgical procedure.

The *gastric bubble* is the newest approach to weight loss. In this procedure, an uninflated balloon is inserted into the stomach with a catheter and then inflated. Once in place, the inflated bubble simulates the distention associated with having eaten, and the person consumes less food. The bubble remains in place for 3 months (see Figure 6-3). The procedure can be repeated. Only a small percentage of patients experience deflation of the bubble while it is in place. Interestingly, recent studies suggest that the gastric bubble may be effective not because of a physical influence, but because of its psychological influence.

Liposuction (lipoplasty)

One of the newest forms of surgical weight loss management is *liposuction* (see Figure 6-4). During this expensive procedure, a physician inserts a small tube through the skin, and a vacuum machine literally sucks away fat cells. This procedure is generally used for stubborn, localized pockets of fat and is usually appropriate for people under the age of 40. After this procedure some patients report rippled skin in the location of the procedure and some complain of pain for months.

In 1986 approximately 99,300 lipoplasty procedures were performed. The average amount of adipose tissue removed was 3.3 pounds.[16] Clearly, liposuction is more of a cosmetic procedure than a general approach to weight loss. Along with unrealistic expectations, the risks of infection, pain and discomfort, bruising, swelling, discoloration, abscesses and unattractive changes in body contours are possible outcomes of liposuction. Consequently, individuals seeking to undergo this procedure need to carefully investigate all aspects of the procedure to determine whether it is the appropriate avenue for them.

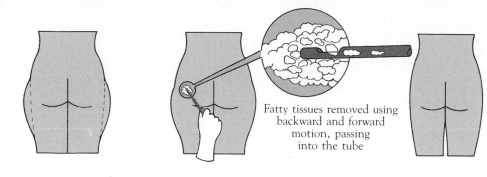

Fatty tissues removed using
backward and forward
motion, passing
into the tube

Figure 6-4
Suction-assisted lipectomy.
Liposuction is a new and
controversial method for
removing body fat.

Acupuncture

Acupuncture is being used as a treatment for obesity as well as for a variety of other health problems. The appearance of acupuncture rings and earrings in drugstores and novelty shops suggests that the procedure is moving into the non-professional domain. The majority of persons receiving acupuncture for the treatment of obesity are, fortunately, receiving treatment from more skilled practitioners.

Data on the effectiveness of this treatment method are not yet readily available and will probably not reflect large-scale studies.

acupuncture
process that attempts to alter the electroenergy fields of the body for the purpose of curing diseases.

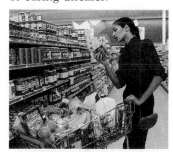

Has this woman chosen to eat wisely?

Behavior Intervention

In addition to dietary alterations and physical intervention approaches to weight reduction, several additional approaches have been tried by persons desiring to lose weight. Because of the relatively small number of people involved in many of these approaches and the limited extent to which they have been scientifically studied, it is difficult to assess their long-term effectiveness. Nevertheless, they remain as alternatives to the approaches already described.

Behavior modification

To the behavioralist, learned behavior can be "unlearned." If people have learned to eat in an inappropriate manner and as a result have difficulty maintaining their weight, then that pattern can be replaced by a more sensible pattern. *Behavior modification* is an approach to accomplishing this more desirable pattern.

In the standard behavioral modification approach to weight loss, the individual would be taught to (1) recognize the environmental factors associated with the faulty eating pattern, (2) identify the reward system that accompanies that pattern, (3) establish a new environment in which to develop the new dietary pattern, and (4) institute a new reward system to support the newly adopted dietary pattern. Behavior modification programs can be undertaken in both group and individual formats. The box on p. 152 gives some approaches to behavior modification.

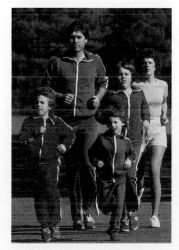

Weight management is a family affair.

Weight Loss Strategies

A number of strategies may be involved in a behavior modification approach to weight loss. Some of these approaches include the following:

- Keeping a log of the times, settings, reasons, and feelings associated with your eating
- Setting realistic, long-term goals (for example, loss of a pound per week instead of 5 pounds per week)
- Avoiding the total deprivation of enjoyable foods (occasionally reward yourself with a small treat)
- Eating slowly and realizing that the sacrifices you are making are what *you* feel are important for *your* health and happiness
- Putting more physical activity into your daily routine (taking stairs instead of elevators, or parking in the distant part of a parking lot, for example)
- Rewarding yourself when you reach your goals (with new clothes, sporting equipment, a vacation trip)
- Sharing your commitment to weight loss with your family and friends (then they can support your efforts)
- Keeping careful records of daily food consumption and weight change
- Being prepared to deal with occasional plateaus and setbacks in your quest for weight loss

Hypnosis

Hypnosis appears to hold some promise as an effective weapon in the obesity battle. Studies involving hypnosis have appeared in the literature for at least 20 years. Many of these have reported excellent success rates, but most involve small numbers of patients and little has been reported on long-term success rates.

More recently, "private practitioners" of hypnosis are applying their skills in many nonprofessional settings such as motel rooms. Claims made for these programs have been extremely high. The cost of treatment is also high. We would be cautious of using hypnosis on this basis.

Physical activity

Another important behavioral component of weight loss programs is regular physical activity. Physical activity can be a major factor in achieving weight loss or maintenance because activity expends Calories. This is a simple but highly predictable process. (See Table 6-1 for a list of caloric expenditures for various activities.)

For years, a consensus of scientific opinion indicated that physical activity can stimulate a 12- to 24-hour period of sustained, elevated basal metabolism rate. This elevated BMR was thought to provide for the expenditure of Calories even after moderate exercise was completed. Investigators now seriously question whether this elevation in basal metabolism is sustained for such a long period.

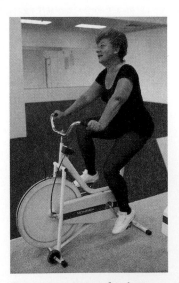

Exercise to expend calories.

A more likely interval of BMR elevation (after moderate exercise) seems to be 2 or 3 hours.[17]

An additional benefit derived from physical activity is that proportionally more fat is lost than occurs through dieting alone. Studies suggest that the loss achieved through physical activity is 95% adipose and 5% lean mass, in comparison to a loss of 75% fat and 25% lean mass when only dieting is used.

A Combination Approach

If we were to recommend a single approach to weight reduction that would, in theory, offer the maximum chance for success, we would suggest a program combining Calorie reduction and aerobic exercise. Specifically, the program would be (1) planned by a team of professionals (physician, nutritionist, fitness expert) in consultation with the individual and his or her family, (2) managed by the individual, and (3) strongly family-centered. This approach would offer the following features:

- A varied, balanced diet emphasizing portion control and low Calorie food items would be developed; with necessary modifications, the diet would be adopted by the entire family.
- Reasonable short-term weight loss goals and weight loss maintenance goals would be established at the beginning of the program and assessed during and following the program.
- A professionally planned aerobic fitness component would be developed and implemented as a part of the total program format.
- The family would actively participate and serve as a source of encouragement for the overweight person.

As encouraging as we would like to be in regard to success in losing weight and maintaining loss, the picture is not exceptionally bright. To the extent that valid data are available, even carefully structured programs using dietary and group-support components rarely report success rates above 15%. When longer-term loss (1 year plus) data are analyzed, the success figure drops to 3% to 5%. Programs that report figures much higher than these are more probably based on small numbers of subjects and thus are suspect.

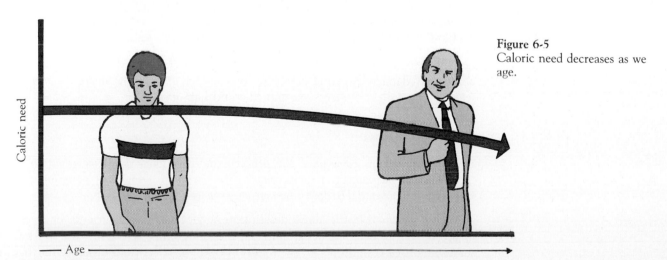

Figure 6-5
Caloric need decreases as we age.

Successful Weight Management: Tips to the Wise

FOR WEIGHT LOSS

1 You probably didn't gain your excessive weight alone. Seek the encouragement and support of family and friends in your weight loss efforts.

2 Eat only at the table. Leave the table immediately after finishing your meal. And by all means never take your meal with you into other rooms of the house.

3 Stop eating after one serving. A second helping contributes more Calories than your diet can afford.

4 If you must snack between meals, choose nutritious, low-calorie snacks. Make them small too.

5 Stay away from the kitchen. An innocent look into the refrigerator will almost certainly lead to a taste, a snack, or even a meal.

FOR WEIGHT GAIN

1 Make certain that there is no medical reason for your thinness.

2 Have your current dietary practices evaluated so that appropriate modifications can be made.

3 Begin a moderate exercise program to enhance your physical fitness.

4 Incorporate the following recommendations into your dietary practice:
- Substitute juice, soup, or hot chocolate for coffee.
- Eat a healthy breakfast.
- Learn appropriate portion sizes.
- Replace junk foods with healthier foods.

Unfortunately we cannot support with data our belief that a combined approach format would be significantly more successful than programs using only diet and group support. The only real alternative to an eventual weight problem is to maintain a lifelong commitment to a dietary and exercise program that can prevent problems from developing.

EATING DISORDERS

Perhaps it is not surprising to find that some people have medically identifiable, potentially dangerous eating patterns. Two serious disorders that are sometimes seen among college students are anorexia and bulimia.

Anorexia Nervosa

A young woman, competitive and perfectionistic by nature, determines that her weight (and appearance) is unacceptable. She sets upon a course of disregarding hunger and appetite. Her food consumption virtually ceases.

The young woman in the above description may be seen by her friends or roommates as active and intelligent, and simply dieting and exercising with an unusual amount of commitment. Eventually, however, you would observe that her

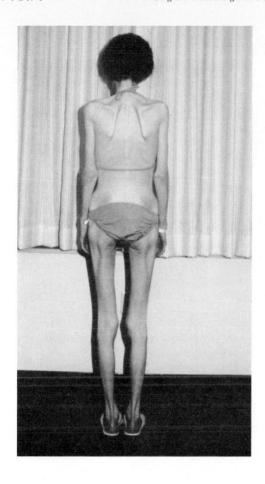

Anorexia can be a life-threatening disorder.

food consumption had virtually ceased. Her weight loss would continue beyond the point that is aesthetically pleasing—at least to you. Nevertheless, her activity level might remain high. When questioned about her weight loss she would probably indicate that she still needed to lose more weight.

This person is suffering from a medical condition referred to as **anorexia nervosa.** This self-induced starvation is life-threatening in about 10% of cases.[18] The stunning amount of weight that some anorexics lose—up to 50% of their body weight—eventually leads to cardiovascular collapse.

Anorexia nervosa appears to be increasing among women, particularly from white, middle-class to upper-middle-class families. Some experts believe that the incidence of anorexia is on the rise because our society expects young women to be as glamorous, sexy, and thin as the women seen on television, in newspapers, and on billboards. Indeed, anorexia patients typically come from families that "place a heavy emphasis on high achievement, perfection, eating patterns, and physical appearances."[19]

Fortunately for the anorexic, psychological intervention in combination with medical and dietary support can return the victim to a more life-sustaining pattern of eating. However, the anorexic needs to seek professional help. Your obligation when you observe this condition in a friend is to secure immediate assistance for this person.

anorexia nervosa
psychogenic disorder in which appetite and hunger are suppressed, and marked weight loss occurs.

Symptoms of Anorexia

20% to 25% body weight loss
Lack of menstrual period
Hyperactivity
Distorted body image
Food binges followed by fasting, vomiting, laxative use

Resources for Anorexia and Bulimia

LOCAL RESOURCES

College/university health centers

College/university counseling centers

Comprehensive mental health centers

Crisis intervention centers

Mental health associations

NATIONAL RESOURCE

American Anorexia/Bulimia Association, Inc.
133 Cedar Lane
Teaneck, NJ 07666
1-201-836-1800

TELEPHONE HOTLINES

BASH (Bulimia and Anorexia Self-Help): St. Louis, Mo (800) 762-3334
ANAD (National Association of Anorexia Nervosa and Associated Disorders): Highland Park, Ill (312) 831-3438

Interestingly, only 6% to 10% of all anorexics are males. Furthermore, whereas the female anorexic displays tendencies toward orderliness and perfectionism, male anorexics are less inclined to do so.

Bulimia Nervosa

bulimia
psychogenic disorder in which binge eating patterns are established; usually accompanied by purging.

purging
using vomiting or laxatives to remove undigested food from the body.

Bulimia reflects a dietary practice pattern in which people gorge themselves with food. When people practice a pattern of massive eating followed by **purging,** they are said to suffer from *bulimarexia,* or bulimia nervosa. This condition, like anorexia, can lead to weight loss, but it differs in terms of the victim's personality and specific behavioral patterns and the prospects for successful treatment. As with anorexia nervosa, most bulimarexics are young women.

Bulimarexics lose weight or maintain weight not because they stop eating but because they eat and then purge their digestive system by vomiting or using laxatives. Syrup of ipecac, a product used to help poisoning victims vomit, is so frequently abused by bulimics that some efforts are underway to make this a prescription drug. Compared with anorexics, bulimarexics tend to be extroverted, socially active, and less perfectionistic. Your primary awareness of a bulimarexic's condition may be the paradox between high food intake and resultant weight loss. Medical experts estimate that as many as 19% of 18- to 22-year old women develop all the principal symptoms of bulimia.[20]

People with bulimarexia may gorge themselves with food (up to 10,000 Calories or more at a sitting) and then quietly disappear, only to return later seemingly unaffected by the foods they recently ate. In all likelihood, they have quickly and quietly regurgitated the food they just ate. Unlike the anorexic, people with bulimia nervosa may demonstrate an extreme sensitivity to food. Thus they have many food likes and dislikes. This suggests that they have not

Symptoms of Bulimia

Inconspicuous binge eating

Menstrual irregularities

Swollen salivary glands

Frequent significant weight fluctuations caused by alternating binging and fasting

Fear or inability to voluntarily stop eating

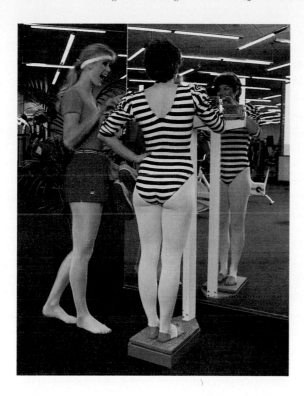

managed to suppress their hunger. Bulimarexics feel hungry, overeat, and then resolve any guilt by vomiting.

Treatment for Eating Disorders

The treatment of anorexia nervosa and bulimia nervosa is a complex and demanding undertaking. The components of therapy, drawn from medical and behavioral sciences, involve the cooperation of several health care providers. Each case of anorexia or bulimia must be approached from an individual perspective.

The initial, physical care for anorexia most often begins with hospitalization of the individual to stabilize the physical deterioration associated with starvation. Nasogastric tubes and intravenous feedings are sometimes necessary, particularly when the patient will not (or cannot) eat. Additionally, drug therapy to decrease hyperactivity and stimulate appetite is often used.

The psychological and familial components underlying anorexia require a variety of therapeutic approaches. Behavioral modification, including eating contracts, is employed, as is psychotherapy in both individual and group formats. Nutritional counseling and family therapy counseling complete the therapy.

Treatment for bulimia involves individual, family, and nutritional counseling. Unlike anorexia, however, bulimia treatment does not so frequently involve hospitalization. Drugs used in the treatment of bulimia include a variety of antidepressive agents.

People with eating disorders are in desperate need of professional assistance. Unfortunately, the assistance available for treating bulimia nervosa appears to be less effective than that available to the victim of anorexia nervosa.[19] Nevertheless, as an observer of this condition, your obligation is to assist in securing help for its victims. (See the box on p. 156 for resources that offer help.)

SUMMARY

Weight management is an important health concern that relates to each of the five dimensions of health. Overweight and obesity represent the most prevalent form of malnutrition in the United States. Obesity is the condition in which there is an abnormal accumulation of fat in the body tissues. Obesity and overweight can be measured in a variety of ways. The principal factor, however, in obesity determination is the percentage of body fat.

Many theories about the cause of obesity emphasize the complexity of this condition. Theories focus on factors from within the individual as well as from the environment. Although much of obesity may be genetically based, other theories are also quite plausible. These theories reflect differences in appetite center functioning, infant and adult feeding patterns, externality, endocrine influences, basal metabolic rates, family dietary patterns, and inactivity.

Weight gain is caused when energy input exceeds energy output. Energy needs vary with each individual and are based upon three factors: activity level, basal metabolism, and the dietary thermogenesis of food.

Weight loss occurs when energy input is less than the energy output of the body. There are a number of approaches to weight management, including dietary alterations, physical interventions, and behavior interventions. Though no approach offers an easy solution, the approach that seems to offer the best chance for successful weight reduction is a combination approach using calorie reduction and aerobic exercise.

The incidence of eating disorders such as anorexia nervosa and bulimia nervosa appears to be increasing. Treatment of eating disorders involves individual, family, and nutritional counseling.

REVIEW QUESTIONS

1 Explain what is meant by the statement, "Malnutrition may be a disease of plenty."
2 Define obesity. How can we differentiate between overweight and obesity? How is obesity determined? What is the key to obesity determination? How is it measured?
3 Define somatotype. Explain how this concept relates to the genetic basis for obesity. Identify and briefly describe the other theories about the origin of obesity presented in this chapter.
4 What three factors determine an individual's specific energy needs? Explain each factor.
5 Describe several approaches to weight management as prersented in this chapter. List some advantages and disadvantages of each approach.
6 What is the most highly recommended weight reduction approach? What are the four main components of this approach? How is this plan better than the other approaches presented?
7 What are the signs and symptoms of anorexia nervosa? How are they different from the signs and symptoms of bulimia?

QUESTIONS FOR PERSONAL CONTEMPLATION

1 What ways have you used to determine whether you were underweight, overweight, or obese? If you have used different methods, did your results differ? Which method do you think was most accurate? Why?

2 What are your own attitudes toward people with weight control problems? Do you treat them differently than you treat other people? In what ways? How might you change these attitudes?

3 Do the attitudes our society has toward underweight people differ from those it has for overweight people? Do you believe that being underweight is as psychologically traumatic as being overweight?

4 If you have ever attempted to lose weight, what methods have you used? Which methods were most successful? Why do you think they were successful when other methods failed? Were any of your methods potentially dangerous?

5 If you have a weight control problem, identify your behavioral or personality traits that you consider positive. Determine how you can emphasize these traits to help achieve a more productive and satisfying life.

6 If you are a person with a weight problem, do you agree or disagree that you have a responsibility to yourself and other people to adjust your weight?

REFERENCES

1 Whitney, E, and Hamilton, E: Understanding nutrition, ed 4, St. Paul, 1987, West Publishing Co.

2 Treichel, J: A new weight-height chart: it's OK to weigh a little more than before, Science News 23:123, 1983.

3 Those new height and weight tables, Nutrition Today 18:16-17, 1983.

4 Kiefer, NC: Less than meets the eye, Nutrition Today 18:18-26, 1983.

5 Manson, E, et al: Body weight and longevity: a reassessment, Journal of the American Medical Association 257:353-358, 1987.

6 Prentice, WE, and Bucher, CA: Fitness for college and life, ed 2, St. Louis, 1988, Times Mirror/Mosby College Publishing.

7 Sheldon, W, Stevens, S, and Tucker, W: The varieties of human physique, New York, 1940, Harper & Row, Publishers Inc.

8 Mayer, J: Overweight, Englewood Cliffs, NJ, 1968, Prentice-Hall.

9 Kemnitz, J: Body weight set point theory, Contemporary Nutrition 10:1-2, 1985.

10 Guthrie, H: Introductory nutrition, ed 7, St. Louis, 1989, Times Mirror/Mosby College Publishing.

11 Food and Nutrition Board: Recommended dietary allowances, Washington DC, 1980, National Academy of Sciences, National Research Council.

12 Guyton, A: Human physiology and mechanisms of disease, ed 4, Philadelphia, 1986, WB Saunders Co.

13 Wurtman J: The carbohydrate craver's diet, New York, 1984, Ballantine/Del Rey/Fawcett Books.

14 Brownell, K: Obesity and weight control: the good and bad of dieting, Nutrition Today 11:4-9, 1987.

15 Ray, O, and Ksir, C: Drugs, society, and human behavior, ed 6, St. Louis, 1987, Times Mirror/Mosby College Publishing.

16 Lipolysis Society of America: Telephone interview, June 10, 1987.

17 Kolata, G: Metabolic catch-22 of exercise regimens, Science 236:146-147, 1987.

18 McNab, W: Anorexia and the adolescent, Journal of School Health 53:427-430, 1983.

19 Dove, J: Facts about anorexia nervosa, Bethesda, MD, National Institute of Child Health and Human Development, U.S. Department of Health and Human Services.

20 Eating disorders: anorexia nervosa and bulimia, Nutrition Today 10:29-33, 1987.

ANNOTATED READINGS

Cross, A: Nutrition for the working woman, St. Louis, 1986, Fireside Books.

    A nondiet diet book that focuses on a balanced diet and exercise approach to healthful nutrition. Suggestions are made for food selection and preparation.

Darden, E: The Nautilus diet: ten weeks to a brand-new body, Boston, 1987, Little, Brown & Co, Inc.

    Outlines a 1,000 Calorie a day diet to be combined with a physical conditioning program. Persons with Nautilus-type equipment may find the book of particular interest.

Katahn, M: The rotation diet, New York, 1986, WW Norton & Co, Inc.

    A detailed dietary plan involving a 600 Calorie diet for 3 days, 900 Calories for 4 days, and 1,200 Calories for a week is presented.

Mastering Tasks

It is our hope that the information you have mastered in Unit II will be helpful as you work on the four developmental tasks this book addresses. Of course, you must remember that all people work on these tasks in different ways and at varying speeds. However, it is through the completion of these developmental tasks that you will have a satisfying and productive life.

■ **Forming an Initial Adult Self-Identity** Developmentally speaking, traditional-age students have as one of their major responsibilities the establishment of an initial adult self-identity. Even nontraditional students (and professors) find that they are often working on their adult identities. In forming these identities, we are expected to blend those traits currently possessed with those that are desired. What are the roles for fitness, nutrition, and weight management in forming and reforming of our identities?

Your enhanced fitness level, interest in nutrition, and body weight will be evident to you and transmitted to others as a sense of your personal self-acceptance. In a sense, you are telling the world, "I like what I am and I hope you like it too."

Your interest in these areas is also a commitment to your future—as you plan for your adult years and as others plan theirs with you in mind. You will be likely to become a person who is more capable of living a productive and satisfying life.

■ **Establishing a Sense of Relative Independence** Independence, a much-desired freedom for those nearing the end of their formal education, will be achieved by the majority of adults regardless of whether they are interested in the health information presented in this unit. However, the quality of your independence can be enhanced by a reasonable level of fitness and an interest in nutrition and weight management. Particularly in terms of your ability to cope with the new demands of independence, a well-developed state of fitness and a sound diet will help you reduce stress and increase the level of alertness you will need to master the demands of adulthood.

For nontraditional students whose independence is already well-established, continued interest and involvement in physical activity, nutrition, and weight management can add a measure of renewal to your demanding life as an employee, single person, spouse, or parent.

■ **Assuming Increasing Levels of Responsibility** As people move through adulthood, to whom should they be most responsible? As we mentioned earlier, people should probably be most responsible to themselves. But the responsibility for oneself does not limit the need to be responsible for others. The reasons compelling you to appreciate your health and to promote it to the fullest extent extend beyond yourself to include others with whom you come into contact. For this reason, your fitness level, nutritional status, and weight management can affect your ability to perform optimally.

Beyond this rather philosophical connection between high-level health and responsibility is another more concrete connection: Your motivation to maintain good cardiorespiratory fitness, nutrition, and weight management will be an indicator of your willingness and ability to assume responsibility. By being faithful to your fitness program and well-rounded diet, you assure yourself that you are a responsible person.

■ **Developing the Skills for Social Interaction** As your social interaction increases with entry into or movement through the adult years, the relationship between this unit's content and your developing social skills becomes evident. Much of our social contact with other adults centers around food and physical activity. Exercise classes, parties, cycling groups, cafeteria meals, outdoor cookouts, an evening with friends, reunions, and athletic teams represent some social groups that cater to our fitness or food desires.

Through your participation in these common social groupings, you will have a great opportunity to practice and improve your social skills. We would encourage you to cherish these opportunities. Indeed, social interactions will form a principal basis for a kind of personal enjoyment that will last a lifetime.

UNIT III

There is little doubt in the minds of health professionals that the use, misuse, and abuse of many substances can negatively influence your health. These substances not only alter the function of the body and the mind, but also have an impact on the social, intellectual, and spiritual dimensions of health as well.

■ **Physical Dimension of Health** The relationship between substance use and the physical dimension of health is reasonably well understood, especially in relation to the long-term use of alcohol and tobacco. These substances clearly increase human morbidity and mortality.

The misuse of beverage alcohol produces destructive changes in the structure and function of a variety of systems. Chemical imbalances and inflammation of the liver, inflammation to tissues of the digestive system, and cardiomyopathy are among the most persistently found destructive effects of alcohol abuse.

Tobacco's damaging influence on physical health centers mainly on effects to the cardiovascular system and the tissues lining the air passages. Damage to the red blood cells, heart irregularities, and lung cancer represent some serious effects of tobacco use.

Chronic misuse and abuse of most psychoactive drugs alter an array of central nervous system functions. Even the experimental use of psychoactive drugs presents the possibility of toxic overdose.

■ **Emotional Dimension of Health** Why do some people use alcohol, other drugs, and tobacco so extensively?

Our understanding of these areas is far from complete. It is known, however, that psychoactive substances are capable of altering the normal function of the central nervous system. For individuals who seem predisposed to dependent relationships, chemical substances can become a readily available crutch. When growing emotional dependency combines with a physical dependency, major detrimental effects begin to surface.

■ **Social Dimension of Health** The use of many psychoactive substances is associated with social interaction. In the minds of some people, the use of these substances seems like a prerequisite for enjoying the company of others. However, little social support exists for inappropriate substance use. In fact, the majority of society is disenchanted with the use of psychoactive drugs, misuse of beverage alcohol, and passive smoking.

Perhaps the most serious social consequence of these substances is the dulling effect they have on the learning of desirable social interaction skills. Successful social interaction demands discrimination and dissemination of a variety of cues and responses. The misuse of drugs, alcohol, and tobacco is likely to interfere with increased growth.

■ **Intellectual Dimension of Health** Intellectual impairment is one part of the gradual decline of the body attributable to chemical abuse. People cannot perform up to their potential when they feel extremely high, extremely low, or are incapacitated by sensory impairment.

One pertinent issue in the intellectual dimension centers on the disregard some people have for valid information related to the use, misuse, and abuse of chemical substances. This is an especially perplexing issue when it concerns college students— people whose education and intellectual abilities would suggest they can fully comprehend the dangers of drug use.

■ **Spiritual Dimension of Health** Although the use of psychoactive substances has a role in the religious practices of many people throughout the world, the nonceremonial misuse or abuse of chemical substances seems in conflict with the tenets of stewardship and service to others. The misuse of these substances seems an affront to the ideals of self-worth associated with many aspects of spiritual maturation. It is unlikely that growth and development in the depth and breadth of one's spiritual life is fostered by the misuse of these substances.

Products of Dependency
A Focus for Responsible Use

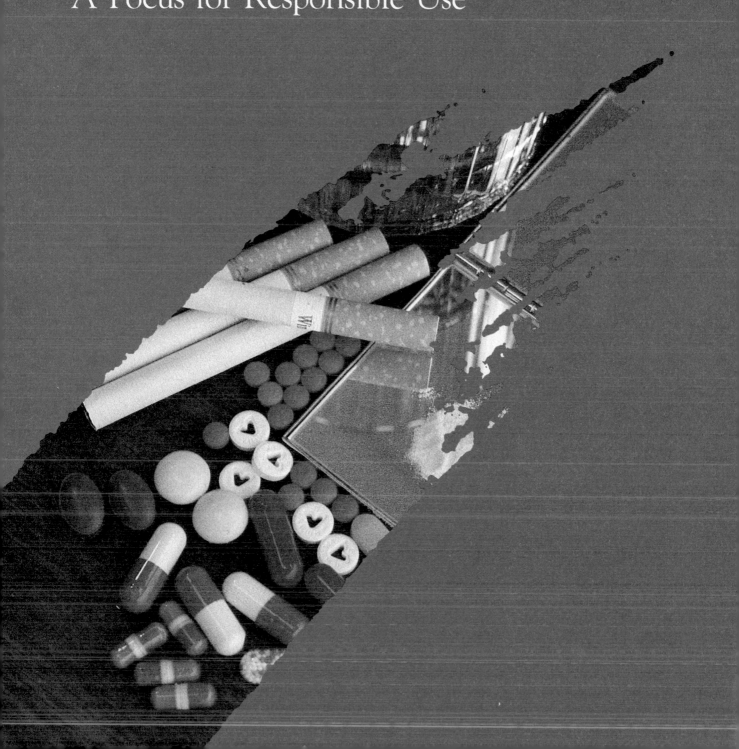

Psychoactive Drugs
Use, Misuse, and Abuse

Key Concepts

Familiarity with drug-related terminology is essential to understanding drug-related issues.

People use, misuse, and abuse drugs to fulfill unmet human needs.

Psychoactive drugs alter neurotransmitter functioning.

Drugs are classified by the nature of the physiological effects they exert on users.

The lethal effects of many drugs are well recognized.

A number of resources exist for college students who seek assistance with drug abuse problems.

Each of us is capable of achieving personally satisfying "highs" through nondrug methods.

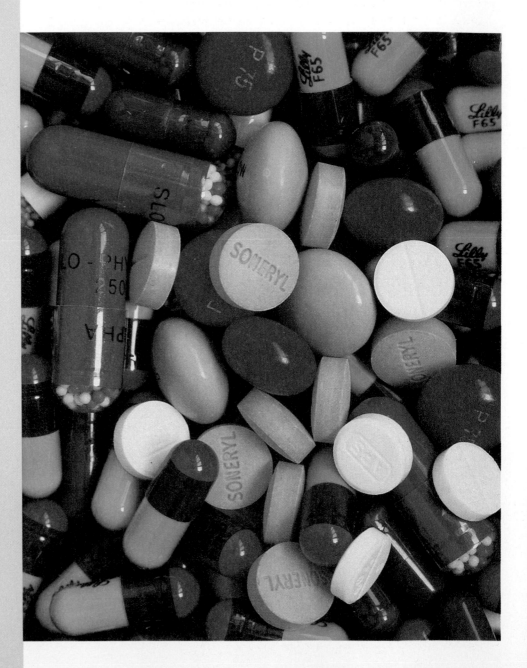

For many of our own students, a chapter on drug use, misuse, and abuse (other than alcohol use) is less than exciting and stimulating. Since junior high school our students have been warned of the "evils of drug abuse." Furthermore, most of our college students rarely misuse or abuse **psychoactive drugs** other than alcohol and marijuana. So what's the big deal about drugs?

To begin with, drugs still play a major role in many people's lives. The tragic deaths of Len Bias, John Belushi, and Don Rogers have pointed this out clearly in the past few years. Although we might not be drug misusers or abusers, perhaps some of our college friends, hometown friends, or even relatives use drugs inappropriately or dangerously. By understanding some of the dynamics of drug use we can better come to grips with the behavior of these friends or relatives.

Second, an academic view of drug use can give you a better idea about how psychoactive drugs function in relationship to the central nervous system. Such a study can give you a much better appreciation of the intricacies of your own body. This understanding may either alter or reaffirm your opinion that misuse or abuse of drugs can only negatively interfere with the quality of your life.

Last, despite the fact that overall drug abuse among college students has dropped in the last few years,[1] cocaine abuse remains unacceptably high,[2] and marijuana recently surpassed corn as our nation's number one cash crop.[3] Also, numerous accidents and crimes are committed daily by persons under the influence of drugs. Even though you may not be a drug misuser or abuser, drug abuse is very likely to have an impact on your life. This is why educated adults need information about drug use, misuse, and abuse.

DRUG TERMINOLOGY

Before you can discuss drug actions or drug behavior, you must first be familiar with some basic terminology. This terminology has been developed by scientists who specialize in *pharmacology*, or the "study of the interaction of chemical agents with living material."[4]

What does the term *drug* mean? Each of us may have different ideas about what a drug is. Although a number of definitions are available, we will consider a drug to be "any substance, other than food, that by its chemical or physical nature alters structure or function in the living organism."[4] Included in this broad definition are a variety of psychoactive drugs, medicines, and substances many people do not usually consider to be drugs.

Psychoactive (or *psychotropic*) drugs have the ability to alter the user's feelings, behaviors, perceptions, or moods. Psychoactive drugs include stimulants, depressants, hallucinogens, opiates, and inhalants. *Medicines* are drugs whose primary function is to heal unhealthy tissue. Medicines are also used to ease pain, prevent illness, and diagnose health conditions. Although some psychoactive drugs are consumed for medical reasons, as in the case of tranquilizers and some narcotics, the most commonly prescribed medicines are antibiotics, sulfa drugs, diuretics, oral contraceptives, and antihypertensive drugs. Substances not usually considered to be drugs (but which certainly are drugs) include caffeine, tobacco, alcohol, aspirin, and other over-the-counter (OTC) preparations. These common substances are used so frequently in our society that they are rarely perceived as true drugs.

For organizational reasons, we will primarily discuss psychoactive drugs in this

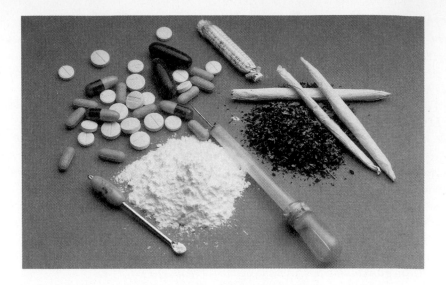

chapter. Alcohol, the most frequently abused drug, will be covered in Chapter 8. The effects of tobacco will be delineated in Chapter 9. Prescription and OTC drugs and medicines are discussed at length in Chapter 17. Environmental pollutants are covered in Chapter 18.

Dependency

dependency
general term that reflects the need to keep consuming a drug for psychological or physical reasons, or both.

Psychoactive drugs have a strong potential for the development of a **dependency.** When users take a psychoactive drug, the patterns of neural function are altered. If these altered neural functions provide perceived benefits for the user, drug use may continue, perhaps at increasingly larger dosages. If persistent use continues, the abuser can develop a dependency on the drug. Pharmacologists have identified two types of dependencies—physical and psychological.

Persons can be said to have developed a *physical dependency* when their body cells have become reliant on a drug. Once this phenomenon has occurred, continued use of the drug is required, because body tissues have adapted to its presence.[5] Said in another way, the person's body needs the drug to maintain homeostasis, or dynamic balance. If the drug is not taken or is suddenly withdrawn, the abuser develops a characteristic **withdrawal illness** or abstinence syndrome. The symptoms of the abstinence syndrome reflect the attempt by the body's cells to regain normality without the drug. Withdrawal symptoms are always unpleasant (ranging from mild to severe irritability, depression, nervousness, digestive difficulties, and abdominal pain) and can be life threatening, as in the case of abrupt withdrawal from barbiturates or alcohol. The term *addiction* is often used interchangeably with physical dependency.

withdrawal illness
uncomfortable, perhaps toxic response of the body as it attempts to maintain homeostasis in the absence of a drug; also called abstinence syndrome.

Persons who possess strong desires to continue the use of a particular drug are said to have developed *psychological dependency*. People who are psychologically dependent on a drug think they need to consume the drug to maintain a sense of well-being. They crave the drug for emotional reasons. Abrupt withdrawal of a drug by these persons would not initiate the complete abstinence syndrome, although minor symptoms of withdrawal might be experienced. The term *habituation* is often used interchangeably with psychological dependency.

Continued use of most drugs can lead to the phenomenon of tolerance. *Tolerance* is an acquired reaction to a drug in which continued intake of the same dose has diminishing effects.[5] Said in another way, the user needs more of a drug to receive previously felt sensations. The continued use of stimulants, depressants, and the opiates can cause users to quickly develop a tolerance to the drug.

College seniors who have engaged in 4 years of beer drinking can usually recognize tolerance occurring in their own bodies. Many such students can vividly recall their initial and subsequent sensations after drinking. For example, five beers consumed during a freshman social gathering might well have resulted in inebriation, but if these same students continued to drink beer regularly for 4 years, five beers would probably fail to produce the response they remembered as freshmen. Perhaps seven or eight beers would be needed to produce such a response. Clearly they have developed a tolerance to alcohol.

Furthermore, tolerance developed for one drug may carry over to another drug within the same general category. This phenomenon is known as **cross-tolerance.** The heavy abuser of alcohol might require a larger dose of a preoperative sedative to become relaxed before surgery. The tolerance to alcohol "crosses over" to the other depressant drug.

cross-tolerance
transfer of tolerance from one drug to another within the same general category.

Drugs whose misuse or abuse can relatively quickly lead to both physical and psychological dependency are the depressants (barbiturates, tranquilizers, and alcohol), narcotics (the opiates: derivatives of the Oriental poppy—heroin, morphine, and codeine), and synthetic narcotics (Demerol and Methadone). Drugs whose misuse or abuse can lead only to various degrees of psychological dependency are the stimulants (amphetamines, caffeine, and, perhaps, cocaine), hallucinogens (LSD, peyote, mescaline, and marijuana), and inhalants (glues, gases, and petroleum products).

Drug Misuse and Abuse

When drugs are inappropriately consumed or are administered in improper amounts, drug misuse has occurred. *Drug misuse* generally is considered a short-term condition. Drug misuse can be either intentional or accidental. The following list gives examples of drug misuse:

Borrowing a friend's prescription to treat yourself

Sharing a prescription medicine among family members

Consuming alcohol concurrently with any other drug

Consuming alcohol immediately before driving an automobile

Consuming any combination of prescription drugs without consulting a physician

Self-medication—not following label directions

Experimentation with any illegal drug

The prescribing of an inappropriate drug by a physician

Writing the incorrect dosage by a physician

A nurse's inappropriate administration of a drug

Drug abuse, however, is the chronic, deliberate, and excessive use of any drug. Drug abuse implies a longer term, more persistent use of a drug without regard to any established medical practice. A further implication is that drug abuse is in some way detrimental to the abuser, persons around the abuser, or to society in general.

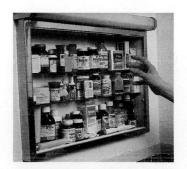

Drug misuse can lead to drug abuse.

DYNAMICS OF DRUG USE—WHY PEOPLE USE DRUGS

The reasons people give when asked why they use drugs are about as varied as the number of drugs people consume. One publication lists over 20 common reasons why people use drugs[6] (see the margin). We would like to focus on four reasons why we think people choose to use drugs.

Society tells us that we should avoid pain whenever possible. Since early childhood we have been behaviorally programmed to believe that substances are available that can reduce and even prevent pain. Now we are living in a "Rolaids generation." Relief from our pain can readily be found in drug products. The field of dentistry provides a good example. Many dentists are able to drill and fill a cavity with virtually no pain to the patient. Procaine (Novocain) is used to numb the appropriate location. Even before the Novocain is used, a topical anesthetic is used to reduce the small pain noticed when the Novocain is injected.

Perhaps the effectiveness of drugs in relieving physical pain has led us to the belief that they can also alleviate psychological pain. We gradually learn that the pain of an unhappy home life, the pressure of athletic competition, a broken relationship, or a boring job need not be tolerated. We learn to escape from stressors by chemically altering the function of our central nervous system. Unfortunately this alteration is usually temporary and fails to help us cope effectively with the roots of such problems.

Drugs are so widely available. Despite the efforts of law enforcement officials, most people have little trouble finding chemical substances that will alter their feelings, moods, and perceptions. Easy availability promotes the notion that nearly everyone uses drugs. For some curious people it is especially difficult to resist peer influence when drugs are so widely available.

The pleasurable effects of drug use are reinforcing. Psychoactive drugs alter feelings and perceptions. Many times these alterations produce a high level of temporarily pleasurable feelings (euphoria). Whether taken for escape or pleasure, drug use tends to reinforce future drug use. Unfortunately a significant number of users are not aware that many similar pleasurable sensations can be achieved through physical exercise, relaxation, or meditation.

People are inherent risk takers. The thrill of taking a risk is especially exciting. More importantly, being successful at taking a risk can be exhilarating. When we were small children, our first ride on a merry-go-round was so exciting that we begged for another ride. Many people continue a lifelong search for thrills and kicks—through daredevil activities or drug experimentation.

THE ADDICTIVE PERSONALITY

Experts in the field of chemical dependency have sought explanations as to why persons develop dependency relationships with a variety of drugs. Factors investigated include genetic predispositions, altered neurophysiological processes, familial influences, and personality traits. Chapter 8 will explore the role of inheritance in the development of alcohol dependency, whereas this section will consider the role of personality in use of drugs, particularly marijuana.

In an excellent review of studies on the topic of the role of personality in the use of marijuana, Ray[4] reported that a pattern of deviance-related traits emerges

Why People Use Drugs

Medication
To get high (a buzz)
To be cool
To get rid of pain
To experiment
Peer pressure
Family problems
To calm nerves
To get down
To escape
Because of friends
Because they like it
Because they are addicted
To work better
To be alert
Because they are bored
To hurt themselves
To hurt someone else
To get in a good mood
For a dare
Fear of stopping
To commit suicide

in those who use marijuana. The adolescents most likely to begin marijuana use, or perhaps use of other drugs, will be more noncomformist in their outlook on life than others of their age. These adolescents will have tendencies to deny religion, have lower grades in school, reject the importance of education, be politically nonconforming, and reject social values such as the work ethic and conformity.

If these traits are interpreted as the "addictive personality," then such a personality may well exist. If, on the other hand, these traits are seen as personality factors that may only correlate with drug use, then there may not be a truly addictive personality.[7] It is clear that carefully structured longitudinal studies designed to determine causation need to be done in greater numbers in the future.

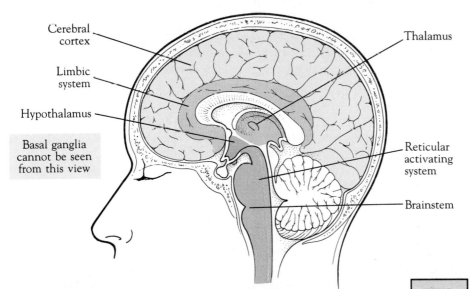

Cerebral cortex

Limbic system

Hypothalamus

Basal ganglia cannot be seen from this view

Thalamus

Reticular activating system

Brainstem

Figure 7-1
Psychoactive drugs alter the function of the brain and nervous system. (Refer to the key at the bottom of the chart for the corresponding drug agents.)

NEUROANATOMY	FUNCTION	DRUG AGENTS
Reticular activating system	Old sensory system—activates cortex in response to incoming stimuli	1+ 2− 3−
Hypothalamus	Control center for autonomic nervous system—interfaces CNS/ANS with endocrine system via pituitary	2− 3−
Brainstem	Control of vital functions (respiration, cardiac, blood pressure)—houses reticular activating system, sleep/wake center, coordination of motor functions	1+ 2− 3−
Cerebral cortex	Higher intellectual function, learning higher motor functions, elaboration (association) of sensory information	1+ 2− 4+
Basal ganglia	Execution of semiautomatic motor activity (body language)	3−
Thalamus	Two-gate controlling interchange among all CNS centers	2− 3− 4+
Limbic system	Connects cortex to thalamus—control of emotional states	3− 4−

Key: 1 Stimulants; 2 Depressants; 3 Opiates; 4 Hallucinogens; 5 Inhalants*; + Enhances normal level of function; − Decreases normal level of function.
*Because of the variety of pharmacological agents delivered as inhalants (anesthetics, toxic solvents), no general influence can be assigned.

DRUG IMPACT ON THE CENTRAL NERVOUS SYSTEM

To the *neuroscientist,* human behavior is explained on the basis of nervous system function. A behavior results when a stimulus from the internal or external environment is received by *sensory receptors,* transmitted to the brain for interpretation, and transformed into mental, muscular, or glandular activity. The continuous function of your nervous system allows you to monitor the environment and respond appropriately. Psychoactive drugs alter the quality of the monitoring, interpreting, and responding processes. (See Figure 7-1).

To better understand the disruption caused by the actions of psychoactive drugs, a general knowledge of the normal functioning of the nervous system's basic unit, the *neuron,* is required. As depicted in Figure 7-2, stimuli from the internal or external environment are received by the appropriate sensory receptor, perhaps an organ, such as an eye or an ear.

Once sensed, these stimuli are converted into electrical impulses. These impulses are then directed along the neuron's **dendrite** and **axon** toward the *synaptic junction* near an adjacent neuron. On arrival at the **synapse,** the electrical impulses stimulate the production and release of chemical messengers called *neurotransmitters.*[8] These neurotransmitters "transfer" the electrical impulses from one neuron to the dendrites of adjoining neurons. Thus step-by-step neurons composing the nervous system function in a coordinated fashion to send information to the brain for interpretation and to relay appropriate response commands outward to the tissues of the body.

Because the nervous system is not a continuous system (as is the circulatory system) but is fragmented at each synaptic junction, the role of neurotransmitters is critically important to the transfer of information within the system. A substance that has the ability to alter some aspect of transmitter function holds the potential for causing a major disruption to the otherwise normally functioning system. Psychoactive drugs are capable of exerting these disruptive influences on the neurotransmitters.

Since the function of neurotransmitters is not yet completely understood and an in-depth discussion of what is understood lies beyond the scope of this textbook, we will present only a brief list of the possible influences that a psychoactive drug can have on neurotransmitter function. Any psychoactive drug can potentially have the following effects.

- *Block the synthesis of the chemical neurotransmitters,* thus slowing or even stopping the transfer of specific stimuli within the nervous system
- *Produce an altered neurotransmitter that mimics the normally occurring transmitter,* thus allowing a distorted view of the stimuli or an inappropriate response to be transmitted to the brain
- *Allow a continuous, slow release of the neurotransmitter,* thus delaying the transfer of a particular stimulus within the nervous system
- *Alter the deactivation of the neurotransmitter,* thus allowing the receptors of the postsynaptic neuron to remain in the excited or inhibited state for a prolonged period

Undoubtedly no single psychoactive drug causes all four dimensions of neurotransmitter alteration to occur, yet each psychoactive drug has some specific influence on neurotransmitter function. In this sense mind-altering drugs are not mystical substances; they are predictable agents that alter the nervous system.

---

dendrite
portion of a neuron that receives electrical stimuli from adjacent neurons; neurons typically have several such branches or extensions.

axon
portion of a neuron that conducts electrical impulses to the dendrites of adjacent neurons; neurons typically have one axon.

synapse (synaptic junction)
location at which an electrical impulse from one neuron is transmitted to an adjacent neuron.

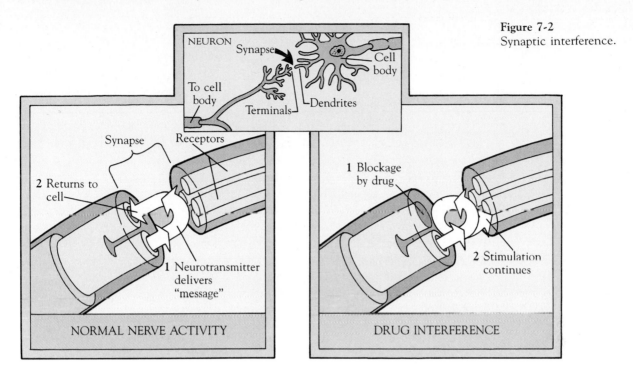

Figure 7-2
Synaptic interference.

The degree to which these changes in the complex chemical environments of the nervous system are harmful has not been fully assessed, but clearly the behaviors that result from drug use potentially can seriously alter your health and your productive, satisfying life.

DRUG CLASSIFICATIONS

Drugs can be categorized by the nature of the physiological effect they exert. Most drugs fall into one of five general categories: stimulants, depressants, hallucinogens, narcotics, and inhalants (see Table 7-1).

Stimulants

In general **stimulants** excite or increase the activity of the central nervous system (CNS). Also called "uppers," stimulants alert the CNS by increasing heart rate, blood pressure, and brain function. Users feel uplifted and less fatigued. Examples of stimulant drugs include caffeine, amphetamines, and cocaine. Stimulants produce psychological dependency and tolerance relatively quickly, but seem incapable of producing significant physical dependency when judged by life-threatening withdrawal symptoms.

stimulants
psychoactive drugs that stimulate the function of the central nervous system.

Caffeine

Caffeine, the tasteless drug found in chocolate, some soft drinks, coffee, tea, some aspirin products, and over-the-counter "stay-awake" pills is a relatively harmless stimulant when consumed in moderate amounts (see Table 7-2). Many coffee drinkers could not start their days successfully without the benefit of a cup or two of coffee in the morning.

Table 7-1   **Psychoactive Drug Categories**

Drugs	Trade or Other Names	Medical Uses	Physical Dependence	Psychological Dependence
Stimulants				
Cocaine*	Coke, flake, snow, crack	Local anesthetic	Possible	High
Amphetamines	Biphetamine, Delcobese, Desoxyn, Dexedrine, Mediatric	Hyperkinesis, narcolepsy, weight control	Possible	High
Phenmetrazine	Preludin			
Methylphenidate	Ritalin			
Other stimulants	Adipex, Bacarate, Cylert, Didrex, Ionamin, Plegine, PreSate, Sanorex, Tenuate, Tepanil, Voranil			
Depressants				
Chloral hydrate	Noctec, Somnos	Hypnotic	Moderate	Moderate
Barbiturates	Amobarbital, Phenobarbital, Butisol, Phenoxbarbital, Secobarbital, Tuinal	Anesthetic, anticonvulsant, sedative, hypnotic	High-moderate	High-moderate
Glutethimide	Doriden	Sedative, hypnotic	High	High
Methaqualone	Optimil, Parest, Quaalude, Somnafec, Sopor	Sedative, hypnotic	High	High
Benzodiazepines	Ativan, Azene, Clonopin, Dalmane, Diazepam, Librium, Serax, Tranxene, Valium, Verstran	Anti-anxiety, anticonvulsant, sedative, hypnotic	Low	Low
Other depressants	Equanil, Miltown, Noludar Placidyl, Valmid	Anti-anxiety, sedative, hypnotic	Moderate	Moderate
Hallucinogens				
LSD	Acid, microdot	None	None	Degree unknown
Mescaline and peyote	Mesc, buttons, cactus	None	None	Degree unknown
Amphetamine variants (designer drugs)	2,5-DMA, PMA, STP, MDA, MDMA, TMA, DOM, DOP	None	Unknown	Degree unknown
Phencyclidine	PCP, Angel Dust, Hog	Veterinary anesthetic	Degree unknown	High
Phencyclidine analogs	PCE, PCPy, TCP	None	Degree unknown	Degree unknown

*Designated a narcotic under the Controlled Substances Act.

Tolerance	Duration of Effects (in hours)	Usual Methods of Administration	Possible Effects	Effects of Overdose	Withdrawal Syndrome
Possible	1-2	Sniffed, injected, smoked	Increased alertness, excitation, euphoria, increased pulse rate and blood pressure, insomnia, loss of appeitite	Agitation, increase in body temperature, hallucinations, convulsions, possible death	Apathy, long periods of sleep, irritability, depression, disorientation
Yes	2-4	Oral, injected			
		Oral			
Possible	5-8	Oral	Slurred speech, disorientation, drunken behavior without odor of alcohol	Shallow respiration, cold and clammy skin, dilated pupils, weak and rapid pulse, coma, possible death	Anxiety, insomnia, tremors, delirium, convulsions, possible death
Yes	1-16	Oral, injected			
Yes	4-8	Oral, injected			
Yes	4-8	Oral, injected			
Yes	4-8	Oral, injected			
Yes	4-8	Oral, injected			
Possible	8-12	Oral	Illusions and hallucinations, poor perception of time and distance	Longer, more intense "trip" episodes, psychosis, possible death	Withdrawal syndrome not reported
Possible	8-12	Oral, injected			
Possible	Up to days	Oral, injected			
Possible	Variable	Smoked, oral, injected			
Possible	Variable	Smoked, oral, injected			

Continued.

Table 7-1   **Psychoactive Drug Categories—cont'd**

Drugs	Trade or Other Names	Medical Uses	Physical Dependence	Psychological Dependence
Hallucinogens—cont'd				
Marijuana	Pot, Acapulco gold, grass, reefer, sinsemilla, Thai sticks	Under investigation	Degree unknown	Moderate
Tetrahydrocannabinol	THC	Under investigation	Degree unknown	Moderate
Hashish	Hash	None	Degree unknown	Moderate
Hashish oil	Hash oil	None	Degree unknown	Moderate
Other hallucinogens	Bufotenine, Ibogaine, DMT, DET, psilocybin, psilocyn	None	None	Degree unknown
Narcotics				
Opium	Dover's Powder, Paregoric, Parepectolin	Analgesic, antidiarrheal	High	High
Morphine	Morphine, Pectoral Syrup	Analgesic, antitussive	High	High
Codeine	Codeine, Empirin Compound with Codeine, Robitussin A-C	Analgesic, antitussive	Moderate	Moderate
Heroin	Diacetylmorphine, horse, smack	Under investigation	High	High
Hydromorphone	Dilaudid	Analgesic	High	High
Meperidine (pethidine)	Demerol, Pethadol	Analgesic	High	High
Methadone	Dolophine, Methadone, Methadose	Analgesic, heroin substitute	High	High
Other narcotics	LAAM, Leitine, Levo-Dromoran, Percodan, Tussionex, Fentanyl, Darvon*, Talwin*, Lomotil	Analgesic, antidiarrheal, antitussive	High-low	High-low
Inhalants				
Anesthetic gases	Petroleum products, solvents, aerosols	Surgical anesthesia	No	Possible
Vasodilators (amyl nitrite, butyl nitrite)	Petroleum products, solvents, aerosols	None	No	Possible

*Not designated a narcotic under the Controlled Substances Act.

Tolerance	Duration of Effects (in hours)	Usual Methods of Administration	Possible Effects	Effects of Overdose	Withdrawal Syndrome
Yes	2-4	Smoked, oral	Euphoria, relaxed inhibitions, increased appetite, disoriented behavior	Fatigue, paranoia, possible psychosis	Insomnia, hyperactivity, and decreased appetite occasionally reported
Yes	2-4	Smoked, oral			
Yes	2-4	Smoked, oral			
Yes	2-4	Smoked, oral			
Possible	Variable	Oral, injected, smoked, sniffed			
Yes	3-6	Oral, smoked	Euphoria, drowsiness, respiratory depression, constricted pupils, nausea	Slow and shallow breathing, clammy skin, convulsions, coma, possible death	Watery eyes, runny nose, yawning, loss of appetite, irritability, tremors, panic, chills and sweating, cramps, nausea
Yes	3-6	Oral, injected, smoked			
Yes	3-6	Oral, injected			
Yes	3-6	Injected, sniffed, smoked			
Yes	3-6	Oral, injected			
Yes	3-6	Oral, injected			
Yes	12-24	Oral, injected			
Yes	Variable	Oral injected			
Unlikely	Variable (minutes to hours)	Inhaled	Intoxication, excitation, disorientation, aggression, hallucination, variable effects	Cardiac or respiratory failure, shock, possible death	None reported
Unlikely	Variable (minutes to hours)	Inhaled	Intoxication, excitation, disorientation, aggression, hallucination, variable effects	Cardiac or respiratory failure, shock, possible death	None reported

Table 7-2   Caffeine Content of Selected Beverages, Foods, and Drugs

	Mean (mg)	Range (mg)
Coffee (5 oz)		
Automatic drip	137	110-164
Nonautomatic drip	124	106-145
Instant	60	47-68
Instant, decaffeinated	3	2-5
Percolated, automatic	117	99-134
Percolated, nonautomatic	108	93-130
Tea (5 oz)		
Brewed 5 minutes	46	39-50
Imported, brewed 5 minutes	65	63-67
Decaffeinated, brewed 5 minutes	1	
Soft drinks (12 oz)		
Cola		30-46
Decaffeinated cola	tr	
Jolt	72	
Mountain Dew	54	
Chocolate		
Chocolate Kisses (6 pieces)	5	
Milk chocolate (1.02 oz bar)	5	
Chocolate ice cream (2/3 cup)	5	
Cocoa beverage (6 oz)	5	2-8
Nonprescription drugs		
Anacin	64	32
Cope		32
Dexatrim	200	200
Dietac	200	200
Dristan	32	16
Excedrin	130	65
Midol	64	32
No Doz	200	100
Vanquish	66	33
Vivarin	200	200

One recent scholarly summary of research on caffeine consumption said, "There is no persuasive evidence that moderate amounts of caffeine are harmful to the average adult."[9] However, the report also indicated that excessive consumption (equivalent to 10 or more cups of coffee daily) could lead to anxiety, diarrhea, restlessness, delayed onset of sleep or frequent awakening, headache, and heart palpitations.

Widespread concerns in the 1970s about a possible link between caffeine consumption and the development of birth defects, ulcers, heartburn, cardiovascular disease, cancer, and fibrocystic breast disease have moderated considerably. Studies completed in the 1980s have been unable to find positive correlations between caffeine consumption and these diseases in human subjects.[9]

Amphetamines

Amphetamines have recently come under attack for their ineffectiveness as weight loss aids. Their value as appetite suppressants appears to diminish after a few weeks of use. Occasionally amphetamines are used medically in the treatment of **narcolepsy** and **hyperactivity.** Amphetamines assist in the management of hyperactivity by stimulating the reticular activating system to filter out nonsignificant stimuli. By not being bombarded with visual or auditory stimuli, the person is better able to focus on a given task. College students during final exam week and truck drivers on long hauls have been known to procure amphetamines to help them combat fatigue and to increase alertness.

Cocaine

Cocaine, perhaps the strongest of the stimulant drugs, has received much media attention. The effects of cocaine are of short duration—from 5 to 30 minutes (see Figure 7-3). Regardless of the form in which it is consumed, cocaine produces an immediate near-orgasmic "rush," or feeling of exhilaration. This euphoria is quickly followed by a period of marked depression. Used occasionally

narcolepsy
sleep-related disorder in which a person has a recurrent, overwhelming, and uncontrollable desire to sleep.

hyperactivity
above-normal physical movement; often accompanied by an inability to concentrate well on a specified task; also called hyperkinesis.

Figure 7-3
Cocaine's effect on the body.

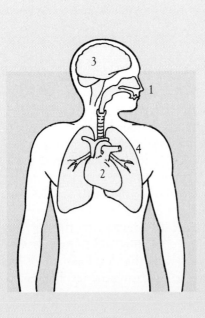

1 | As cocaine is snorted, nasal vessels immediately constrict and prohibit about 40% of the drug from entering the body. The remaining 60% enters the bloodstream.

2 | Electrical impulses that regulate rhythmic pumping are impaired. Beating becomes irregular (arrhythmia). The heart will no longer supply itself with enough oxygenated blood.

3 | Dopamine and norepinephrine are released into the brain, producing a feeling of euphoria and confidence. Electrical signals to the heart are distorted; heart rate and pulse increase. A seizure may occur, causing coma and breathing stoppage.

4 | Blood circulation is out of control. The heart may simply flutter and stop, or it can be pumping so little oxygenated blood to the brain that the brain dies and the heart stops beating.

Snorting lines of cocaine.

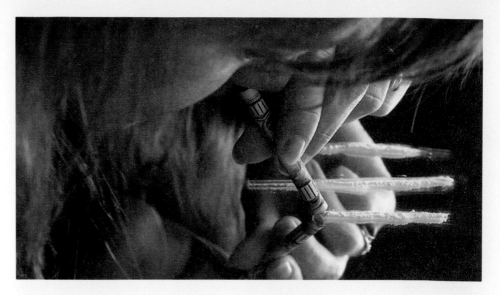

as a topical anesthetic, today cocaine is generally inhaled (snorted), injected, or smoked (as freebase or crack). There is much scientific evidence to indicate that users quickly develop a strong psychological dependency to cocaine. There is increasing, though not conclusive, evidence that physical dependency is also quickly developed.

Cocaine is extracted from the leaves of the coca plant, a small bush that grows in Bolivia and Peru. The Indian natives in these high-altitude regions commonly chew the leaves as a stimulant in the oxygen-weak environment. Yes, it is true, as you may have heard, that the original Coca-Cola beverage did contain minute amounts of coca bush extracts. However, cocaine was removed from Coca-Cola in 1903, and cocaine became an illegal drug in 1914 in the United States.[4]

Freebasing *Freebasing* and the use of *crack* cocaine represent the most recent techniques for maximizing the psychoactive effects of the drug. Freebasing first requires the common form of powdered cocaine (cocaine hydrochloride) to be chemically altered (alkalized). This altered form is then dissolved in a solvent, such as ether or benzene. This liquid solution is heated to evaporate the solvent. The heating process leaves the freebase cocaine in a powder form that can then be smoked, often through a waterpipe. Because of the large surface area of the lungs, smoking cocaine facilitates fast absorption into the bloodstream.

One danger in freebasing cocaine is the risk related to the solvents used. Ether is a highly volatile solvent capable of exploding and causing serious burns. Benzene is a known carcinogen associated with the development of leukemia. Clearly, neither solvent can be used without increasing the level of risk normally associated with cocaine use.

Crack In contrast to freebase cocaine, crack is obtained by combining cocaine hydrochloride with common baking soda. When this pastelike mixture is allowed to dry, a small rocklike crystalline material remains. This crack is heated in the bowl of a small pipe, and the vapors are inhaled into the lungs. Currently a single dose of crack sells for $10 to $20. Some crack users spend $100 or more a day to maintain their habit.

The influence of crack is almost instantaneous. Within 10 seconds after inhalation, cocaine reaches the central nervous system and influences the action of several neurotransmitters at specific sites in the brain. As with other forms of cocaine use, convulsions, seizures, respiratory distress, and cardiac failure have been reported with this sudden, extensive stimulation of the nervous system.

Within about 6 minutes, the stimulating effect of crack is completely expended and users frequently enter into a state of depression. Dependency develops within a few weeks as users consume more crack in response to the short duration of stimulation and rapid onset of depression.

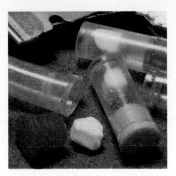

Vials of crack cocaine.

Depressants

Depressants (or sedatives) are those drugs that tend to sedate or slow down CNS function. Drugs included in this category are alcohol, barbiturates, and tranquilizers. Depressants produce tolerance in abusers, as well as strong psychological and physical dependence. (For a discussion of alcohol, see Chapter 8.)

Barbiturates

Barbiturates are the so-called sleeping compounds. They depress the CNS to the point where the user drops off to sleep or—as is the case with surgical anesthetics—the patient becomes anesthetized. Medically barbiturates are used in widely varied dosages as an anesthetic and for treatment of anxiety, insomnia, and epilepsy.[4] Regular use of a barbiturate drug quickly produces tolerance—even to the point where such a high dosage is required that the user finds the drug effects linger through the next morning. Some abusers then begin to alternate barbiturates with stimulants, producing a vicious cycle of dependency. Other misusers combine alcohol and barbiturates or tranquilizers, inadvertently producing toxic, even lethal results—witness the fates of Marilyn Monroe and Karen Quinlan. Abrupt withdrawal from barbiturate use frequently produces a deadly withdrawal syndrome.

Methaqualone (Quaalude, "ludes," Sopor) was developed as a sedative that supposedly would not have the dependency properties of other barbiturates.[4] While this did not happen, Quaaludes were occasionally prescribed for anxious patients. Today compounds resembling Quaaludes are manufactured in home laboratories and illegally sold as products to combine with small amounts of alcohol for an inexpensive, drunklike effect.

Tranquilizers

Tranquilizers are depressants that are intended to reduce anxiety and to relax persons who are having problems coping with the stressors of life. They are not specifically designed to produce sleep, but rather to help people cope during their waking hours. Such tranquilizers are termed *minor tranquilizers,* of which diazepam (Valium) and chlordiazepoxide (Librium) may be the most commonly prescribed examples.

Some tranquilizers are further designed for controlling hospitalized psychotic patients who may have suicidal tendencies or who are potential threats to others.[10] These *major tranquilizers* subdue people physically but permit them to remain conscious. Their use is generally limited to institutional settings. All tranquilizers hold the potential to produce both physical and psychological dependency and tolerance, but not as quickly as barbiturates.

Marijuana.

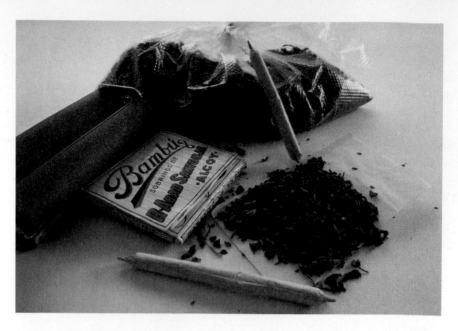

Hallucinogens

As the name suggests, hallucinogenic drugs produce hallucinations—perceived distortions of reality. Also known as *psychedelic* drugs or *phantasticants*, **hallucinogens** reached their height of popularity during the 1960s.[10] At that time young people were encouraged to use hallucinogenic drugs to "expand the mind," "reach an altered state," or "discover reality." Not all of the reality distortions, or "trips," were pleasant. Many users reported "bummers," or trips of negative, frightful distortions.

Hallocinogenc drugs include laboratory-produced lysergic acid diethylamide (LSD), mescaline (from the peyote cactus plant), and psilocybin (from a particular genus of mushroom). Consumption of hallucinogens seems not to produce physical dependency but rather mild levels of psychological dependency. The development of tolerance is questionable. **Synesthesia,** a process in which users report "hearing a color, smelling music, or touching a taste," is sometimes produced in hallucinogen use.

The long-term effects of hallucinogenic drug misuse and abuse are not fully understood. Questions about genetic abnormalities in offspring, *fecundity*, sex drive and performance, and the development of personality disorders have not been fully answered. One phenomenon that has been identified and documented is the development of *flashbacks*—the unpredictable return to a psychedelic trip that occurred months or even years earlier. Flashbacks are thought to result from the accumulation of a drug within body cells.

LSD

The most well-known hallucinogen is lysergic acid diethylamide (LSD). This laboratory-produced drug was the focus of a great deal of research and recreational use in the 1960s and early 1970s. LSD's ability to produce a psychedelic (mind-viewing) effect was scientifically investigated in conjunction with therapy for mental disorders, the treatment of alcoholism, and as an aid to persons with

hallucinogens
psychoactive drugs capable of producing hallucinations (distortions of reality).

synesthesia
perceptual process in which a stimulus produces a response from a different sensory modality.

terminal illnesses. Illicit use of LSD formed the basis of the "turn on, tune in, and drop out" drug-based religion of Dr. Timothy Leary in the 1960s.

As a pharmacologic agent, LSD is an extremely potent hallucinogen—only a small amount of the drug is required to produce a maximal response. How the drug exerts its influence on the central nervous system is not fully understood. It appears, however, to influence the action of serotonin, a neurotransmitter associated with the sympathetic actions of the autonomic nervous system. Excitatory responses observed in conjunction with LSD use include dilation of the pupils and hypertension. Interestingly, LSD can also generate inhibitory responses which slow the body's processes. Tolerance develops rapidly with daily LSD use, but addiction does not occur.

The most important pharmacological property of LSD is its altering of the perceptual processing abilities of the nervous system. Altered perceptions of shapes, images, time, sound, and body form occur in people during an LSD trip. These altered perceptions occur within several minutes of ingestion of the drug and generally subside within 6 to 9 hours. The qualitative nature of these experiences varies from person to person. In well-adjusted individuals the LSD trip is most often perceived to be expansive, or regarded as having been positive and enjoyable. The bad trip is more often observed in a person whose level of emotional stability is suspect even during periods of nondrug use. Flashbacks occur in some persons following LSD use.

Marijuana

Marijuana has been labeled a mild hallucinogen for a number of years. It is also known to produce mild effects like those of stimulants and depressants. However, the recent implications of marijuana in a large number of traffic fatalities make this drug one whose consumption should be carefully considered. Marijuana is actually a wild plant (*Cannabis sativa*) whose fibers were originally used in the manufacture of hemp rope. When the leafy material and small stems are crushed and dried, users often smoke the mixture in rolled cigarettes (joints) or pipes. The resins collected from scraping the flowering tops of the plant yield a marijuana product called *hashish*, or simply hash, commonly smoked in a pipe.

Smoking pot.

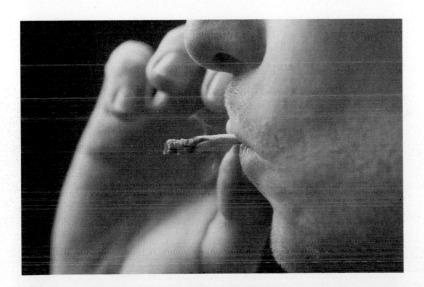

The potency of marijuana's hallucinogenic effect is determined by the percentage of the active ingredient THC, or tetrahydrocannabinol, present in the product. Hashish contains a higher percentage of THC; thus its psychoactive effects are much greater than an equivalent amount of marijuana. Through selective plant breeding, the percentage of THC in marijuana today is estimated to be considerably higher than in the 1960s, when "pot" began to soar in popularity among young people. According to the director of the National Institute on Drug Abuse Marijuana Project, today's marijuana averages 3% to 4% THC (with some samples exceeding 10%), whereas earlier marijuana averaged less than 0.5% THC.[11] THC is a fat soluble substance and thus is absorbed and retained in fat tissues within the body. Before being excreted, THC can remain in the body for up to a month. With the sophistication of today's drug tests, trace amounts of THC can be detected in the bloodstream for as long as 6 months after consumption. It is possible that the THC that comes from passive inhalation (for example, during an indoor rock concert) can be detected.

Once marijuana is consumed, its effects vary from person to person. Being "high" or "stoned" or "wrecked" means different things to different persons. Many persons report heightened sensitivity to music, cravings for particular foods, and a relaxed mood. Widespread consensus about marijuana's behavioral effects includes four probabilities: (1) users must learn to recognize what a marijuana high is like, (2) marijuana impairs short-term memory, (3) users overestimate the passage of time, and (4) users lose the ability to maintain focused attention on a task.[4]

The long-term effects of marijuana use are still being studied. Chronic abuse may lead to an *amotivational syndrome* in some people. The irritating effects of the marijuana smoke on lung tissue are more pronounced than those of cigarette smoke, and some of the over 400 chemicals in marijuana are now linked to lung cancer development. Long-term marijuana use is also associated with damage to the immune system, damage to both male and female reproductive systems, and an increase in birth defects in babies born to parents who smoke marijuana.[4] The effect of long-term marijuana use on sexual behavior is not fully understood. Since the drug clearly can distort perceptions and thus perceptual ability (especially when combined with alcohol), its misuse or abuse by automobile drivers clearly jeopardizes the lives of many innocent persons.

In recent years, the only medicinal uses for marijuana have been (1) to relieve the nausea from chemotherapy and (2) to lower the buildup of pressure in the eyes of glaucoma patients. However, a variety of other drugs, many of which are considered more effective, are also used for these two purposes.

Phencyclidine (PCP)

Phencyclidine (PCP, Angel Dust) is a drug that has been classified variously as a hallucinogen, a stimulant, a depressant, and an anesthetic. PCP was studied for years during the 1950s and 1960s and found to be an unsuitable animal and human anesthetic. PCP is now known to be an extremely unpredictable drug. Easily manufactured in home laboratories in tablet or powder form, PCP can be injected, inhaled, taken orally, or smoked. The effects vary. Some users report mild euphoria, although most users report bizarre perceptions, paranoid feelings, and aggressive behavior. PCP overdose may cause convulsions, cardiovascular collapse, and damage to the brain's respiratory center.

In a number of cases, the aggressive behavior caused by PCP has led users to commit violent, brutal crimes against both friends and innocent strangers. PCP accumulates in cells and may stimulate bizarre behaviors months after initial use.

Narcotics

True **narcotics** (also called **opiates**) are derived from extracts of the Oriental poppy plant. Medically opiates are used to relieve pain and induce sleep. The unripe poppy pod produces a cream-colored juice called *opium.* Oriental users first dry the opium and then usually smoke it to achieve the psychoactive effects of euphoric relaxation. Additional narcotics include morphine, the active ingredient in opium. Medically, morphine is an extremely powerful painkiller.

narcotics (opiates)
psychoactive drugs derived from the Oriental poppy plant; narcotics serve to relieve pain and induce sleep.

Heroin

Heroin, a drug synthesized from morphine, is the most frequently abused narcotic. Once injected into a vein or "skin-popped" beneath the skin surface, heroin produces dreamlike euphoria in users and, like all narcotics, produces strong physical and psychological dependency and tolerance. As with other forms of illicit injectable drugs, the practice of sharing needles increases the likelihood of transmission of various communicable diseases, including hepatitis and AIDS (see Chapter 12). Abrupt withdrawal from narcotic use rarely produces death in abusers, but the discomfort during **cold turkey** withdrawal is reported to be overwhelming.

cold turkey
withdrawal discomfort associated with abrupt discontinuance of a drug.

Black tar, an extremely pure and powerful form of Mexican heroin that looks like roofing tar, has become available in recent years. In comparison to the powdered heroin normally available on the street with a purity of approximately 2% to 6%, black tar has a purity of 60% to 90%. Additionally, this heroin is considerably cheaper than other forms, selling for about $2 per dose. Drug enforcement agencies are concerned that this more affordable heroin may make current problems with heroin even worse.

Synthetic narcotics

Meperidine (Demerol), a common postsurgery painkiller, and Methadone, the drug prescribed during the rehabilitation of heroin addicts, are both *synthetic narcotics.* These opiate-like drugs are manufactured in medical laboratories. They are not true narcotics because they do not originate from the Oriental poppy plant. Like true narcotics, however, these drugs can rapidly cause physical dependency to develop. One major criticism of Methadone rehabilitation programs is that they merely shift the addiction from heroin to methadone. Over the last 20 years, heroin abuse has remained at a fairly constant level in the United States, although many new abusers appear to be from the middle to upper social strata.

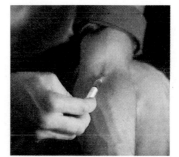

IV drug use increases the risk of contracting diseases, including AIDS.

Inhalants

This drug classification includes a variety of volatile (quickly evaporating) compounds that generally produce unpredictable, drunklike effects in users. Users of **inhalants** may further experience some degree of delusionary and hallucinogenic effects. Some users may become quite aggressive. Drugs in this category include anesthetic gases (chloroform, laughing gas, and ether), vasodilators (amyl nitrite and butyl nitrite), petroleum products and commercial solvents (gasoline, kero-

inhalants
psychoactive drugs that enter the body through inhalation.

sene, plastic cement, glue, typewriter correction fluid, paint, and paint thinner), and certain aerosols (found in some propelled spray products, fertilizers, and insecticides).

Frequently children misuse or abuse volatile substances to achieve a psychoactive effect. They find other drugs difficult to obtain. One example of a common inhalant is butyl nitrite, a vasodilator sometimes used in the management of coronary artery disease. This product can be legally sold as a room odorizer. Children purchase these "poppers" and inhale the gas to achieve a variety of psychoactive effects.

Most of the danger in using inhalants lies with the damaging, sometimes fatal, effects on the respiratory system. Furthermore, users may unknowingly place themselves in potentially dangerous situations because of the drunklike hallucinogenic effects. Aggressive behavior might also make users dangerous to themselves and others.

Designer drugs

FDA Schedule 1
list comprising drugs that hold a high potential for abuse but have no medical use.

In recent years, chemists who produce many of the illicit drugs in home laboratories have managed to design versions of drugs listed on **FDA Schedule 1.** These *designer drugs* are similar to the controlled drugs on the FDA Schedule 1 but are sufficiently different that they escape governmental control. Designer drugs are said to produce effects similar to their controlled drug counterparts.

People who consume designer drugs do so at great risk, because the manufacturing of these drugs is an unknown process. The neurophysiological impact of these homemade drugs can be quite dangerous. So far, a synthetic heroin product (MPPP) and several amphetamine derivatives with hallucinogenic properties have been designed for the unwary drug consumer.

STP (DOM), MDA, and MDMA (Ecstasy) are examples of types of hallucinogenic designer drugs. These drugs produce mild LSD-like hallucinogenic experiences. Experts are particularly concerned that MDMA can produce strong psychological dependency and deplete serotonin, an important excitatory neurotransmitter associated with a state of alertness.[4]

PSYCHOACTIVE DRUG POSTULATES

A *postulate* is an underlying hypothesis or statement that can safely be accepted as valid. The following six postulates refer to general responses that take place when people consume drugs. Obviously every effect or response to a drug depends on which drug is consumed, the nature of the user, and the environmental setting in which the drug is consumed. With this introduction, one noted drug educator believes these six postulates can safely be said about all psychoactive drugs.[12]

1 *A drug's effect on a person will depend on the influence the drug makes on the user's brain and spinal cord.* The regions of the brain that are targeted by the particular drug will reflect the functions that will be altered. The user's coordination, mood, perceptions, respirations, heart rate, nerve pathways, and body temperature may be changed if control centers in the central nervous system are influenced.

2 *Psychoactive drug effects vary with the dose.* Generally the higher the quantity of a drug consumed, the greater the response or effect exhibited by the user.

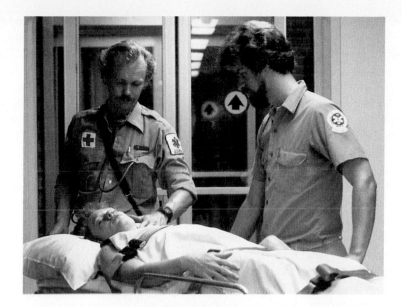

Drug overdoses are potentially life threatening.

Furthermore, drugs taken in various combinations and dosages can alter and perhaps intensify the effects.

A **synergistic drug effect** is a dangerous consequence that can occur when different drugs in the same general category are taken at the same time. The combined effect produces an exaggeration of each individual drug's effects. For example, the combined use of alcohol and tranquilizers will produce a synergistic effect greater than the total effect of each of the two drugs taken separately. In this instance a much-exaggerated, perhaps fatal sedation will occur. In a simplistic sense, "one plus one equals four or five."

When taken at or near the same time, drug combinations produce a variety of effects. Some drug combinations produce an additive effect, other combinations produce a potentiating effect,[5] and still others produce an antagonistic effect. When two or more drugs are taken and the result is merely a combined total effect of each drug, the result is an **additive effect.** The sum of the effects is not exaggerated. In a sense, "one plus one plus one equals three."

When one drug produces an intensified action of a second drug, the first drug is said to have a **potentiated effect** on the second drug. One popular drug-taking activity in the 1970s was the consumption of Quaaludes and beer. Quaaludes potentiated the inhibition-releasing, sedative effects of alcohol. This particular drug combination produced an inexpensive, but potentially fatal, drunklike euphoria in the user.

An **antagonistic effect** is an opposite effect one drug can have on another drug. One drug may be able to reduce or nullify another drug's influence on the body. Knowledge of this principle has been useful in the medical treatment of certain drug overdoses, as in the use of tranquilizers to relieve the effects of LSD or other hallucinogenic drugs.

3 *For each psychoactive drug, there is an effective dose, a toxic dose, and a lethal dose.* Each drug has a dose that a user will find achieves the desired effect. Of course, this **effective dose** will vary with each user and is usually difficult to pinpoint. Inaccurate estimation of this effective dose by the user can result in a **toxic dose** or a **lethal dose.**

synergistic drug effect
heightened, exaggerated effect produced by the concurrent use of two or more drugs.

additive effect
combined (but not exaggerated) effect produced by the concurrent use of two or more drugs.

potentiated effect
phenomenon whereby the use of one drug intensifies the effect of a second drug.

antagonistic effect
effect produced when one drug nullifies (reduces, offsets) the effects of a second drug.

effective dose
dose level that produces a desired effect.

toxic dose
dose level that produces a poisonous effect.

lethal dose
dose level capable of causing death.

4 *The higher the dose, the less important the nondrug factors become in determining a drug's effects.* The mind-set of the user and the user's environmental surroundings will have less bearing on a drug's effects as the dose is increased. For example, the consumption of eight tranquilizer capsules would surely produce a depressive effect (perhaps a lethal effect) on a person, even if that person were to be standing in front of a firing squad! In such an instance the nondrug (stimulating) factor of standing in front of a firing squad would be entirely offset by the large dose of tranquilizer.

Of course, the opposite phenomenon is equally true. At low dose levels, the more important the nondrug factors become in determining a psychoactive drug's effects. For example, when you are in a comfortable setting with close friends, the consumption of just one alcoholic beverage may make you feel and act rather inebriated. You can probably recall a group of high school students who, after having shared just one bottle of beer, appeared quite intoxicated. At this low dose level, the nondrug factors in the lives of these adolescents had more bearing on the resultant behavior than did the alcohol itself.

5 *At high dose levels, and for some individuals at much lower dose levels, all psychoactive drugs may be dangerous.* Although individual tolerance to drug use is highly variable, the dangerous consequences are most common when the user consumes high dosages. However, some persons may have a major tragic result during the first experimentation with a drug. Clearly each person's body chemistry is unique.

6 *The individual and social consequences of psychoactive drug use escalate with the frequency and duration of drug use.* This postulate supports the concept that increased involvement with drug use only serves to be a personal detriment or a detriment to society in general. Over the course of a person's life, increased psychoactive drug abuse cannot be shown to enhance a person's productivity, personal satisfaction, or relationships with others. In the final analysis the advancement of society is doubtful when increasing numbers of people continue to become dependent on psychoactive drugs, whether the drug is cocaine, alcohol, or nicotine.

SOCIETY'S RESPONSE TO DRUG USE

In the last 20 years society's response to illegal drug use has been one of growing concern. For the vast majority of adults, drug abuse has been seen as a clear danger to the fabric of society. This position has been supported by the development of community, school, state, and national organizations interested in the ultimate reduction of illegal drug use. These organizations have included such diverse groups as Parents Against Drugs, Parents for a Drug-Free Youth, Mothers Against Drunk Drivers (MADD), Drugs Anonymous, and the federal Drug Enforcement Administration. Certain groups have concentrated their efforts on education, others on enforcement, and still others on the development of laws and public policy.

The Omnibus Drug Enforcement Education and Control Act (signed into law in 1986) reflects a recent focus of society's concern about drug use. This act requested that $1.7 billion be spent for drug enforcement and education in 1987. Specific areas to be supported included penalties and fines for major traffickers, enforcement against the manufacturing and distribution of certain drugs, funding

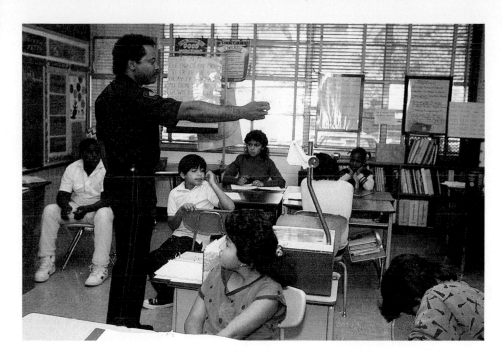

Drug education efforts often include law enforcement personnel.

of various federal and state programs, educational programs in local schools, military surveillance of drug trafficking, and international help for countries that cooperate with U.S. drug enforcement efforts.

Whereas the 1970s witnessed a reduction in penalties for recreational drug users and a drive to locate and prosecute pushers, the late 1980s is seeing renewed interest in curtailing even recreational drug use. Perhaps because drug use continues to flourish, some believe that greater legal action must be taken against those who create the demand for drugs. If this is the direction in which drug enforcement is headed, today's recreational users may find themselves at greater legal risk than is currently the case. The message is clear: If you are caught abusing illegal drugs, you can expect the full impact of the judicial system.

Unless significant changes in society's response to drug use take place soon, the disastrous effects of virtually uncontrolled drug abuse may continue. Families and communities will continue to be plagued by drug-related tragedies. Law enforcement officials will be pressed to the limit in their attempts to reduce drug flow. Our judicial system will be heavily burdened by thousands of court cases. Health care facilities could face overwhelming numbers of clients.

Without attempting to be overly dramatic, it is safe to say that drug use may continue to play an increasingly negative role in virtually all aspects of our society. This would be a sad legacy for us to leave our children.

Drug Testing

One clear response of society to the concern over drug use is the development and growing use of drug tests. At the present time, drug tests are available that detect the presence of over 150 different chemical compounds, including virtually all of the illicit drugs, alcohol, over-the-counter drugs, and many prescription medications in the user's body. Using urine samples, these tests can detect

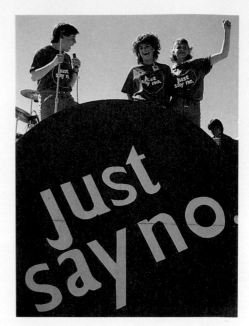

Will this approach reduce drug abuse?

the presence of various drugs for periods of time ranging from a few days to 4 weeks, as in the case of marijuana.

Interestingly, in 1987 the sixth most important employment criterion for graduating college seniors was the ability to pass a preemployment drug-screening test. Only verification of education, verification of past employment, physical examinations, personal references, and faculty references were given higher priority.[13] Most Fortune 500 companies, the armed forces, various government agencies, and nearly all athletic organizations have already implemented mandatory drug testing.

Do you think that the possibility of having to take such a drug test will have any impact on college students' use of drugs?

COLLEGE AND COMMUNITY SUPPORT SERVICES FOR DRUG DEPENDENCY

If students have drug problems and realize they need assistance, they can turn to various sources for help (see the box on p. 189). The assistance one might select could depend on the services available on campus or in the community near the university and the costs one is willing to pay for treatment services.

One recent approach to convince drug-dependent people to enter treatment programs is the use of *confrontation.* People who live or work with chemically dependent persons are being encouraged to confront them directly about their problems. Direct confrontation helps chemically dependent persons realize the impact of their behaviors on others. Once chemically dependent persons realize that others will no longer tolerate their behaviors, the likelihood of their entering treatment programs is increased significantly. Although effective, this approach is very stressful for family members and friends and may require the assistance of professionals in the field of chemical dependence. These professionals can be contacted at a drug treatment center in your area.

National Groups and Hotlines

NATIONAL GROUPS

- PRIDE (Parents' Resource Institute for Drug Education): Atlanta, (800) 241-7946, in Georgia (404) 658-2548
- National Federation of State High School Associations Target Programs: Kansas City, Mo, (816) 464-5400
- National Health Information Clearinghouse: (800) 336-4797
- National Drug Information Clearinghouse: (301) 443-6500
- National Federation of Parents for Drug-Free Youth: Silver Spring, Md (800) 554-KIDS
- National Clearinghouse for Alcohol Information: (301) 468-2600
- Narcotics Anonymous: Van Nuys, Calif, (818) 780-3951
- ToughLove, Doylestown, Pa (215) 348-7090

HOTLINES

- Action/PRIDE Drug information system: (800) 241-7946, 9 AM and 5 PM EDT (taped message after 5)
- National Institute on Drug Abuse Cocaine Hotline: (800) 662-HELP
- National Cocaine Hotline: (800) COCAINE
- Alcohol Hotline: (800) ALCOHOL

COCAINE ANONYMOUS (central offices)

- National Office: Culver City, Calif, (213) 839-1141
- California: Los Angeles: (213) 553-8306, (213) 937-7250, (213) 839-1141; Los Angeles area: (818) 447-2887; San Diego: (619) 275-3078; San Francisco: (415) 563-2358
- Connecticut: (203) 378-4364
- Georgia: Atlanta: (404) 255-7787
- Illinois: Chicago: (312) 278-7444
- New Jersey: Summit: (201) 273-4530
- New York: Manhattan: (212) 496-4266; Westchester: (914) 941-6800
- Pennsylvania: Willow Grove: (215) 657-4010
- Tennessee: Nashville: (615) 327-8990

Services

Comprehensive drug treatment programs are found in very few college or university health centers. College settings for drug dependency programs are more commonly found in the university counseling center. At such a center the emphasis will probably not be on the medical management of dependency but on the behavioral dimensions of drug abuse. Trained counselors and psychologists who specialize in chemical dependency counseling will work with students to (1) analyze their particular concerns, (2) establish constructive ways to cope with stress, and (3) search for alternative ways to achieve new "highs."

Medical treatment for the management of drug problems may need to be obtained through the services of a community treatment facility administered by a local health department, community mental health center, private clinic, or local hospital. Treatment may be on an inpatient or outpatient basis. Medical management might include detoxification, treatment of secondary health complications and nutritional deficiencies, and therapeutic counseling related to chemical dependency.

Although specific formats differ, a typical comprehensive program follows a version of the program described below:

Intake
Detoxification
Physical, psychological, and psychiatric evaluation
Inpatient services (averaging 30-40 days)
Psychological and spiritual lectures
Group therapy sessions
Recreational activities
Individually structured "therapeutic tasks"
Individual counseling sessions
Counseling for family members
Outpatient services (averaging several weeks)
May be in a halfway house
Entry into a community-based self-help program
Stress management training
Aftercare
Continued involvement in a local self-help group
Periodic return trips to the treatment center
Continued counseling for family members

Some communities have voluntary health agencies that deliver services and treatment programs for drug-dependent persons. Check your phonebook for listings of drug treatment facilities. Some communities have drug hotlines that offer advice for persons with questions about drugs. From this hotline you may find all the information necessary about locally available programs (see the box on p. 189).

Costs of Treatment for Dependency

sliding scale
method of payment by which patient fees are scaled according to income levels.

Drug treatment programs that are administered by colleges and universities for faculty and students generally require no fees. Local agencies may provide either free services or services based on a **sliding scale.** Private hospitals, physicians, and clinics are the most expensive forms of treatment. Inpatient treatment at a private facility may cost as much as $300 per day. Since the length of inpatient treatment averages about a month, a patient can quickly accumulate a very large bill. However, with many types of health insurance policies now providing coverage for alcohol and other drug dependencies, even these services may not require additional out-of-pocket expenses.

FUTURE TRENDS IN DRUG USE

Making predictions is not something that college professors are likely to do with great certainty. Regarding the future misuse and abuse of drugs among college students, we can suggest that current drug-taking behaviors do seem to provide a glimpse of what might happen in the future.

We predict that with the exception of alcohol, psychoactive drugs will meet with increasing disfavor from most of America's college students. Our students have shown us that education—in schools and through the media—about the

Personal Assessment

Nonchemical High Challenge

Experts agree that drug use provides only short-term, ineffective, and often destructive solutions to problems. We will challenge you on p. 193 to seek innovative, invigorating nondrug experiences that might make your life more exciting. Circle the number for each activity that reflects your intention to try that activity. Use the following guide:

1 No intention of trying this activity
2 Intend to try this within 2 years
3 Intend to try this within 6 months
4 Already tried this activity
5 Regularly do this activity

1 Learn to juggle	1 2 3 4 5	11 Parachute from a plane	1 2 3 4 5
2 Go backpacking	1 2 3 4 5	12 Go rockclimbing	1 2 3 4 5
3 Complete a marathon race	1 2 3 4 5	13 Take a role in a theater production	1 2 3 4 5
4 Start a vegetable garden	1 2 3 4 5	14 Build a piece of furniture	1 2 3 4 5
5 Ride in a hot air balloon	1 2 3 4 5	15 Solicit funds for a worthy cause	1 2 3 4 5
6 Snow ski or water ski	1 2 3 4 5	16 Learn to swim	1 2 3 4 5
7 Donate a unit of blood	1 2 3 4 5	17 Overhaul your car engine	1 2 3 4 5
8 Go river rafting	1 2 3 4 5	18 Compose a song	1 2 3 4 5
9 Learn to play a musical instrument	1 2 3 4 5	19 Travel to a foreign country	1 2 3 4 5
10 Cycle 100 miles	1 2 3 4 5	20 Write the first chapter of a book	1 2 3 4 5

Your total points _____

Interpretation

61-100   You participate in many challenging experiences
41-60   You are willing to try some challenging experiences
20-40   You take few challenging risks described here

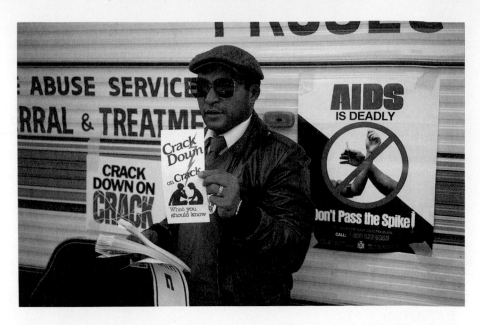

complicated problems of abuse of psychoactive drugs appears to have influenced the decision-making processes of most young adults. After nearly 20 years of experimentation, people have discovered that dependency relationships with drugs fail to give long-term solutions for personal conflicts. Drugs cannot make you more attractive or more interesting. Drugs cannot make you more productive, more contributive, or more scholarly. Drugs cannot even make you pain free. Instead drugs seem only to be insidiously destructive.

A second prediction is that concurrent with a reduction in drug misuse and abuse will be an increase in the use of nondrug ways "to get high." More college students will reach for "altered states" through fitness programs, relaxation training, and a wide range of activities that promise to "take you to the limit." Positive risk-taking activities will take precedence in the lives of more and more college students (see the box on p. 193). Rock climbing, rafting, skiing, hang gliding, and skydiving will attract more people than ever.

On the negative side, however, is our prediction that overall societal drug use may very well increase. Drugs will continue to pour into this country in quantities equal to the demand. Drug enforcement will have little impact in controlling drug availability. Furthermore, this demand for drugs may be disproportionately high among segments of our society where drug education efforts are ignored or are poorly advanced and where social and political strife continue to exist. It is within these parts of society where hope has faded over the last 15 years. For many, drugs will provide a form of escape that helps mask the absence of upward mobility.

SUMMARY

Chapter 7 emphasized the concept that drug abuse in our society has a significant impact on each of us, regardless of whether we personally use or abuse drugs. Because of this it is important to learn about psychoactive drugs, including such basic terms as dependency, tolerance, drug misuse, and drug abuse.

Challenge to Readers

In Chapter 2 we offered a strategy for personal growth and development. One major component in this strategy was for people to attempt new activities—to try new experiences. This strategy supports our contention that personal growth requires effort on your part. Sometimes this effort resembles real work. Such work is a prerequisite if you are to achieve the satisfying feeling and moods that psychoactive drugs can so easily (and dangerously) provide.

Our challenge is for you to work to find the ways that you can best reach your own "highs," whether those highs come from physical activities, creative strategies, artistic expressions, or through helping others.

Although there may be many reasons why people decide to consume drugs, this chapter focuses on four encompassing reasons: (1) a desire to avoid pain, (2) the widespread availability of drugs, (3) the reinforcing pleasurable effects drugs produce, and (4) the fact that people are inherent risk takers.

Most people realize that drugs can alter human perceptions and behaviors, yet few actually understand the basis for these changes. These alterations stem from one of four impacts that a drug may have on the chemical neurotransmitters produced by the neurons.

Psychoactive drugs are classified by the nature of the physiological effects they produce. Almost all drugs fall into one of five categories: stimulants, depressants, hallucinogens, narcotics, and inhalants. The development of designer drugs complicates the control of drugs and adds to the risk of abuse.

Significant attempts have been made to reduce illegal drug use, yet the misuse and abuse of drugs continues to be a complex, widespread problem. Drug testing is becoming increasingly prevalent within certain occupational groups. Fortunately for most college students who need help for drug-related problems, a variety of resources exist.

Students are challenged by this chapter to search for nondrug ways to achieve highs.

REVIEW QUESTIONS

1 How is the term *drug* defined in this chapter? What are psychoactive drugs? How do medicines differ from drugs?
2 Explain what is meant by dependency. Identify and explain what the two types of dependencies are. What term is often used interchangeably with physical dependence? What term is often used interchangeably with psychological dependence?
3 Define the word *tolerance*. What is meant by cross-tolerance? Give an example of cross-tolerance.
4 Differentiate between drug misuse and drug abuse. Identify at least five examples of drug misuse.
5 Identify some reasons commonly given for why people use psychoactive drugs. What are the four reasons we think people are willing to choose to use drugs? What traits may be related to an addictive personality?

6 Describe the normal function of the neuron as discussed in this chapter. What are the four possible influences that a psychoactive drug could have on neurotransmitter function?

7 Specify the five general categories of drugs. For each category, identify several examples of drugs and explain the effects they would have on the user. What are designer drugs?

8 What is the active ingredient in marijuana? What are its common effects on the user? What is known about the long-term effects of marijuana use?

9 What are some of the many ways that dose levels affect users of psychoactive drugs? Why, at low dose levels, does the overall environment play such a significant role in the response drugs produce?

10 What is meant by synergistic effect, additive effect, potentiated effect, and antagonistic effect?

QUESTIONS FOR PERSONAL CONTEMPLATION

1 Considering this chapter's definition of a drug, evaluate your own status as a user of drugs, including caffeine, tobacco, and aspirin. Do you consider your use of drugs to be a problem? Can you identify any drugs to which you may have developed either a physical or psychological dependence?

2 Have you ever experienced (in your own body) drug tolerance? Do you find that you now require a larger dose of a particular drug to reach a high or low that you once felt with a smaller dose? How long did it take for this level of tolerance to develop?

3 This chapter listed a number of examples of drug misuse. Have any of these examples applied to you? If so, were you aware that your actions reflected drug misuse? Would you repeat such an activity knowing now that it might be considered drug misuse? Why or why not?

4 What are your feelings about your friends or relatives who might be drug abusers? What responsibilities, if any, do you feel toward these people?

5 This chapter discussed nondrug ways of getting high. Think about your own life experiences. What things have you done that have produced nondrug highs? What activities do you think might produce continued highs for you as you move through the life cycle?

REFERENCES

1 National Institute on Drug Abuse: Drug use among American high school students, college students, and other young adults: national trends through 1985, US Department of Health and Human Services DHHS Pub no (ADM) 86-1450, Washington DC, 1986, US Government Printing Office.

2 National Institute on Drug Abuse: Cocaine use in America, Prevention Networks DHHS Pub no (ADM) 86-1433, Washington DC, 1986, US Government Printing Office.

3 Meddis, S: Report: pot—USA's top cash crop, USA Today January 10, 1986, p 3a.

4 Ray, O, and Ksir, C: Drugs, society, and human behavior, ed 4, St Louis, 1987, Times/Mirror Mosby College Publishing.

5 Carroll, CR: Drugs in modern society, Dubuque, IA, 1985, Wm C Brown Group.

6 Interagency Drug Alcohol Council: Why people use drugs, Ft Wayne, Ind, The Council.

7 A psychiatrist's view of addiction: an interview with Dr Mark Gold, USA Today September 16, 1986, p 4d.

8 Thibodeau, G: Anatomy and physiology, St Louis, 1987, Times Mirror/Mosby College Publishing.
9 Mermelstein, NH: Caffeine, Contemporary Nutrition 9:1-2, 1984.
10 Schlaadt, RG, and Shannon, PT: Drugs of choice: current perspectives on drug use, Englewood Cliffs, NJ, 1986, Prentice-Hall.
11 Sperling, D: Pot: more punch than in the '60s, USA Today March 31, 1986, p 1a.
12 Jones, HL: Psychopharmacological postulates, Adapted from health science course handout materials, Muncie, Ind, 1988, Ball State University.
13 Greene, E: Job outlook for 1987's graduating seniors: level hiring, lagging pay, and drug tests, The Chronicle of Higher Education 33, 1987.

ANNOTATED READINGS

Bargmann, E, et al: Stopping Valium: and Ativan, Centrax, Dalmane, Librium, Paxipam, Restoril, Serax, Tranxene and Xanax, New York, 1982, Warner Books, Inc.
> The full story of the dangers of these "harmless" tranquilizers, their side effects, and the dangers of addiction.

Britt, DR: The all-American cocaine story, Minneapolis, 1984, CompCare Publishers.
> A guide to the realities of cocaine; intent is to give basic information to recreational users and their friends and families. The first half of the book is devoted to the author's own experiences with cocaine.

Gold, MS: 800-Cocaine, New York, 1984, Bantam Books, Inc.
> Gold is the founder of the toll-free national hotline for cocaine users and victims; the book includes the warning signs of addiction, the typical user, and the life-changing effects of cocaine abuse.

Harkness, R: Drug interactions handbook, Englewood Cliffs, NJ, 1984, Prentice Hall, Inc.
> This handbook will help you avoid potentially harmful side effects from combining prescription or over-the-counter medications, vitamins, alcohol, and food.

Johnson, VE: Intervention: how to help someone who doesn't want help, Minneapolis, 1986, Johnson Institute.
> Written by the founder of the well-known Johnson Institute in Minneapolis, this book is a step-by-step guide for friends and family members of chemically dependent people. Describes the behavioral patterns of chemically dependent persons and shows how concerned people can initiate help for those they care about.

Larson, E: Stage II recovery: life beyond addiction, San Francisco, 1985, Harper & Row, Publishers.
> Discusses how sustained abstinence from addiction is only the first step in the overall process of recovery. Larson indicates that real recovery starts when the person learns how to identify and change the behaviors that are self-defeating.

Mothner, I, and Weitz, A: How to get off drugs, New York, 1984, Simon & Schuster (Rolling Stone Press).
> By the editors of *Rolling Stone* magazine; what it costs you physically and psychologically to use drugs; all that you need to know to help someone get off and stay off drugs; where to go for help.

Reilly, P: A private practice, New York, 1984, MacMillan Publishing Co.
> A pediatrician's story of how the pressure of being a doctor can result in drug abuse and his successful battle against prescription drug addiction.

Schaef, AW: When society becomes an addict, San Francisco; 1987, Harper & Row, Publishers.
> Examines dependency from its broadest perspective. Schaef, a psychotherapist and lecturer, describes our society as an addictive system that traps many of us into dependency relationships involving drugs, eating, spending, and sex. The author shows readers how to think and act more independently.

Weil, A, and Rosen, W: Chocolate to morphine: understanding mind active drugs, Boston, 1983, Houghton Mifflin Co.
> Discussions of each substance's nature, how it is likely to affect the body, and what precautions are necessary to limit any potential harm; neither condones nor condemns drug use.

CHAPTER 8

Alcohol
Responsible Choices

Key Concepts

Heavy drinking is a common practice among a large percentage of college students.

■

Many factors influence the rate of absorption of alcohol.

■

A continuous increase in the blood alcohol concentration produces a predictable sequence of depressive effects.

■

Responsible drinking patterns can foster satisfying and socially integrative behavior.

■

Safe party hosting, avoiding drunk driving, and recognizing the rights of nondrinkers reflect responsible drinking patterns.

■

Denial and enabling are common factors seen in alcoholism.

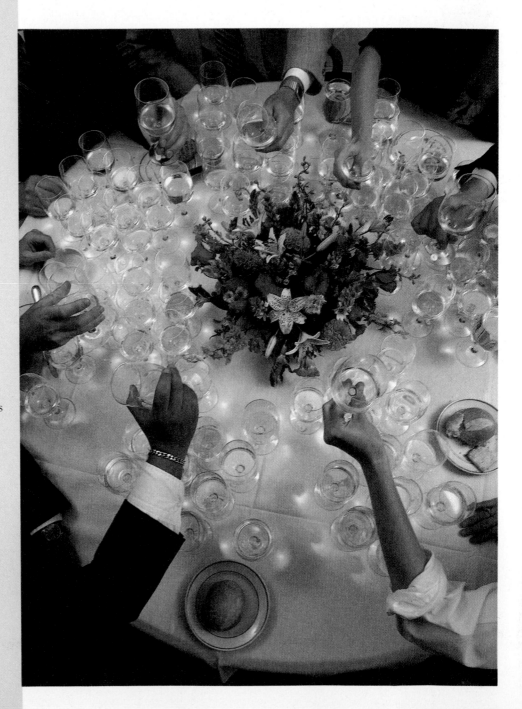

The raising of legal drinking ages, the tightening of standards for determining legal intoxication, and the emergence of national groups concerned with alcohol misuse indicate that our society is more sensitive than ever to the growing misuse of alcohol. People are asking questions about the consequences of drunk driving, alcohol-related crime, and lowered job productivity. Alcohol use remains the preferred form of drug use for the majority of adults, but as a society we are increasingly uncomfortable with the ease with which alcohol can be misused.

The alcohol use patterns of many people are irresponsible. Frequent heavy drinking, drinking to get drunk, drinking on the job, and drinking while driving are but a few of the irresponsible ways in which adults drink. The use patterns being formed today by young adults may tip the delicate balance that now exists between alcohol as an agent for achieving satisfaction and social integration and alcohol as an agent for disruptive and life-threatening behavior. We think responsible drinking patterns can be developed, and it is to this end that this chapter is directed.

CHOOSING TO DRINK

As plausible as all of the explanations in the box on p. 199 are in explaining why people might choose to drink, we believe that the last choice listed is ultimately the only reason most people drink alcohol: they drink to feel the effects of alcohol. Although most people will not admit it, they find alcohol an effective, affordable, and legal substance for altering the normal function of the central nervous system. As one's restraints are removed by the influence of the alcohol, behaviors that are generally held in check by **inhibitions** are expressed. At least temporarily they become a different version of themselves—more outgoing, relaxed, and adventuresome. If alcohol did not make these changes in people, little alcohol would be consumed.

People hold different views about the appropriateness of alcohol use. Some people may view the use of alcohol (or the behaviors that its use generates) as being so morally wrong that they cannot accept the person. Then there are those who strongly support the use of alcohol by others, who encourage drinking—even to the point where lives may be endangered.

A 1983 Indianapolis incident illustrates this. A popular local "watering hole" offered a special for Professional Secretaries Day and persuaded several young women to participate in a "chug-a-lug" contest. Several of the contestants had to be taken to a hospital intensive care unit, suffering from acute alcohol intoxication.[1] As a result the bartenders lost their licenses, and their merchant's license was restricted. This represented the first case prosecuted in Indiana in which managers of a tavern were held legally responsible for endangering their customers by encouraging virtually unlimited drinking.

Between these two extremes are persons who are generally willing to judge the appropriateness of alcohol use on the basis of behavior after drinking. When use is moderate and the consequences of that use do not generate problems for others or for the drinker, these individuals usually remain nonjudgmental. However, when the use of alcohol results in destructive behavior, their reactions may become unexpectedly forceful. For example, many townspeople near college campuses tolerate "normal" levels of campus alcohol misuse, until a certain level of disruption has been reached. At that point they begin to defend their property

inhibitions
inner controls that prevent a person's engaging in certain types of behavior.

Do you see this behavior frequently on your campus?

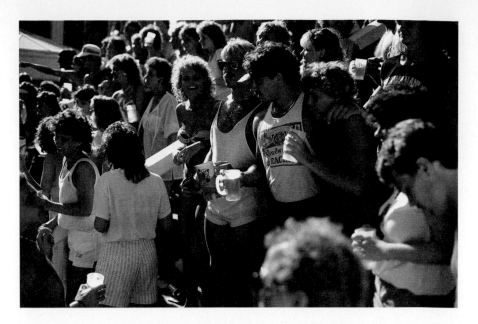

and peace of mind with overt, forceful measures. Even roommates can respond in this manner when drinking leads to behaviors they cannot accept.

Persons on this large center segment of the continuum believe that misuse of alcohol has no place in our society. These individuals perceive clear differences in the acceptability of behaviors associated with alcohol use. They will continue to feel comfortable when alcohol use is satisfying and integrative, yet clearly not compromising to other users and nonusers. Their response to compromising behavior could be spirited and harsh. They will recognize alcohol use as a source of problems for which they will want resolution.

In the remainder of the chapter you will find the information necessary to develop an alcohol use pattern that could foster the *satisfying and integrative use of alcohol.* By thoughtfully considering this information, you can (if you choose to drink) begin to establish the type of alcohol use pattern that is in keeping with the high expectations you hold for yourself as an adult.

ALCOHOL USE PATTERNS

From magazines to billboards to television, alcohol is one of the most heavily advertised consumer products in the country.[2] You cannot watch television, listen to a radio, or read a newspaper without being encouraged to buy a particular brand of beer, wine, or liquor. The advertisements create a warm aura about the nature of alcohol use. The implications are clear: alcohol use will bring you good times, handsome men or seductive women, exotic settings, and a chance to forget the hassles of hard work.

The advertisements further seem to imply that we live in a two-dimensional society. One aspect of living centers on work, the other on play. There appears to be no true middle ground; we either work or play. After a hard day as a lumberjack, office manager, reporter, businesswoman, coach, firefighter, or college student, we are told that we deserve to move directly into play. No longer are we expected to stop work and move slowly into other personally productive

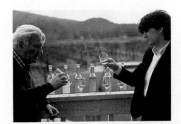

The alcohol industry caters to our tastes.

Why Do I Choose an Alcoholic Beverage Instead of a Nonalcoholic One?

Alcoholic beverages are more thirst quenching than nonalcoholic alternatives.

Alcoholic beverages taste better—their flavor is unique and satisfying.

My friends always choose alcoholic beverages—I've learned to do the same.

Alcoholic drinks form an important part of the larger statement that I am making about myself. They reflect the fact that I am an adult.

Drinking alcoholic beverages causes me to feel different—I like the changes that come about when I drink.

activities. Suddenly it is not "quitting time," or "time to go home." It's "Miller time!" It's time to party!

Perhaps as a consequence of the many pressures to drink, it is not surprising that most adults drink alcoholic beverages. Two thirds of all American adults are classified as drinkers. Yet one in three adults does not drink. In the college environment, where surveys indicate that 90% of all students drink, it is difficult for many students to imagine that every third adult is an abstainer.

Of the two thirds who do drink alcoholic beverages, approximately 15% are classified as infrequent drinkers, 41% as light to moderate drinkers, and 12% as heavy drinkers. These figures for adult drinking come from studies reported by the National Institute on Alcohol Abuse and Alcoholism (NIAAA) and do not seem to surprise many of the students in our health classes.[3] Students who drink in college generally tend to classify themselves as light to moderate drinkers. It comes as a shock to our students, though, when they read the criteria for each drinking classification. According to the combination of quantity of alcohol consumed per occasion and the frequency of drinking, these criteria are established as shown in Table 8-1.

In a recent unpublished survey of our undergraduate health science classes, we found that 42% of the 210 students met the criteria for heavy drinking, 25% met the criteria for moderate drinking, 15% met the criteria for light drinking, 11% were infrequent drinkers, and 7% were abstainers. It is not surprising that in a national survey over half the students questioned believed that alcohol abuse was a problem on their campuses.[4]

For large numbers of students who drink, the college years represent a time when they will drink more heavily than at any other period during their lifetime. Unfortunately, for some students these years will also be the entry years into a lifetime of problem drinking.

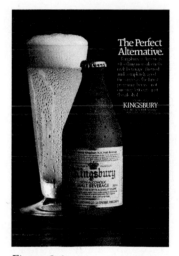

Figure 8-1
Recently, many low- and non-alcoholic malt beverages have entered the marketplace. Do you believe these products will have much influence on the beer industry? Would you consider using these beverages as alternatives to alcoholic beverages at a party you would host? Why or why not?

THE NATURE OF ALCOHOLIC BEVERAGES

Alcohol (also known as ethyl alcohol or ethanol) is the principal product of **fermentation.** In this process *yeast* cells act on the sugar content of fruits and grains to produce alcohol and carbon dioxide. Alcohol was probably first discovered in prehistoric times when people consumed the juices of a berry mash that

fermentation
chemical process whereby plant products are converted into alcohol by the action of yeast cells on carbohydrate materials.

Table 8-1 Criteria for Drinking Classifications	
Classification	**Alcohol-Related Behavior**
Abstainers	Do not drink or drink less than once a year
Infrequent drinkers	Drink once a month at most and drink small amounts per typical drinking occasion
Light drinkers	Drink once a month at most and drink medium amounts per typical drinking occasion, or drink no more than three to four times a month and drink small amounts per typical drinking occasion
Moderate drinkers	Drink at least once a week and small amounts per typical drinking occasion or three to four times a month and medium amounts per typical drinking occasion or no more than once a month and large amounts per typical drinking occasion
Moderate/heavy drinkers	Drink at least once a week and medium amounts per typical drinking occasion or three to four times a month and large amounts per typical drinking occasion
Heavy drinkers	Drink at least once a week and large amounts per typical drinking occasion

NOTE: Small amounts = One drink or less per drinking occasion
Medium amounts = Two to four drinks per drinking occasion
Large amounts = Five or more drinks per drinking occasion
Drink = 12 fluid oz of beer, 4 fluid oz of wine, or 1 fluid oz of distilled spirits

was exposed to airborne yeast cells.[5] When this product produced more physical effects than the mere satisfaction of thirst, early man began the purposeful production of this crude wine. Alcohol became a celebrated elixir in a slowly developing world. Fermented juices have been consumed for at least 4,000 years, and have been used medically for hundreds of years as an analgesic and a sedative.

Until about 500 years ago, the principal beverages made with alcohol were wine (from fruit sources) and beer (from grain sources). These beverages were similar in their rather low percentage of alcohol concentration. At most, the early alcoholic beverages contained 10% to 14% pure alcohol. Any greater concentration seemed to destroy the yeast cells. Not until the European development of the process of **distillation** in the fifteenth century did alcoholic beverages contain a higher percentage of alcohol. By gathering the alcohol vapors from a fermented mixture that was heated in a device called a *still*, early distillers learned they could process a much more potent product. These vapors were then cooled and condensed to form distilled liquids, or spirits. Even after the addition of water and flavoring ingredients, the alcohol concentration of these new beverages exceeded 50%. Through the years, whiskey, rum, vodka, and gin were further developed to contain even higher concentrations of alcohol.

distillation
production of alcoholic beverages by the vaporization and condensation of the alcohol component of plant material; the process that produces liquor.

The alcohol concentration in distilled beverages today is expressed in the term *proof,* a number that is twice the percentage of alcohol by volume in a beverage. Thus 70% of the fluid in a bottle of 140 proof gin is pure alcohol. Most proofs in distilled beverages range from 80 to 160. The familiar, pure *grain alcohol* that is often added to fruit punches and similar beverages has a proof that approaches 200.

In its purest form, ethyl alcohol has little taste. This clear fluid, when consumed alone, usually produces an initial burning sensation of the oral cavity and esophagus. The various flavors that you notice in alcoholic beverages are by-products of the sugar source (the type of fruit or grain) and any additional flavorings added to the fermenting mixture. Whereas wine and beer are generally not mixed with other nonalcoholic liquids, distilled spirits are frequently combined with fruit juices, colas, and prepared mixes. (See Table 8-2 for the categories of alcoholic beverages and the box on p. 202 for types of alcoholic beverages.)

Table 8-2   Categories of Alcoholic Beverages

Alcoholic Beverages	Alcohol Content (%)	Normal Measures Dispensed
Beer		
Ale	5	12-oz bottle
Malt beverage	7	12-oz bottle
Lite beer	4	12-oz bottle
Regular beer	4	12-oz bottle
Low-alcohol beer	1.5	12-oz bottle
Wines		
Fortified: port, muscatel, etc.	18	3-oz glass
Natural: red/white	12	3-oz glass
Champagne	12	4-oz glass
Wine cooler	6	12-oz bottle
Cider (hard)	10	6-oz glass
Liqueurs		
Strong: sweet, syrupy	40	1-oz glass
Medium: fruit brandies	25	2-oz glass
Distilled spirits		
Brandy, cognac, rum, scotch, vodka, whiskey	45	1-oz glass
Mixed drinks and cocktails		
Strong martini, manhattan	30	3½-oz glass
Medium: old-fashioned, daiquiri, alexander	15	4-oz glass
Light: highball, sweet and sour mixes, tonics	7	8-oz glass

Types of Alcoholic Beverages

In all major alcoholic beverages—beer, table wines, cocktail and dessert wines, liqueurs and cordials, and distilled spirits—the significant ingredient is identical: alcohol. The typical drink, half an ounce of alcohol, is provided by:

- A shot of spirits (1.5 ounces of 40% alcohol—80 proof whiskey or vodka)
- A glass of fortified wine (3 ounces of 20% alcohol)
- A larger glass of table wine (5 ounces of 12% alcohol)
- Beer (12 ounces of 4.5% alcohol)

In addition, these beverages contain other chemical constituents. Some come from the original grains, grapes, or other fruits; others are produced during the chemical processes of fermentation, distillation, and storage. Some are added as flavoring or coloring.

These nonalcoholic substances contribute to the effects of certain beverages either by directly affecting the body or by affecting the rates at which alcohol is absorbed into the blood.

The nutritional value of alcohol is extremely limited. Although the crude, early fermented mixtures of alcoholic beverages did contain moderate amounts of vitamins and minerals, alcoholic beverages produced today through modern processing methods contain nothing but empty Calories—about 100 Calories per fluid ounce of 100 proof distilled spirits and about 150 Calories per each 12 ounce bottle or can of beer.[5] Alcohol contains few minerals and no vitamins, fats, or protein.

As a chemical compound, alcohol exists in many forms. Among the more familiar of these are methyl (wood alcohol), ethyl (grain alcohol), isopropyl (rubbing alcohol), and butyl. Only ethyl alcohol can be consumed safely by humans. All other forms are toxic and thus unsafe for use in beverages. Consumption of alcohols other than ethyl has resulted in serious injury and death.

The addition of denaturing substances to nonethyl alcohols prevents many persons from ingesting a lethal dose. This is because a nauseating effect is produced once the denaturing chemicals are ingested. Be careful never to consume alcohol unless you are certain of its form. Too frequently, beverages purported to be "home brew" or "moonshine" have proven to be dangerously concocted from nonethyl alcohols.

The introduction of "lite" beer and low-calorie wines has been in response to concerns over the empty Calories that alcoholic beverages provide. Be certain to remember that these "lite" beverages are not low-alcoholic beverages—merely low-calorie beverages. Only beverages marked "low-alcohol" contain a lower concentration of alcohol than the usual beverages of that type.

Cold Weather and Alcohol

Did you know that drinking alcohol in cold weather actually causes heat loss? The feeling of warmth results from the loss of body heat related to the dilation of blood vessels under the skin. In effect you may feel warm but are actually getting colder.

THE PHYSIOLOGICAL EFFECTS OF ALCOHOL

During certain periods of our lives, we want only to see the world in clear, uncomplicated terms. We have good days or bad days; we like certain people, and we don't like others. And sometimes we tend to oversimplify complex ideas, lending a "bumpersticker slogan" flippancy to serious concerns.

When we talk about the effect of alcohol on body function, we sometimes reduce the impact of many complex interactions by merely saying, "Alcohol makes you silly," "It messes you up," or "It calms your nerves." We further make light of the effects of alcohol when we say, "I got bombed," "We got loaded," or "She got wasted." Perhaps we forget that alcohol's impact on the human body is much more complicated than we generally admit.

The knowledge of how alcohol affects the body may help you understand the social behaviors of others who are under the influence of alcohol. An understanding of alcohol's pharmacological properties may help you discover some of the roots of problem drinking and alcoholism. Furthermore, an intellectual examination of how alcohol functions in your body can assist you in analyzing your own use of alcohol.

First and foremost, alcohol is classified as a drug—a very strong *central nervous system depressant*. The primary depressant effect of alcohol is observed in the

How Do You Use Alcoholic Beverages?

Answer the following questions in terms of your own alcohol use. Record your number of YES and NO responses in the box at the end of the questionnaire.

Do you: YES   NO

1 Drink more frequently than did a year ago?   _____ _____

2 Drink more heavily than you did a year ago?   _____ _____

3 Plan to drink, sometimes days in advance?   _____ _____

4 Gulp or "chug" your drinks, perhaps in a contest?   _____ _____

5 Set personal limits on the amount you plan to drink but then   _____ _____
   consistently disregard these limits?

6 Drink at a rate greater than two drinks per hour?   _____ _____

7 Encourage or even pressure others to drink with you?   _____ _____

8 Frequently want a nonalcoholic beverage but then end up   _____ _____
   drinking an alcoholic drink?

9 Drive your car while under the influence of alcohol or ride   _____ _____
   with another person who has been drinking?

10 Use alcoholic beverages while taking prescription or OTC   _____ _____
   medications?

11 Forget what happened while you were drinking?   _____ _____

12 Have a tendency to disregard information about the effects of   _____ _____
   drinking?

13 Find your reputation fading because of alcohol use?   _____ _____

                                                          Total   _____ _____

Interpretation

If you indicate a "yes" response on any of these questions, you may be demonstrating aspects of irresponsible alcohol use. Two or more "yes" responses indicates an unacceptable pattern of alcohol use and may reflect problem drinking behavior.

Personal
Assessment

brain and spinal cord. Many people think of alcohol as a stimulant because of the way most users feel after consuming a serving or two of their favorite drink. Any temporary sensations of jubilation, boldness, or relief must be attributed to alcohol's ability as a depressant drug to release personal inhibitions and provide temporary relief from tension.[6]

Factors Related to the Absorption of Alcohol

absorption
passage of nutrients or alcohol through the walls of the stomach or intestinal tract into the bloodstream.

The basic principle of *diffusion,* or the movement of a substance from an area of greater concentration to an area of lesser concentration, applies to the movement of alcohol from the digestive tract into the bloodstream. This **absorption** of alcohol is influenced by several factors, most of which are capable of being controlled by the individual. These factors include:

- *Strength of the beverage.* The stronger the beverage, the greater the amount of alcohol that will accumulate within the digestive tract.
- *Number of drinks consumed.* The greater the number of drinks that are consumed, the more alcohol that must be absorbed. If consumed in a relatively short period of time, a concentration gradient will develop that will foster the rapid movement of alcohol into the bloodstream.
- *Rapidness of consumption.* If consumed rapidly, even relatively few drinks will result in a large concentration gradient that will foster high blood alcohol concentrations.
- *Presence of food.* Food can compete with alcohol for absorption into the bloodstream thus slowing the absorption of alcohol. By slowing alcohol absorption, oxidation of the alcohol already in the bloodstream can occur. Slow absorption favors better control of blood alcohol concentrations.
- *Body chemistry.* Each person has an individual pattern of physiological functioning that may affect the ability to process alcohol. For example, in some conditions such as that marked by the "dumping syndrome," the stomach empties more rapidly than is normal, and alcohol seems to be absorbed more quickly. The emptying time may be either slowed or quickened by anger, fear, stress, nausea, and the condition of the stomach tissues.

With the exception of the last factor, all other factors that influence absorption can be moderated by the user of alcohol.

Blood Alcohol Concentration

blood alcohol concentration (BAC)
percentage of alcohol in a measured quantity of blood; BACs can be determined directly through the analysis of a blood sample or indirectly through the analysis of exhaled air.

A person's **blood alcohol concentration (BAC)** level rises when alcohol is consumed at a rate faster than it can be oxidized by the liver (see Figure 8-2). A fairly predictable sequence of effects takes place when a person drinks alcohol at a rate faster than one drink every 2 hours. When the BAC reaches 0.05%, initial measurable changes in mood and behavior take place. Inhibitions and everyday tensions appear to be released, while at the same time judgment and critical thinking are somewhat impaired. This BAC level would be achieved by a 160-pound person taking about two drinks in an hour.

At a level of 0.10% (one part alcohol to 1,000 parts blood) the drinker typically loses significant motor coordination. Voluntary motor function becomes quite clumsy. At this BAC level most states consider a drinker legally intoxicated and thus incapable of operating a vehicle within the limits of safety. Al-

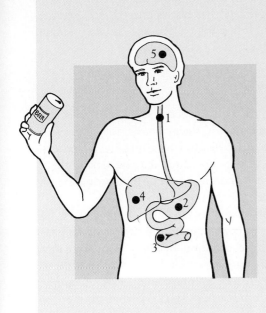

1   When it is swallowed, alcohol travels through the esophagus to the stomach.

2   Absorption of alcohol begins in the stomach. Approximately 20% passes directly into the venous drainage of the stomach wall. Food in the stomach wall will delay passage of the remaining alcohol into the small intestine.

3   The majority of alcohol (80%) is absorbed into the venous drainage of the small intestine. Absorption is proportional to the concentration of alcohol within the small intestine. Once in the venous drainage, alcohol is transported to the liver for oxidation.

4   When it arrives in the liver, alcohol undergoes oxidation. The liver is capable of oxidizing approximately ⅔ oz of alcohol per hour. Surplus alcohol is circulated throughout the body and BAC rises. Blood alcohol concentrations gradually fall as the liver oxidizes the remaining alcohol.

5   As BAC rises in the blood reaching the brain, predictable changes occur. At levels approximating 0.50, central nervous system function can be so depressed that death can occur.

Figure 8-2
The body's absorption and oxidation of alcohol.

though physiological changes associated with this BAC level are occurring, certain users may not feel intoxicated or outwardly appear to be impaired.

As a person continues to elevate the BAC from 0.20% to 0.50%, the health risk of acute alcohol intoxication increases rapidly. A BAC of 0.20% is characterized by the loud, boisterous, obnoxious drunk who staggers. A 0.30% BAC produces futher depression and stuporous behavior, during which time the drinker becomes so confused that he or she may by wholly incapable of understanding external stimuli. The 0.40% or 0.50% BAC produces unconsciousness. Survival at this time may be tenuous, since brain centers that control body temperature, heartbeat, and respiration may be virtually shut down.[5]

An important factor influencing the blood alcohol concentration that results from a given amount of alcohol is the individual's blood volume. The heavier the person, the greater the amount of blood into which alcohol can be distributed. Conversely, the smaller individual has less blood into which alcohol can be distributed and as a result a higher BAC will develop.

Sobering Up

Alcohol is removed from the bloodstream principally through the process of oxidation. Oxidation occurs at a constant rate that cannot be appreciably altered. Although people have attempted to sober up by drinking hot coffee, taking cold showers, or by exercising, the oxidation of alcohol remains unaffected. Thus far the U.S. Food and Drug Administration (FDA) has not approved any commercial product that can help people accomplish sobriety. Passage of time remains the only effective remedy for diminishing alcohol's effects.

First Aid for Acute Alcohol Intoxication

Not everyone who goes to sleep, passes out, or even becomes unconscious after drinking has a high BAC. People who are already sleepy, have not eaten well, are sick, or who are bored may drink a little alcohol and quickly fall asleep. However, people who drink heavily in a rather short time may be setting themselves up for an extremely unpleasant, toxic, potentially life-threatening experience. These people will have problems because of their high BACs.

As you watch people consuming alcohol at a social function, it can be important for you to carefully observe the drinking behavior and the resultant physical signs and symptoms exhibited by those drinking heavily. Although most cases of alcohol intoxication produce only uncomfortable hangovers and bruised egos, some social drinking episodes result in serious injury and death. A number of these deaths occur in college settings, often when inexperienced drinkers are encouraged to drink large amounts of alcohol in a relatively short time. Such behavior is not uncommon during days preceding or following the weekend's big game, during social club gatherings and initiations, and during residence hall parties.

Although responsible drinking would preclude the necessity for first aid knowledge about **acute alcohol intoxication** (poisoning), such responsible drinking will never be a reality for everyone. As caring adults, what should we know about this health emergency that may help us save a life—perhaps even a friend's life?

The first true danger signs we need to recognize are the typical signs of **shock.**[7] By the time these shock signs are evident, a drinker will already have advanced to an unconscious stage. He or she cannot be aroused from a deep stupor. The person will probably have a weak, rapid pulse (over 100 beats per minute). Skin will be cool and damp, and breathing will be increased to once every 3 or 4 seconds. These breaths may be shallow or deep but will certainly be irregular in pattern. Skin color will be pale or bluish. (In the case of a black victim, these skin color changes will be more evident in the fingernail beds or the mucous membranes inside the mouth or under the eyelids.) Whenever any of these signs are present, seek emergency medical help immediately.

Involuntary regurgitation (vomiting) can be another potential life-threatening emergency for a person who has consumed too much alcohol. When a drinker has consumed more alcohol than the liver can oxidize, the pyloric valve at the base of the stomach tends to close. Additional alcohol remains in the stomach. This alcohol irritates the lining of the stomach to the extent that involuntary muscle contractions force the stomach contents to flow back through the esophagus. The body is telling conscious drinkers that they have had too much to drink.

An unconscious victim who regurgitates may be lying in such a position that the airway becomes obstructed with the vomitus from the stomach. This victim can easily die from **asphyxiation.**[7] As a first aid measure, unconscious drinkers should always be rolled on their sides to minimize the chance of airway obstruc-

acute alcohol intoxication
potentially fatal elevation of the blood alcohol concentration, often resulting from heavy, rapid consumption of alcohol.

shock
profound collapse of many vital body functions; evident during acute alcohol intoxication and other serious health emergencies.

asphyxiation
death resulting from lack of oxygen to the brain.

tion. If vomiting occurs when you are with the victim, make certain that the head is positioned lower than the rest of the body. This position minimizes the chance that vomitus will obstruct the air passages.

It is also important to keep a close watch on anyone who "passes out" from heavy drinking. Unfortunately partygoers sometimes make the mistake of carrying these persons to bed and then forgetting about them. By the next morning, these forgotten people may have died. We should do our best to monitor the physical condition of anyone who passes out from heavy drinking. If you really care about these unconscious people, you will observe them at regular intervals until they appear to be clearly out of danger. Although this may mean an evening of interrupted sleep for you, you may save a friend's life.

ALCOHOL-RELATED HEALTH PROBLEMS

The relationship of chronic alcohol use to the structure and function of the body is reasonably well understood. Heavy alcohol use causes a variety of changes to the body that lead to an increase in morbidity and mortality. Table 8-3 describes these changes.

Table 8-3 Alcohol-Related Health Problems

Organ or Body System	Debilitative Change
Liver	Chemical imbalance: altered protein production, blood sugar imbalance, fat accumulation in the liver tissue
	Inflammation: impaired circulation, scar tissue formation, alcohol-related hepatitis
	Cirrhosis: impaired circulation, kidney failure, death
Digestive tract	Oral cavity: when combined with smoking, alcohol use promotes cancer of the mouth, tongue, and throat
	Esophagus: irritation, impaired swallowing
	Stomach: irritation, gastritis, ulceration
	Pancreas: inflammation (pancreatitis)
	Digestion: impaired absorption
	Nausea: diarrhea, vomiting
Cardiovascular	Cardiomyopathy: shortness of breath, heart enlargement, arrhythmias
	Arrhythmias: cardiac insufficiency
	Coronary artery disease: angina pectoris, myocardial infarction
Malnutrition	Faulty dietary practices: empty calories, obesity
Cancer	Prevalence: mouth, larynx, esophagus, liver; alcohol's role as a carcinogenic agent is not clearly understood
Reproductive Women	Dysmenorrhea, infertility, miscarriage, fetal alcohol syndrome
Men	Impotence with heavy, chronic use

In addition to the more specific changes listed in Table 8-3, recently reported research suggests a strong correlation between heavy alcohol consumption and stroke,[8] as well as breast cancer in women.[9] In the case of stroke, the role of alcohol appears to be related to the bursting of small blood vessels. How alcohol affects the development of breast cancer is not clearly understood.

Fetal Alcohol Syndrome

placenta
structure through which nutrients, metabolic wastes, and drugs (including alcohol) pass from the bloodstream of the mother into the bloodstream of the developing fetus.

A growing body of scientific evidence indicates that alcohol use by pregnant women can result in a variety of birth defects in unborn children. When alcohol crosses the **placenta,** it enters the fetal bloodstream in a concentration equal to that in the mother's bloodstream. Because of the underdeveloped nature of the fetal liver, this alcohol is oxidized much more slowly than the alcohol in the mother. During this time of slow detoxification, the developing fetus is certain to be overexposed to the toxic effects of alcohol. This high blood alcohol concentration has a major impact on the developing fetal brain, especially the *reticular formation,* the biological coordinating center of brain impulses. Once impaired during its critical developing stages, the brain seems incapable of normal function; this incapacitation remains for a lifetime.

The exposure to alcohol can produce additional disastrous consequences for the developing fetus. Low birth weight, facial abnormalities (small heads, widely spaced eyes), mental retardation, learning disability, joint problems, and heart problems are often seen in such infants. This combination of birth defects was first identified in 1973 at the University of Washington. It is called **fetal alcohol syndrome.** Recent estimates indicate that the full expression of this syndrome occurs at a rate of between one and two per thousand births. Partial expression can be seen in three to five per thousand live births.[10]

fetal alcohol syndrome
characteristic birth defects noted in the children of some women who consume alcohol during their pregnancies.

Is there a safe limit to the number of drinks one can consume during pregnancy? Although the NIAAA's first recommendation in 1977 was for women to drink no more than two drinks a day, the same agency in 1981 revised its warning to suggest complete abstinence throughout a pregnancy.[11]

Even though the full expression of fetal alcohol syndrome has thus far been seen only in children of heavy drinkers, it is possible that even one drink taken by a pregnant woman (especially during a critical stage of early fetal growth and

Fetal alcohol syndrome.

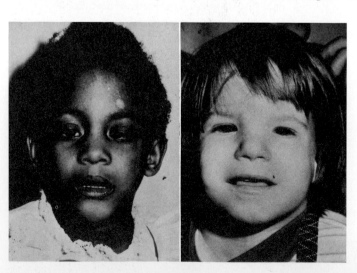

development) can result in fetal impairment. Although such an impairment might never be clinically apparent in a child, the defect could reduce the overall potential of that child. The child who was biologically programmed to be gifted, for example, might just develop to be "above average." The child who was programmed to be average may struggle to be only "below average." Since no one can accurately predict the impact of even small amounts of alcohol during pregnancy, the wisest plan would be to avoid alcohol altogether.

Because of the critical growth and development that occurs during the first months of fetal life, women who have any reason to think they are pregnant should halt all alcohol consumption. Furthermore, women who are planning to become pregnant or women who are not practicing effective contraception must also consider keeping their alcohol use to a minimal level.

ALCOHOL-RELATED SOCIAL PROBLEMS

Beyond personal health problems, the misuse and abuse of alcohol is related to a variety of social problems. These problems encompass changes in the quality of interpersonal relationships, employment stability, and the financial security on which both the individual and family depend.

The impact of alcohol consumption on several of these problems was identified in the recent *Special Report to the U.S. Congress on Alcohol and Health.*[3] This document reported findings in the following areas:

- *Job accidents.* Alcohol misuse was an important contributive factor in approximately 50% of all industrial accidents, and 40% of all industry-related deaths.
- *Domestic violence.* Violence, in the form of violent behavior and abuse within the family, is influenced by alcohol in one third to one half of all cases.
- *Robberies.* Of all robberies committed, approximately 72% were committed by persons using alcohol.
- *Highway accidents.* In approximately 22,360 highway fatalities drinking by the other driver was a contributive factor.
- *Murder.* Alcohol use is a contributive factor in murders for both the victims and the offenders. Approximately 50% of all victims and 85% of all offenders were drinking at the time.
- *Rape.* Alcohol consumption by offenders is involved in over 50% of all rapes.
- *Assaults.* Only 25% of all assault cases did not involve alcohol use on the part of both the victims and the offenders.
- *Drownings.* Nearly 70% of all drowning victims were using alcohol at the time of their accidents.
- *Suicide.* Approximately 65% of all suicide attempts are undertaken by persons under the influence of alcohol.
- *Fire.* Over 80% of fire and burn victims were using alcohol at the time of their accidents.

Clearly, the use of alcohol is frequently a part of serious problems involving life and property. When critical judgment is removed by the influence of alcohol, human behavior can quickly become reckless and antisocial. Because most of us wish to minimize problems associated with alcohol use, hosting a responsible party is a first step in this direction.

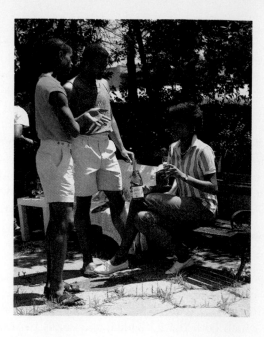

What encourages responsible alcohol use?

HOSTING A RESPONSIBLE PARTY

Some people might say that no party is totally safe when alcohol is served. These people are probably right when you consider the possibility of unexpected **drug synergism,** overconsumption, and the consequences of released inhibitions. Fortunately an increasing awareness of the value of responsible party hosting seems to be permeating college communities in the 1980s.[12] The impetus for this awareness has come from various sources, including the respect for an individual's right to choose not to drink alcohol, the growing recognition of alcohol-related automobile accidents, and the legal threats related to *host negligence.*

For whatever reasons, hosting responsible parties at which alcohol is served is becoming a trend, especially among college-educated young adults. The Education Commission of the State's Task Force on Responsible Decisions about Alcohol has generated a list of guidelines for hosting a social event that includes the use of alcoholic beverages. The list includes the following recommendations[13]:

- Provide other social activities as a primary focus when beverage alcohol is served.
- Respect an individual's decision about alcohol, if that decision is either to abstain or to drink responsibly.
- Recognize the decision not to drink and the respect it warrants by providing equally attractive and accessible nonalcoholic drinks when alcohol is served.
- Recognize that drunkenness is neither healthy nor safe. One should not excuse otherwise unacceptable behavior either for that individual or for others solely because of "too much to drink."
- Provide food when alcohol is served.
- Serve diluted drinks and do not urge that glasses be constantly full.
- Keep the cocktail hour before dinner to a reasonable time and consumption limit.

drug synergism
enhancement of a drug's effect as a result of the presence of additional drugs within the system.

- Recognize a responsibility for the health, safety, and pleasure of both the drinker and the nondrinker by avoiding intoxication and helping others to do the same.
- Make contingency plans for intoxication. If it occurs in spite of efforts to prevent it, assume responsibility for the health and safety of guests—transportation home, overnight accommodations, etc.
- Serve or use alcohol only in environments conducive to pleasant and relaxing behavior.

In addition to these suggestions, we would add that the use of **designated drivers** is an important component of responsible alcohol use. By planning to abstain or carefully limit their own alcohol consumption, designated drivers are able to safely transport friends who have been drinking. Have you noticed an increased use of designated drivers in your community? Would you be willing to be a designated driver?

designated driver
a person who abstains or carefully limits alcohol comsumption to be able to safely transport other people who have been drinking.

ORGANIZATIONS SUPPORTING RESPONSIBLE DRINKING

The serious consequences of the irresponsible use of alcohol have led to the formation of a number of concerned-citizen groups. Although each organization has its specific approach, all attempt to deal objectively with two indisputable facts: alcohol use is part of the fabric of our society, and irresponsible alcohol use can be deadly.

Mothers Against Drunk Drivers (MADD)

As mentioned in Chapter 2, Candy Lightner founded MADD in 1980 after her daughter was killed by a drunk driver. Now a national network of over 200 local chapters in 47 states and several Canadian provinces, MADD attempts to educate people about alcohol's effects on driving and to influence legislation and enforcement of laws related to drunk drivers. MADD clearly had a major impact on the passage of a federal law requiring states to raise the drinking age to 21 or risk the loss of federal highway funds.

Students Against Driving Drunk (SADD)

SADD is an organization composed primarily of high school students whose goal is to reduce drinking deaths among teenagers. In this organization, students help to educate other students about the consequences of combining drinking and driving. One interesting feature of this organization's effort is the encouragement of a contract between students and their parents to provide transportation for each other if either is unable to drive safely after consuming alcohol. This pact also stipulates that no reprisals are to be discussed until the following day.

Boost Alcohol Consciousness Concerning the Health of University Students (BACCHUS)

BACCHUS is an acronym for Boost Alcohol Consciousness Concerning the Health of University Students. Run by student volunteers, this college-based organization promotes responsible drinking among university students who choose to drink. BACCHUS supports responsible party hosting, including providing quantities of food and nonalcoholic beverages. The individual chapters of BACCHUS (now totaling well over 100) are encouraged to use a number of innovative educational approaches to promote alcohol awareness.

Other Approaches

Other responsible approaches to alcohol use are surfacing on a nearly daily basis. Even among college fraternity organizations, attitudes toward the indiscriminate use of alcohol are changing. In December 1983 the National Interfraternity Conference (the governing body of 57 of the 62 national fraternities) approved a resolution that "condemns all-campus drinking parties and contests in which prizes are awarded according to the volume of alcohol consumed."[14] Furthermore, many fraternity rush functions are now conducted without the use of alcohol.

Another encouraging sign seen on college campuses is the increasing number of "alcohol use task forces." Although each of these study committees has its own focus and title, many of these groups are meeting to discuss alcohol-related concerns on their particular campus. These task forces often attempt to formulate detailed, comprehensive policies for alcohol use across the entire campus community. Membership on these committees often includes students (on-campus and off-campus, graduate and undergraduate), faculty and staff members, academic administrators, residence hall advisors, university police, health center personnel, alumni, and local citizens. Does your college have such an ongoing committee?

PROBLEM DRINKING AND ALCOHOLISM

Problem Drinking

The line separating **problem drinking** from alcoholism is difficult to distinguish. In fact, there may be no true line with the exception that an alcoholic is unable to stop drinking. Problem drinking can be recognized when "anyone drinks to such an excess that he loses the ability to control his actions and maintain a socially acceptable life adjustment."[5] One federal government publication lists criteria against which one might judge a problem drinker. Such a person is:

Anyone who must drink in order to function or "cope with life"
Anyone who by his own personal definition or that of his family and friends frequently drinks to a state of intoxication
Anyone who goes to work intoxicated
Anyone who is intoxicated and drives a car
Anyone who sustains bodily injury requiring medical attention as a consequence of an intoxicated state
Anyone who, under the influence of alcohol, does something he contends he would never do without alcohol

Other warning signs that often indicate problem drinking are the need to drink before facing certain situations, frequent drinking sprees, a steady increase in intake, solitary drinking, early morning drinking, and the occurrence of blackouts. For a heavy drinker, a **blackout** is not "passing out" but a period of time in which he [or she] walks, talks, and acts but does not remember. Such blackouts may be one of the early signs of the more serious form of alcoholism.[5]

Sidebar

Tips to Help You Keep Drinking Under Control

Do not drink before a party.
Avoid drinking when you are anxious, mad, or depressed.
Measure the liquor you put in mixed drinks (1-1½ oz).
Eat ample amounts of food before and during your drinking.
Avoid salty foods that may make you drink more than you had planned.
Drink slowly.
Avoid drinking games.
Do not drive after drinking; use a "designated" nondrinking driver.
Consume only a preplanned number of drinks.
Stop alcohol consumption at a preplanned hour.

problem drinking
alcohol use pattern in which a drinker's behavior creates personal difficulties or difficulties for other persons.

blackout
temporary state of amnesia experienced by an alcoholic; an inability to remember events that occurred during a period of alcohol use.

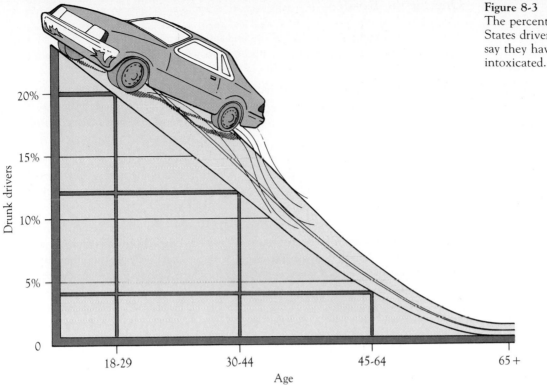

Figure 8-3
The percentage of United States drivers, by age, who say they have driven while intoxicated.

In problem drinking, alcohol seems to interfere with one's adjustment to day-to-day activities. Although perhaps not physically dependent on alcohol to maintain homeostasis, the problem drinker either uses alcohol too frequently to cope with life stressors or uses alcohol in a totally inappropriate or socially unacceptable manner. Alcohol use reduces the quality of a productive life for the drinker and for those who come in contact with the drinker.

Problem drinkers may or may not fit the definition of heavy drinkers presented earlier in this chapter. Yet when they do drink, they lose a major element of control in their lives. They become problems for themselves and others. Do you consider people who abstain during the week but *binge drink* on the weekend to be problem drinkers?

Alcohol and Driving

Although some reports indicate that the percentage of traffic deaths resulting from alcohol use has dropped to below 50% in recent years, the annual number of alcohol-related traffic deaths remains high. In recent years, state legislatures have enacted over 430 new laws designed to reduce the scope of this problem.[15]

In addition to these measures, all states have raised the legal drinking age to 21 years. Further, laws banning open containers of alcohol in cars have now been enacted in 15 states.

Other programs and policies are being used that are designed to prevent intoxicated people from driving. Included among these are efforts to educate bartenders to recognize intoxicated customers, to establish designated drivers, to use

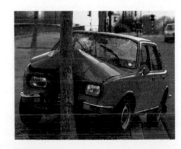

Drinking drivers frequently hurt themselves as well as others.

One for the Road?

Test your knowledge about alcohol use and safe driving. Circle T for true or F for false; then check your response against the answers at right. Knowing the right answers may save your life or the life of a friend.

T F **1** Alcohol is a factor in one half of all highway fatalities.

True **1** Over 53,000 persons were killed in U.S. traffic accidents in 1980. Over half of these deaths were alcohol-related.

T F **2** One and one-half ounces of 86-proof whiskey contains as much alcohol as 12 ounces of beer or 5 ounces of wine.

True **2** Many alcoholic beverages are of the same approximate strength.

T F **3** A blood-alcohol concentration (BAC) of 0.10% is considered legal evidence of intoxication while operating a motor vehicle in most states.

True **3** Even more importantly, at 0.10% BAC the chances of your having an accident are seven and one-half times greater than when you are sober. These chances increase to 25 times if your BAC reaches 0.15%.

T F **4** A 150-pound drinker (male or female) having four drinks per hour would be considered legally drunk if stopped while operating a motor vehicle.

True **4** Using the blood-alcohol chart in Figure 8-4, you can determine your own safe drinking-driving blood-alcohol concentration.

T F **5** Having one to two drinks per hour will cause intoxication within a 4-hour period.

False **5** The body metabolizes one to two drinks per hour. Therefore, if you have only one to two drinks per hour you will not become intoxicated.

T F **6** Drinking large amounts of coffee or taking a cold shower will "sober up" a drinker.

False **6** Absolutely nothing but time will "sober up" an intoxicated person.

T F **7** If your friend has been drinking heavily, your kindest act may be to hide his or her car keys.

True **7** A friend who drives while intoxicated may not be a friend for long. Hide your friend's car keys if he or she drinks too much.

T F **8** Eating before drinking or while drinking is a good idea.

True **8** Alcohol enters the bloodstream rapidly because it requires no digestion. Eating slows the absorption of alcohol, also, providing high-protein snacks at a drinking party may prevent a friend from becoming intoxicated.

Friends Don't Let Friends Drive Drunk!

off-duty police officers as observers in bars, to use police roadblocks, and to develop mechanical devices that prevent intoxicated drivers from starting their cars.

In spite of the efforts described above, a recent study suggests that at least once a month, over 7% of all drivers are under the influence of alcohol[16] (see Figure 8-3). It is these drinking drivers who not only cause the injury and death of others, but who also tax our jails, courts, and liability insurance industry. As a result, society bears the burden of increased monetary expenses for the damage caused.

Alcoholism

Bill consumes alcohol to experience some level of intoxication, while Susan drinks to escape sobriety. For Bill alcohol alters inhibitions, builds his sense of self-confidence, and in his own mind makes him appear to be like those around him who are using alcohol. Susan, on the other hand, has learned that the more negative and unpleasant aspects of her life can be hidden under a blanket of alcohol intoxication. To become sober is to see too much of what is negative and undesirable in her life. Both drink, but for vastly different reasons.

Who is more likely to be labeled an alcoholic—Bill or Susan? Can you distinguish which person is more likely to be the alcoholic? If you identified Susan as the likely alcoholic, then you recognize a subtle difference that exists between the person with **alcoholism** and other alcohol users, including the problem drinker. Alcoholics drink, not for the pleasurable effects of alcohol, but as a response to the stressful events in their lives. For many alcoholics, merely being sober is a stressful experience.

In addition to its behavioral components, alcoholism involves a physical addiction to alcohol. For the true alcoholic, when the body is deprived of alcohol, physical and mental withdrawal symptoms become evident. These withdrawal symptoms can be life threatening. Uncontrollable shaking can progress into nausea, vomiting, hallucinations, shock, and ultimately to cardiac and pulmonary

alcoholism
pattern of alcohol use characterized by emotional and physical dependence as well as a general loss of control over the use of alcohol.

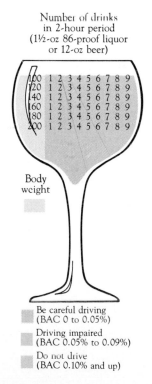

Number of drinks in 2-hour period (1½-oz 86-proof liquor or 12-oz beer)

Body weight

Be careful driving (BAC 0 to 0.05%)

Driving impaired (BAC 0.05% to 0.09%)

Do not drive (BAC 0.10% and up)

Figure 8-4
For most states, a BAC of 0.10% represents legal intoxication. However, a BAC as low as 0.05% can impair functioning enough to lead to a serious accident.

Progressive Stages of Alcohol Dependence

Early	Middle	Late
Escape drinking	Loss of control	Prolonged binges
Guilt feelings	Self-hate	Alcohol used to control withdrawal symptoms
Sneaking drinks	Impaired social relationships	Alcohol psychosis
Difficulty stopping once drinking has begun	Changes in drinking patterns	Nutritional disease
Increased tolerance	Temporary sobriety	
Preoccupation with drinking	Morning drinking	
Blackouts	Dietary neglect	

arrest. Uncontrollable shaking combined with irrational hallucinations represents *delirium tremens* (DTs), an occasional manifestation during an alcoholic's withdrawal.[6]

The physical and emotional dependency encompassed by the term *alcoholism* has a complex and poorly understood cause. Why, when more than 100 million adults use alcohol without establishing a dependency relationship with it, do 10 million or more individuals lose their ability to control its use?

Could alcoholism be an inherited condition? The answer to this question remains unresolved.[17] A number of studies using children of alcoholic parents who were adopted into nonalcoholic homes suggests that a genetic predisposition exists for two forms of alcoholism.[18]

Type I alcoholism, or milieu-limited alcoholism, is a relatively mild form seen in adults who were reared in home environments characterized by an adoptive father of low socioeconomic status and whose biological parents were alcoholics. In this form of alcoholism both genetic and environmental factors are required for the condition to be expressed.[18]

The second form of alcoholism in which a genetic predisposition is required is type II alcoholism (or male-limited alcoholism.) This type of alcoholism is a severe form found only in males and accounts for approximately 25% of all alcoholism found in the general population. Male-limited alcoholism is most often seen in the biological children of fathers with severe alcoholism. Neither the alcoholism status of the biological mother nor the environment provided in the adoptive home seem to be important factors in the expression of this form of alcoholism. Abstinence by male children appears to be the only preventive factor for those who have inherited this predisposition to alcoholism.

In addition to the genetic basis of the forms of alcoholism described above, genetics may account for some alcoholism seen in Oriental people. In this condition, low levels of aldehyde dehydrogenase (an enzyme necessary for the metabolism of alcohol) may account for an intolerance to alcohol. Genetic factors pertaining to the absorption rates of alcohol in the intestinal tract have been hypothesized to predispose American Indians to alcoholism. It is likely that more

Most alcoholics do not fit this stereotype.

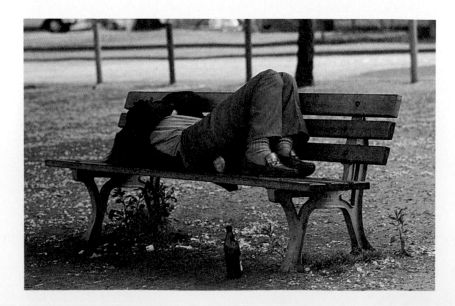

The Disease of Alcoholism

Exactly what is alcoholism? And why do alcoholics act the way they do—seemingly insane while not really insane, predictable in their nonsensical behavior, notoriously insensitive to others' feelings and needs, and most importantly, fanatic in their persistence in continuing to drink a liquid that is killing them?

There are over 100 million consumers of alcohol beverages in the United States. Some drinkers become alcoholics in their teens, some not until their sixties. Roughly 85% to 90% of these drinkers can take in alcohol without becoming alcoholic. If alcohol caused alcoholism, then *all* these drinkers would be alcoholics. But they aren't. This means, as anyone can plainly see, that people who become alcoholics are in some ways different from drinkers who are not. Alcoholism is chronic; it does not go away. Alcoholism is progressive; it gets worse in its effects as the alcoholic keeps drinking. Alcoholism is incurable; there is no cure, but a halt to drinking can arrest the disease—if the drinker stays dry.

A peculiar characteristic of the disease is that even if the alcoholic stops drinking for many years, then takes it up again, usually within 30 days or less the drinker is right back where he was when he quit, and almost always worse.

When alcohol enters the system it puts the part of the brain governing reason and judgment to sleep. That's why grown men and women act childish and emotional when they have had a few drinks: it's a physiological fact.

Alcoholics are allergic to alcohol and all other sedative drugs such as tranquilizers and sleeping pills. One prominent physician in the alcoholism/drug abuse field wants to call the disease "sedativism."

Scientists have learned that the alcoholic's brain chemistry is different from a nonalcoholic's. The alcoholic's brain, through a complicated biochemical process, takes in alcohol and produces a substance called THIQ, which is more addicting than morphine. The nonalcoholic's brain does not produce THIQ. Years of sobriety do not eliminate the THIQ process for the luckless alcoholic; if he or she starts drinking again after 25 years, there it is waiting.

Because alcohol is addictive, alcoholics drink *against* their will. This is difficult for nonalcoholics to understand. They may ask, "Why don't you just quit?" Alcoholics wish they could.

research will be undertaken concerning the role of genetic factors in all forms of chemical dependency.

The role of personality traits as conditioning factors in the development of alcoholism has received considerable attention. Factors ranging from unusually low levels of self-esteem to an antisocial personality have been described. Additional factors making persons susceptible to alcoholism may include excessive reliance on denial, hypervigilance, compulsiveness, and chronic levels of anxiety. Always complicating the study of personality traits is the uncertainty of whether the personality profile is a predisposing factor (perhaps from inheritance) or is caused by alcoholism itself.

Aside from the causes of alcoholism, there are nevertheless many specific behaviors that can be seen in individuals who are progressing through the stages of becoming an alcoholic. The characteristics listed in the box on p. 215 are not all inclusive. They are, however, behaviors that you can observe in the drinking patterns of others, including those who may soon be identified as alcoholics. The box above gives more information on alcoholism.

Denial and Enabling

Problem drinkers and alcoholics frequently use the psychological defense mechanism of *denial* to maintain their drinking behavior. By convincing themselves

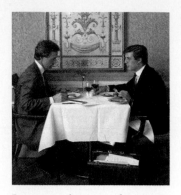

Important business decisions could be compromised by the use of alcohol.

that their lives are not affected by their drinking behavior, problem drinkers and alcoholics are able to maintain their drinking patterns. A person's denial is an unconscious process that is apparent only to rational observers.

Formerly, it was up to alcoholics to admit that their denial was no longer effective before they could be admitted to a treatment program. This is not the case today. Currently, family members, friends, or co-workers of alcohol dependent persons are encouraged to intervene and force an alcohol-dependent person into treatment.

During treatment, it is important for chemically dependent persons to break through the security of denial and to admit that alcohol controls their lives. This process will be demanding and often time consuming, but no alternative exists if recovery is to be achieved.

For family and friends of chemically dependent people, denial can be evident in a process known as *enabling*. In this process, people close to the problem drinker or alcoholic inadvertently support their behaviors by denying that a problem really exists. Enablers unconsciously make excuses for the drinker, try to keep the drinker's work and family life intact, and (in effect) make the continued abuse of alcohol possible. Alcohol counselors contend that enablers are an alcoholic's own worst enemy because they can significantly delay the onset of effective therapy. Do you know of a situation in which you or others have enabled a person with alcohol problems?

The processes of denial and enabling are major disruptive influences on family life. These family influences may be most keenly felt when the alcoholic persons are mothers. In a study of families in which the mother is an alcoholic, these patterns were observed[19]:

- Children were more likely to use drugs, be disinterested in school, and to run away from home.
- Marital problems were more likely to be present, but also denied by the husbands.
- Family members engaged in little social life outside the family.

Clearly, delaying the treatment of alcoholism is not in the best interest of the alcoholic or the family.

Alcoholism and the Family

Because the alcoholic individual is afflicted and subsequently affects the entire family, there is considerable disruption in the families of alcoholics. Families are disrupted not only by the consequences of the drinking behavior (such as violence, illness, unemployment), but also by the uncertainty of their role in causing and prolonging the situation. Frequently, family members begin to adopt a variety of new roles that will allow them to cope with the presence of the alcoholic in the family. Among the more commonly seen roles are the family hero, the lost child, the family mascot, and the scapegoat.[20] Unless family members receive appropriate counseling, these roles may remain intact for a lifetime.

Once an alcoholic's therapy has begun, family members are encouraged to participate in many aspects of the recovery. This will also help them to better understand the ways in which they were affected by alcoholism. Should therapy and aftercare include participation in Alcoholics Anonymous, family members will be encouraged to affiliate with related support groups.

HELPING THE ALCOHOLIC: REHABILITATION

Once an alcoholic realizes that alcoholism is not a form of moral weakness but rather a clearly defined illness, the chances for recovery are remarkably good. It is estimated that as many as two thirds of the victims of alcoholism can recover.[21] Recovery is especially enhanced when the victim has a good emotional support system, including concerned family members, friends, and employer. When this support system is not well established, the alcoholic's chances for recovery become considerably lessened.

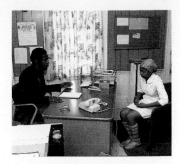

Problem drinkers and alcoholics need professional help.

Treatment methods for alcoholism will vary according to the specific needs of the individual. Following are three general steps in the treatment of alcoholism[22]:

1 *Managing acute episodes of intoxication* to save a life and overcome the immediate effects of excess alchohol. This step usually includes inpatient medical care for the person suffering from severe intoxication or acute alcohol withdrawal. Depending on the severity of the acute medical problem, the alcoholic may spend up to 2 weeks receiving this medical care. Common procedures might include proper *hydration,* use of tranquilizers to cope with withdrawal symptoms, and close supervision of food intake and **electrolyte balance.**

    Some therapists prescribe the deterrent drug disulfiram (Antabuse) in the initial weeks following detoxification. This drug is taken daily and produces an array of unpleasant symptoms if the patient should subsequently consume alcohol. These symptoms include nausea, vomiting, and pounding headaches. Used temporarily as an aid to other forms of supportive treatment, Antabuse can help the patient make the critical decision not to drink.*

2 *Correcting chronic health problems* associated with alcoholism. During this stage of treatment, attempts are made to medically manage established diseases such as **cirrhosis,** *polyneuropathy,* and even psychiatric disorders that have an origin in alcoholism.

3 *Changing long-term behavior* of alcoholic individuals so that destructive drinking patterns are not continued. Through individual and group counseling, the alcoholic learns to focus on behaviors that can produce positive effects in a person's life. No one plan is effective for everyone. Attempts are often made to encourage the development of skills in assertiveness, stress management, problem solving, and relaxation. Some recent behavioral programs have included the use of biofeedback machines to help alcoholics monitor their physiological responses during stressful and relaxing experiences.

electrolyte balance
proper concentration of various minerals within the blood and body fluids.

cirrhosis
pathological changes to the liver resulting from chronic, heavy alcohol consumption; a frequent cause of death among heavy alcohol users.

These three general steps to the treatment of alcoholism can be undertaken in various settings, including hospitals, clinics, and detoxification centers.

Alcoholics Anonymous (AA) is a voluntary support group of recovering alcoholics who meet regularly to help each other get sober and stay sober. Over 19,000 groups are in existence in the United States. AA encourages alcoholics to admit their lack of power over alcohol and to turn their lives over to a higher power (although the organization is nonsectarian). Members of AA are encouraged not to be judgmental about the behavior of other members. They support anyone with a problem caused by alcohol.

Al-Anon and Alateen are parallel organizations that give support to persons

---

*Recent research indicates that Antabuse may be more effective in helping a person maintain sobriety than it is in initially helping a person stop drinking.[23]

Resources for Children of Alcoholics

Many experts agree that adult children of alcoholics who believe they have come to terms with their feelings sometimes face lingering problems. It can prove worthwhile to seek help if you:

- Experience difficulty in identifying your needs
- Are always angry or sad
- Cannot enjoy your successes
- Tolerate inappropriate behavior
- Are regularly afraid of losing control

Support groups to contact for more information include the following:

- Al-Anon Adult Children Group
  One Park Avenue
  New York, NY 10016
  (212) 302-7240

- Children of Alcoholics Foundation, Inc.
  200 Park Avenue, 31st Floor
  New York, NY 10010
  (212) 351-2680

- National Association for Children of Alcoholics (NACoA)
  31706 Coast Highway
  Suite 201
  South Laguna, CA 92677
  (714) 499-3889

- National Council on Alcoholism
  12 West 21st Street
  New York, NY 10010
  (212) 206-6770
  Hotline: 1-800-NCA-CALL (1-800-622-2255)

who live with alcoholics. Al-Anon is geared for spouses and other relatives, while Alateen focuses on children of alcoholics. Both organizations help members realize that they are not alone and that successful adjustments can be made to nearly every alcoholic-related situation. AA, Al-Anon, and Alateen chapter organizations are usually listed in the telephone book or in the classified sections of local newspapers.

CURRENT ALCOHOL CONCERNS

Adult Children of Alcoholic Parents

In recent years a new dimension of alcoholism has been identified—the unusually high prevalence of alcoholism in the adult children of alcoholic parents.[24] Estimates are that these children are about four times more likely to develop alcoholism than children whose parents are not alcoholics. In response to this concern, support groups have been formed to assist the adult sons and daughters from developing the condition that afflicted the parents (see the box on p. 220). Should a stronger link for an inherited genetic predisposition to alcoholism be found, these groups may play an even greater role in the prevention of alcoholism.

SUMMARY

Alcohol is the drug of preference in most of Western society. For a significant number of people, including many college students, alcohol use is quite high. Heavy alcohol use and sporadic alcohol misuse are related to a variety of potentially serious problems, many of which include the entire family.

Alcohol in its purest form has little taste and negligible nutritional value. Most users of alcohol consume varieties of beer, wine, or distilled spirits. An understanding of alcohol's pharmacological properties may help one realize how problem drinking patterns can start and how difficult they are to resolve.

There are many factors that affect the rate of absorption of alcohol into the bloodstream. Some of these include food in the stomach, strength and amount of beverage, and the rate of consumption. When alcohol is consumed at a rate faster than it can be oxidized by the liver, the blood alcohol concentration rises and produces a fairly predictable sequence of depressive effects, which may have serious or even fatal consequences. For these reasons, it is important to be aware of the signs and symptoms of heavy alcohol use and to know first aid procedures for acute alcohol intoxication.

Alcohol use that interferes with one's adjustment in day-to-day activities is usually classified as problem drinking. Alcohol use that also involves physical dependency is usually classified as alcoholism. Although it is not known exactly what causes alcoholism, genetic links and specific behaviors leading to alcoholism have been identified. Denial and enabling are common defense mechanisms in alcoholism. Treatment and rehabilitation methods for the alcoholic include a variety of approaches.

Two current alcohol-related concerns are adult children of alcoholic parents and fetal alcohol syndrome. Though the misuse of alcohol appears to be an ever-increasing and unacceptable problem in our society, it is possible for one to develop responsible drinking patterns that can foster the satisfying and integrative use of alcohol.

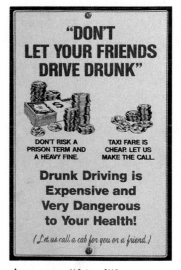

Are you a "friend"?

REVIEW QUESTIONS

1 What percentage of American adults consume alcohol? What percentage are classified as heavy drinkers? Approximately what percentage of adults are classified as abstainers? What percentage of college students drink?

2 What is meant by the term *proof*? What is the nutritional value of alcohol? How do distilled spirits differ from beer and wine? How do light- and low-alcoholic beverages compare?

3 Identify and explain the various factors that influence the absorption of alcohol. Why is it important to be aware of these factors?

4 What is BAC? Describe the general sequence of physiological effects that takes place when a person drinks alcohol at a rate faster than the liver can oxidize it.

5 What are the signs and symptoms of acute alcohol intoxication? What are the first aid steps you should take to help a person with this problem?

6 Explain the differences between problem drinking and alcoholism.

7 List five ways in which a host can serve alcohol responsibly.

8 What roles do denial and enabling play in alcoholism?

9 What types of alcoholism treatment programs are available in most communities?

10 Describe the characteristics of fetal alcohol syndrome and explain how it can be prevented.

QUESTIONS FOR PERSONAL CONTEMPLATION

1 Whether or not you use alcohol, consider how others react to your use or nonuse. Are they supportive of your decision? Do they encourage you to drink or not drink when you would rather do otherwise? How much is your decision influenced by those around you?

2 This chapter refers to data indicating that about one third of college drinkers can be considered heavy drinkers. Do you feel that this is true at your college?

3 Review the criteria for drinking levels and identify the classification that fits your current drinking pattern. Are you comfortable with this description? Do you think your drinking pattern will change when you are out of college?

4 How can you tell whether you and your friends are drinking in a responsible manner? How often do you use alcohol only as a social lubricant?

5 How frequently do you drive a car while under the influence of alcohol? What risks are you taking? What might you do to avoid these situations in the future? Do you feel it is your responsibility to make sure friends do not drink and drive?

6 Do you feel any sense of responsibility for a woman's fetus when you see her drink alcohol? What role should men play in the prevention of fetal alcohol syndrome?

REFERENCES

1 Drinking spree sponsor may face charges, The Indianapolis Star April 30, 1983, p 23.

2 US Bureau of the Census: Statistical abstract of the United States: 1986, ed 106, Washington DC, 1985, US Department of Commerce.

3 US Department of Health and Human Services: Alcohol and health: special report to the US Congress, DHHS Pub no (ADM) 87-1519, Washington DC, 1987, US Government Printing Office.

4 On campus poll: drugs and health, Newsweek: On Campus April, 1987, p 23.

5 US Department of Health and Human Services: Facts about alcohol and alcoholism, Rockville, Md, 1980, National Institute on Alcohol Abuse and Alcoholism.

6 Ray, O, and Ksir, C: Drugs, society, and human behavior, ed 4, St Louis, 1987, Times Mirror/Mosby College Publishing.

7 Parcel, GS: Basic emergency care of the sick and injured, ed 3, St Louis, 1986, Times Mirror/Mosby College Publishing.

8 Donahue, RP, et al: Alcohol and hemorrhage stroke, Journal of the American Medical Association 255:2311-2314, 1986.

9 Schatzkin, A, et al: Alcohol consumption and breast cancer in the epidemiologic follow-up study at the first national health and nutrition examination survey, The New England Journal of Medicine 316, 1169-1123.

10 Ouelette, E: The fetal alcohol syndrome, Contemporary Nutrition 9:1, 1984.

11 Alcohol in perspective, Consumer Reports July, 1983, pp. 354, 378.

12 College awareness program provides range of activities, NIAAA Information and Feature Services IFS no 107, May 3, 1983.

13 Task Force on Responsible Decisions About Alcohol: Interim report no 2, Denver, 1975, Education Commission of the States.

14 Witt, H: Temptation vs temperance: a battle over college alcohol, Chicago Tribune March 4, 1984, p 4.

15 Crackdown needed to stop this carnage, USA Today December 31, 1986, p 8a.

16 Anda, RF, Remington, PL, and Williamson, DF: A sobering perspective on a lower blood alcohol limit, Journal of the American Medical Association 256:3213, 1986.

17 Peele, S: The implications and limitations of genetic models of alcoholism and other addicitons, Journal of Studies on Alcohol 47:63-73, 1986.

18 US Department of Health and Human Services: Alcohol and health: fourth special report to the US Congress, DHHS Pub no ADM 281-85-0009, 1987.

19 Ames, GM: Middle-class protestants: alcohol and family. In The American experience with alcohol: contrasting cultural perspectives, New York, 1985, Plenum Publishing Corp.

20 Kinney, J, and Leaton, G: Loosening the grip: a handbook of alcohol information, ed 3, St Louis, 1987, Times Mirror/Mosby College Publishing.

21 Moore, J: Director, Middletown Center for Chemical Dependency, personal interview, July 10, 1987.

22 Alcohol, Drug Abuse, and Mental Health Administration: Treating alcoholism: the illness, the symptoms, the treatment, DHHS Pub no ADM 82-128, 1982, The Administration.

23 Fuller, RK, et al: Disulfiram treatment of alcoholism, Journal of the American Medical Association 256:1449-1455, 1986.

24 Woititz, JG: Adult children of alcoholics, Pompano Beach, Fla, 1983, Health Communications, Inc.

ANNOTATED READINGS

Elkin, M: Families under the influence: changing alcoholic patterns, New York, 1984, WW Norton & Co, Inc.
   Written especially for those who work with alcoholics and their families; also suggested for anyone interested in the problem of alcoholism.

Gross, L: How much is too much? New York, 1983, Random House, Inc.
   The effects of social drinking; a report on the most authoritative findings about the risks and rewards of social drinking; will help people decide how much is too much.

Meyer, M: Drinking problems—family problems, Claremont, Calif, 1982, Momenta Publishing, Hunter House, Inc, Publishers.
   Helps the reader learn to cope better with both the problem drinker and his or her own problems.

Mumey, J: The joy of being sober: a book for recovering alcoholics and those who love them, Chicago, 1984, Contemporary Books, Inc.
   A practical handbook that offers advice and insight into the new horizons that await the recovering alcoholic.

Pinkham, ME: How to stop the one you love from drinking, New York, 1986, The Putnam Publishing Group, Inc.
   Describes the relationships within an alcoholic family. The process of how to confront the alcoholic is explained.

Woititz, JG: Adult children of alcoholics, Pompano Beach, Fla, 1983, Health Communications, Inc.
   Best-selling book that describes the tendency for alcoholism to occur in the grown children of alcoholic parents.

CHAPTER 9

Tobacco Use
A Losing Choice

Key Concepts

Tobacco use has a major impact on a person's health.

The use of cigarettes among adults is declining, while the use of smokeless tobacco is only beginning to decline.

Tobacco is a source of many physiologically active chemicals.

Physiological and psychosocial factors underlie tobacco dependency.

A high degree of personal motivation is required to quit smoking.

The issues of smokers' and nonsmokers' rights are complex.

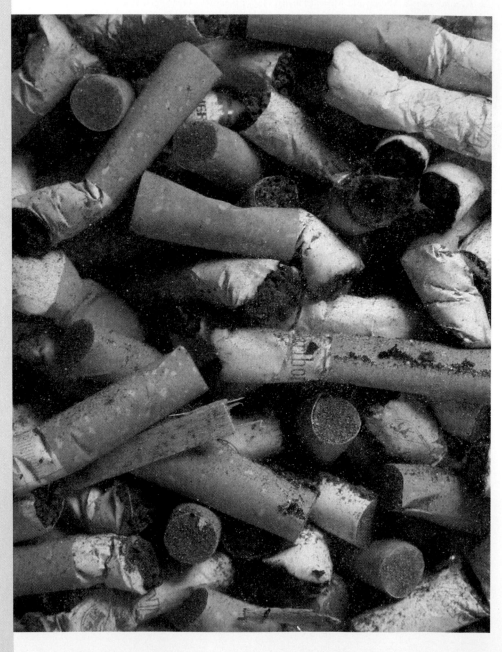

In May 1984, Dr. C. Everett Koop, the U.S. Surgeon General, called for a smoke-free society by the year 2000. This directive came as no real surprise, since an earlier report by the Surgeon General stated: "Cigarette smoking should be considered the most important of the known modifiable risk factors for coronary heart disease in the United States."[1]

Most health professionals are in complete agreement that "cigarette smoking is the single most preventable cause of death."[2] Apparently our legislators feel the same way. President Ronald Reagan's signing of the Comprehensive Smoking Education Act in October 1984 indicated a greater congressional awareness of the hazards of smoking. One major provision of this act required new warning labels on cigarette packages and advertisements. These new warnings, which are used on a 3-month rotating cycle, are listed below[3]:

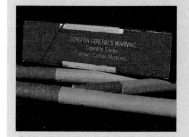

SURGEON GENERAL'S WARNING:
Smoking causes lung cancer, heart disease, emphysema, and may complicate pregnancy.

SURGEON GENERAL'S WARNING:
Quitting smoking now greatly reduces serious risks to your health.

SURGEON GENERAL'S WARNING:
Smoking by pregnant women may result in fetal injury, premature birth, and low birth weight.

SURGEON GENERAL'S WARNING:
Cigarette smoke contains carbon monoxide.

Today the evidence linking tobacco use to impaired health is beyond serious challenge. The regular user of tobacco products, particularly cigarettes, will be more likely to become sick, remain sick for extended periods, and die prematurely. Any contention to the contrary made by the tobacco industry is little more than a rationalization that ignores the growing weight of scientific evidence.

THE PHYSIOLOGICAL EFFECTS OF TOBACCO

The above warnings exist because of tobacco's ability to alter the normal function of the body and produce a variety of disease processes. Throughout this chapter we will describe these tobacco-related illnesses. Before doing so, however, it is necessary to describe some of the basic changes in physiological function that occur in conjunction with tobacco use, even short-term use. Particularly important are those changes brought about because of the presence of **nicotine** in tobacco smoke.

The changes listed in Table 9-1 should seem familiar to you, because they are the changes associated with the stress response described in Chapter 3. Nicotine functions as a powerful stressor to the body, and its presence stimulates the production of epinephrine from the adrenal medulla and adrenocorticotropic hormone (ACTH) from the pituitary gland. The cardiovascular, respiratory, and endocrine systems of the body are, of course, primarily involved in the stress response. Chronic exposure to nicotine produces additional functional and structural changes that serve as the basis for specific disease processes and illnesses.

In addition to nicotine's important role, the presence of **carbon monoxide** and many **carcinogens** in tobacco smoke also influences physiological function. These agents and their specific influences will be presented in later sections of this chapter.

nicotine
physiologically active, dependency-producing drug found in tobacco.

carbon monoxide (CO)
chemical compound that can "inactivate" red blood cells.

carcinogens
substances that stimulate the development of cancer.

Table 9-1   Physiological Changes in Response to Tobacco Smoke

Body Process	Effect
Peripheral vascular circulation	Restricts
Heart rate	Increases
Heart rhythm (pattern of beat)	Alters
Blood pressure	Increases
Clotting time	Decreases
Bronchial (airway) diameter	Decreases
Respiratory rate	Increases
Mucus production (in airways)	Increases
Gastric motility	Decreases
Hunger (sensation of)	Decreases
Urinary output	Decreases
Excitatory neurotransmitter activity	Increases
Inhibitory neurotransmitter activity (with high doses)	Increases
Mobilization of energy stores (including blood lipids)	Increases

TOBACCO USE IN AMERICAN SOCIETY

If you were to visit certain businesses, entertainment spots, or sporting events in your community, you might leave convinced that virtually every adult is a tobacco user. Certainly, for some segments of the society, tobacco use is the rule rather than the exception. You may be quite surprised to find out that the great majority of adults do not use tobacco products.

On the basis of a variety of currently available statistics,[4] less than 30% of all adults smoke cigarettes. Further, data on smoking reveal that since 1964 the percentages of men and women who smoke cigarettes have declined steadily. For example, in 1965, 52.4% of adult males (age 20 and over) smoked compared to 29.5% in 1987. Among women (age 20 and over), 34.1% smoked in 1965 compared to 23.8% in 1987.[5]

Among younger persons, 1985 national statistics indicated that 18.7% of high school seniors were regular cigarette smokers.[6] By contrast, 1986 statistics indicated that approximately 14% of college students smoke cigarettes.[7] Clearly, college-educated people are not as likely to smoke as those who do not go to college. Furthermore, college students at prestigious schools and black college students represent the populations of college students least likely to smoke.[6]

In contrast to the general population, where higher percentages of men smoke than women, college women are more likely to smoke than are college men. Approximately 18% of college women smoke, whereas only 10% of college men smoke.[7] Why do you think more women than men smoke cigarettes?

Although the total percentage of the population using tobacco is lower now than it has been, the total number of persons using tobacco is at an all-time high. This finding reflects the continuing expansion of our population. Some evidence suggests that smokers are smoking more heavily than before, yet the production of cigarettes dropped from 711 billion cigarettes in 1982 to 652 billion in 1986.[8] Cigarette sales are projected to begin a gradual decline as the number of young persons reaching "smoking age" declines and as more smokers stop. In 1983 about one of every eight cigarette smokers actually quit smoking.[8]

In addition to the trend changes already discussed, preference for various types of tobacco products is also undergoing change. For over 400 years, cigars, pipes, and *smokeless tobacco* dominated the tobacco market. Cigarettes then rose greatly in popularity in the early 1900s and have remained the most popular tobacco item. Since 1970, however, a significant resurgence in the use of smokeless tobacco has been noted. Snuff and chewing tobacco, unfortunately, are thought by some users to represent safer alternatives to cigarettes.

In recent years the type of cigarettes preferred by smokers has changed. Today only a small percentage of all cigarette smokers prefer the small unfiltered cigarettes that were popular before and after World War II. Even the king-sized filtered cigarettes popular during the 1960s are losing popularity. High tar, high nicotine, high carbon monoxide cigarettes are rapidly being replaced by low and ultralow tar and nicotine brands. Today *low tar and nicotine* brands (15 mg of tar or less) and *ultralow tar and nicotine* brands (less than 4 mg of tar) have cornered over 65% of the total cigarette market.[9]

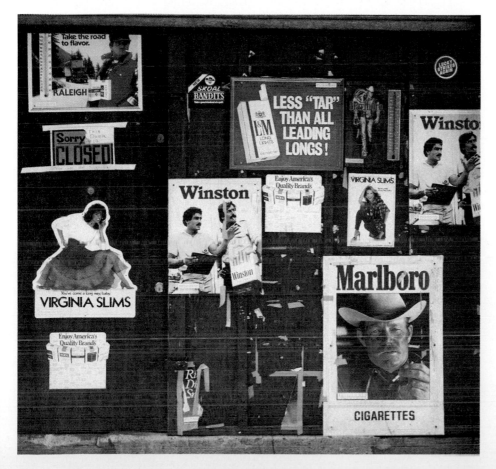

Cigarette advertising delivers a persuasive message for some.

Tobacco production is declining.

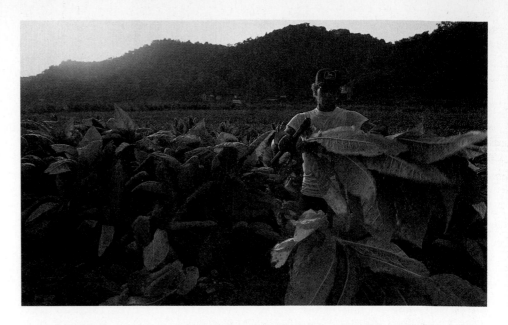

Beyond the statistics and trends discussed, a few additional changes seem likely in the cigarette industry. Included among these are the following:

- *More cigarettes per package.* An attempt by some tobacco companies to out-market their fewer-per-pack competitors.
- *Higher federal and state taxes per package.* Revenue sources are important to government, and cigarette taxation is a proven source of revenue.
- *Increased popularity of generic brands.* Most major manufacturers of cigarettes have several brands on the market at the same time, some of which are generic.
- *Decreased emphasis on taste and an increased emphasis on status.* Since smokers lose their ability to taste, an emphasis on taste becomes a meaningless focus. Cigarette marketing will focus on status, including the introduction of "designer cigarettes." Indeed, cigarette marketing is expensive (see Figure 9-1).

Thus tobacco use remains dynamic—and, as it has always been—dangerous.

Pipe and Cigar Smoking

Many persons believe that pipe or cigar smoking is a safe alternative to cigarette smoking. Unfortunately, this is not the case. All forms of tobacco present users with a series of health threats.

When compared to cigarette smokers, pipe and cigar smokers have cancer of the mouth, throat, larynx (voice box), and esophagus at the same frequency. Cigarette smokers are more likely than pipe and cigar smokers to have lung cancer, chronic obstructive lung disease (COLD), and heart disease. However, the incidence of respiratory disease and heart disease in pipe and cigar smokers is greater than among nonusers of tobacco.

In addition to the health risks described above, pipe and cigar smokers, like cigarette smokers, are not immune from the legal and social prohibitions against smoking. Whether pipe and cigar smoking even represents an "improvement" over cigarette smoking is open to debate.

TOBACCO USE AND THE DEVELOPMENT OF DEPENDENCY

Dependency can imply both a physical and psychological relationship. Particularly for the cigarette smoker, *physical dependency,* with its associated tolerance, withdrawal, **titration,** and *psychological dependency,* with its accompanying psychological **compulsion,** and **indulgence,** are frequently seen. Research has, in fact, determined that dependency on tobacco is far more easily established than is dependency on alcohol, cocaine, or heroin. Eighty-five percent of all persons who experiment with cigarettes develop a dependency relationship.[10] Typical cigarette smokers develop *addiction* to some aspect of the tobacco's chemical composition, while at the same time they become emotionally dependent on its consistent availability.

Physiological and psychosocial factors identified as possible causes of this dependency will be discussed next.

Physiological Factors Related to Dependency

Russell's bolus model[11] suggests that tobacco use is conditioned by the periods of neurohormonal arousal produced by each *bolus* (ball) of nicotine reaching the brain. Wanting to maintain this feeling of arousal, the smoker inhales again and again. Several hundred puffs per day (approximately eight per cigarette) quickly establish the schedule necessary to maintain the desired effect. Unique differences in smoking behavior (including the number of puffs per cigarette, the depth of inhalation, and the length of time the smoke is held in the lungs) and

titration
particular level of a drug within the body.

compulsion
compelling emotional desire to engage in a particular behavior.

indulgence
strong emotional desire to engage in a particular behavior solely for one's own enjoyment or benefit.

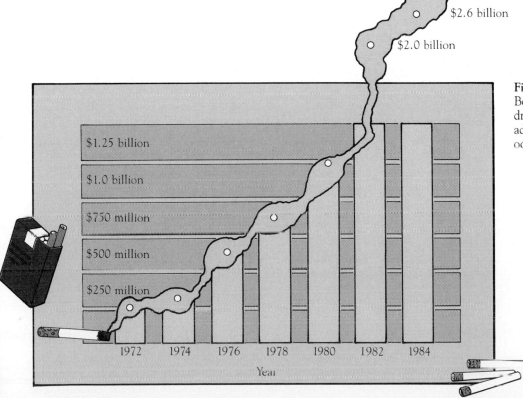

Figure 9-1
Between 1974 and 1984, dramatic growth in cigarette advertising expenditures occurred.

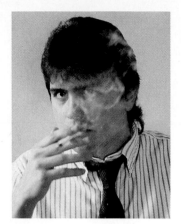

Dependency can last a lifetime.

a variance in genetic predisposition to dependency account for the differing degrees of dependency noted among smokers. The speed at which dependency is established is also likely to be *dose related.*

As tolerance to nicotine develops, the person's smoking behavior is adjusted to maintain titration and prevent the occurrence of withdrawal symptoms. At some point the desire for constant arousal is probably negated by the smoker's desire not to experience withdrawal. Thus people smoke to protect themselves from the withdrawal effects, rather than for the pleasure of being aroused.

As with any other psychoactive drug, cessation of nicotine can result in withdrawal symptoms. These symptoms are described in Chapter 7, p. 166, in more detail.

The importance of nicotine as the primary factor in establishing dependency on tobacco is supported by research that demonstrates that smokers will not select a nontobacco cigarette if a tobacco cigarette is available. Even tobacco cigarettes with a very low level of nicotine seem to be unacceptable to most smokers, as do cigarettes with very low nicotine but with high tar content. Interestingly, users of low nicotine cigarettes tend to inhale more frequently and deeply to obtain as much nicotine as possible.

In many regards, a *high nicotine–low tar cigarette* might be a "safer" cigarette than those currently recommended (low nicotine–low tar) as being safer. The high nicotine would more quickly satisfy the dependency needs of the smoker and fewer cigarettes would be smoked. The low tar content would somewhat protect the smoker from the concentrated carcinogenic environment associated with a higher tar brand.

Although not burned, snuff and chewing tobacco deliver nicotine effectively through the mucous membranes of the mouth and nose. Cigar and pipe smoke, when not inhaled, manage to transmit some nicotine to the smoker but in amounts considerably below those associated with cigarettes.

A relatively recent theory of the pharmacological basis of tobacco dependency is that nicotine is a stimulant for the release of the hormone **ACTH.** Once released from the pituitary gland, ACTH stimulates the release of *beta endorphins.* These endorphins are opiate-like chemicals found within the nervous system that produce feelings of euphoria. Should this biological opiate link with nicotine be substantiated, smoking could be seen as accomplishing through negative addiction what jogging and meditation accomplish through positive addiction. Considerably more research remains to be done in this area.

ACTH
adrenocorticotropic hormone.

Psychosocial Factors Related to Dependency

In the view of behavioral scientists, dependency to tobacco can also be explained on the basis of psychosocial factors. Both research and general observation support many of the powerful influences these factors have on the beginning smoker.

Modeling

Because tobacco use is a learned behavior, it is reasonable to accept the role that *modeling* plays as a stimulus to experimental smoking. Modeling suggests that adolescents smoke to emulate smokers whom they admire. Because of this, teachers, coaches, actors, athletes, and even rock stars need to consider the

How Much Do You Know About Smoking?

SMOKERS DIE YOUNGER

The death rate of cigarette smokers at all ages is higher than that of non-smokers. It climbs in proportion to the number of cigarettes smoked, the number of years the smokers have smoked, and the earlier the age at which they started. According to the British Royal College of Physicians, "Cigarette smoking is now as important a cause of death as the great epidemics of typhoid, cholera and tuberculosis, in the past." The reason for the deadliness of cigarettes is the many different diseases they cause.

CIGARETTE-RELATED CANCERS IN MEN

Men who smoke less than half a pack a day have a death rate about 60% higher than that of nonsmokers; a pack to two packs a day, about 90% higher; and two or more packs a day, 120% above normal. Male cigarette smokers have about five times the normal risk of dying of mouth cancer as nonsmokers. Larynx cancer is six to nine times as frequent among cigarette smokers as among nonsmokers. Deaths from urinary bladder cancer are two to three times as numerous among cigarette smokers as among nonsmokers. They are also more likely to get pancreatic cancer.

CIGARETTE-RELATED CANCERS IN WOMEN

The lung cancer death rate of women has almost tripled in 15 years. Lung cancer is now the leading cause of cancer deaths in women. Pregnant women who smoke have a greater number of stillbirths than nonsmoking women; and their infants are more likely to die within the first month. Their babies more often weigh less than 5½ pounds (which is considered premature) and are exposed to more risk of disease and death.

SMOKING AND FIRES

In 1981, a total of 65,000 fires were specifically traced as being smoking related, resulting in 2,300 deaths, 5,000 victims suffering from burns, and a total property loss of more than $300 million in the United States. About 9% of all U.S. fires are caused by smokers.

FILTER CIGARETTES

Ninety-five percent of American smokers have switched to filter tips. Recent studies have shown that smokers who smoke low tar–low nicotine cigarettes have a lower lung cancer death rate than those who smoke high tar–high nicotine cigarettes. But these rates are still far higher than for those who have never smoked.

INVOLUNTARY SMOKING

The health effects of smoking do not apply only to smokers. A number of studies have shown that nonsmoking women married to smokers have an increased risk of lung cancer and that the risk increased with the number of cigarettes their husbands smoked.

Does smoking make young people appear older?

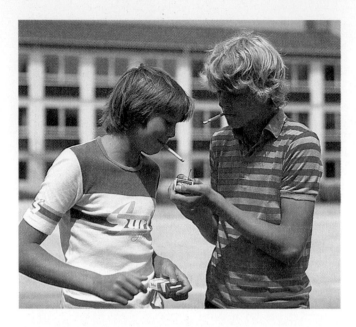

powerful but subtle impact they have on young people. The smoking behavior of adolescents does correlate with the smoking behavior of their parents, older siblings, and school friends. It is true that smoking behavior is reinforced by the actions of others. The tobacco industry has capitalized on this process by showing only attractive, successful, healthy people in its advertisements.

For those of you who are both smokers and parents of young children, you should remember this relationship between smoking and modeling when you think about your children's use or nonuse of tobacco. With tobacco use, parents can be excellent teachers of bad behavior.

Manipulation

In addition to modeling as a psychosocial link with tobacco use, tobacco use may meet the beginning smoker's need to manipulate something and at the same time provide the manipulative "tool" necessary to offset boredom or social immaturity. Clearly the availability of affordable smoking paraphernalia provides smokers with ways to reward themselves. A new cigarette lighter, a status brand of tobacco, or a beach towel with a cigarette's logo are all reinforcements to some smokers. For others, the ability to take out a cigarette or fill a pipe adds a measure of structure and control to situations in which they might otherwise feel somewhat ill at ease. The cigarette becomes a readily available and dependable "friend" to turn to during stressful moments.

Self-indulgence

The images of the smoker's world portrayed by the media can be particularly attractive. For young adolescents, few ways are available to experience the "real world." Sexual activity can establish a kind of instant adulthood, as can alcohol use and driving. Nothing, however, is as readily available as the cigarette for accomplishing this magical transition from the powerless world of childhood to the desired status of being "grown-up." Young smokers wish to emulate tobacco users, and the world depicted by tobacco advertisements is clearly better than the world in which they must live as children. Thus another strong motive is present for experimentation.

In Chapter 7 the human need to take risks was offered as a reason why many people turn to psychoactive drugs. Smoking also involves great personal risks, some of which might be characterized as self-indulgent. Since beginning smokers have been frequently informed of these risks, it is possible that it is the exciting opportunity to "beat the odds" that encourages them to start smoking in the first place.

With this multiplicity of forces at work, it is possible to understand why so many who experiment with tobacco use find that they quickly become tobacco dependent. Human needs, both physiological and psychosocial, are many and complex. Tobacco use meets these needs on a short-term basis, while dependency, once established, replaces these needs with a different, more immediate set of needs.

In spite of self-indulgence, approximately 90% of adult smokers have on at least one occasion expressed a desire to quit and 80% have actually attempted to become nonsmokers; therefore, tobacco use is a source of **dissonance.** This dissonance stems from the need to deal emotionally with a behavior that is both enjoyable and dangerous. The degree that this dissonance exists and the extent to which it negates the effectiveness of tobacco use as a coping technique probably varies greatly from user to user.

dissonance
feeling of uncertainty that occurs when a person believes two equally attractive but opposite ideas.

TOBACCO: THE SOURCE OF PHYSIOLOGICALLY ACTIVE COMPOUNDS

When burned, the tobacco in cigarettes, cigars, and pipe mixtures is a source of an array of physiologically active chemicals, many of which are closely linked to significant changes in normal body structure and function. At the burning tip of the cigarette the 900° C (1,652° F) heat oxidizes tobacco (as well as paper, wrapper, filler, and additives). With each puff of smoke, the body is exposed to over 2,000 chemical compounds, 200 of which are currently suspected to be *carcinogenic.* An annual 50,000 puffs taken in by the one-pack-a-day cigarette smoker result in a regularly occurring environment that makes the most polluted urban environment seem mild by comparison.

Cigarette, cigar, and pipe smoke can be described on the basis of two phases or components. These phases include a particulate phase and a gaseous phase. The **particulate phase** includes a variety of powerful compounds, including nicotine, phenol, cresol, pyrene, DDT, and a benzene-ring group of compounds that includes benzo[a]pyrene. The majority of the carcinogenic compounds are located in the particulate phase.

The **gaseous phase** of tobacco smoke, like the particulate phase, is composed of a variety of physiologically active compounds, including carbon monoxide, carbon dioxide, ammonia, hydrogen cyanide, isoprene, acetaldehyde, and acetone. *Carbon monoxide* is the most damaging compound found in this component of tobacco smoke. Its impact will be discussed shortly.

particulate phase
portion of the tobacco smoke composed of small suspended particles.

gaseous phase
portion of the tobacco smoke containing carbon monoxide and many other physiologically active gaseous compounds.

Nicotine

Nicotine is the powerful chemical agent found in the particulate phase of tobacco smoke. When drawn into the lungs, about one fourth of the nicotine in

Personal Assessment

Test Your Knowledge About Cigarette Smoking

Assumption

1 There are now safe cigarettes on the market.

2 A small number of cigarettes can be smoked without risk.

3 Most early changes in the body resulting from cigarette smoking are temporary.

4 Filters provide a measure of safety to cigarette smokers.

5 Low tar–low nicotine cigarettes are safer than high tar–high nicotine brands.

6 Mentholated cigarettes are better for the smoker than are nonmentholated brands.

7 It has been scientifically proved that cigarette smoking causes cancer.

8 No specific agent capable of causing cancer has ever been identified in the tobacco used in smokeless tobacco.

9 The cure rate for lung cancer is so good that no one should fear developing this form of cancer.

10 Smoking is not harmful as long as the smoke is not inhaled.

11 The "smoker's cough" reflects underlying damage to the tissue of the airways.

12 Cigarette smoking does not appear to be associated with damage of the heart and blood vessels.

13 Because of the design of the placenta, smoking does not present a major risk to the developing fetus.

Discussion

F Depending on the brand, some cigarettes contain less tar and nicotine; none are safe, however.

F Even a low level of smoking exposes the body to harmful substances in tobacco smoke.

T Some, however, cannot be reversed—particularly changes associated with emphysema.

T However, the protection is far from adequate.

T Many persons, however, smoke low tar–low nicotine cigarettes in a manner that makes them just as dangerous as stronger cigarettes.

F Menthol simply makes cigarette smoke feel cooler. The smoke contains all of the harmful agents found in the smoke from regular cigarettes.

T Particularly for lung cancer and cancers of the larynx, esophagus, oral cavity, and urinary bladder.

F Unfortunately, smokeless tobacco is no safer than the tobacco that is burned. The user of smokeless tobacco swallows much of what the smoker inhales.

F Approximately 10% of those persons having lung cancer will live the 5 years required to meet the medical definition of "cured."

F Because of the toxic material in smoke, even its contact with the tissue of the oral cavity introduces a measure of risk in this form of cigarette use.

T The "cough" occurs in response to an inability to clear the airway of mucus as a result of changes in the cells which normally keep the air passages clear.

F Cigarette smoking is, in fact, the single most important risk factor in the development of cardiovascular disease.

F Children born to women who smoked during pregnancy show a variety of health impairments, including smaller birth size, premature birth, and more illnesses during the first year of life. Smoking women also have more stillbirths.

Assumption	Discussion
14 Women who smoke cigarettes and use an oral contraceptive should decide which they wish to continue, because there is a risk in using both.	T Women over 35 years of age, in particular, are at risk of experiencing serious heart disease should they continue using both cigarettes and an oral contraceptive.
15 Air pollution is a greater risk to our respiratory health than is cigarette smoking.	F Although air pollution does expose the body to potentially serious problems, the risk is considerably less than that associated with smoking.
16 Addiction, in the sense of physical addiction, is found in conjunction with cigarette smoking.	T Dependency, including true physical addition, is widely recognized in cigarette smokers.
17 The best "teachers" a young smoker has are his or her parents.	T There is a strong correlation between cigarette smoking of parents and the subsequent smoking of their children. Parents who do not want their children to smoke should not smoke.
18 Nonsmoking and higher levels of education are directly related.	T The higher one's level of education, the less likely one is to smoke.
19 About as many women smoke cigarettes as do men.	T Although in the past more men smoked than did women, the trend is changing. In the future cigarette smoking could become a woman's pastime.
20 Fortunately, for those who now smoke, stopping is relatively easy.	F Unfortunately, relatively few smokers can quit. The best advice is never to begin smoking.

the inhaled smoke passes into the systemic circulation, through the brain barrier, and into the brain. *Nicotine receptors* within the brain are activated and produce a variety of responses, the majority of which are stimulating. The effects of low to moderate levels of nicotine include altered **EEG patterns** and behavior arousal as a result of the increased production of neurotransmitters, including norepinephrine, dopamine, acetylcholine, and serotonin. High levels of nicotine, however, depress the central nervous system and result in the relaxation associated with heavy smoking. These phenomena suggest that nicotine is a neurotransmitter blocking agent as well as a neurotransmitter stimulant. (Refer to Chapter 7 for a more detailed discussion of neurotransmitter function.)

The remaining nicotine absorbed into the blood travels throughout the body to nicotinic receptors located in a variety of tissues. Among the presently understood additional effects of nicotine are the reduction of intestinal motility, the release of epinephrine from the adrenal glands, the release of **norepinephrine** from peripheral nerves, increase in heart rate, the constriction of peripheral blood vessels, and the dilation of airways within the respiratory system.

EEG patterns
patterns reflecting the type and extent of electrical activity occurring in the cerebral cortex of the brain.

norepinephrine
adrenalin-like chemical produced within the nervous system.

Tar

When nicotine and water are removed from tobacco, the remainder of the particulate phase forms the *tar* we are familiar with through today's cigarette advertisements. This dark-brown residue is a rich, chemically active substance that potentially can cause detrimental changes within the tissues of the respiratory system. The relationship of tar's carcinogenic compounds to cancer of the cells lining the air passages will be discussed later in the chapter.

Carbon Monoxide

Like every inefficient engine, a cigarette, cigar, or pipe burns (oxidizes) its fuel with less than complete conversion into carbon dioxide, water, and heat. As a result of this incomplete oxidation, burning tobacco forms carbon monoxide gas. Carbon monoxide is one of the most harmful components of tobacco smoke.

Carbon monoxide is a colorless, odorless, tasteless gas that possesses an affinity for hemoglobin, the oxygen-carrying pigment on each red blood cell. When carbon monoxide is inhaled, it quickly bonds with hemoglobin and reduces the red blood cell's ability to transport oxygen.[9] This leads to shortness of breath and lowered endurance. Recall that adequate oxygen supply to all body tissues is critical for normal functioning. Any oxygen reduction can have a serious impact on a person's body. Brain functioning may be reduced, reactions and judgments dulled, and circulation impaired. Fetuses are especially at risk to this oxygen deprivation, since the fetal development is so critically dependent on sufficient oxygen supply from the mother.[12]

ILLNESS, PREMATURE DEATH, AND TOBACCO USE

For the person who begins tobacco use as an adolescent or young adult, smokes heavily, and continues to smoke, the likelihood of living significantly fewer years is virtually assured. Current data suggest that the two-pack-a-day cigarette smoker can expect to die 7 to 8 years earlier than his or her nonsmoking peers.[1] If one wishes to translate this decrease in life expectancy into a shorter term perspective, then for each cigarette, subtract approximately 6 minutes from the normal life expectancy. Ten cigarettes—half a pack—will reduce life expectancy by an interval equal to the length of a college class period. A full pack takes two lecture periods' worth of time. It is certainly true that smoking a cigarette can make time fly.

More recent evidence suggests that the 7- to 8-year reduction in life expectancy attributed to cigarette smoking may be a grossly underestimated interpretation of the impact of smoking. If life expectancy statistics were based solely on causes of death directly related to smoking (such as lung cancer, cardiovascular disease, and emphysema), smokers would be projected to die 23 years earlier than nonsmokers.[13] Clearly the seriousness of cancer, cardiovascular disease, and respiratory disease in smokers contributes to this remarkable statistical projection.

The smoker is 70% more likely to die prematurely than is the nonsmoker. According to one authoritative estimate, smoking is directly related to 485,000 deaths per year in the United States.[14] Included in this estimate are 147,000 cancer deaths, 240,000 cardiovascular deaths, 61,000 noncancer deaths from diseases of the respiratory system, 14,000 deaths from digestive system diseases, 4,000 infant deaths related to mother's smoking, 4,000 deaths from fires and accidents, and nearly 15,000 deaths from miscellaneous and ill-defined diseases.

CARDIOVASCULAR DISEASE AND TOBACCO USE

Cardiovascular disease is the leading cause of death among all adults, accounting for 986,370 deaths in the United States in 1984.[15] Tobacco use, and cigarette smoking in particular, is clearly one of the major factors contributing to this cause of death. While overall progress is being made in reducing the incidence of cardiovascular-related deaths, tobacco use affects these efforts. So important is tobacco use as a contributing factor in deaths from cardiovascular disease that the cigarette smoker doubles the risk of experiencing a **myocardial infarction,** the leading cause of death from cardiovascular disease (see Figure 9-2). Smokers also increase their risk of **sudden cardiac death** by two to four times.[15] Fully one third of all cardiovascular disease can be traced to cigarette smoking.

The relationship between tobacco use and cardiovascular disease is centered on two major components of tobacco smoke: nicotine and carbon monoxide.

Nicotine and Cardiovascular Disease

The influence of nicotine on the cardiovascular system occurs when it stimulates the nervous system to release norepinephrine. This powerful stimulant increases the rate at which the heart contracts. In turn an elevated heart rate increases cardiac output, thus increasing blood pressure. The extent to which an elevated heart rate is dangerous depends in part on the coronary circulation's ability to supply blood to the rapidly contracting heart muscle. The development of **angina pectoris** and the possibility of sudden heart attack are heightened by this sus-

myocardial infarction
heart attack; the death of heart muscle as a result of a blockage in one of the coronary arteries.

sudden cardiac death
immediate death resulting from a sudden change in the rhythm of the heart.

angina pectoris
chest pain that results from impaired blood supply to the heart muscle.

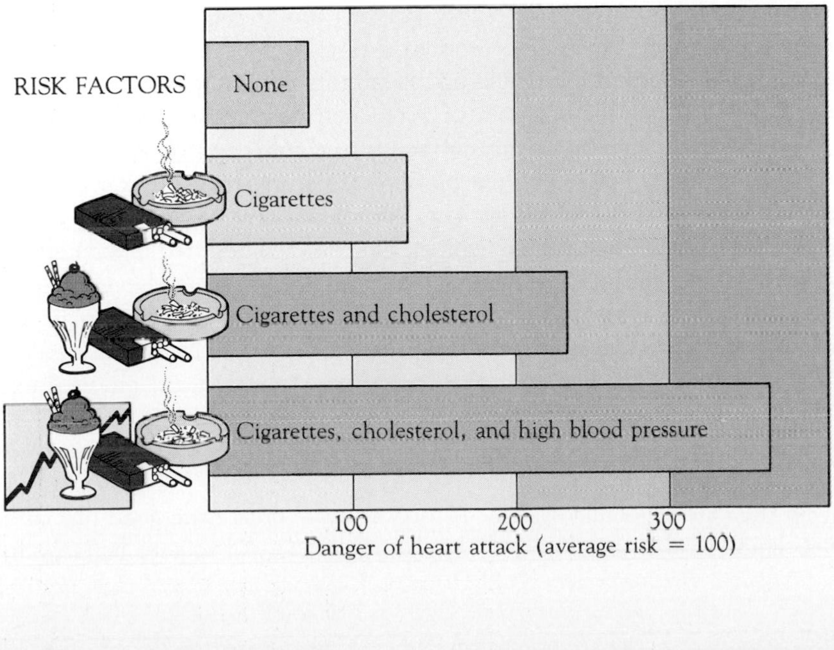

Figure 9-2
The danger of heart attack increases with the number of risk factors present. Smoking is the most significant of the three risk factors listed.

RISK FACTORS

None

Cigarettes

Cigarettes and cholesterol

Cigarettes, cholesterol, and high blood pressure

100   200   300
Danger of heart attack (average risk = 100)

tained elevation of heart rate, particularly in those individuals with existing coronary artery disease (see Chapter 10).

The ability of the general circulation to accommodate the elevated blood pressure generated by the increased cardiac output reflects the overall health of the vascular system. In persons with atherosclerotic disease, elevated blood pressure could result after only a slight increase in cardiac output. In such persons *cerebrovascular accidents* and kidney damage are intensified by prolonged periods of hypertension. Clearly persons with atherosclerosis are not well served by the effects of nicotine on heart rate.

In addition to its influence on heart rate, nicotine is also a powerful vasoconstrictor of the peripheral blood vessels. As these vessels are constricted by the influence of nicotine, the pressure against their walls increases. The resultant hypertensive change elevates blood pressure, thus compounding any existing hypertension.

platelet adhesiveness
tendency of platelets to clump together, thus enhancing speed at which the blood clots.

Nicotine also increases blood **platelet adhesiveness.**[16] As the platelets become more and more likely to "clump," an individual will be more likely to develop a blood clot. In persons already prone to cardiovascular disease, more rapidly clotting blood is an unwelcomed liability. Heart attacks occur when clots form within the coronary arteries or are transported to the heart from other areas of the body.

A relatively recent insight about the influence of nicotine on cardiovascular disease is that of nicotine's ability to decrease the proportion of high-density lipoproteins (HDLs) and to increase the proportion of low-density lipoproteins (LDLs).[17] Low-density lipoproteins appear to support the development of atherosclerosis and are clearly increased in the bloodstreams of smokers.

Carbon Monoxide and Cardiovascular Disease

A second substance contributed by tobacco influences the type and extent of cardiovascular disease found among tobacco users. Carbon monoxide interferes with oxygen transport within the circulatory system.

As described earlier in the chapter, carbon monoxide is a component of the gaseous phase of tobacco smoke and readily joins with the hemoglobin of the red blood cells. Carbon monoxide has an affinity for hemoglobin 200 times that of oxygen. Once the hemoglobin of a red cell has accepted carbon monoxide molecules, the hemoglobin is transformed into *carboxyhemoglobin*. Thereafter the carboxyhemoglobin makes the red blood cell permanently weaker in its ability to transport oxygen. In heavy smokers approximately 5% of all red blood cells have hemoglobin in this carboxyhemoglobin form.[9] These red blood cells remain relatively useless during the remainder of their 120-day life. Levels of carboxyhemoglobin in heavy smokers are associated with significant increases in the incidence of myocardial infarction.

When a person has impaired oxygen-transporting abilities, physical exertion becomes increasingly demanding on both the heart and the lungs. The cardiovascular system will attempt to respond to the body's demand for oxygen, but these responses are themselves impaired as a result of the influence of nicotine on the cardiovascular system. If tobacco does create the good life, as advertisers claim, it also unfortunately lowers ability to participate actively in that life.

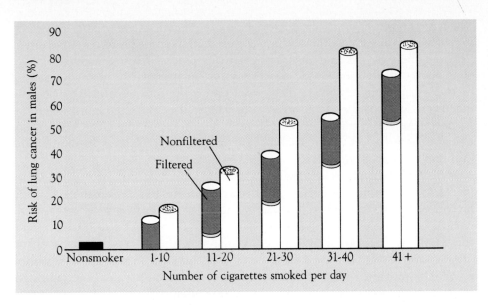

Figure 9-3
How important is cigarette smoking in the development of lung cancer? As the number of cigarettes smoked per day increases, the relative risk of developing lung cancer increases dramatically.

CANCER DEVELOPMENT AND TOBACCO USE

Over the past 35 years, research from the most reputable institutions in this country and abroad has consistently concluded that tobacco use is a significant factor in the development of virtually all forms of cancer and the most significant factor in cancers involving the respiratory system[18] (see Figure 9-3).

In describing cancer development, the currently used reference is *20 pack-years,* or an amount of smoking equal to smoking one pack of cigarettes a day for 20 years. Thus the two-pack-a-day smoker can anticipate cancer development as early as 10 years, while the half-pack-a-day smoker may have to wait 40 years. Regardless, the opportunity is there for all people to confirm these data. We hope that most people will think twice before disregarding this evidence.

Data supplied by the American Cancer Society (ACS) indicate that during 1987 an estimated 965,000 Americans developed cancer.* These cases were nearly equally divided between the sexes and resulted in approximately 483,000 deaths. In the opinion of the ACS, 30% of all cancer cases are heavily influenced by tobacco use. Lung cancer alone accounted for about 150,000 of the new cancer cases and 136,000 deaths in 1987. Fully 85% of male lung cancer victims were cigarette smokers. Cancer of the respiratory system, including lung cancer and cancers of the mouth and throat, accounted for about 195,900 new cases of cancer and 150,650 deaths.[18]

Chapter 11 will present a more detailed discussion of oncogenesis as the basis for cancer formation. Carcinogens, including those in tobacco smoke, will be seen in terms of their relationship to the formation of cancer. At this time, however, we will simply describe the way carcinogens are delivered through smoking to the tissues of the respiratory system and other sites.

Recall that tobacco smoke produces both a gaseous phase and a particulate phase. The particulate contains the tar fragment of tobacco smoke. This rich chemical environment contains over 2,000 known chemical compounds, 200 of

*Excluding about 500,000 cases of nonmelanoma skin cancer.

which are known or possible carcinogens. Other chemical compounds in tar strip the tissues lining the respiratory system of their normal protective properties. This sets the stage for carcinogens to begin the process leading to cancer.

In the normally functioning respiratory system, particulate matter suspended in the inhaled air settles on the tissues lining the airways and is trapped in **mucus** produced by specialized *goblet cells*. This mucus with its trapped impurities is continuously swept upward by the beating action of hairlike **cilia** of the *ciliated columnar epithelial cells*. On reaching the throat, this mucus is swallowed and eventually removed through the digestive system.

When tobacco smoke is drawn into the respiratory system, however, its rapidly dropping temperature allows the particulate matter to accumulate. This brown, sticky tar contains compounds known to have adverse effects on the ciliated columnar epithelial cells, goblet cells, and the *basal cells* of the respiratory lining. In the case of the ciliated columnar epithelial cells, *phenol,* a chemical in tobacco tar, is suspected of being the chemical that alters control and coordination of the cilia. As this control is lost, the cilia become less effective in sweeping mucus upward to the throat. Eventually the cilia are so damaged that they stop their sweeping motions entirely. When cilia can no longer clean the airway, tar accumulates on the surfaces and brings carcinogenic compounds into direct contact with the tissues of the airway.

At the same time that the ciliary action of the columnar cells is being reduced, substances in the tar are stimulating the goblet cells to increase the amount of mucus they normally produce. As a result of the combination of decreased ciliary action and increased mucus production, the overall accumulation of mucus within the airways becomes pronounced. The "smoker's cough" is an attempt to remove this excess mucus.

With prolonged exposure to the carcinogenic materials in tar, predictable changes will begin to occur within the respiratory system's *basal cell layer* (see Figure 9-4). The basal cells begin to display changes in their nuclei that are characteristic of all cancer cells. In addition to these changes, *hyperplasia,* or an

mucus
clear, sticky material produced by specialized cells within the mucous membranes of the body; mucus traps much of the suspended particulate matter within tobacco smoke.

cilia
small, hairlike structures that extend from cells that line the air passages

Bronchogenic carcinoma.

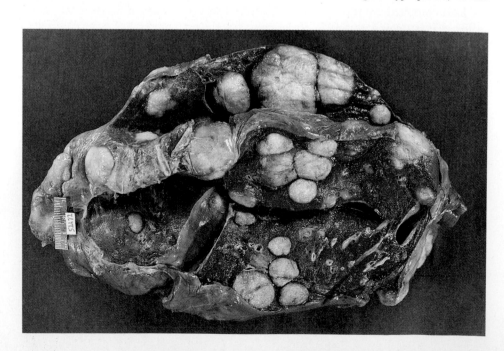

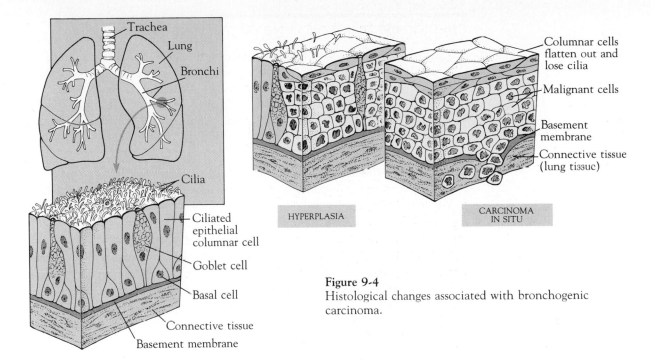

Figure 9-4
Histological changes associated with bronchogenic carcinoma.

abnormal accumulation of cells, occurs as the life expectancy of the cells is extended. Collectively these changes in the basal cell layer signal the beginning of lung cancer.

In the time elapsed between the onset of basal cell changes and the first clinical expression of lung cancer (about 30 *doublings*), cancerous cells will have invaded the *basement membrane.* The cancerous activity will have spread from airways into the adjoining tissues of the lung. This represents bronchogenic carcinoma, or lung cancer.[19]

By the time bronchogenic carcinoma is usually diagnosed, its development is so advanced that the prognosis for recovery is very poor. Only 13% of all lung cancer victims survive for 5 years or more after diagnosis.[18] Most die in a very agonizing, painful way.

Cancerous activity in other areas of the respiratory system, including the *larynx,* and within the oral cavity follows a similar course. In the case of oral cavity cancer, carcinogens found within the smoke and within the saliva are involved in the cancerous changes. Tobacco users such as pipe smokers, cigar smokers, and the users of smokeless tobacco are particularly susceptible to malignancy in the oral cavity.

In addition to drawing smoke into the lungs, tobacco users inadvertently swallow saliva that contains an array of chemical compounds extracted from tobacco. As this saliva is swallowed, carcinogens are absorbed into the circulatory system and transported to all areas of the body. The filtering of the blood by the liver, kidneys, and bladder may account for the higher than normal levels of malignancy in these organs among smokers.

Although the tobacco industry may take some comfort in the difficulty that the scientific community has in proving that tobacco products "cause" many of these cancers, the degree of association between tobacco use and the incidence of many cancers is too great to be dismissed.

CHRONIC OBSTRUCTIVE LUNG DISEASE AND TOBACCO USE

I passed him going the other way in a slow-moving line of traffic. The first thing that I remember seeing was the green plastic tubing flapping against the door on the driver's side of his old truck. A second later, I saw the large oxygen tank chained in an upright position to the bed of the truck. Finally, I saw the oxygen mask he was wearing. Without even knowing him, I knew he was once a heavy smoker and now emphysema controlled his life.

alveoli
thin, saclike terminal ends of the airways; the site at which gases are exchanged between the blood and inhaled air.

chronic bronchitis
persistent inflammation and infection of the smaller airways within the lung.

pulmonary emphysema
irreversible disease process in which the alveoli are destroyed.

sputum
mucus-based material that can be expectorated from the lungs and airways.

Cardiovascular disease and cancer are not the only effects that tobacco use has on a person's physical health. In addition, serious and often irreversible changes to the respiratory system are eventually found in all smokers. Chronic irritation and narrowing of the airways followed by eventual destruction of the **alveoli** are among the most incapacitating damages resulting from tobacco use.

Chronic obstructive lung disease (COLD, sometimes called chronic obstructive pulmonary disease, or COPD) is the gradual blockage of the airways within the lungs. The collective term COLD encompasses two related, yet distinct disease processes: **chronic bronchitis** and **pulmonary emphysema.** Chronic bronchitis predisposes the heavy smoker to emphysema, but emphysema is not, fortunately, an automatic consequence of having chronic bronchitis.

In the progression from normal airway tissue, through chronic bronchitis, to pulmonary emphysema, three levels of impairment are typically observed. Because these changes are dose related, the longer one has smoked, the more heavily one smokes, and the deeper one inhales, the sooner the changes will become evident. However, among smokers who have remarkably similar smoking histories, differences in the development of COLD are observed. This suggests a possible genetic predisposition to more or less involvement with COLD.

One first indicator of the development of COLD is the familiar *smoker's cough.* This condition, often seen within months of beginning regular smoking, reflects a combination of enlargement of the goblet cells and the deactivation of the cilia of the ciliated epithelial cells. Mucus laden with tar accumulates along the walls of the airways. The smoker tries to cough out what the cilia are no longer capable of sweeping out. Particularly noticeable on arising in the morning, this cough should alert the smoker that tissue damage is already occurring.

The second level in the progression toward COLD is that of persistent bacterial infections. **Sputum** taken from the smoker at this stage of the disease process consistently shows the presence of pathogenic bacteria. The presence of these organisms indicates that the lung's immune defenses are markedly deficient.

Persistent narrowing of the airways marks the third stage of COLD. In this stage the effects of chronic irritation and infection result in the narrowing and closure of the bronchi leading into the deepest recesses of the lung tissue—the alveoli. Concurrently an enzyme is produced that destroys the elastic tissue in the alveolar wall.[20] As these changes progress, chest pressure builds when air can no longer be freely exchanged. The thin-walled alveoli swell and eventually rupture. This damage to the alveoli characterizes pulmonary emphysema. A person with emphysema can breathe in but cannot exhale completely. This creates the "barrel chest" and suffocating feeling associated with emphysema. (Emphysema literally means "barrel chest.") Tissue damage has reached a stage at which not even cessation of smoking will return the tissue to normal.

The smoker who has reached this advanced state of pulmonary disease is likely to display additional structural and functional changes, including enlargement of the chest and obvious breathing impairment. Additionally, the circulatory system is under stress as the right side of the heart attempts to send blood to lungs that are themselves increasingly impaired. A general collapse of normal cardiopulmonary function can occur resulting in *congestive heart failure*. For the person with emphysema, life is truly threatened, and any physical activity above a minimal level is virtually impossible.

SMOKING AND REPRODUCTION

In all of its dimensions, the reproduction process is impaired by the use of tobacco, particularly cigarette smoking. Problems can be found in association with infertility, problem pregnancy, breastfeeding, and the health of the newborn.

Infertility

Recent research indicates that cigarette smoking by both males and females can reduce levels of fertility.[21] Among men, smoking adversely affects sperm motility and sperm shape and can inhibit sperm production. Among women, lower levels of estrogen (a hormone necessary for uterine wall development), a reduced ability to conceive, and a somewhat earlier onset of menopause appear to be related to cigarette smoking.

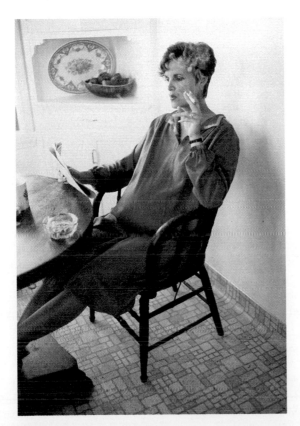

Tobacco use during
pregnancy is dangerous.

Problem Pregnancy

The harmful effects of tobacco smoke on the course of pregnancy are principally the result of the carbon monoxide and nicotine to which the mother and her fetus are exposed. Carbon monoxide from the incomplete oxidation of tobacco is carried in the maternal blood to the placenta, where it diffuses across the placental barrier and enters the fetal circulation. Once in the fetal blood, the carbon monoxide bonds with the *fetal hemoglobin* to form *fetal carboxyhemoglobin*. As a result of this exposure to carbon monoxide, the fetus is deprived of normal oxygen transport and literally suffocates.

In the same manner that carbon monoxide enters the fetal circulation, nicotine exerts its influence on the developing fetus. Thermographs of the placenta and fetus show signs of marked vasoconstriction within a few seconds after inhalation by the mother. This constriction further reduces oxygen supplies. Additionally, nicotine stimulates the mother's stress response, placing the mother and fetus under the potentially harmful influence of elevated epinephrine and corticoid levels (see Chapter 3). Any fetus exposed to all of these agents is more likely to be *miscarried* or be *stillborn*.

Breastfeeding

For women who decide to breastfeed their infants, smoking during this period will continue to expose their children to the harmful effects of tobacco smoke. It is well recognized that nicotine appears in breast milk and thus is capable of exerting its vasoconstricting and stress-response influences on nursing infants. Mothers who stop smoking during pregnancy should be encouraged to continue to refrain from smoking while they are breastfeeding.

Neonatal Health Problems

Babies born to women who smoked during pregnancy will, on the average, be shorter and have a lower birth weight than children born to nonsmoking mothers. Statistics also show that infants of smoking mothers are more likely to develop bronchitis, pneumonia, or middle ear infections. These problems are caused by the effects of passive smoke.[22]

Parenting, in the sense of assuming responsibility for the well-being of children, does not begin at birth. In the case of smoking, this is especially true. Pregnant women who continue smoking are disregarding the well-being of the children they are carrying. Other family members, friends, and co-workers who subject pregnant women to cigarette, pipe, or cigar smoke are in a sense contributing a measure of their own disregard for the health of the next generation.

ORAL CONTRACEPTIVES AND TOBACCO USE

Women who smoke and use oral contraceptives are, in comparison to women who smoke but do not use oral contraceptives or women who use the oral contraceptive but do not smoke, placing themselves at a much greater risk of experiencing a fatal cardiovascular accident (heart attack, stroke, **embolism**). This risk of cardiovascular complications is further increased for oral contraceptive users 25 years of age or older.[23] Women who both smoke and use oral contraceptives are four times more likely to die from myocardial infarction (heart attack) than women who only smoke.[24] Because of this adverse relationship, *it is strongly recommended that women who smoke should not use oral contraceptives.*

embolism
potentially fatal situation in which a circulating blood clot lodges itself in a smaller vessel.

SMOKELESS TOBACCO USE

Chewing Tobacco and Snuff

What do "Red Man," "Skoal," and "Copenhagen" have in common? The answer? They have all served to introduce 22 million Americans to a bit of the past—the use of smokeless tobacco.

Thanks to the resurgence of smokeless tobacco use, no longer are professional baseball players the only Americans to know the value of an empty coffee can or an empty soft drink cup. These discarded containers are becoming standard equipment for people who dip and chew smokeless tobacco.

As the term implies, smokeless tobacco is not burned; rather, it is placed into the mouth. Once in place, the physiologically active nicotine and other soluble compounds are absorbed through the mucous membranes and into the blood. Within a few minutes, chewing tobacco and snuff generate blood levels of nicotine in amounts equivalent to those seen in cigarette smokers. The user of smokeless tobacco experiences the effects of nicotine without being exposed to the carbon monoxide and tar generated by burning tobacco.

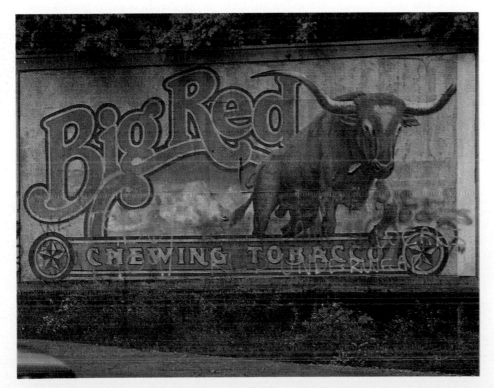

Smokeless tobacco use presents its own risks.

Chewing tobacco is taken from its foil pouch, formed into a small ball (called a "wad," "chaw," or "chew"), and placed into the mouth. Once in place, the bolus of tobacco is sucked and occasionally chewed, but not swallowed. Some users develop great skill at spitting the copious dark brown liquid residue into an empty coffee can, out a car window, or on the sidewalk.

Snuff, a more finely shredded smokeless tobacco product, is marketed in small round cans. Snuff is formed into a small mass (or "quid") for dipping. The quid is placed between the jaw and the cheek; the user sucks the quid, then spits out the brown liquid—in cans, on the street, or next to urinals. Snuff, as once used, was actually a powdered form of tobacco that was inhaled through the nose.

periodontal disease destruction to soft tissue and bone that surround the teeth.

Although smokeless tobacco would seem to free the tobacco user from many of the risks associated with smoking, both chewing and dipping are not without their own substantial risks. The formation of *precancerous leukoplakia* and *erythroplakia* (precursors to oral cancer), the increase in **periodontal disease** (with the pulling away of the gum from the teeth and later tooth loss), the abrasive damage to the enamel of the teeth, and the high concentration of sugar in processed tobacco all contribute to health problems seen among users of smokeless tobacco.[25,26] In those individuals who develop oral cancer, the risk is dramatically heightened if the cancer metastasizes from the site of origin in the mouth to the brain. In addition to changes associated with cancer, users should be aware of any of the following indicators of the damage being done by their use of smokeless tobacco:

- Lumps in the jaw or neck area
- Color changes or lumps inside the lips
- White, smooth, or scaly patches in the mouth or on the neck, lips, or tongue (precancerous leukoplakia)
- A red spot or sore on the lips or gums or inside the mouth that does not heal in 2 weeks (erythroplakia)
- Repeated bleeding in the mouth
- Difficulty or abnormality in speaking or swallowing

When any of the above indicators of smokeless tobacco damage are noted, users should promptly notify a dentist or physician.

In addition to the damage done to the tissues of the mouth, the need to process the inadvertently swallowed saliva that contains dissolved carcinogens places both the digestive and urinary systems at risk of cancer.

In the opinion of health experts, the use of smokeless tobacco and its potential for life-threatening disease is presently at the place cigarette smoking was 40 years ago. Just as television advertising for cigarettes was banned in the early 1970s, television advertising for smokeless tobacco products is now banned. President Reagan signed the Comprehensive Smokeless Tobacco and Health Education Act in February 1986. This act requires that the rotation of the following warnings be placed on all smokeless tobacco products:

WARNING: THIS PRODUCT MAY CAUSE MOUTH CANCER.

WARNING: THIS PRODUCT MAY CAUSE GUM DISEASE AND TOOTH LOSS.

WARNING: THIS PRODUCT IS NOT A SAFE ALTERNATIVE TO CIGARETTE SMOKING.

Clearly, those who use smokeless tobacco have chosen a dangerous product. There is little doubt that continued use of tobacco in this form is a serious affront to health in all of its dimensions.

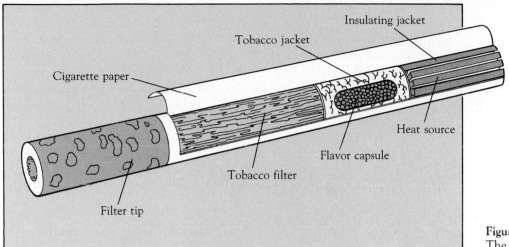

Figure 9-5
The smokeless cigarette.

Smokeless Cigarettes

The development of the "smokeless" cigarette reflects the tobacco industry's most recent attempt to counter the antismoking movement (see Figure 9-5). Instead of igniting tobacco, the smokeless cigarette lights a carbon heat source. As the smoker uses the cigarette, warm air flows through the flavor capsule, which is surrounded by tobacco. Although the "smoke" flows through two filters before being inhaled, carbon monoxide and nicotine compounds remain at the same strength as in low-tar cigarettes. However, because the tobacco is warmed and not burned, no smoke, odor, and ash result. As to whether this product is safer for the cigarette user and/or less irritating to nonsmokers remains to be seen. The "heated tobacco" technology that makes this product possible may prove to be only a smoke screen.

CLOVE CIGARETTES

During the last 10 years a segment of the adolescent population has experimented with a cigarette composed of two thirds tobacco and one third ground raw cloves. Imported from Indonesia, these "clove cigarettes" are of growing concern to health experts as they begin to better understand the effects that smoking these cigarettes can have on health.

In comparison to American cigarettes, clove cigarettes are made of low-quality, high-nicotine tobacco. The high nicotine, tar, and carbon monoxide content makes these cigarettes every bit as dangerous and dependency producing as regular cigarettes. Furthermore, cloves contain eugenol, a chemical used in dental anesthesia and perfumes. Eugenol produces localized deadening of airway tissues, which can lead to deeper and longer inhalations. Also, a variety of reactions including fevers and labored breathing, coughing up blood, fluid accumulation in the lungs, chest pain, muscle sensitivity, and vomiting have been reported in persons who smoke clove cigarettes.

In light of an increasing incidence of serious illness associated with regular use of clove cigarettes, these cigarettes present smokers with a new and no less serious group of insults to health.

STOPPING WHAT YOU STARTED

Theories in the area of health behavior suggest to us five steps through which the smoker must progress to join the ranks of the nonsmoker. These progressions include the following:

1 *Knowledge* about the health risks associated with tobacco use—particularly cigarette smoking
2 *Recognition* that these health risks are applicable to all smokers
3 *Familiarity* with steps that can be taken to eliminate or reduce these risks
4 *Belief* that the benefits to be gained by no longer using tobacco will outweigh the pleasures gained through the use of tobacco
5 *Certainty* that one can initiate and maintain the behaviors required to stop or reduce the use of tobacco

When you study these five steps more closely, you can see that the initial steps are primarily based on having information, whereas the latter steps are a reflection of self-confidence. In other words, it requires you to be motivated. You must really want to be a nonsmoker and be willing to pay the price. Knowledge alone may not generate the high level of motivation required to change many persons' smoking behaviors. The high failure rate associated with most smoking cessation programs (70% and higher) suggests that motivation is certainly not as easy to maintain as many people initially believe.

As is the case with weight reduction programs, smoking cessation programs are available in a variety of formats, including educational programs, behavior modification, aversive conditioning, hypnosis, acupuncture, and various combinations of these approaches. Programs are offered in both individual and group formats and are operated by a variety of organizations and practitioners, including hospitals, universities, health departments, voluntary health agencies, churches, and private practitioners.

Programs vary in their level of effectiveness, and individuals within the same program will experience differing levels of success. Perhaps the best that can be said is that the better programs will have limited success—a 20% to 30% success rate as measured over 1 year—while the remainder will have even poorer levels of success. And since the majority of programs rely on the self-reporting of smoking behavior, success rates may be routinely inflated.

A new product designed to be used with smoking cessation programs is the nicotine-impregnated chewing gum (trade name Nicorette).[27] When the gum is chewed slowly, the nicotine is released and absorbed through the mucous membranes of the mouth. Proper use of the gum results in nicotine levels sufficiently high to discourage a return to cigarette use.[28] Studies in both the United States and England have demonstrated a long-term success rate of 40% or more when used in conjunction with other smoking cessation therapies.[29] This gum is available only in prescription form.

Although nicotine gum is not a panacea for those who wish to quit smoking, it is an important advancement. Relatively few adverse side effects have been noted. Contraindications are limited to people with certain forms of cardiovascular disease.

For those wishing to stop smoking without turning to an organized program, a **cold turkey** approach can be very effective, especially for those who are highly

Now's the Time

Instead of reaching for a cigarette, reach out for life and health. Start with the following steps suggested by the American Cancer Society:

- Pick a quit day, sometime within the next 2 weeks. Plan either to stop cold turkey or to cut down gradually.
- Plan ahead for how you will handle tough times in your first few days off cigarettes.
- Think of one sentence that expresses your personal reason for wanting to quit smoking. Repeat the sentence to yourself often.
- Stock up on low- or no-calorie snacks.
- On your quit day, drink a lot of water and keep busy.
- Call the American Cancer Society for more information about quitting: self-help, how-to's, and group sessions in your community.

cold turkey
immediate, total discontinuation of tobacco use or other addictive substances.

motivated to quit. For those less motivated, or at least less certain about this drastic approach, commercial products are available that promise to help break the cigarette habit. However, the effectiveness of these products is highly questionable.

An alternative to total cessation is, of course, to reduce one's exposure to tobacco. This reduction can be accomplished through one or more of the following approaches:

- Reduce the consumption of your present high tar and nicotine brand by smoking fewer cigarettes, inhaling less often and less deeply, and by smoking the cigarette only halfway down.
- Switch to a low tar and nicotine brand of cigarette. Your smoking behavior, other than the brand change, must remain the same, however; do not compensate by inhaling more deeply and frequently.
- Switch to a low tar and nicotine brand of cigarette and, in addition, reduce the number smoked, the depth and number of inhalations, and smoke only a limited portion of the cigarette.
- Switch to a smokeless form of tobacco, but be prepared for potential problems (discussed earlier in this chapter).

For low tar and low nicotine cigarettes to be of value, it appears important that the smoker reduces the level of nicotine very gradually. When nicotine is reduced too quickly, the smoker is likely to smoke more cigarettes, puff more frequently, or inhale more deeply. By engaging in these compensatory smoking behaviors, one is less likely to be able to achieve the desired health benefits.

Smokeless tobacco provides the nicotine that the smoker desires without exposing the respiratory system to the smoke from cigarettes, pipes, or cigars. Unfortunately, the user of smokeless tobacco, like the smoker, still must deal with the problems that nicotine and other dangerous chemicals may produce.

Although stopping smoking is difficult, 30 million adults have managed to do so. Many former smokers report that they feel better about themselves and they believe their futures will be much healthier. As the positive benefits become more apparent over time, few former smokers will wish to return to the smoking habit.

PASSIVE SMOKING

In the next section we will discuss the important topic of smokers' versus nonsmokers' rights. Central to the conflict that exists between these groups is the issue of passive smoking by nonsmokers as they inhale smoke from the cigarettes, pipes, and cigars of smokers with whom they live, work, and spend leisure time with.

The smoke generated by the smoking of tobacco can be classified as either *mainstream* (the smoke inhaled and then exhaled by the smoker) or *sidestream* (the smoke that comes from the burning end of the cigarette, pipe, or cigar). When either form of tobacco smoke is diluted and stays within a common source of air, it is referred to as *environmental tobacco smoke*. All three forms of tobacco smoke can present health problems for nonsmokers.

Mainsteam smoke (MS) is, of course, the smoke that generates the significant health problems for smokers. Although much of the nicotine, carbon monoxide, and particulate matter are retained in smokers, exhaled mainstream smoke contributes substantial quantities of carbon monoxide, ammonia, nicotine, cyanide, and highly carcinogenic N-nitrosamines for the nonsmoker to inhale.[30]

Sidestream smoke (SS) is the smoke from the burning end of the cigarette, cigar, or pipe that is not inhaled by the smoker. Because it is not filtered by the tobacco, filter, or the smoker's lungs, sidestream smoke contains more free nicotine in the vapor phase than mainstream smoke and produces high yields of both carbon dioxide and carbon monoxide. Much to the detriment of nonsmokers, sidestream smoke has 20 to 100 times the quantity of highly carcinogenic N-nitrosamines as mainstream smoke.[30]

Current scientific opinion suggests that smokers and nonsmokers are exposed to very much the same smoke when tobacco is used within a common air source. The important difference is the quantity of smoke inhaled by smokers and nonsmokers. It is likely that for each pack of cigarettes smoked by a smoker, nonsmokers who must share a common air supply with the smoker will passively smoke the equivalent of three to five cigarettes. Because of the small size of the particles produced by burning tobacco, environmental tobacco smoke (ETS) cannot be completely removed from the worksite by even the most effective ventilation system.[30]

According to the 1986 report of the Surgeon General, *The Health Consequences of Involuntary Smoking,* epidemiological studies examining passive smoking in the worksite and in public places have *not* found strong evidence that passive smoking creates significant health risks for most nonsmokers. Although it probably creates significant annoyance problems for nonsmokers, worksite passive smoking may not be as dangerous as many people think. Of course, this scientific opinion may change with further study.

However, it is clear that passive smoking poses major threats to nonsmokers within residential settings. Spouses and children of smokers are at greatest risk from passive smoking. Scientific studies over the past decade suggest that nonsmokers married to smokers are three times more likely to experience heart attacks than nonsmoking spouses of nonsmokers, and have a 30% greater risk of lung cancer than nonsmoking spouses of nonsmokers.[30]

The children of parents who smoke are twice as likely as children of nonsmoking parents to experience bronchitis or pneumonia during the first year of life. Additionally, throughout childhood, these children will experience more wheezing, coughing, and sputum production than children whose parents do not smoke. Of course, the impact on children who have two parents who smoke is greater than on children who have only one parent who uses tobacco. Is it possible that in light of our current concern over child abuse and neglect, a court of law might someday determine that parental smoking is, in fact, a form of child abuse?

TOBACCO USE: A QUESTION OF RIGHTS

Let us offer two simple questions concerning the issues of smokers' versus nonsmokers' rights:

- To what extent should the smoker be allowed to pollute the air and endanger the health of the nonsmoker?
- To what extent should nonsmokers be allowed to restrict the personal freedom of the smoker?

At this time answers to these questions are only partially available, but one trend is developing: the tobacco user is being forced to give ground to the nonsmoker. The health concerns of the majority are prevailing over the dependency needs of the minority.

Several distinct approaches have been employed by the antismoking forces in their attempt to shift the weight of law and public sentiment in the direction of controlling the smoker's use of cigarettes, including the following:

Public education programs designed to educate the population concerning the destructive effects of smoking on health

Laws restricting smoking in public places, including buses, trains, and planes

Bans on cigarette advertisements on television and radio

More forceful warnings on cigarette packages and on the advertising of cigarettes in the print media

Recent court decisions that define smoking within the work place as being a privilege rather than a right

Today it is becoming more a matter of when the smoker will be allowed to smoke, rather than a matter of when smoking will be restricted. Increasingly, smoking is less and less tolerated. As an example, many office buildings are beginning to indicate where smoking is permitted rather than prohibited.

Airline Bans

Following the banning of smoking on all flights in the continental U.S. by a major airline carrier, FAA regulations now prohibit any smoking on all flights within the continental U.S. of 2 hours or less.

ENHANCING COMMUNICATION BETWEEN SMOKERS AND NONSMOKERS

The Nonsmoker's Bill of Rights (see Figure 9-6) is another indicator of the division that is occurring between those who smoke cigarettes and those who do not. Exchanges between smokers and nonsmokers are sometimes strained and, in many cases, friendships are damaged beyond the point of repair. As you have more than likely observed on your campus, roommates are changed, dates are refused, and memberships in study groups are withheld or rejected because of the opposing rights of these two groups.

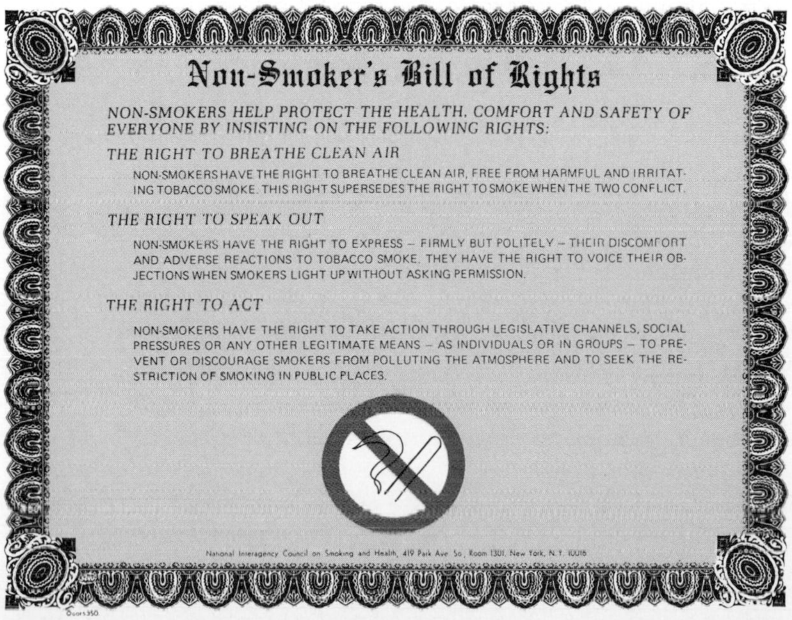
Non-Smoker's Bill of Rights

NON-SMOKERS HELP PROTECT THE HEALTH, COMFORT AND SAFETY OF EVERYONE BY INSISTING ON THE FOLLOWING RIGHTS:

THE RIGHT TO BREATHE CLEAN AIR

NON-SMOKERS HAVE THE RIGHT TO BREATHE CLEAN AIR, FREE FROM HARMFUL AND IRRITATING TOBACCO SMOKE. THIS RIGHT SUPERSEDES THE RIGHT TO SMOKE WHEN THE TWO CONFLICT.

THE RIGHT TO SPEAK OUT

NON-SMOKERS HAVE THE RIGHT TO EXPRESS — FIRMLY BUT POLITELY — THEIR DISCOMFORT AND ADVERSE REACTIONS TO TOBACCO SMOKE. THEY HAVE THE RIGHT TO VOICE THEIR OBJECTIONS WHEN SMOKERS LIGHT UP WITHOUT ASKING PERMISSION.

THE RIGHT TO ACT

NON-SMOKERS HAVE THE RIGHT TO TAKE ACTION THROUGH LEGISLATIVE CHANNELS, SOCIAL PRESSURES OR ANY OTHER LEGITIMATE MEANS — AS INDIVIDUALS OR IN GROUPS — TO PREVENT OR DISCOURAGE SMOKERS FROM POLLUTING THE ATMOSPHERE AND TO SEEK THE RESTRICTION OF SMOKING IN PUBLIC PLACES.

National Interagency Council on Smoking and Health, 419 Park Ave. So., Room 1301, New York, N.Y. 10016

Goes 350

Figure 9-6
Nonsmoker's Bill of Rights.

Recognizing that social skill development is an important task for young adults, we offer several simple considerations or approaches we believe can reduce some conflict presently associated with smoking. We hope they will also become skills for the social dimension of your health that can be applied to other social conflicts. Remember that as a smoker you are part of a statistical minority living in a society which often makes decisions and resolves conflict based on majority rule.

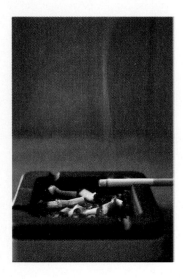

- Ask whether smoking would bother others in close proximity to you. Some nonsmokers are intimidated by the authority with which you reach for your cigarettes and are reluctant to stop you from doing something that seems so natural to you.
- When in a neutral setting, seek physical space in which you will be able to smoke and in a reasonable way not interfere with nonsmokers' comfort.
- Accept the validity of the nonsmoker's statement that your smoke "smells up everything and everyone." Your loss of olfactory sensitivity has occurred gradually, and, more than likely, you are grossly insensitive to your own smoke.
- Respect stated prohibitions against smoking. Laws have been passed and policies have been established that restrict smoking in many public and private places. If you choose to smoke in spite of these prohibitions, then accept the legal and social consequences of your decision.
- If a nonsmoker requests that you refrain from smoking, respond with courtesy, regardless of whether you intend to comply. Nonsmokers can better accept your refusal to comply when it is accompanied with a rational explanation of why the request is unwarranted or unnecessary.
- Practice "preventive smoking" by applying a measure of restraint when you recognize that smoking is offensive to others. Particularly, respect the esthetics that should accompany any act of smoking—ashes on dinner plates and cigarette butts in flower pots are hardly "winners" with others.

For those of you who are nonsmokers, we would suggest several approaches we believe will make you more sensitive and skilled in dealing with smoking behavior:

- Attempt to develop a feeling for or a sensitivity to the power of the dependence that smokers have on their cigarettes. Imagine something you truly feel you "could not live without," and then envision how hard you would defend your right to keep that possession. That is how smokers feel about cigarettes.
- Accept the reality of the smoker's sensory insensitivity—an insensitivity that is so profound that the odors you complain about are not even recognized. Further, realize that this insensitivity to smell is joined with an insensitivity to taste that produces an inability to enjoy the world of tastes to which you are accustomed.
- When in a neutral setting, allow smokers their fair share of physical space in which to smoke. So long as the host does not object to smoking, you, as a guest, do not have the right to infringe on a person's right to smoke. You may have more obligation to compromise than does the smoker, in this situation.
- Request relief from a person's smoke in a manner that reflects social consideration and skill. State your request clearly and accept a refusal gracefully.

Are You Ready to Try?

As powerful as a dependency on cigarettes can be, many people have been able to quit smoking. Hopefully, the suggestions appearing below will assist you in making a concerted effort to stop.

1 Get mad at yourself for having become less fully self-directed than you could be. Few smokers can contend that they are fully self-directed when they can barely function in the absence of their cigarettes.

2 Observe nonsmokers. Note that nonsmokers are not missing out on anything as the result of not smoking. Recognize that the price you will pay for no longer smoking is not as high as it might have first appeared.

3 Limit your contact with other cigarette smokers. Keep in mind that once you quit, smokers won't go out of their way to assist you in your efforts.

4 Stay clear, as much as possible, of the locations and activities that are now associated with your smoking. Old habits will be hard to break, but, at least, you do not have to be constantly reminded by their presence.

5 Establish a series of rewards that you will bestow upon yourself as you progress through your smoking cessation program.

Having done the above, you are now ready to make an attempt at quitting. Good luck.

■ Respond with honesty to inquiries from the smoker as to whether the smoke is bothering you. Do not assume that your response, "It's all right with me," should really be interpreted in any way other than the way you state it.

For those who are contemplating smoking, we ask you to explore closely whether the social isolation that appears to be more and more common for smokers will be offset by the benefits you might receive from cigarettes. The developmental task of developing the skills for social interaction cannot be taken lightly. The ability to find satisfaction through social contact may be one of the most important dimensions in a productive and satisfying adult life.

SUMMARY

Cigarette smoking is clearly identified as the chief preventable cause of death in our society—and perhaps the most important public health issue of our time. Tobacco use produces few positive influences on a person's health. This concept is supported by data indicating that the percentage of adults who smoke is lower now than it has been at any time in the last 25 years.

The reasons people begin to smoke and continue to smoke are complex and multifaceted. Chapter 9 explored many of the factors that lead to tobacco use. Once smoking has begun, many factors also play roles in the development of a dependency relationship with tobacco.

To date the physiological role of nicotine has received the majority of the public's attention. Psychosocial causes of tobacco dependency might include such factors as role modeling, manipulation, and self-indulgence.

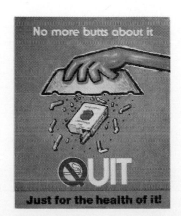
No more butts about it

QUIT

Just for the health of it!

The impact of tobacco use on mortality is evident through tobacco's role in the development of several seriously debilitating disease processes. The major diseases directly associated with tobacco use are cardiovascular disease, cancer, and chronic obstructive lung disease. Tobacco use is also associated with other health risks. The fetus of a pregnant women who smokes may suffer harmful effects, the user of oral contraceptives who smokes increases her risk of serious complications, and the user of smokeless tobacco also incurs certain health risks. Passive smoking is a major health concern currently being explored.

Health behavior theory suggests five steps through which smokers must progress to join the ranks of the nonsmoker. For smoking cessation to be successful, a large measure of motivation is required. Alternatives to total cessation include approaches that reduce exposure to tobacco's harmful components, including smoking fewer cigarettes, inhaling less often, inhaling less deeply, and smoking a cigarette only halfway down.

The issue of smokers' versus nonsmokers' rights is complex. Those who oppose smoking can cite a good deal of research that suggests that their complaints against sidestream and secondhand smoke are valid. Smokers and nonsmokers are encouraged to deal with smoking behavior with sensitivity and an understanding of individual rights.

REVIEW QUESTIONS

1 What percent of adult men are smokers? Adult women? What is the relationship between men *nonsmokers* and employment level? Between *smokers* and education? What are the smoking trends among college students?

2 Identify the two phases or components of tobacco smoke. Describe each phase.

3 Describe the paths of nicotine, tar, and carbon monoxide once they are inhaled. How does each substance affect the body?

4 Define *dependency* as it relates to tobacco use. What are the mechanisms that have been identified as possible causes of a dependency relationship? Which one of these causes has received the most attention?

5 How important is modeling in the development of smoking behaviors? Identify other psychosocial factors that play a role in dependency development.

6 What role does tobacco use play in the development of cardiovascular disease? Describe the influence of nicotine and carbon monoxide on the cardiovascular system.

7 What is meant by the term *20 pack-years?* How does this relate to tobacco use? What is the role of tobacco use in cancer development?

8 What is the role of tobacco use in the development of chronic obstructive lung disease? What are the three levels of impairment that are typically observed in the progression of COLD?

9 What harmful effects does tobacco use have on a fetus?

10 What are the risks associated with smoking and oral contraceptive use?

11 What is smokeless tobacco? How is it used? What health risks are associated with its use?

12 Define mainstream smoke (MS), sidestream smoke (SS), and environmental tobacco smoke (ETS). Who is most likely to be affected by passive smoking?

13 Beyond total smoking cessation, what are some ways smokers can reduce their exposure to tobacco?

QUESTIONS FOR PERSONAL CONTEMPLATION

1 Do you think the warnings on cigarette packages affect the decisions people make about smoking? In what ways? If you are a smoker, do these warnings affect your decision to smoke? Do you think the warnings are fair? Why or why not?

2 What are your feelings about the facts concerning college women and smoking? Do you think this trend will change in the next decade?

3 If you smoke, considering the large amount of information available on the risks associated with smoking, why do you continue to smoke?

4 Observe those people you know who smoke. Aside from the health risks, what impact does smoking have on their general appearance? Do you think that they are aware of these influences? Would you be willing to discuss these matters with them?

5 Do you feel a pregnant woman who smokes is being a responsible parent? Knowing the effects this behavior may have on the fetus, might this not be considered a form of child abuse?

6 If you are a smoker, have you ever been asked to extinguish your cigarette because it was annoying someone else? How did you react? How did you feel about this situation? Did you feel your rights were being violated? After reading this chapter, will you react any differently the next time this happens?

REFERENCES

1 Healthy people: the Surgeon General's report on health and disease prevention, DHEW (PHS) Pub no 79-55071, Washington, DC, 1979, US Government Printing Office.

2 Health consequences of smoking: cardiovascular disease, Smoking and Health Reporter 2:1, 1984.

3 Comprehensive Smoking Education Act signed into law, Smoking and Health Reporter 2:7, 1985.

4 Seffrin, J: Editor of *Tobacco-Free Young American Reporter*, Personal interview, August 21, 1987.

5 New surveys show that smoking rates continue to drop, Tobacco-Free Young American Reporter 4:4, 1987.

6 Astin, A: The American freshman: national norms for 1985, Los Angeles, 1985, UCLA Higher Education Research Institute.

7 Johnson, L, et al: Drug use among American high school students, college students, and other young adults: national trends through 1985, National Institute on Drug Abuse, DHHS (PHS) Pub No (ADM) 86-1450, 1986, US Government Printing Office.

8 US Bureau of the Census: Statistical Abstract of the United States, ed 108, Washington DC, 1988, The Bureau.

9 Ray, O, and Ksir, C: Drugs, society, and human behavior, ed 4, St Louis 1987, Times Mirror/ Mosby College Publishing.

10 Russell, M: Tobacco dependence: is nicotine rewarding or aversive? In Krasnegor N, editor: Cigarette smoking as a dependency process, NIDA Research Monograph, Rockville, Md, 1979, Department of Health, Education and Welfare.

11 Russel, M: Cigarette smoking: natural history of a dependency disorder, British Journal of Medical Psychology 44:1-16, 1971.

12 Martin, J: Maternal nicotine and caffeine consumption and offspring outcome, Neurobehavioral Toxicology and Teratology 4:421–427, 1982.

13 Warner, K, and Murt, A: Premature deaths avoided by the antismoking campaign, Journal of Public Health 76:672-677, 1983.

14 Ravenholt, R: Addiction mortality in the United States, 1980: tobacco, alcohol, and other substances, Population and Development Review 10:697-724, 1984.

15 American Heart Association: 1987 Heart Facts, Dallas, 1986, The Association.

16 Nowak, J, et al: Biochemical evidence of a chronic abnormality in platelet and vascular function in healthy individuals who smoke cigarettes, Circulation 76:1, 6-14, 1987.

17 Hopkins, P, and Williams, R: A survey of 246 suggested coronary risk factors, Atherosclerosis 40:1, 1-52, 1981.
18 American Cancer Society: Cancer facts and figures: 1987, New York, 1987, American Cancer Society, p 9.
19 Fisher, W: Oncologist, Personal interview, August 18, 1987, Muncie, Ind.
20 Surgeon General's 1984 report addresses chronic obstructive lung disease, Smoking and Health Reporter 1:4, 1984.
21 Tobacco profoundly affects reproduction, HE-XTRA 12:1, 1984.
22 Cunningham, D, et al: Smoking and pregnancy (Letters), American Journal of Diseases of Children 136:82, 1982.
23 Population Reports, Oral contraceptives population information program, series A, no 6, Baltimore, 1982, The Johns Hopkins University.
24 Rosenberg, L, et al: Myocardial infarction and cigarette smoking in women younger than 50 years of age, Journal of the American Medical Association 253:20, 2965-2969, 1985.
25 Oral snuff, a preventable carcinogenic hazard, The Lancet II:8500, 198-200, 1986.
26 Health implications of smokeless tobacco use, Public Health Reports 101:4, 349-354, 1986.
27 Merrell Dow releases nicotine chewing gum in US—new tool to help smokers quit, Smoking and Health Reporter 1:4, 1984.
28 McCusker, K: A physician's view of Nicorette, Smoking and Health Reporter 1:4, 1984.
29 Pharmacological adjuncts in smoking cessation, Research Monograph Series, Department of Health and Human Services, DDHS Pub no (ADM) 85-1333, Washington, DC, 1985, US Government Printing Office.
30 The health consequences of involuntary smoking: A report of the Surgeon General, Department of Health and Human Services, DHHS (CDC) 87-8393, Washington, DC, 1986, US Government Printing Office.

ANNOTATED READINGS

Ferguson, T: The smoker's book of health, New York, 1987, GP Putnam's Sons.
  Basic information about smoking and strategies for improving health through quitting. Steps for preventing postsmoking weight gain are presented.

Harris, RW: How to keep smoking and live, New York, 1978, St. Martin's Press.
  This book is touted as being for the smoker who has tried to quit smoking and failed. By using a variety of personal inventories, amusing historical information, and quasi-current news stories, this book encourages smokers to reexamine their smoking habits and change the manner in which they smoke. Emphasis is on low-tar and low-nicotine cigarettes. The author encourages quitting as the next logical step.

Miles, RH: Coffin nails and corporate strategies, Englewood Cliffs, NJ, 1982, Prentice-Hall, Inc.
  The health implications of tobacco use have posed major threats for the economic survivability of the "Big Six" corporations that produce tobacco products. This book describes how corporate strategies were developed to offset the momentum generated by the antismoking organizations. An interesting insight into the way this industry has adapted to public policy and values.

Troyer, RJ, and Markle, GE: Cigarettes; the battle over smoking, New Brunswick, NJ, 1983, Rutgers University Press.
  Chronicles the growth of tobacco use in our society and how this practice has led to major confrontations between prosmoking and antismoking forces. The roles of government, social movement organizations, and other resources are examined. The way society establishes deviance rules is also explored.

Understandably, relationships could exist between your decisions concerning substance use and all four of the developmental tasks of growth and development. Look within the chapters of this unit for specific information to support our contentions about alcohol, drugs, and tobacco use and their effects on developmental task mastery.

- **Forming an Initial Adult Self-Identity** For most of you, this period of life will be a time when you will discover more about yourself—about who you really are. All of life's experiences will help you find out who you are. In conjunction with these experiences, you will begin to take on a self-identity that probably differs somewhat from the one you had a few years ago when you were younger and less independent. The relative freedom you now have allows you to develop a unique self-identity that might carry you through all of your adult life.

Your decision to use or avoid alcohol, drugs, and tobacco will reflect your uniqueness and how you view yourself. Some people will judge you either positively or negatively solely on your use or misuse of these substances. Will patterns of use established now support or hinder your self-identity as you wish it to be 15 years hence?

- **Establishing a Sense of Relative Independence** Living where you want, pursuing a career for which you have prepared yourself, and marrying the person of your choice are among the more obvious dimensions of the independence enjoyed by adults. There are, however, less obvious dimensions of independence that can also be important. Substance use, such as that seen in conjunction with smoking, can influence independence in these subtle dimensions.

You may have seen a substance abuser experience a partial loss of independence—not the absence of independence to reside, work, or marry as you choose—but rather the independence to make decisions unencumbered by the substance addiction. While none of us is totally independent, the user of dependency-producing substances is relatively less independent.

- **Developing Skills for Social Interaction** Not only is the use or misuse of substances such as alcohol, psychoactive drugs, and tobacco detrimental to the user, but it also compromises the health and sense of well-being of others with whom the user has contact. Alcohol abusers and drugs users frequently find themselves unable (physically and psychologically) to interact socially with a wide range of people. As a result, the user may cease social communication. With tobacco use in particular, we see substance abuse having an insidious impact on others.

For those who are contemplating using dependency-producing substances, explore closely whether the social isolation that appears to be more and more common for users will be offset by the benefits you might receive from the substance. The importance of social acceptance cannot be taken lightly.

- **Assuming Increasing Levels of Responsibility** College requires students to accept increasing levels of academic responsibility. Adult life in general demands additional responsibilities—everything from paying taxes to managing a growing family. Job requirements force us to assign priorities to schedules and personal activities. Clearly, adulthood is marked by our assumption of more and more responsibility.

Will you be able to accept these complex responsibilities if you find yourself incapable of functioning because of substance abuse? If you recognize now that your preferred method of coping with stress is to rely on alcohol or drugs, then you need to explore alternatives in light of the level of responsibility that lies ahead.

UNIT IV

Unit IV consists of three chapters that focus on disease processes. Throughout your lifetime, each illness you contract or develop has the potential to influence your overall health status and each of its five dimensions.

■ **Physical Dimension of Health** We usually associate illness with pain, fear, discomfort, and limitations. While many of these factors do go hand in hand with illness, it is also possible that health problems can contribute positively to the physical dimension of health. Exposure to certain infectious diseases may allow your body to develop immunity. This is a very beneficial effect. Illness can also force you to rest, reduce your work load, reconsider your health behaviors, and stimulate you to take better care of yourself. Weight loss, smoking cessation, improved dietary practices, genetic counseling, or a renewed commitment to physical fitness may follow your recovery from an illness.

■ **Emotional Dimension of Health** Emotionally healthy people feel good about themselves and other people and are generally able to cope with most of the demands of life. Being diagnosed as having some form of illness or disease can seriously jeopardize emotional resources. Until the disease is under control, we can feel frightened, depressed, anxious, isolated, and vulnerable. Fortunately, as you will discover in this unit, medical science has enhanced the prospects of recovery from many diseases.

■ **Social Dimension of Health** Rarely do people face an illness or chronic health condition alone. Friends, family members, physicians, nurses, and therapists often interact with you when you have health problems. In fact, it is possible that health problems may lead you to meet many new people who might challenge and reward your social skills and insights. People who have heart disease, cancer, diabetes, or AIDS often establish relationships with others who have the same condition or with members of support groups.

Illnesses can test your ability to be a friend. When friends are ill, you have an opportunity to practice the friendship skills you have sharpened over the years. Occasionally, however, your social interactions with friends who are ill might expose you to unnecessary risks of disease. It may be in your best interests to temporarily avoid close contacts with these persons until they are no longer infectious.

■ **Intellectual Dimension of Health** Our ability to use the various intellectual processes of reasoning, analysis, interpretation, synthesis, creativity, and memory is best accomplished when we are free from health problems. When we are ill, we may not even want to exercise our higher reasoning powers. In some cases, diseases or medications affect our bodies in ways that make some intellectual processes impossible.

For some people, however, illnesses and other health problems can prove to be important learning experiences. Ill people can learn much about their bodies, their personalities, and health care technology. In fact, most physicians encourage their patients to learn as much as possible about managing their conditions. Although health problems frequently cause short-term decreases in intellectual function, they can also help people grow intellectually.

■ **Spiritual Dimension of Health** What relationships exist between the spiritual dimension of health and illness? Certainly, our ability to serve others can be compromised by a major health problem. A person can easily feel victimized after being diagnosed with a serious illness. This feeling may be the first testing that one experiences about the nature of life and the purpose of living. Some persons who believe in the existence of a loving God may begin to question that belief.

It is also evident that many people who have never held deep spiritual feelings may attempt to establish contact with a higher power when they are diagnosed with a serious illness. Many ill persons pray to their God to work through their physicians and through their own healing powers to accomplish a recovery. Indeed, serious illness is often the single most powerful factor that tests faith.

Diseases

Obstacles to a Healthy Life

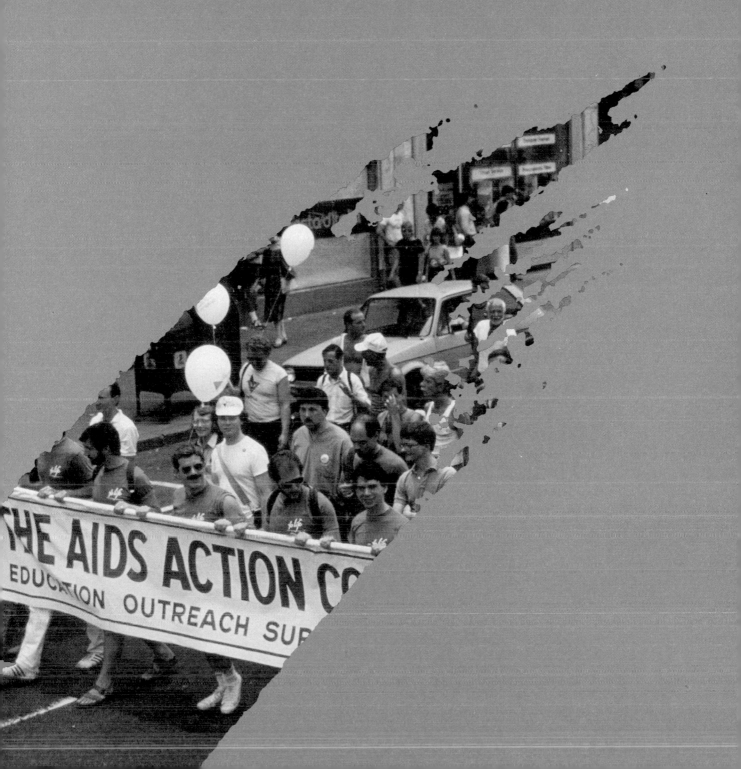

CHAPTER 10

Cardiovascular Disease
Turning the Corner

Key Concepts

Positive lifestyle changes appear to be important factors in reducing cardiovascular disease.

∎

The cardiovascular system, consisting of the heart, blood, and blood vessels, performs a variety of functions.

∎

A healthy cardiovascular system exists when four important physiological requirements are met.

∎

There are five major forms of cardiovascular disease.

∎

Cardiovascular risk factors increase the likelihood of cardiovascular disease.

∎

A person may be able to reduce the impact of certain risk factors.

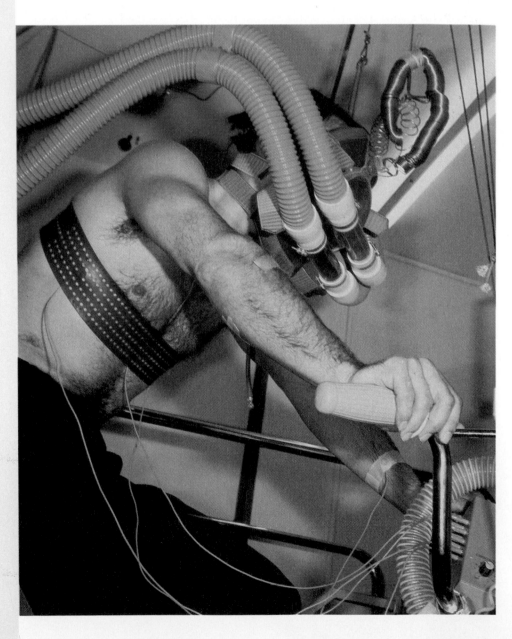

The title of this chapter implies that medical science is making steady advances in its efforts to reduce the deaths and disabilities that result from heart and blood vessel disorders. Indeed, over the last two decades, deaths from heart disease have declined by 30%.[1] With combined efforts in medicine, technology, research, and education, we are finally turning the corner on these dreaded diseases. Although we will probably never reach the point where all of us are free from heart disease, the incidence of heart disorders should continue to decline through this century. Surely we will all eventually succumb to some health condition, but it may be possible that persons who study the current literature in this area and then apply suggested preventive measures will be least likely to develop **cardiovascular** disease.

cardiovascular
pertaining to the heart (cardio) and blood vessels (vascular).

PERVASIVENESS OF CARDIOVASCULAR DISEASE

Cardiovascular diseases are directly related to over 50% of deaths in the United States and indirectly related to a large percentage of additional deaths. Heart disease, stroke, and related blood vessel disorders combined to kill nearly 1 million Americans in 1984 (see Figure 10-1). This figure represents more deaths than were caused by cancer, accidents, pneumonia, lung disease, influenza, and all other causes combined.[2]

The odds are better than 50/50 that the heart you feel beating in your chest right now, the blood vessels you can see in your arms and legs, and the lungs you can feel transporting air will someday simply stop functioning well enough for you to continue to live. This is indeed the gloomy side of the cardiovascular picture. The brighter side shows us that recent advances in medical science, including early detection and innovative treatment methods, have helped reduce the numbers of premature deaths and disabilities. Successful educational efforts have created a better public awareness about cardiovascular disease. Furthermore, the realization that it is possible to prevent the development of certain forms of heart disease has also encouraged many of us to consider positive lifestyle changes in diet, exercise, and smoking behaviors. All of these new efforts have contributed to a brighter outlook for the potential victims of cardiovascular disease.

Who are these potential victims of cardiovascular disease? We all are potential victims of some form of heart or blood vessel disease. Young and old, rich and poor, black and white, athlete and nonathlete, male and female—we are all susceptible to one or more of the many forms of cardiovascular disease. You need only read newspapers or national news magazines to realize the pervasiveness of heart-related disorders in our population. We are stunned to hear of famous people having a stroke or heart attack, coronary bypass surgery, or perhaps a crisis related to hypertension. On a more personal level, almost everyone in your present health class could report that a member of their family has some form of heart disease.

Any academic understanding of cardiovascular diseases must begin with basic anatomical and physiological considerations. This information will be presented next, then the various forms of cardiovascular disease will be specifically discussed. The risk factors that predispose people to cardiovascular disease will follow. Finally, we will discuss specific ways that people might reduce the impact of certain risk factors in their lives.

Figure 10-1
Of the nearly 1 million deaths in the United States each year resulting from cardiovascular diseases, over half are attributable to heart attack.

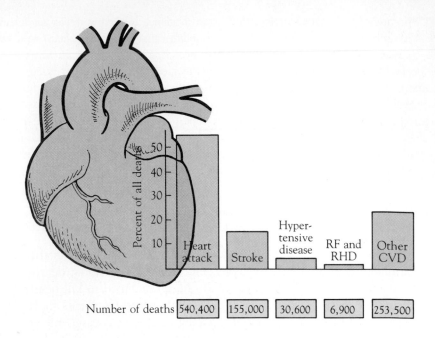

NORMAL CARDIOVASCULAR FUNCTION

The cardiovascular or circulatory system is a transportation system that uses a muscular pump to send a complex fluid on a continuous trip through a closed system of tubes. The pump is, of course, the heart, the fluid is blood, and the closed system of tubes is the network of blood vessels.

The Vascular System

Vascular System
_____

Arteries
Arterioles
Capillaries
Venules
Veins

The **vascular system** refers to the body's blood vessels. Although we might be familiar with the arteries (vessels that carry blood away from the heart) and the veins (vessels that carry blood toward the heart), arterioles, capillaries, and venules are also included in the vascular system. Arterioles are the farther, smaller diameter extensions of arteries. These arterioles lead eventually to capillaries, the smallest extensions of the vascular system. The tiny capillaries, measuring 7 to 9 microns in diameter (about one eighth the diameter of a human hair), function as the vessels through which exchanges of oxygen, food, and waste products occur between the cell and the blood. The vast surface area of the capillaries reduces the speed of the blood flow, thus permitting sufficient time for these critical exchanges to take place.

Once the blood leaves the capillaries and begins its return to the heart, it drains into small veins, or venules. The blood in the venules flows into increasingly larger vessels called veins. Blood pressure is highest in arteries and lowest in veins, especially the largest veins, which empty into the right atrium.

Generally arteries carry blood that has been oxygenated in the lungs. Veins usually carry deoxygenated blood and cellular waste products. Exceptions are the pulmonary arteries and pulmonary veins. The pulmonary arteries carry deoxygenated blood from the heart to the lungs for oxygenation, whereas the pulmonary veins transport oxygenated blood from the lungs back to the left atrium.

The Heart

The heart is a four-chambered pump designed to create the pressure required to circulate blood throughout the body. Usually considered to be about the size of a person's clenched fist, this organ lies slightly tilted between the lungs in the central portion of the **thorax.** The heart does not lie completely in the center of the chest. Rather, approximately two thirds of the heart is to the left of the body midline and one third to the right.[3]

Two upper chambers called *atria* and two lower chambers called *ventricles* form the heart. The thin-walled atrial chambers are considered collecting chambers, while the thick-walled muscular ventricles are considered pressure chambers, or pumping chambers. The right and left sides of the heart are divided by a partition called the *septum* (see Figure 10-2).

Blood is circulated through the heart in a continuous, predictable fashion. Deoxygenated blood enters the right atrium from the **superior vena cava** and the **inferior vena cava.** On contraction of the right atrium, blood is forced through the **tricuspid valve** into the right ventricle. When the right ventricle contracts, the blood is forced through the **pulmonary valve** into the pulmonary arteries for distribution to the right and left lungs. In the smallest branches of the lungs, the alveoli, the blood is reoxygenated and its carbon dioxide exchanged.

The oxygen-rich blood returns to the heart by means of four pulmonary veins that empty into the left atrium. When the left atrium contracts, blood is forced

thorax
the chest; portion of the torso above the diaphragm and within the rib cage.

superior vena cava
body's largest vein; the vessel that brings blood from the upper body regions back to the right atrium of the heart.

inferior vena cava
large vein that returns blood from lower body regions back to the right atrium of the heart.

tricuspid valve
three-cusp (leaves) valve that regulates blood flow between the right atrium and the right ventricle of the heart.

pulmonary valve
valve that controls the flow of blood into the pulmonary arteries from the right ventricle of the heart.

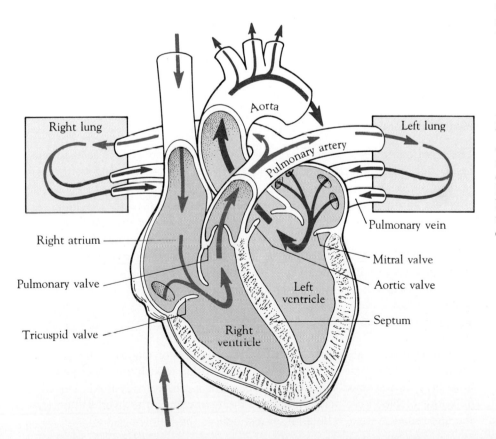

Figure 10-2
The heart functions like a complex double pump. The right side of the heart pumps deoxygenated blood to the lungs. The left side of the heart pumps oxygenated blood through the aorta to all parts of the body.

Aorta

Right lung

Left lung

Pulmonary artery

Pulmonary vein

Right atrium

Mitral valve

Pulmonary valve

Aortic valve

Left ventricle

Septum

Tricuspid valve

Right ventricle

Evaluating cardiovascular function.

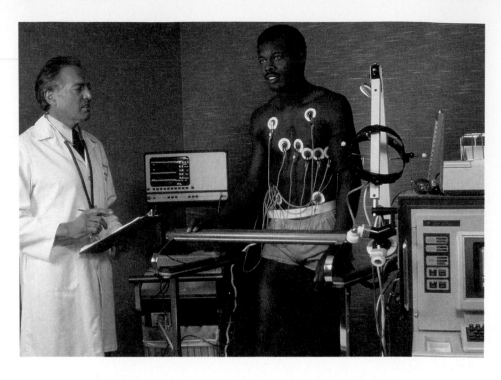

mitral (bicuspid) valve
two-cusp valve that regulates blood flow between the left atrium and the left ventricle of the heart.

aortic valve
valve that controls the blood flow into the aorta from the left ventricle of the heart.

cardiac muscle
specialized, smooth muscle tissue that forms the middle (muscular) layer of the heart wall.

through the **mitral (bicuspid) valve** into the left ventricle. The left ventricle has a muscular wall about three times as thick as that of the right ventricle. This larger size results from the greater pressure that is required to send oxygenated blood throughout the entire body. When the left ventricle contracts, blood is pushed or forced under great pressure through the **aortic valve** into the *aorta*, the largest artery of the body. The aorta quickly branches into smaller arteries, which supply blood to heart muscle, the brain, and the rest of the body.

Heart Stimulation

The heart contracts and relaxes through the delicate interplay of **cardiac muscle** tissue and cardiac electrical centers called *nodes*. Nodal tissue, developed from cardiac tissues during the embryonic stage, generates the electrical impulses necessary to contract heart muscle. The *pacemaker,* also called the *sinoatrial* or *SA node,* provides the depolarization necessary for establishing the electrical current required first to contract the two atria simultaneously, and then to simultaneously contract the two ventricles.[3] The heart's electrical activity is measured by an electrocardiograph (ECG). This instrument provides a printout (electrocardiogram), which can be evaluated to determine cardiac electrical functioning.

Blood

The average-sized adult has approximately 6 quarts of blood in the circulatory system. From the time when we were small children with cuts and scrapes, we have been conditioned to realize that blood is a critical body fluid. Indeed, the functions of blood are many. They are quite similar to the overall functions of the circulatory system. These functions include the following:

- Transportation of nutrients, oxygen, wastes, hormones, and enzymes
- Regulation of water content of body cells and fluids
- Buffering to help maintain appropriate pH balance of body fluids
- Regulation of body temperature; the water component in the blood absorbs heat and transfers it
- Prevention of blood loss; by coagulating or clotting, the blood can alter its form to prevent blood loss through injured vessels
- Protection against toxins and microorganisms, accomplished by chemical substances (antibodies) and specialized cellular elements circulating in the bloodstream.

Your blood accomplishes all of these functions on a daily, full-time basis.

REQUIREMENTS FOR OVERALL CARDIOVASCULAR HEALTH

To promote overall good health, the cardiovascular system must be maintained in its own state of optimal health. Four primary functions can be used as indicators of the system's own health status. Should these functions be impaired, then the system itself is no longer a dependable transportation system.

The first of the four indicators is heart muscle that is adequately nourished and oxygenated. This condition is met when the heart muscle can receive a blood supply capable of transporting nutrients, oxygen, and removing metabolic wastes. Failure by the heart to supply itself with sufficient blood because of damage to its own coronary vascular system results in a less than fully functional pump. Fortunately, physical exercise helps promote cardiovascular fitness by enhancing our *collateral circulation*. Thus when a coronary artery is blocked, nearby blood vessels are better able to enlarge and distribute blood to the heart muscle deprived of normal blood flow.

A second characteristic of an efficiently working cardiovascular system is the heart's ability to maintain a rhythm compatible with a particular level of demand. Because heart rate is an important component of overall cardiac output,

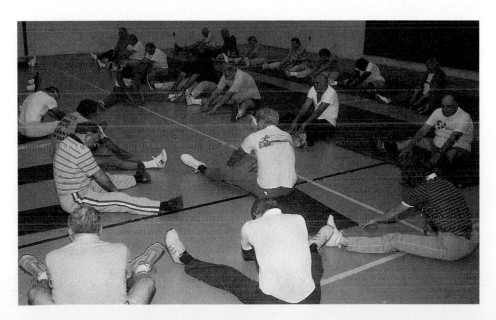

Maintaining cardiovascular health.

failure of the heart to maintain an appropriate beating rhythm will reduce the cardiovascular system's ability to meet the body's demand for blood.

The third factor that is important in overall efficiency of the cardiovascular system is the ability of all blood vessels to adjust to increased cardiac output without experiencing excessive increases in blood pressure. Our blood vessels need the ability to dilate when our heart rate increases, such as when we exercise or find ourselves stressed. If our blood vessels cannot accommodate these changes well, our blood pressure might elevate dangerously.

The last important factor is oxygen transport. Hemoglobin, a pigment found on the surface of red blood cells, is the compound whose natural affinity for oxygen makes this transport possible. Should any substance or process (carbon monoxide, for example) interfere with hemoglobin's affinity for oxygen, then transport activity will be altered and cells will be deprived of the oxygen needed for conversion of nutrients into energy.

Estimated Prevalence of Major CVDs

Coronary heart disease	4,810,000
Hypertension	57,710,000
Stroke	1,960,000
Congenital heart disease	506,800
Rheumatic heart disease	2,120,000
TOTAL CVD*	63,400,000

*The sum of the individual estimates exceeds 63,400,000, since many persons have more than one cardiovascular disorder.

coronary arteries
vessels that supply oxygenated blood to heart muscle tissues.

atherosclerosis
buildup of plaque on the inner walls of arteries.

myocardial infarction
heart attack; the death of heart muscle as a result of a blockage in one of the coronary arteries.

FORMS OF CARDIOVASCULAR DISEASE

The American Heart Association[2] describes the five major forms of cardiovascular disease (CVD) as coronary heart disease, hypertension, stroke, congenital heart disease, and rheumatic heart disease. A person may have just one of these five diseases or a combination of forms at the same time. Each form exists in varying degrees of severity. All forms are capable of providing secondary damages to other body organs and body systems.

Coronary Heart Disease

This form of CVD, also known as coronary artery disease, involves damage to the vessels that supply blood to the heart muscle. The bulk of this blood is supplied by the **coronary arteries.** Any damage to these important vessels can cause a reduction of blood (and its vital oxygen and nutrients) to specific areas of heart muscle. The ultimate result of inadequate blood supply is a heart attack.

Atherosclerosis

The principal culprit in the development of coronary heart disease is a condition known as atherosclerosis (see Figure 10-3). **Atherosclerosis** is a condition that produces a narrowing of the coronary arteries. This narrowing stems from the long-term buildup of fatty deposits (plaque) on the inner walls of the arteries. This buildup reduces the blood supply to specific portions of the heart. Some arteries of the heart can become so blocked (occluded) that all blood supply is stopped. Heart muscle tissue begins to die when it is deprived of oxygen and nutrients. This damage is known as **myocardial infarction.** In lay terms, this event is called *heart attack.* The box on p. 268 discusses the signals and action of a heart attack. (Arteriosclerosis, a dangerous condition of the arteries that is distinctly different from atherosclerosis, is discussed on pp. 274-275.)

A myocardial infarction can also result from a blood clot or a fatty clot that occludes a coronary artery. These clots might be circulating clots (*emboli*) that form in a distant artery, travel, and eventually lodge themselves in a narrowed coronary artery. Clots may also form at a site directly in the coronary artery.

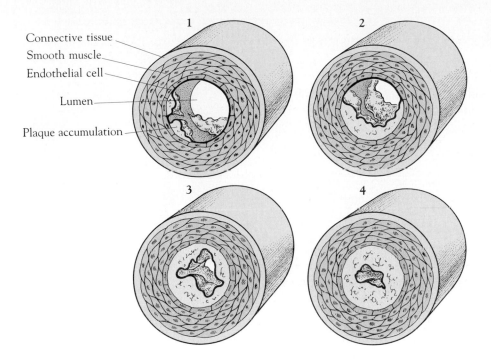

Connective tissue
Smooth muscle
Endothelial cell
Lumen
Plaque accumulation

Figure 10-3
Progression of atherosclerosis. This diagram shows how plaque deposits gradually accumulate to reduce the amount of lumen (space) within an artery.

Such stationary clots are called *thrombi*. Heart crises produced by clots are appropriately labeled coronary embolism, coronary thrombosis, or coronary occlusion, depending on the nature of the origin of the blockage.

Cholesterol and lipoproteins For many years, scientists have known atherosclerosis as a complicated disease that has many causes. Some of these causes are not well understood but others are clearly understood. *Cholesterol*, a fatty substance in alcohol form, is manufactured in the liver and small intestine and is a necessary element in the formation of sex hormones, bile salts, and nerve fibers. Elevated levels of serum cholesterol (above 200 milligrams per deciliter) are known to be associated with an increased risk for developing atherosclerosis. This knowledge has helped us learn to control serum cholesterol by limiting our intake of foods high in saturated fats and cholesterol. Today, many people make a conscious effort to read food labels and avoid foods high in saturated fats and oils containing monounsaturated fats like palm oil and coconut oil.

Another probable factor related to the development of atherosclerosis concerns structures called *lipoproteins*. Lipoproteins are chemical structures that circulate in the bloodstream and transport fatty material, including cholesterol. Two main varieties of lipoproteins exist—low density lipoproteins (LDLs) and high density lipoproteins (HDLs). People have both varieties of lipoproteins, but in varying proportions. We now know that having a higher percentage of HDLs than LDLs seems to protect against the development of atherosclerosis and resultant coronary heart disease. HDLs are able to transport more cholesterol from the bloodstream than LDLs. Thus the bloodstream does not accumulate as much fatty material to clog the arteries. Smoking, a poor diet, and lack of exercise may contribute to an increase in the proportion of LDLs. Fortunately, one of

Heart Attack—Signals and Action

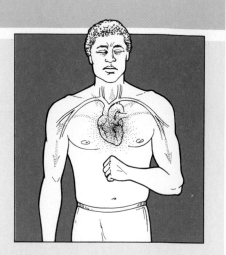

KNOW THE WARNING SIGNALS OF A HEART ATTACK

- Uncomfortable pressure, fullness, squeezing, or pain in the center of your chest lasting 2 minutes or longer.
- Pain spreading to your shoulders, neck, or arms.
- Severe pain, dizziness, fainting, sweating, nausea, or shortness of breath.

    Not all of these warning signs occur in every heart attack. If some start to occur, however, don't wait. Get help immediately!

KNOW WHAT TO DO IN AN EMERGENCY

- Find out which hospitals in your area have 24-hour emergency cardiac care.
- Determine (in advance) the hospital or medical facility that is nearest your home and office, and tell your family and friends to call this facility in an emergency.
- Keep a list of emergency rescue service numbers next to your telephone and in your pocket, wallet, or purse.
- If you have chest discomfort that lasts for 2 minutes or more, call the emergency rescue service.
- If you can get to a hospital faster by going yourself and not waiting for an ambulance, have someone drive you there.

BE A HEART SAVER

- If you are with someone experiencing the signs of a heart attack—and the warning signs last for 2 minutes or longer—act immediately.
- Expect a "denial." It is normal for someone with chest discomfort to deny the possibility of something as serious as a heart attack. Don't take "no" for an answer. Insist on taking prompt action.
- Call the emergency rescue service, or
- Get to the nearest hospital emergency room that offers 24-hour emergency cardiac care.
- Give CPR (mouth-to-mouth breathing and chest compression) if it is necessary and if you're properly trained.

the best ways to improve your lipoprotein profile (ratio of HDL to LDL) is to exercise regularly.

A controversy exists among scientists as to whether a group of fatty acids found in cold-water fish, whales, and seals protects against atherosclerosis. Some claim that these omega-3 fatty acids (now available in stores as "fish oil" capsules) reduce serum cholesterol and increase the proportion of HDLs in the bloodstream.

Several studies have, however, called attention to some increased risks associated with the use of fish oil capsules. These concerns include an unacceptable increase in the proportion of LDLs, the development of vitamin A toxicity, and the consumption of unnecessary saturated fats.

Angina pectoris

Most of the circulation insufficiencies to heart muscle precipitate some degree of chest pain or *angina pectoris*. This pain results from a diminished supply of oxygen to heart muscle tissue. Usually angina is felt when the patient exercises too strenuously. Angina reportedly can range from a feeling of mild indigestion to a severe viselike pressure in the chest. The pain may radiate from the center of the chest to the arms and even up to a person's jaw. Generally the more severe the occlusion, the more pain is felt. Some cardiac patients relieve angina with the drug *nitroglycerin,* a powerful vasodilator. This prescription drug, available in slow-release skin pads or small pills placed under a person's tongue, causes the coronary arteries to dilate and allow for more flow of blood into heart muscle tissue.

When a person's angina has been primarily caused by spasms of the coronary arteries, relatively new drugs, the **calcium channel blockers,** may prove to be beneficial.[4] Calcium channel blockers prevent calcium ions from passing through the thin walls of the coronary arteries and causing the muscular layers of the vessels to contract. By preventing these contractions, adequate blood flow can be maintained and angina symptoms will be diminished.

calcium channel blockers drugs that prevent arterial spasms; used in the long-term management of angina pectoris.

In addition to their primary effect, calcium channel blockers may in some cases lower blood pressure and slow the heart rate. These two alterations in cardiac function provide additional relief to an already overstressed cardiovascular system.

Beta blockers are another class of drugs used in the management of angina pectoris.[5] These drugs block some of the heart muscle's sensitivity to nervous impulses that tell it to "beat harder and faster." Thus during periods of activity a person's heart is kept somewhat "uninformed" of the demand for greater output. As a consequence the coronary arteries do not become stressed and angina symptoms are minimized. Beta blockers, like calcium channel blockers, are taken to prevent the restricted blood flow that may precede a coronary crisis in patients with diagnosed coronary artery disease.

beta blockers drugs that prevent overactivity of the heart, which results in angina pectoris.

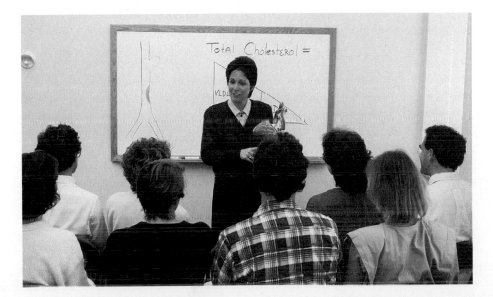

Learning about cholesterol's role in cardiovascular disease.

Could you provide help during a cardiac emergency?

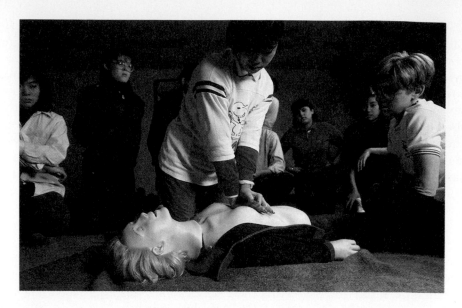

Emergency response to heart crises

Heart attacks are not always fatal. The consequences of any heart attack depend on the location of the damage, the extent to which heart muscle is damaged, and the speed at which adequate circulation is restored. Injury to the primary pumping chambers (ventricles) may very well prove fatal unless medical countermeasures are immediately undertaken.

Cardiopulmonary resuscitation (CPR) has been demonstrated to be one of the most important immediate countermeasures that trained people can use when confronted with a victim of heart attack. Public education programs sponsored by the American Red Cross and the American Heart Association teach people how to recognize, evaluate, and manage heart attack emergencies. CPR trainees are taught how to restore breathing (through mouth-to-mouth resuscitation) and circulation (through external chest compressions) in victims who require such emergency countermeasures. Frequently colleges offer CPR classes through health science or physical education departments. We would encourage each student to enroll in a CPR course.

In the event of a coronary crisis, medical therapies available to aid the victim include both drug and nondrug-centered approaches. Drugs can be used to enlarge coronary arteries (thus improving blood flow), to lower blood pressure (reducing the heart's work load), and to regulate the heart rate (reducing **arrhythmias**). Anticoagulant drugs may also be administered to help dissolve clots and prevent the formation of new clots.

In 1987 the FDA granted final approval for the distribution of tissue plasminogen activator (TPA) under the brand name Activase.[6] TPA is administered to victims of heart attack over a 3-hour period following their attacks. The drug works by dissolving blood clots, thus minimizing the extent of the damage and reducing the likelihood of a subsequent attack. The use of TPA is expected to save thousands of lives. However, long-term evaluation will resolve the extent to which this drug should be administered.[7]

A second and more rapidly acting "clot busting" drug is nearing approval by the FDA. Eminase (APSAC) can be administered more quickly than TPA and

---

Coronary Crisis Priorities

Establish:
Airway
Breathing
Circulation

---

arrhythmias
irregularities of the heart's normal rhythm or beating pattern.

thus further minimizes the damage of the attacks. When available, this drug will further decrease the likelihood of persons dying from heart attack. Both TPA and APSAC are very expensive but effective drugs.

Although not a drug therapy, electric shock pads can also be used in emergency situations to stimulate the return of a normal heart rate, especially in victims of *ventricular fibrillation*, a condition in which the ventricles are merely fluttering in a weak, nonproductive manner. Recent evidence suggests that arrhythmias, including ventricular fibrillation, may be responsible for the majority of sudden deaths once attributed to myocardial infarction.

Diagnosis and coronary repair

Once a victim's vital signs have stabilized, further diagnostic examinations can reveal the type and extent of damaged heart muscle. Included among these examinations is a procedure called *heart catheterization*. Also called coronary arteriography, this minor surgical procedure starts with the introduction of a thin plastic tube in an arm or leg vein. This tube, or catheter, is guided through the vein until it reaches coronary circulation, where a *radiopaque dye* is then released. X-ray pictures called angiograms then record the progress of the dye through the coronary arteries.[8] Areas of occlusion are relatively easily identified. More recently echocardiography (the use of **ultrasound** procedures[9]) and highly specific blood enzymes studies are being employed as diagnostic tools.

ultrasound
use of high-intensity sound waves to create an image of internal body structures.

Once the extent of damage is identified, a physician or team of physicians can decide on a medical course of action. Currently popular is an extensive form of surgery called **coronary artery bypass surgery.** An estimated 202,000 bypass surgeries were performed in 1984.[2] The purpose of such surgery is to detour (bypass) areas of coronary artery obstruction. This is achieved by using sections of a vein from the patient's leg (often the saphenous vein) and grafting it from the aorta to a location just beyond the area of obstruction. Multiple areas of obstruction result in double, triple, or quadruple bypasses. Each operation costs about $30,000.

coronary artery bypass surgery
surgical procedure designed to improve blood flow to the heart by providing alternate routes for blood to take around points of blockage.

Coronary bypass surgery requires a highly specialized team of surgeons, anesthesiologists, and nurses. Doctors perform delicate procedures that include a major incision directly through the sternum (breastbone), procedures to connect the patient's heart to the **heart-lung machine,** microsurgery to complete the vessel grafting procedures, and techniques to restimulate the normal heartbeat. Within a few months after surgery, patients often report reduced chest pain, increased physical activity, and the feeling of a "new lease on life."

heart-lung machine
device that oxygenates and circulates blood during bypass surgery.

However, there is increasing evidence that coronary bypass surgery does not prolong survival in most cardiac patients.[10] Thus there is some concern among health professionals that too many bypass operations are being performed. This concern should be lessened, however, by the recent development of the Cardio-pulmonary Support System (CSS) that will allow thousands of patients facing bypass surgery to undergo less demanding angioplasty. The CSS is a portable pump similar to the heart-lung machine.

Angioplasty

Angioplasty, an alternative to bypass surgery, involves the surgical insertion of a doughnut-shaped "balloon" directly into the narrowed coronary artery. When this balloon is inflated, plaque and fatty deposits are compressed against the artery walls.[11] The open center of the balloon allows for adequate blood flow. These balloons usually remain within the artery for less than 1 hour. Although one might expect the compression of plaque to provide only short-term relief, only 5% of angioplasty patients elect to have bypass surgery. It is predicted that renarrowing of the artery will occur in about one third of angioplasty patients. About 125,000 angioplasty procedures were performed in 1986.[12]

For victims of occlusions resulting primarily from blood clots forming in the extremities, an experimental technique may prove beneficial in the coming years. This technique uses a laser beam to dissolve blood clots. This futuristic, surgical procedure is currently being carefully scrutinized by medical researchers.

Peripheral artery disease

Peripheral artery disease (PAD), also called peripheral vascular disease (PVD), is a blood vessel disease characterized by serious changes to the arteries and arterioles in the extremities (primarily the legs and feet, but sometimes in the hands). These changes result from years of atherosclerotic and arteriosclerotic damage to the blood vessels. The result of PAD is severely restricted blood flow to the extremities. The reduction in blood flow is responsible for leg pain or cramping during exercise, numbness, tingling, coldness, and loss of hair in the affected limb. The most serious consequence of PAD is the increased likelihood of developing ulcerations and tissue death. These conditions can lead to gangrene and eventually necessitate amputation.

A likely candidate for PAD is someone over the age of 50 who smokes and has diabetes or other cardiovascular problems, does not exercise much, has hypertension, is significantly overweight, and has a poor blood lipid profile (low ratio of HDL to LDL). The management of PAD consists of multiple approaches and may include efforts to improve lipid profiles (through diet, exercise, or drug therapy), reduce hypertension, reduce body weight, and eliminate smoking. Blood vessel surgery may be a possibility, but only after other approaches (in-

Cardiovascular surgery.

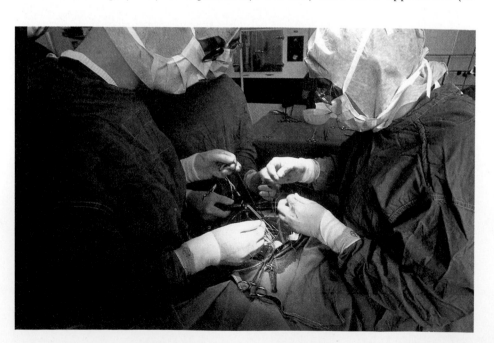

cluding the use of drugs that dilate the affected blood vessels) are first explored. The likelihood of developing PAD in later life can be reduced by sound diet, regular aerobic exercise, the avoidance of cigarette smoking, and proper weight maintenance.

Congestive heart failure

Congestive heart failure is a condition in which the heart lacks the strength to continue to circulate blood normally throughout the body. During congestive heart failure, the heart continues to work, but it just cannot function well enough to maintain appropriate circulation. Venous blood flow starts to "back up." Swelling occurs, especially in the legs and ankles. Fluid can collect in the lungs and cause breathing difficulties and shortness of breath, and kidney function may be damaged. Without medical care, congestive heart failure can be fatal.[2]

Congestive heart failure can result from heart damage caused by congenital heart defects, rheumatic fever, heart attack, atherosclerosis, or high blood pressure. Generally, congestive heart failure is treatable through a combined program of rest, proper diet, modified daily activities, and the use of appropriate drugs. Diuretics, vasodilators, and drugs that maintain normal heart beating patterns are used with patients of congestive heart failure. If a specific cause for heart failure, such as hypertension or heart valve damage, can be corrected or managed, further complications will be minimized.[2]

Hypertension

Just as your car's water pump recirculates water and maintains water pressure, your heart recirculates blood and maintains blood pressure. When the heart contracts, blood is forced through your arteries and veins. Your blood pressure is a measure of the force that your circulating blood exerts against the interior walls of your arteries and veins.

Blood pressure is measured by a *sphygmomanometer*. A sphygmomanometer is attached to an arm-cuff device that can be inflated to stop the flow of blood temporarily in the brachial artery. This artery is a major supplier of blood to the lower arm. It is located on the inside of the upper arm, between the biceps and triceps muscles.

A physician, nurse, or technician using a stethoscope will listen for blood flow as the pressure in the cuff is released. Two pressure measurements will be recorded. The **systolic pressure** is the blood pressure against the vessel walls when the heart contracts. The **diastolic pressure** is the blood pressure against the vessel walls when the heart relaxes (between heart beats). Expressed in millimeters of mercury displaced on the sphygmomanometer, blood pressure is recorded in the form of a fraction, 115/82, for example. Since blood pressure drops when the heart relaxes, the systolic pressure is always higher than the diastolic pressure.

Although many persons still consider 120/80 as a "normal" or safe blood pressure for a young adult, variances from this figure do not necessarily indicate a medical problem. In fact, many young college women of average weight will indicate blood pressures that seem to be relatively low (105/65 for example), yet these lowered blood pressures are quite "normal" for them. Any major deviation from 120/80 in your blood pressure should be discussed with a physician.

systolic pressure
blood pressure against blood vessel walls when the heart contracts.

diastolic pressure
blood pressure against blood vessel walls when the heart relaxes.

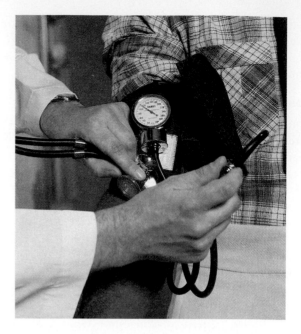

Hypertension screening.

Hypertension refers to a consistently elevated blood pressure. Generally, concern about a young adult's high blood pressure begins when he or she has a systolic reading of 140 or above or a diastolic reading of 90 or above. Nearly 58 million American adults have hypertension.[2]

It is estimated that in 90% of the cases of hypertension, the cause is not clearly known. This form of hypertension is called *essential hypertension.*[2] Essential hypertension does appear to be statistically related to age, heredity, and diet, since epidemiological studies have indicated that this disease tends to strike older persons, to run in families (especially black families), and to afflict persons who eat a diet high in saturated fat and salt. Unresolved stress may be a factor in essential hypertension, but the relationship has not been clearly established. (Two important points are worth remembering. First, persons under a lot of tension do not necessarily have hypertension. Second, hypertension and hyperactivity are two completely different conditions.)

A second form of hypertension is called *secondary hypertension.* This is a logical term, since this form of hypertension appears to be triggered by a specific cause. **Arteriosclerosis,** endocrine gland disorders, and kidney diseases may all be causes of secondary hypertension. Scientific research also implicates unresolved stress as another possible contributor to secondary hypertension.

The cardiovascular health risks produced by unmitigated hypertension are many. Hypertension accelerates atherosclerosis (see p. 266). Thus the heart is required to work much more forcefully to pump blood through narrowed vessels. This requirement places too much demand on the coronary arteries and the ventricles, which must carry the brunt of the work load. Heart attack and heart failure may result.

Throughout the body, hypertension also accelerates arteriosclerosis. This process makes arteries and arterioles become less elastic and thus incapable of dilating under a heavy work load.[2] Brittle, calcified blood vessels can burst unexpectedly and produce serious strokes (brain accidents), kidney failure (renal

arteriosclerosis
calcification within the artery's wall that makes the vessel less elastic, more brittle and more susceptible to bursting; hardening of the arteries.

accidents), or eye damage **(retinal hemorrhage).** Furthermore, it appears that blood and fat clots are more easily formed and dislodged in a vascular system influenced by hypertension. Clearly hypertension is a potential killer.

Ironically, despite its deadly nature, hypertension is referred to as "the silent killer," because victims of hypertension rarely if ever are aware that they have hypertension. Victims cannot feel the sensation of high blood pressure. Hypertension does not produce dizziness, headaches, or memory loss, unless one is experiencing a medical crisis. Because it is a silent killer, estimates are that over 50% of the people who have hypertension do not realize they have it. Many who are aware of their hypertension do little to control it. Only a small percentage of people who have hypertension control it adequately, generally through dietary control, supervised fitness, relaxation training, and drug therapy. Essential hypertension is not thought of as a curable disease; rather, it is a controllable disease. Once therapy is stopped, the condition returns.

Weight reduction, physical exercise, and sodium restriction are often used to reduce one's hypertension. For heavy or obese persons, a reduction in body weight may produce a significant drop in blood pressure. Physical activity helps lower blood pressure by expending calories (which leads to weight loss) and improving overall circulation. The restriction of sodium (salt) in one's diet also helps some people to reduce hypertension. Interestingly, this strategy is only effective for those who are **salt sensitive**—estimated to be about 20% of the population.[13] Reducing salt intake would have little effect on the blood pressure of the rest of the population. (Nevertheless, since our daily intake of salt vastly exceeds our need for salt, the general recommendation to curb salt intake still makes good sense.)

Many of the stress reduction activities we discussed in Chapter 3 are receiving increased attention in the struggle to reduce hypertension. In recent years behavioral scientists have reported the success of meditation, biofeedback, controlled breathing, and muscle relaxation exercises in reducing hypertension. Look for further research in these areas in the years to come.

Drug therapies for hypertension involve the use of one or two general categories of drugs. *Antihypertensive drugs* dilate the peripheral blood vessels to reduce blood pressure. *Diuretic drugs* work by forcing excess fluid (water) from the bloodstream, thereby reducing blood volume. The most disturbing aspect of drug therapy for hypertension is that many patients refuse to take their medication on a consistent basis, probably because of the mistaken notion that "you must feel sick to be sick."

A number of people taking these medications report uncomfortable side effects, including depression, reduced libido (sex drive), muscle weakness, impotence, dizziness, and fainting. Thus the treatment's side effects may seem worse than the disease. Because of the poor record of patient compliance with hypertension drug therapy, numerous television and radio announcements are geared to the hypertensive patient.

As a responsible adult, you might push yourself to use every opportunity you can find to measure your blood pressure. Ask to have your blood pressure checked when you are in a physician's office or in the student health center. (You may have to pry these measures from the nurse—you do have a right to this information!) You could also check with nursing majors to see whether they might check your blood pressure. Use the free machines that measure blood

retinal hemorrhage
uncontrolled bleeding from arteries within the eye's retina.

salt sensitive
description of people who overreact to the presence of sodium by retaining fluid, and thus increase blood pressure.

cerebrovascular occlusions
blockages to arteries supplying blood to the cerebral cortex of the brain; strokes.

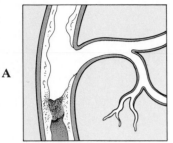

A

Thrombus

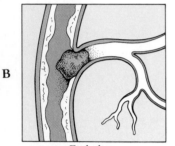

B

Embolism

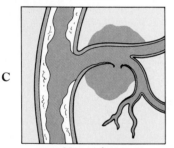

C

Hemorrhage

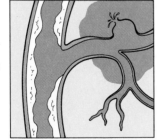

D

Aneurysm (ruptured)

Figure 10-4
Causes of stroke.

transient ischemic attack (TIA)
strokelike symptoms caused by temporary spasm of cerebral blood vessels.

pressure in shopping malls or drug stores. (Do not count on completely accurate measurements from these machines, however.) Become familiar with your own potential silent killer.

Stroke

Stroke is a general term for a wide variety of crises (sometimes called *cerebrovascular accidents* or CVAs) that result from blood vessel damage in the brain. Data for 1984 indicate that nearly 155,000 deaths and half a million new cases of stroke occur each year.[2] Just as heart muscle needs adequate blood supply, so does the brain. Any disturbance in the proper supply of oxygen and nutrients can pose a hazardous situation.

Perhaps the most common form of stroke results from the blockage in a cerebral (brain) artery. Similar to coronary occlusions, **cerebrovascular occlusions** can be initiated by a clot (thrombus) that forms within an artery or by a clot (embolus) that travels from another part of the body to the brain (see Figure 10-4, A and B.) The resultant accidents (cerebral thrombosis or cerebral embolism) both cause strokes. The portion of the brain deprived of oxygen and nutrients can literally die.

The extent of damage depends on the location of the occlusion and the degree of blockage. Thus an occlusion in a portion of brain tissue that serves as a speech center can result in a person's inability to speak. Occlusion in motor coordination areas can result in paralysis. Memory, behavior, and thought patterns can also be affected by stroke. Obviously a massive occlusion or an occlusion in a critical area (such as a center that controls respiration, temperature, or coronary function) can initiate a life-threatening situation.

Strokes can also result from an artery that bursts to produce a crisis called *cerebral hemorrhage* (see Figure 10-4, C). Damaged, brittle arteries can be especially susceptible to bursting when a person has hypertension. Brittle arteries may result from a condition known as arteriosclerosis. In arteriosclerosis, excess calcium deposits are found in the middle layer of the arterial walls. The arteries become less elastic in nature; the arterial walls harden and eventually become brittle. Arteriosclerosis tends to increase as we age or as a consequence of other disease processes, such as diabetes or hypertension. Cerebral hemorrhage produces two key problems: (1) the brain tissue supplied by the damaged artery is deprived of oxygen and nutrients, and (2) the accumulation of blood places added pressure on surrounding brain tissue. Because the skull (cranium) will not expand, this pressure buildup can be enormous and life threatening in itself.

A fourth form of stroke is a *cerebral aneurysm*. An aneurysm is a ballooning or outpouching on a weakened area of an artery. (See Figure 10-4, D.) Aneurysms may occur in various locations of the body and are not always life threatening. The development of aneurysms is not fully understood, although there seems to be a relationship between aneurysms and hypertension. It is quite possible that many aneurysms are congenital defects. In any case, when a cerebral aneurysm bursts, a stroke results. See the box on p. 277 for warning signs of stroke.

A person who reports any warning signs of stroke or any little stroke (**transient ischemic attack [TIA]**) will undergo a battery of diagnostic tests, which could include a physical examination, a search for possible brain tumors, tests to

Warning Signs of Stroke

Although many victims of stroke have little advance warning of an impending crisis, there are some warning signals of stroke that should be recognized. The American Heart Association encourages everyone to be aware of the following signs:

- Sudden, temporary weakness or numbness of the face, arm, and leg on one side of the body
- Temporary loss of speech or trouble in speaking or understanding speech
- Temporary dimness or loss of vision, particularly in one eye
- Unexplained dizziness, unsteadiness, or sudden falls
- Many major strokes are preceded by "little strokes," warning signals like the above, experienced days, weeks, or months before the more severe event

Prompt medical or surgical attention to these symptoms may prevent a fatal or disabling stroke from occurring.

identify areas of the brain affected, use of the electroencephalogram, cerebral arteriography, and the use of the **CAT scan** (computerized axial tomography scanner).[2]

Treatment of stroke patients depends on the nature and extent of the damage. Some patients require surgery (to repair vessels and relieve pressure) and acute care in the hospital. Others undergo drug treatment, especially the use of anticoagulant drugs, including aspirin. Patients with related diseases (atherosclerosis, diabetes, kidney disorders, obesity, and hypertension) must undergo further treatment to minimize the damage these disorders can produce. Some researchers currently believe that the incidence of stroke could be reduced by eating an extra serving of potassium-rich fresh fruits and vegetables on a daily basis.[14] Good examples are a small banana or a cup of orange juice. Potassium tablets or supplements are not recommended.

The advancements made in the rehabilitation of stroke victims are amazing. It is true that some severely damaged patients have little hope of improvement. However, our increasing advancements in the application of computer technology to such disciplines as speech therapy and physical therapy do offer encouraging signs for stroke patients and their families.

CAT scan
computerized axial tomography; x-ray procedure designed to visualize structures within the body that would not normally be seen through conventional x-ray procedures.

Congenital Heart Disease

It is estimated that each year 25,000 babies are born with a congenital heart defect. Over 6,000 died of congenital heart disease in 1984.[2] A congenital defect is one that is present at birth. The cause of congenital heart defects is not clearly understood, although one cause, *rubella*, has been clearly identified. Mothers who contract the rubella virus during the first 3 months of pregnancy place their child at great risk of developing *congenital rubella syndrome (CRS)*, a catchall term for a wide variety of congenital defects, including heart defects, deafness, cataracts, and mental retardation. Other hypotheses about the development of

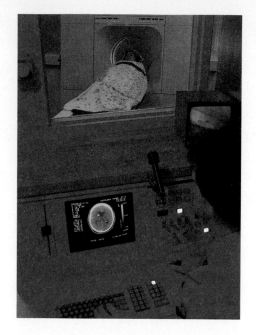

CAT scan.

congenital heart disease implicate environmental pollutants, use of drugs including alcohol, and unknown genetic factors.

A variety of abnormalities may be produced by congenital heart disease, including valve damage, holes in the walls of the septum, blood vessel transposition, and an underdevelopment of the left side of the heart.[2] All of these problems ultimately prevent a newborn baby from adequately oxygenating tissues throughout the body. A bluish skin color (cyanosis) is seen in some infants with such congenital heart defects. These infants are sometimes collectively referred to as "blue babies."

Treatment of congenital defects centers on surgery. Defective blood vessels and certain malformations of the heart can be surgically repaired. So successful is this surgery that many children respond quite quickly to the increased circulation and oxygenation. Many are able to lead normally active lives.*

Rheumatic Heart Disease

rheumatic heart disease chronic damage to the heart (especially heart valves) resulting from a streptococcal infections within the heart; a complication associated with rheumatic fever.

Rheumatic heart disease is the final stage in a series of complications initiated by a streptococcal infection of the throat (strep throat). This bacterial infection, if untreated, can result in an inflammatory disease called *rheumatic fever* (and a corollary condition, scarlet fever). Rheumatic fever is a whole-body (systemic) reaction that can produce fever, joint pain, skin rashes, and possible brain and heart damage. Once having had rheumatic fever, a person is more susceptible to additional attacks. Rheumatic fever tends to run in families.

Damage from rheumatic fever centers on the heart's valves. For some reason, the bacteria prefer to proliferate in the region of the heart valves.

Defective heart valves may fail either to open fully (*stenosis*) or to close fully (*insufficiency*). Diagnosis of valve damage might initially come when a physician

---

*Recently introduced drug therapy can also be used in correcting congenital defects in the hearts of newborns.

hears a backwashing or back flow of blood (a **murmur**). Further tests, including cardiac catheterization or echocardiography, can reveal the extent of valve damage.[2] Once identified, a faulty valve can be replaced surgically with a metal and plastic artificial valve or a valve taken from an animal's heart. The success rate of such surgery is quite high. Patients with only moderate valve damage might forego surgery, instead receiving regular, periodic reexaminations, possible long-term antibiotic treatment, and careful monitoring of physical exercise. Those with mild damage, as evidenced by only a slight murmur, may have no physical restrictions imposed on them. In fact, to the relief of most parents, most murmurs initially identified by physicians are labeled "innocent murmurs," because they are not related to streptococcal damage and will never impair a child's normal development.

Rheumatic heart disease is best prevented by recognizing that *any* sore throat might be strep throat. Although most sore throats are not caused by streptococcal bacteria, any unusually sore throat of sudden onset, especially in children aged 5 to 15, should be examined by a physician.[2] A throat culture and possibly a strep antibody test would determine the causative agent or at least rule out strep as a probable cause.

Besides the cardiovascular diseases already discussed, the heart and blood vessels are also subject to other pathological conditions. Tumors of the heart, although rare, are known to occur. Infectious conditions involving the pericardial sac that surrounds the heart (*pericarditis*) and the innermost layer of the heart (*endocarditis*) are more commonly seen. Additionally, inflammation of the veins (*phlebitis*) is troublesome to some people.

murmur
atypical heart sound that suggests a backwashing of blood into a chamber of the heart from which it just left.

CARDIOVASCULAR RISK FACTORS

A *cardiovascular risk factor* is an attribute that a person has or is exposed to that increases the likelihood that he or she will develop some form of cardiovascular disease. However, merely having one or even a few risk factors does not always mean that a person will develop a disease. You may even know some at-risk people who never seem to develop clinical symptoms of heart disease.

"Big Three" Risk Factors
for Cardiovascular Disease

Cigarette smoking
Hypertension
High cholesterol

Risk Factors for Coronary Artery Disease, Hypertension, and Stroke

Even though research methods for cardiovascular disease determination have improved, medical science can only predict that our chances of developing disease are significantly enhanced if we have multiple risk factors. Some scientists believe that we really understand only about half of the risk factors that may cause cardiovascular disease.

Risk factors for cardiovascular disease can be categorized as follows: (1) those a person cannot change, or (2) those a person can change or control. The box on pp. 280-281 lists ways to reduce risk factors of cardiovascular disease from the American Heart Association 1987 *Heart Facts.*

Many of the risk factors mentioned in the box are more specifically discussed in other chapters of this text.

Most health professionals are convinced that *now* is the best time for people to take a close look at the risk factors they can control. They are convinced that cardiovascular diseases are lifestyle diseases—diseases that closely parallel the

Factors That Cannot Be
Changed

Heredity
Sex
Race
Age

Reducing Risk Factors for Cardiovascular Disease

Extensive clinical and statistical studies have identified several factors that increase the risk of heart attack and stroke. The most significant factors are heredity, male sex, increasing age, smoking, high blood pressure, and elevated blood cholesterol. Other (contributing) factors are diabetes, obesity, and lack of exercise. Stress may also be a contributing factor.

The more risk factors present, the greater the chance a person will develop heart disease. Some risk factors can't be changed; other factors can be changed under a doctor's direction; and still others can be controlled without a doctor's supervision.

MAJOR RISK FACTORS THAT CAN'T BE CHANGED
HEREDITY

A tendency toward heart disease or atherosclerosis appears to be hereditary, so children of parents with cardiovascular disease are more likely to develop it themselves. Race is a consideration, too. Black Americans have moderate hypertension twice as often as whites and severe hypertension three times as often. Consequently, their risk of heart disease is greater.

MALE SEX

Men have a greater risk of heart attack than women. Even after menopause, when women's death rate from heart disease increases, it's not as great as men's.

INCREASING AGE

Fifty-five percent of all heart attack victims are age 65 or older; of those who die, almost 4 out of 5 are over 65.

MAJOR RISK FACTORS THAT CAN BE CHANGED
CIGARETTE SMOKING

Smokers have more than twice the risk of heart attacks as nonsmokers. In fact, cigarette smoking is the biggest risk factor for sudden cardiac death: smokers have 2 to 4 times the risk of nonsmokers. A smoker who has a heart attack is more likely to die from it and is more likely to die suddenly (within an hour) than a nonsmoker.

Smoking is also the biggest risk factor for peripheral vascular disease (narrowing of blood vessels carrying blood to leg and arm muscles). In fact, this condition is almost exclusively confined to smokers. Smokers with peripheral vascular disease are also more likely to develop gangrene and require leg amputation than nonsmokers. The benefits from corrective surgery are also reduced when patients continue to smoke.

When people stop smoking, regardless of how long or how much they've smoked, their risk of heart disease rapidly declines. Ten years after quitting smoking, the risk of death from heart disease for people who have smoked a pack a day or less is almost the same as for those who have never smoked. It's important to stop smoking before the signs of heart disease appear, so if you don't smoke, don't start, and if you do smoke, quit. STOP SMOKING NOW!

HIGH BLOOD PRESSURE

High blood pressure usually has no specific symptoms and no early warning signs. It truly is a "silent killer."

High blood pressure adds to the heart's work load, causing the heart to enlarge and become weaker over time. It also increases the risk of stroke, heart attack, kidney failure, and congestive heart failure. When high blood pressure is combined with obesity, smoking, high blood cholesterol levels, or diabetes, the risk of heart attack or stroke increases several times.

High blood pressure can be detected by a simple, quick, and painless test. People who have high blood pressure should work with their doctor to control it. Proper diet, weight reduction, regular exercise, restricting salt (sodium) intake, and sticking with a program of medication may all be prescribed to lower blood pressure and keep it within healthy limits.

BLOOD CHOLESTEROL LEVELS

The risk of coronary heart disease rises with increasing levels of blood cholesterol. When other risk factors (such as high blood pressure and smoking) are present, this risk increases even more. A person's cholesterol level is also affected by age, sex, heredity, and diet.

Based on large population studies, a cholesterol concentration below 200 mg/dl in middle-aged adults appears to indicate a relatively low risk of coronary heart disease. A level over 240 mg/dl approximately doubles the risk; 20 to 25 percent of the U.S. population falls into this category. Blood cholesterol values between 200 to 240 mg/dl are in a zone of moderate and increasing risk.

Blood cholesterol and triglyceride levels should be measured at least once every 5 years in healthy adults. People with cholesterol levels greater than 200 mg/dl should have a second cholesterol test to confirm the results of the first test. If cholesterol remains elevated in the second test, dietary modification or other treatment may be recommended.

A certain amount of cholesterol in the body is necessary to build cell walls, etc., but the liver produces enough cholesterol to meet these needs. That's why it is important to monitor the amount of cholesterol and saturated fats in the diet—that's where some of the excess cholesterol usually comes from. A diet high in saturated fat and cholesterol tends to raise the level of cholesterol in the blood; a diet low in saturated fat and cholesterol usually results in lower levels of blood cholesterol.

On the whole, Americans should reduce the amount of fat and cholesterol in their diet. For information about the various types of dietary fat (saturated, polyunsaturated, monounsaturated) and how to reduce dietary fat and cholesterol, see *The American Heart Association Diet*. It's available from local AHA offices.

By watching their diet, people with low levels of blood cholesterol will help minimize the tendency for cholesterol levels to rise with age. People with higher levels of blood cholesterol will benefit even more. First, controlling their diet will help reduce their blood cholesterol levels. Second, if drugs are still needed to reduce their blood cholesterol, the diet will improve their effectiveness.

OTHER CONTRIBUTING RISK FACTORS
DIABETES

Diabetes most often appears during middle age, and among people who are overweight. In a mild form, diabetes can go undetected for many years. When a person has diabetes, controlling other risk factors becomes even more important because diabetes can sharply increase the risk of heart attack. This occurs because diabetes affects cholesterol and triglyceride levels.

When a doctor detects diabetes, he or she may prescribe changes in eating habits, programs for weight control and exercise, and even drugs (if necessary) to keep it in check.

OBESITY

Recent evidence indicates that where fat is located on the body may affect the risk of coronary heart disease. A waist/hip ratio greater than 1.0 for men indicates a significantly increased risk. The corresponding value for women is 0.8. This means that a man's waist measurement should not exceed his hip measurement, and a woman's waist measurement should not be more than 80% of her hip measurement.

Obesity is unhealthy because excess weight puts an added strain on the heart. It's linked with coronary heart disease primarily because of its influence on blood pressure and blood cholesterol, and because it can lead to diabetes.

Obesity is generally defined as 20% or more over ideal body weight.

PHYSICAL INACTIVITY

Physical inactivity hasn't been clearly established as a risk factor for heart disease. When a lack of exercise is combined with overeating, however, excess weight can result—and excess weight is unquestionably a contributing factor in heart disease. Overweight individuals should consult a doctor to learn which physical activities best suit people of their age and physical condition.

STRESS

It's almost impossible to define and measure someone's levels of emotional stress. There's no way to measure the psychological impact of different experiences. All people feel stress, but they feel it in different amounts and react in different ways. Life would be dull without stress, but excessive amounts of stress over a long time may create health problems in some people.

Some scientists have noted a relationship between risk for coronary heart disease and a person's life stress, behavior habits, and socioeconomic status. These factors may influence established risk factors. For example, people in stressful situations may start smoking or smoke more than they otherwise would.

While the factors just listed aren't as significant as high blood pressure, smoking, or high blood cholesterol in their impact on heart disease, they still shouldn't be ignored.

way people live their lives. We also support the concept that positive lifestyle changes can reduce an individual's chances of developing certain cardiovascular diseases.

Although no one can promise you freedom from heart and blood vessel diseases, we think your conscious efforts to control the "big three" risk factors (cigarette smoking, hypertension, and high cholesterol) can pay healthful benefits throughout your lifetime. By managing these three risk factors successfully, you will undoubtedly be paying the kind of attention to your body that will also help you manage the contributing factors to cardiovascular disease—obesity, lack of exercise, and chronic, unresolved stress.

In the 1970s and early 1980s skeptics argued that there was not enough scientific evidence to indicate that lifestyle changes had much influence on cardiovascular disease. At the time these conclusions were reasonably valid, since *longitudinal studies* on this topic were not frequently published in the scientific literature. Now, however, a growing body of scientifically controlled longitudinal studies are reporting that lifestyle changes do make a difference. For example, the 10-year, $100 million study for the National Heart, Lung, and Blood Institute confirmed the value of lowering blood cholesterol on the subsequent development of heart disease.[15] A more recently completed 30-year longitudinal study also confirmed this finding.[16] Additionally, an extensive review of 43 studies on the association between physical activity and coronary heart disease concluded that physical activity provides a protective effect against heart disease.[17]

In the future we expect other longitudinal studies to further substantiate the value of managing the various risk factors. We have little control over our genetic background, race, gender, or age, but we must as a society convince ourselves that our lifestyles can make a difference.

Risk Factors for Congenital Heart Disease and Rheumatic Heart Disease

It may already be apparent to you that the risk factors for stroke, coronary artery disease, and high blood pressure differ considerably from the factors that appear to be correlated with the development of congenital heart disease and rheumatic heart disease. Most of the causal factors of congenital heart disease are not well understood. Only the mother's contraction of rubella during pregnancy has been specifically linked to congenital heart abnormalities, although other maternal insults during pregnancy (alcohol or drug abuse, exposure to other disease processes or environmental pollutants) are thought to potentially contribute to heart defects in newborn children.

These risk factors can be minimized by a woman's careful control of her body before conception and during pregnancy, including being immunized before becoming pregnant, reducing exposure to environmental pollutants and tobacco smoke, and limiting drug and alcohol use during pregnancy. Appropriate obstetrical supervision and proper nutrition are other factors that might enhance the birth of a healthy baby—one who is free of congenital heart maladies.

The greatest risk factor related to rheumatic heart disease is the failure to control the streptococcal (bacterial) infection commonly called strep throat. Administration of appropriate antibacterial drugs (primarily penicillin) before bacteria spread to the heart valves is the best way to check the spread of this potentially serious disease.

Factors That Can Be Changed

Cigarette smoking
High blood pressure
Blood cholesterol levels
Diabetes
Obesity
Lack of exercise
Stress

Risk Factors for Congenital Heart Disease

Exposure to rubella, pollutants, or tobacco smoke during pregnancy
Strep throat

Risk Factors for Rheumatic Heart Disease

Streptococcal infection

Since this disease most commonly strikes children aged 5 to 15, it is important for parents to be reasonably concerned about children's sore throats.[2] For people of all ages, high-level health can reduce susceptibility to a wide variety of infections, including strep infection. Adequate sleep, regular exercise, and proper diet (factors that are sometimes difficult for college students to control) can all contribute to your high level of physical health.

ASPIRIN

Studies released in 1988 highlighted the role of aspirin in reducing the risk of heart attack in men who had no history of previous attacks. Specifically, the studies concluded that for men with hypertension, elevated cholesterol, or both, taking one aspirin per day was a significant factor in reducing their risk of myocardial infarction. Presently there is differing opinion regarding the age at which this preventive action should begin. Some researchers have suggested that men with known risk factors should begin taking one aspirin per day by age 35.

HEART TRANSPLANTS AND ARTIFICIAL HEARTS

For approximately 25 years, surgeons have been able to surgically replace (transplant) a person's damaged heart with that of another human being. Although very risky, such an operation has added years to a number of patients who otherwise would have lived only a short time. Aside from the seriousness of this surgery, two major difficulties must be overcome in the process of heart transplantation: (1) finding a suitable donor heart, and (2) coping with the recipient's possible rejection of the newly transplanted heart.

With an increased national awareness for the importance of organ donations, it is hoped that more hearts will become available for transplantation. Donor

Common Symptoms of Strep Throat

Sudden onset of sore throat, particularly with pain when swallowing

Fever

Swollen, tender glands under the angle of the jaw

Headache

Nausea and vomiting

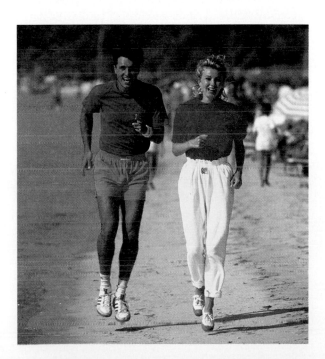

Exercise can reduce the risk of cardiovascular disease.

Personal Assessment

RISKO

Study each risk factor and its row. These are medical conditions and habits associated with an increased danger of heart attack. *Not all risk factors are measurable enough to be included.* Circle the number in the box applicable to you. For example, if you are 37, circle the number in the box labeled 31-40.

    After checking all the rows, total the circled numbers. This score is an estimate of your chances of suffering a heart attack.

HEREDITY
Count parents, grandparents, brothers, and sisters who have had a heart attack and/or stroke.

TOBACCO SMOKING
If you inhale deeply and smoke a cigarette down to the filter, add 1 to your classification. Do not subtract because you think you do not inhale or smoke only a half inch on a cigarette.

EXERCISE
Lower your score one point if you exercise regularly and frequently.

Age	1 10 to 20	2 21 to 30	3 31 to 40	4 41 to 50	6 51 to 60	8 61 and over
Heredity	1 No known history of heart disease	2 1 relative with cardiovascular disease Over 60	3 2 relatives with cardiovascular disease Over 60	4 1 relative with cardiovascular disease Under 60	6 2 relatives with cardiovascular disease Under 60	7 3 relatives with cardiovascular disease Under 60
Weight	0 More than 5 lb below standard weight	1 −5 to +5 lb standard weight	2 6 to 20 lb overweight	3 21 to 35 lb overweight	5 38 to 50 lb overweight	7 51 to 65 lb overweight
Tobacco smoking	0 Nonuser	1 Cigar and/or pipe	2 10 cigarettes or less a day	4 20 cigarettes a day	6 30 cigarettes a day	10 40 cigarettes a day or more
Exercise	1 Intense occupational and recreational exertion	2 Moderate occupational and recreational exertion	3 Sedentary work and intense recreational exertion	5 Sedentary occupational and moderate recreational exertion	6 Sedentary work and light recreational exertion	8 Complete lack of all exercise

CHOLESTEROL OR SATURATED FAT INTAKE LEVEL

If you can't get your cholesterol blood level from your doctor, then estimate honestly the percentage of solid fats you eat. These are usually of animal origin—lard, cream, butter, and beef and lamb fat. If you eat much of this, your cholesterol level probably will be high. The United States average, 40% cholesterol, is too high for good health.

BLOOD PRESSURE

If you have no recent reading but have passed an insurance or industrial examination, chances are your blood pressure is 140 or less.

SEX

This takes into account the fact that men have from 6 to 10 times more heart attacks than women of childbearing age.

	1	2	3	4	5	7
Cholesterol or fat % in diet	Cholesterol below 100 mg % Diet contains no animal or solid fats	Cholesterol 181 to 205 mg % Diet contains 10% animal or or solid fats	Cholesterol 206 to 230 mg % Diet contains 20% animal or solid fats	Cholesterol 231 to 255 mg % Diet contains 30% animal or solid fats	Cholesterol 256 to 280 mg % Diet contains 40% animal or solid fats	Cholesterol 281 to 305 mg % Diet contains 50% animal or solid fats
	1	2	3	4	6	8
Blood pressure	100 upper reading	120 upper reading	140 upper reading	160 upper reading	180 upper reading	200 or over upper reading
	1	2	3	5	6	7
Sex	Female under 40	Female 40 to 50	Female over 50	Male	Stocky male	Bald stocky male

For meaningful interpretation of RISKO only the official RISKO directions should be used.

Interpretation

6-11	Risk well below average	25-31	Risk moderate
12-17	Risk below average	32-40	Risk at a dangerous level
18-24	Risk generally average	41-62	Danger. See your doctor now

Reduce Your Risk of Heart Attack

The American lifestyle—high-fat diets, lack of regular exercise, being over-weight, and cigarette smoking—is a major contributor to heart attacks. To reduce your risks of suffering a heart attack you should:

- Have your blood pressure checked regularly. If it's high, cooperate with your doctor to keep it under control.
- Not smoke cigarettes.
- Eat foods that are low in saturated (animal) fats and cholesterol.
- Maintain proper weight. If you are overweight, follow the Heart Associa-tion's suggestions to reduce weight while maintaining a balanced and nutri-tious diet.
- Exercise regularly to maintain cardiovascular fitness. Check with your doctor before beginning an exercise program.
- Have regular medical checkups and follow your doctor's advice about reduc-ing your risks of heart attack.

hearts must be removed immediately from the bodies of deceased donors and transported to the recipient's hospital as quickly as possible. This can be a com-plicated process. Once transplant surgery is completed, tissue rejection by the recipient is possible. However, with the use of the antirejection drug cyclospor-ine, it is estimated that about 70% of heart transplant recipients will be able to live at least 5 years.[18] Although not to be considered a wonder drug, cyclospor-ine does offer heart recipients a more optimistic future.

Artificial hearts have also been developed and implanted in humans. These mechanical devices have extended the lives of patients (as in the well-publicized cases of Barney Clark and William Schroeder). Artificial hearts have also served as temporary hearts while patients are waiting for a suitable donor heart.[19] One of the major difficulties with artificial heart implantation has been the control of blood clots which may form, especially around the artificial valves. At the time of this writing, federal funds supporting artificial heart development have been reduced. Perhaps the era of the internal artificial heart is over.

SUMMARY

Although we will probably never reach the point where we are free from heart disease, the combined efforts of medicine, technology, research, and education are working to reduce the incidence of cardiovascular diseases in our country. Everyone is a potential victim of some form of heart or blood vessel disease, yet advances in medical science, educational efforts, and positive lifestyle changes are reducing our odds of becoming a victim of this number one killer.

The cardiovascular system consists of the heart, blood, and blood vessels. The system performs a variety of functions, including transportation of food, oxygen, and cellular waste products, regulation of body temperature, protection against diseases, and circulation of hormones. Our overall health depends on the health of the cardiovascular system. Four primary physiological functions reflect a healthy cardiovascular system.

The major forms of cardiovascular diseases include coronary artery disease, high blood pressure, stroke, congenital heart disease, and rheumatic heart disease. Each disease develops in a specific way and may require a highly specialized form of treatment.

A relationship exists between cardiovascular diseases and a variety of risk factors. A risk factor is an attribute that a person has or is exposed to which increases the likelihood of disease. Heredity, gender, race, and age are risk factors that cannot be changed. Cigarette smoking, hypertension, blood cholesterol levels, and diabetes are risk factors that can be controlled. The contributing risk factors of obesity, lack of exercise, and stress can be reduced.

The lifestyle decisions you make regarding cardiovascular risk factors may enhance your ability to master some of the developmental tasks of the young adult years and the years that follow.

REVIEW QUESTIONS

1 What are some of the factors that are helping to reduce the deaths from cardiovascular diseases?

2 Describe a potential victim of cardiovascular disease.

3 Identify the principal components of the cardiovascular or circulatory system. Trace the path of blood through the cardiovascular system.

4 How much blood does the average adult have? What are some of the major functions of blood?

5 What four important physiological requirements reflect a healthy cardiovascular system?

6 What are the major forms of cardiovascular disease? For each of these diseases, describe what the disease is, its cause (if known), and its treatment. What role does atherosclerosis play in each of these diseases? How does arterosclerosis differ from atherosclerosis?

7 Why is hypertension referred to as "the silent killer"?

8 What are the warning signals of stroke?

9 Define cardiovascular risk factor. What relationship do risk factors have to cardiovascular disease? Describe the role of cholesterol and lipoproteins as risk factors in cardiovascular disease.

10 Identify those risk factors for cardiovascular disease that cannot be changed. Identify those risk factors that can be changed. Identify those risk factors that are contributing factors.

QUESTIONS FOR PERSONAL CONTEMPLATION

1 Before reading this chapter, how did you perceive your own risk for cardiovascular disease? Has this perception changed at all now that you have read this chapter?

2 Taking into consideration the important functions of the cardiovascular system, have you paid enough attention to your own cardiovascular health? In the past week, what have you done that might have been either beneficial or detrimental to your cardiovascular system?

3 Cardiopulmonary resuscitation (CPR) can be very effective in saving the victim of a heart attack. Are you trained in CPR? What resources are available on your campus or in your community to train you for CPR? Can you see a relationship between your CPR certification and any of the four developmental tasks?

4 When was the last time you had your blood pressure checked? Were you told what your reading was? Do you think you have the responsibility to ask for the reading if you are not told? What are your opportunities for having your blood pressure checked on your campus?

5 Considering the cardiovascular risk factors presented in this chapter, decide which ones apply to you. List the ones you can control or change. Are you doing anything now about these risk factors?

6 Since cardiovascular diseases are so prevalent in our society, many people close to you may be at high risk for these diseases. What are your responsibilities for informing these people of their risk status and for helping them lower their risks?

REFERENCES

1 Wallis, C: Hold the eggs and butter, Time March 6, 1984, p 60.

2 The American Heart Association: 1987 Heart Facts, Dallas, 1986, The Association.

3 Thibodeau, G: Anatomy and physiology, St Louis, 1987, Times Mirror/Mosby College Publishing.

4 Putting the squeeze on angina: calcium channel blockers, The Harvard Medical School Health Letter 9:1-2, 1984.

5 Putting the squeeze on angina: beta blockers, The Harvard Medical School Health Letter 9:2, 1984.

6 Findlay, S: Heart attack victims get new hope, USA Today May 27, 1987, p 1d.

7 Sherry, S: Recombinant tissue plasminogen activator (rt-PA): is it the thrombolytic agent of choice for an evolving acute myocardial infarction? American Journal of Cardiology 59:984-989, 1987.

8 Naccarelli, G, et al: Patient assessment: laboratory studies. In Andreoli, K, et al: Comprehensive cardiac care, ed 6, St Louis, 1987, The CV Mosby Co.

9 McPherson, DD, Hiratzka, LF, and Lamberth, WC: Delineation of the extent of atherosclerosis by high frequency epicardial echocardiography, The New England Journal of Medicine 316:304-309, 1987.

10 Angina update: the surgical alternative, The Harvard Medical School Health Letter 9:5-6, 1984.

11 Council on Scientific Affairs: Percutaneous transluminal angioplasty, Journal of the American Medical Association 251:764-768, 1984.

12 Findlay, S: Balloon heart surgery saving more lives, USA Today March 10, 1987, p 1a.

13 Holden RA: Dietary salt intake and blood pressure, Journal of the American Medical Association 251:764-768, 1983.

14 Teekhaw, K, and Barret-Conner, E: Dietary potassium and stroke-associated mortality: a 12-year prospective study, The New England Journal of Medicine 316:235-240, 1987.

15 The Lipid Research Clinics coronary primary prevention trial results: (1) Reduction in incidence of coronary heart disease. (2) The relationship of reduction in incidence of coronary heart disease to cholesterol lowering, Journal of the American Medical Association 251:351-373, 1984.

16 Anderson, KM, Castelli, WP, and Levy, D: Cholesterol and mortality: 30 years of follow-up from the Framingham study, Journal of the American Medical Association 257:2176-2180, 1987.

17 Centers for Disease Control: Protective effect of physical activity on coronary heart disease, Morbidity and Mortality Weekly Report 36:426-430, 1987.

18 Mayfield, M: Cyclosporine is a boon to heart transplants, USA Today March 11, 1986, p 1d.

19 Griffith, BP, Hardesty, RL, and Kormos, RL: Temporary use of the Jarvik-7 total artificial heart before transplantation, The New England Journal of Medicine 316:130-134, 1987.

ANNOTATED READINGS

Bennett, CM: Control your high blood pressure without drugs, Garden City, New York, 1984, Doubleday & Co.
   Presents an approach for hypertensive patients to learn to take control of their own lives with a regimen of proper diet, exercise, and stress management.

Caris, T: Understanding hypertension, New York, 1986, Warner Books, Inc.
   Explains the types of high blood pressure and their causes, health consequences, and treatments.

Froman, J: How to save a heart attack victim, New York, 1984, Bantam Books.
   An easy-to-follow book that describes how to provide basic life support until professional assistance arrives.

Goor, R, and Goor, N: A food lover's guide to lower cholesterol, New York, 1987, Houghton Mifflin Co.
   Outlines a sound step-by-step process for lower cholesterol levels through the control of saturated fats in the diet. A variety of healthy recipes are included.

Kaplan, NM: Prevent your heart attack, New York, 1987, Pinnacle Books.
   Includes the latest research and preventive measures. This book helps you to determine your risk profile and provides medically proven strategies to prevent heart attack.

Kushi, M: Diet for a strong heart, New York, 1985, St Martin's Press, Inc.
   Describes cardiovascular function and the disease processes that influence the cardiovascular system. Modified eating practices are described. A distinct Eastern orientation is associated with risk-reduction guidelines.

Mincar, RE: The joy of living salt-free, New York, 1984, MacMillan Publishing Co.
   One approach to breaking the salt habit and staying healthy while enjoying what you eat.

CHAPTER 11

Cancer and Other Noninfectious Conditions

Key Concepts

Cancer is the second leading cause of death among adults.

■

Current cancer research focuses on the relationship between protooncogenes, oncogenes and carcinogens.

■

The chances for recovery from cancer are best enhanced when cancer is diagnosed in its early stages of development.

■

A number of significant health problems may confront the young adult.

■

The successful management of any health problem starts with an understanding of the factors that cause the condition.

■

Treatment of noninfectious conditions generally combines proven therapies with promising experimental approaches.

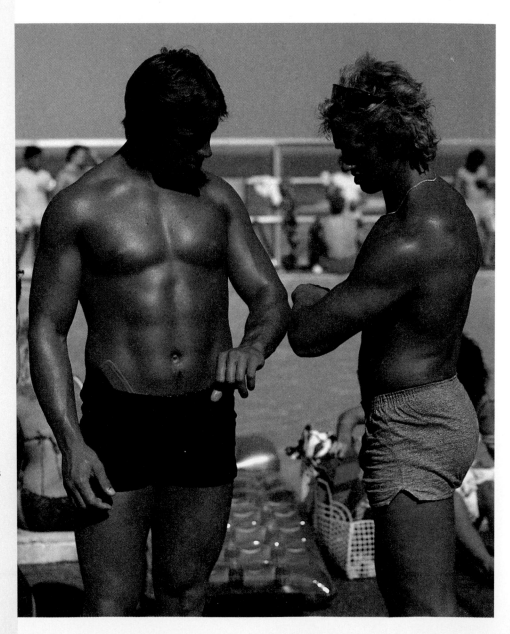

M ost of you can already attest to the disruptive influence an illness can have on your ability to participate in day-to-day activities. When you are sick, your usual school, employment, and leisure activities are replaced by periods in which you feel like doing little more than sleeping. When you are ill, your entire body is in a state of dysfunction, and your usual level of optimal health is compromised.

Noninfectious conditions, particularly cancer, influence all aspects of health. Alterations in a body system's configuration, composition, or physiological activities are the most familiar indicators of a condition's presence. Stress imposed by these conditions on the remaining dimensions of health occurs frequently.

HEALTH CONCERNS: A LIST OF FOURTEEN

Having completed our study of cardiovascular disease in Chapter 10, we will now turn our attention to other important noninfectious conditions. Cancer, the second leading cause of death for adults,[1] will be studied in detail. Other health concerns, however, are significant. The following list includes the additional conditions we will present and our rationale for selection. Among these conditions may be one that you might have or see develop in a friend or family member. Many other health problems could be added to the list, but we selected these conditions as being of special concern to young adults:

cerebral palsy Among the most handicapped students are those with cerebral palsy, yet they are frequently classmates and dormitory neighbors. If you have previously not understood the nature of this condition, we believe that this chapter will be of assistance.

premenstrual syndrome For 22 million young women, premenstrual syndrome might be responsible for making 1 week out of every 4 weeks quite uncomfortable.

type 2 (non-insulin-dependent) diabetes mellitus For some young persons, the occurrence of this condition is the first major health problem that they have seen develop in their **midlife** parents. (The condition was formerly called "adult onset" diabetes mellitus.)

osteoporosis This gradual resorption of calcium from the bones of postmenopausal women and some older men can lead to incapacitation and even death from complications. Dietary practices, including sufficient calcium intake, and an exercise program begun during young adulthood may minimize the impact of this disease process.

allergic disorders Are you hypersensitive to something in your environment—a pet, a type of fabric, or the pollen from a particular type of plant? If so, you can attest to the discomfort that you and others with asthma, hay fever, and other allergies experience.

fibrocystic breast condition When mistaken for breast tumors, the fluid-filled cysts characteristic of fibrocystic breast condition can be a source of anxiety. Breast self-examination at the correct time should reduce the concerns about these cyclic changes to breast tissue.

midlife
between 45 and 60 years of age.

291

endogenous depression   In contrast to the type of depression associated with identifiable stressors, this depression results from changes in brain chemistry. Could you develop endogenous depression someday?

epilepsy   The seizures that characterize epilepsy are neither painful to the victim nor communicable to you, yet many people fear and discriminate against those who have this condition. We hope you are not among those who will continue to misunderstand the nature of this condition.

multiple sclerosis   At no time in your life will you be more likely to be afflicted with multiple sclerosis than you are now. What is the nature of this condition which strikes at the time when young persons have so much to look forward to?

lower back pain   Every year 10 million adults of all ages are "stopped in their tracks" by back pain that has been caused by improper sitting, bending, or lifting. You can do simple activities to minimize the chances of lower back pain.

sickle cell trait and sickle cell disease   These inherited conditions are found in about 10% of the black students on campus. In its fully developed form, the disease is incapacitating and life-shortening. Family planning must be carefully considered by people with these conditions.

arthritis   Like most other body parts, the skeleton can degenerate over the course of time. We hope your adult years will not be seriously compromised by the limitations associated with arthritic changes to the joints.

cirrhosis of the liver   Some medical experts feel that this condition may be the second leading killer of adults. This serious health problem can be caused by a variety of conditions, including chronic heavy alcohol use. Is your current pattern of alcohol use likely to dispose you to this very serious health problem?

Many of these health problems are related to material in other chapters of your textbook. Look for these relationships as you study each condition.

Cancer: A Problem of Cell Regulation

In much the same manner that a corporation depends on competent individuals to staff its various departments, the body depends on its basic units of function—the cells. Cells band together as tissues to perform a prescribed function. Tissues in turn join to form organs, and organs are assembled into the body's several organ systems. Such is the "corporate structure" of the body.

If individuals and cells are the basic units of function for their respective organizations, the failure of either to perform in a prescribed, dependable manner can erode the overall organization to the extent that it might not be able to continue. Cancer, the second leading cause of death among adults, is a condition reflecting cell dysfunction in its most extreme form. In cancer the prescribed behavior of normal cells ceases.

The malignant cell

Contrary to general belief, cancer cells do not divide more quickly than do normal cells; in fact, they divide at the same rate or even more slowly. Cancer

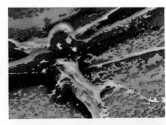

Cancer cell invading normal tissue.

cells' ability to overrun normal cells, however, results from their inability to respond to the negative feedback process that occurs in normal tissue maintenance. Because malignant (cancerous) cells do not possess the *contact inhibition* of normal cells, they accumulate and eventually alter the structure of a body organ. A decrease in **cellular cohesiveness** allows cancer cells to invade surrounding tissues or spread through the circulatory or lymphatic system to distant points *(metastasis).*[2] A malignancy that has metastasized has been present in the body longer than a tissue of the same origin that has not yet spread. Metastasis increases the difficulty of diagnosis and treatment because cancerous cells are no longer localized in a single area of the body.

Because of the relatively slow growth rate of cancer cells, an extended time may be required for a **tumor** mass to reach a size in which normal function of the tissue or organ is impaired. Clinical identification of a malignant mass may not be possible until approximately 30 *doublings* (separate cell divisions) have taken place. Thus if a single doubling in a cancer cell requires 2 or more months, 5 or more years may pass before a tumor is recognized.[2]

Like a normal cell, a malignant cell requires metabolic material to sustain itself. An **angiogenesis factor** is believed to give the malignant cell an advantage over the normal cell in establishing a rich blood supply.[2] Cancer cells, however, are not endowed with an infinite life expectancy, and *necrosis* or cell death is observed within tumors. Furthermore, the slow cell division process increases the length of time that a cancer cell's genetic material is susceptible to the destructive effects of radiation and other treatment methods.

Benign tumors

Noncancerous or **benign** tumors can also form in the body. These tumors are usually encapsulated by a fiberous membrane and do not spread from their point of origin as cancerous tumors can. Benign tumors are dangerous, however, when they crowd out normal tissue within a confined space.

The role of oncogenesis in the development of cancer

If is often possible to recognize what a particular disease process does to the body without understanding why and how that process functions. This is the situation for cancer researchers. However, a new line of reasoning has evolved that holds considerable promise for better understanding of how malignant tumors develop—and as a consequence cancer management and prevention. Oncogenesis, or the role of cancer-causing **oncogenes,** is the focus of current research.

The common observations that cancer "runs in families" and that all persons exposed to a similar environmental carcinogen do not develop cancer has led researchers to theorize that genetic differences may underlie cancer formation. Recent findings in studies of animals and humans concerning the role of cancer-causing genes support this line of investigation.[3,4]

Current theory holds that humans have within each cell a variable number of **protooncogenes** that, if altered, could cause the development of cancer causing oncogenes. Questions concerning the number of protooncogenes, their location on particular chromosomes, and the manner in which they are altered are being intensively studied. It is currently believed that protooncogenes are normal genes that participate in the control of cellular division but can be converted into oncogenes through **mutation** or by recombination with viral genes.

---

cellular cohesiveness
tendency of normal cells to "stick together" rather than to move independently throughout the body.

tumor
mass of cells; may be cancerous (malignant) or noncancerous (benign).

angiogenesis factor
chemical messenger that stimulates the development of additional capillaries into the tumor.

benign
noncancerous, tumors that do not spread

oncogenes
genes that are believed to activate the development of cancer.

protooncogene
normal gene that is altered by mutation or recombination with a viral gene to become an oncogene.

mutation
spontaneous alteration of genetic material.

To date, more than 30 oncogenes have been identified in humans, with the possibility that 100 protooncogenes or more may exist.[5]

Another question under study is the role of *carcinogens* in the conversion of protooncogenes into oncogenes. Current thought holds that this change is a multistep process involving carcinogens acting over an extended period. For example, lung cancer would develop only in those individuals who had a protooncogene converted into an oncogene by actions of the carcinogens from multiple sources such as tobacco smoke, diet, and environmental pollution.

A second possibility concerning the regulatory process of cancer involves the identification of a gene that prevents the development of cancer.[6] The possibility that "antioncogenes" (genes that prevent formation of an oncogene) exist might be another direction that cancer research will take.

Regardless of whether oncogenetic studies or another line of investigation proves to be the breakthrough needed to resolve the problem of cancer, years of research will be required. Every **oncologist** we talked with has expressed the same basic feeling on this matter: until the regulatory mechanisms that control normal cell behavior are fully understood, abnormal cell function (cancer) will never be fully understood. A cure for cancer, should one ever be found, will be based on a better understanding of cell regulation.

Types of cancer and their locations

Malignancies can be categorized by the tissues in which they occur and by the varying rates to which specific organs are subjected to the development of malignancies. Although oncologists and pathologists use a far more extensive nomenclature, the classifications below are used by physicians to describe malignancies to a layperson:

carcinoma Found most frequently in the skin, nose, mouth, throat, stomach, intestinal tract, glands, nerves, breasts, urinary and genital structures, lungs, kidneys, and liver; approximately 85% of all malignant tumors are classified as carcinomas

sarcoma Formed in the connective tissues of the body; bone, cartilage, and tendon are the sites of sarcoma development; only 2% of all malignancies are of this type

melanoma Arises from the melanin-containing cells of skin; found most often in individuals who have sustained extensive sun exposure, particularly, a deep, penetrating sunburn; although rare, it is among the most deadly

neuroblastoma Originates in the immature cells found within the central nervous system; neuroblastomas are rare, usually found in children

adenocarcinoma Derived from cells of the endocrine glands

hepatoma Originates in cells of the liver; although not thought to be directly caused by alcohol use, hepatomas are more frequently seen in individuals who have experienced **sclerotic changes** in the liver

leukemia Found in cells of the blood and blood-forming tissues; characterized by abnormal, immature white blood cell formation; multiple forms found in both children and adults

lymphoma Arises in cells of the lymphatic tissues of other immune system tissues; includes lymphosarcomas and Hodgkin's disease, characterized by abnormal white cell production and decreased resistance

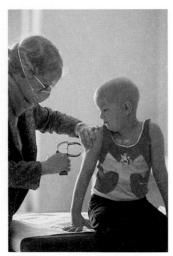

The effects of chemotherapy are carefully monitored.

oncologist
physician who specializes in the treatment of malignancies.

sclerotic changes
thickening or hardening or tissues.

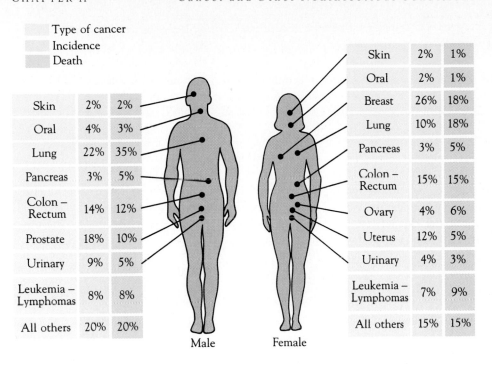

Type of cancer
Incidence
Death

Skin	2%	2%
Oral	4%	3%
Lung	22%	35%
Pancreas	3%	5%
Colon – Rectum	14%	12%
Prostate	18%	10%
Urinary	9%	5%
Leukemia – Lymphomas	8%	8%
All others	20%	20%

Male

Skin	2%	1%
Oral	2%	1%
Breast	26%	18%
Lung	10%	18%
Pancreas	3%	5%
Colon – Rectum	15%	15%
Ovary	4%	6%
Uterus	12%	5%
Urinary	4%	3%
Leukemia – Lymphomas	7%	9%
All others	15%	15%

Female

Figure 11-1
These 1987 estimates of cancer incidence and cancer deaths reveal some significant similarities between men and women. Note that lung cancer is now the leading cause of cancer deaths for *both* genders.

Figure 11-1 presents data on the incidence and deaths from cancer in various sites for both men and women.

CANCER AT SELECTED SITES IN THE BODY

A second and more familiar way to describe cancer is on the basis of the organ (or tissue) site at which it occurs. The American Cancer Society annually reports the incidence and deaths associated with cancer in some 14 sites, comprising nearly 40 organs or tissues.[7] The following discussion relates to some of these more familiar sites. The box on p. 296 describes cancer-related checkups.

Lung

Lung cancer is one of the most lethal forms of cancer, that is frequently diagnosed. Primarily because of the advanced stage at the time symptoms first appear, only 13% of all lung cancer victims survive 5 years beyond diagnosis.[7] By the time victims are sufficiently concerned about their persistent cough, blood-streaked sputum, and chest pain, their fate has too often been sealed.

The tragedy of lung cancer rests in its extremely close association with smoking—including both active and passive smoking (83% of all cases of lung cancer are in smokers). In recent years the incidence of lung cancer has risen markedly for women, paralleling their increased incidence of cigarette smoking.[8] Currently lung cancer exceeds breast cancer as the leading cause of cancer deaths in females. The incidence of lung cancer has shown an encouraging decline in males as their use of tobacco drops. Exposure to asbestos and, perhaps, some forms of radiation contribute to lung cancer in all persons.

Once diagnosed, lung cancer is generally so widely distributed in the body that surgery, radiation, and chemotherapy are combined in an attempt to achieve effective treatment.

Cancer-Related Checkups

Following are guidelines for the early detection of cancer in people without symptoms. Talk with your doctor—ask how these guidelines relate to you. Remember, these guidelines are not rules and only apply to people without symptoms. If you have any of the seven warning signals of cancer, see your doctor or go to your clinic without delay.

AGE 20 TO 40
CANCER-RELATED CHECKUP EVERY 3 YEARS

Should include the procedures listed below plus health counseling (such as tips on quitting cigarettes) and examinations for cancers of the thyroid, testes, prostate, mouth, ovaries, skin and lymph nodes. *Some people are at higher risk for certain cancers and may need to have tests more frequently.*

Breast
- Examination by doctor every 3 years
- Self-exam every month
- One baseline mammogram between ages 35 and 40
  Higher risk for breast cancer: personal or family history of breast cancer, never had children, first child after 30

Uterus
- Pelvic exam every 3 years

Cervix
- Pap test—after two initial negative tests 1 year apart—*at least* every 3 years, includes women under 20 if sexually active
  Higher risk for cervical cancer: early age at first intercourse, multiple sex partners

Testes
- Self-exam every month
- Consult doctor when an abnormality is present
  Higher risk for testicular cancer: personal or family history of testicular cancer, undescended testicles not corrected during early childhood, more prevalent in Caucasians and in men under 35 years of age

AGE 40 AND OVER
CANCER-RELATED CHECKUP EVERY YEAR

Should include the procedures listed below plus health counseling (such as tips on quitting cigarettes) and examinations for cancers of the thyroid, testes, prostate, mouth, ovaries, skin and lymph nodes. *Some people are at higher risk for certain cancers and may need to have tests more frequently.*

Breast
- Examination by doctor every year
- Self-exam every month
- Mammogram every year after 50 (between ages 40 and 50, ask your doctor)
  Higher risk for breast cancer: personal or family history of breast cancer, never had children, first child after 30

Uterus
- Pelvic examination every year

Cervix
- Pap test—after two initial negative tests 1 year apart—*at least* every 3 years
  Higher risk for cervical cancer: early age at first intercourse, multiple sex partners

Endometrium
- Endometrial tissue sample at menopause if at risk
  Higher risk for endometrial cancer: infertility, obesity, failure of ovulation, abnormal uterine bleeding, estrogen therapy

Testes
- Self-exam every month
- Consult doctor when an abnormality is present
  Higher risk for testicular cancer: personal or family history of testicular cancer, undescended testicles not corrected during early childhood, more prevalent in Caucasians, risk declines with increasing age

Colon and Rectum
- Digital rectal examination every year
- Guaiac slide test every year after 50
- Procto exam—after two initial negative tests 1 year apart—every 3 to 5 years after 50
  Higher risk for colorectal cancer: personal or family history of colon or rectal cancer, personal or family history of polyps in the colon or rectum, ulcerative colitis

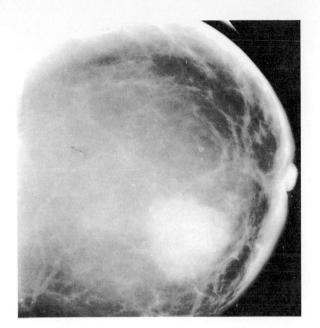

Cancerous tissue can be seen in the dense area of this mammogram.

Breast

Surpassed only by lung cancer, breast cancer is the second leading cause of death from cancer in females.[7] Nearly 1 in 10 women will have this form of cancer at some time in their lives. Countless more will experience stress as they wait to learn that a suspicious lump was a benign mass or fluid-filled cyst.

Although all women (and men) are at some risk for developing breast cancer, females over the age of 50—particularly those with a family history of breast cancer—are at greatest risk. Breast self-examination is recommended for women 20 years of age and older. Annual mammograms are recommended for asymptomatic women 50 years of age and older, although many physicians recommend annual mammograms starting at age 35. The box on p. 298 gives a description of breast self-examination and the symptoms associated with breast cancer. Each woman should consult her physician for specific guidance about breast self-examination and other screening procedures.

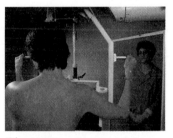

Obtaining a mammogram.

When a localized breast cancer is diagnosed, survival is highly likely (90% to 100%). Treatment will encompass one or a combination of techniques, including surgery, radiation, chemotherapy, and hormonal therapy. Medical opinion regarding surgery for breast cancer is in a process of evolution.[9] Choices range from very limited removal of tissue (the "lumpectomy") to more radical procedures. Second opinions are highly desirable before receiving any type of treatment. Breast reconstruction is a distinct possibility following more radical cancer surgery.

Prostate

Cancer of the prostate is the third most common form of cancer in males and a leading cause of death from cancer in older males. On the basis of current statistics, approximately 1 out of 11 men will develop this form of cancer.[7]

Prostate diseases, including cancer of the prostate, present a variety of symp-

Breast Self-Examination

HOW TO EXAMINE YOUR BREASTS

1 *In the shower:* Examine your breasts during bath or shower; hands glide easier over wet skin. Fingers flat, move gently over every part of each breast. Use right hand to examine left breast, left hand for right breast. Check for any lump, hard knot, or thickening. This self-examination should be done monthly, preferably a day or two following the end of the menstrual period.

2 *Before a mirror:* Inspect your breasts with arms at your sides. Next, raise your arms high overhead. Look for any changes in contour of each breast, a swelling, dimpling of skin, changes in the nipple.

Then rest palms on hips and press down firmly to flex your chest muscles. Left and right breast will not exactly match—few women's breasts do.

3 *Lying down:* To examine your right breast, put a pillow or folded towel under your right shoulder. Place right hand behind your head—this distributes breast tissue more evenly on the chest. With left hand, fingers flat, press gently in small circular motions around an imaginary clock face. Begin at outermost top of your right breast for 12 o'clock, then move to 1 o'clock, and so on around the circle back to 12. A ridge of firm tissue in the lower curve of each breast is normal. Then move in an inch, toward the nipple; keep circling to examine *every part of your breast,* including the nipple. This requires at least three more circles. Now slowly repeat the procedure on your left breast with a pillow under your left shoulder and left hand behind head. Notice how your breast structure feels. Finally, squeeze the nipple of each breast gently between thumb and index finger. Any discharge, clear or bloody, should be reported to your doctor immediately.

Breast cancer can occur in men too. Therefore this examination should be performed monthly by men. Regular inspection shows what is normal for you and will give you confidence in your examination.

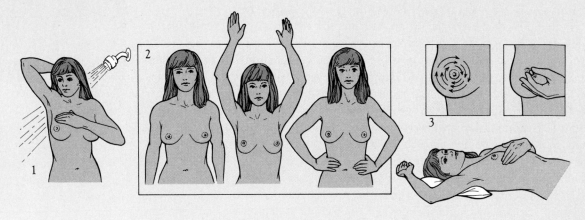

toms that are primarily related to difficulty in urination. Weak or interrupted flow of urine, inability to urinate, the need to urinate frequently, and blood in the urine are symptoms that should alert males to prostate-related problems. Persistent lower back pain or pain in the upper thighs and pelvis should also be reported to a physician.

An annual rectal examination for men over 40 years of age is recommended. Ultrasound examinations of the prostate may soon become a component of male preventive health care.

Should cancer of the prostate be diagnosed, treatment will most likely involve surgery in combination with radiation, chemotherapy, or hormonal therapy. Survival rates have progressed steadily since 1960 and now stand at 50% to 70%.

Colon and Rectal Cancer

Cancer of the colon and rectum has a combined incidence and death rate second only to that of lung cancer. Fortunately, when diagnosed in a localized state, both forms of cancer have relatively high survival rates (86% for colon and 77% for rectal).[7] A pattern in these forms of cancer has been noted among family members, and a strong link is suspected between diets high in saturated fats and low in fiber.

Symptoms associated with colon and rectal cancers include bleeding from the rectum, blood in the stool, or a change in bowel habits. Also a family history of inflammatory bowel disease, polyp formation, or cancer of the colon or rectum should make one more alert to symptoms. Preventive health care that includes digital rectal examination after age 40, a stool blood test after age 50, and proctosigmoidoscopic examination every 3 to 5 years after age 50 is recommended by the American Cancer Society.[7] More extensive studies, including an x-ray examination of the lower bowel, can be done when required.

Treatment for colon and rectal cancer generally combines surgery with radiation. A **colostomy** will be required in 15% of the cases of colon or rectal cancer.

colostomy
surgically created opening on the abdominal wall for the elimination of body wastes.

Skin

Thanks in large part to our desire for a fashionable tan, we are spending more time in the sun (and in tanning booths) than our skin can tolerate. As a result, skin cancer, once common only among those people who had to work in the sun, is occurring with alarming frequency. In 1987, nearly 500,000 Americans developed basal or squamous cell skin cancer and 23,000 cases of highly dangerous malignant melanoma were diagnosed.[7] Severe sunburning during childhood and chronic sun exposure during adolescence and younger adulthood are responsible for these increases in skin cancer.

The key to successful treatment of skin cancer lies in early detection. In the case of basal or squamous cell cancer, the development of a pale, waxlike, pearly nodule or red scaly patch may be the first symptom. For others, skin cancer may be reflected in the changing configuration of an already existing skin mole. If such a change is noted, a physician should be contacted. Melanomas usually

Skin Carcinomas

Basal and squamous cell carcinomas are more common forms of skin cancer that can be cured. Squamous cell cancer can metastasize to adjacent areas if not treated.

**Basal cell carcinoma.
Squamous cell carcinoma.**

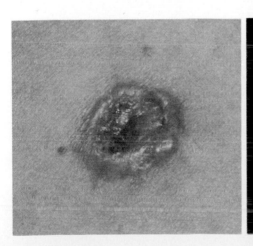
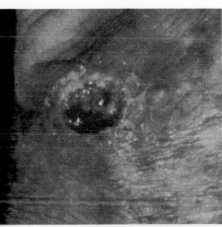

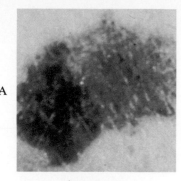

Asymmetry.

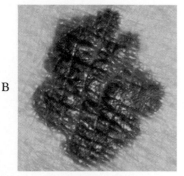

Border irregularity.

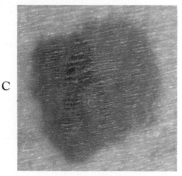

Color change.

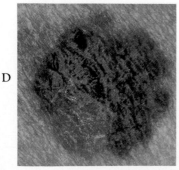

Diameter increase.

begin as a small, molelike growth that grows progressively in size, changes color, ulcerates, and bleeds easily. For use in detecting these melanomas, the American Cancer Society recommends the following set of guidelines[7] (see the figures in the margin):

A is for asymmetry

B is for border irregularity

C is for color (change)

D is for a diameter greater than 6 mm

When skin cancer is detected, various treatment methods can be used. Surgery, radiation, and tissue destruction by heat or by freezing are frequently combined to achieve an almost 100% cure rate. For the more serious and difficult to cure melanomas, more extensive surgery will be required to make certain that the cancerous cells and surrounding lymph nodes have been removed.

Prevention of skin cancers is obviously related to controlling exposure to the sun (see Table 11-1). Information about healthy suntanning and tanning booths can be found in the box on p. 301.

Uterus

In 1987 approximately 48,000 new cases of cancer of the uterus were reported in the United States.[7] Included in this figure were 35,000 cases of endometrial (lining of the uterus) cancer and 13,000 cases of cervical (neck of the uterus) cancer. Fortunately, the death rate for uterine cancer has dropped more than 70% in the last 4 decades, primarily resulting from the widespread acceptance of the Pap test for precancerous changes in the cervix. When diagnosed in its initial stage, cancer of the uterus has an 80% to 90% cure rate, while the precancerous changes identified by the Pap test are virtually 100% curable.

In addition to changes discovered by the Pap test, symptoms suggesting cancer

Table 11-1 Sunscreen Guide

Skin Type	Pigmentation	Sunburn/Tanning History	Sun Protection Factor (SPF)
I	Very fair skin; freckling; blond, red, or brown hair	Always burns easily never tans	15-30
II	Fair skin: blond, red, or brown hair	Always burns easily, tans minimally	15-20
III	Brown hair and eyes, darker skin (light brown)	Burns moderately, tans gradually and uniformly	8-15
IV	Light brown skin; dark hair and eyes (moderate brown)	Burns minimally; always tans well	8-15
V	Brown skin; dark hair and eyes	Rarely burns, tans profusely (dark brown)	Recommend same as Skin Type IV
VI	Brown-black skin; dark hair and eyes	Never burns, deeply pigmented (black)	Recommend same as Skin Type IV

The Dark Side of Tanning Beds and Booths

During the 1950s, 60s, and 70s, people with dark suntans were thought to have a healthy, sexy look. In the early 1980s, thousands of entrepreneurs catered to this image by providing tanning beds and tanning booths to image-conscious consumers. For a fee, customers can now develop and maintain a dark tan year round. In many establishments, customers are assured that they will only be exposed to the longer "safe" ultraviolet alpha (UVA) rays, not the more harmful (burn-producing) shorter ultraviolet beta (UVB) rays. How safe are tanning salons?

Virtually every dermatologist will say that there is nothing healthy about suntanned skin. Despite what operators say about their booths, many UVA ray lights also emit some UVB rays. UVA rays are not safe themselves. UVA rays penetrate the deeper layers of skin more readily than UVB rays, increasing the likelihood of immune system suppression, skin aging, skin cancer, and eye damage.[10]

Besides the skin damage resulting from prolonged exposure to tanning booths, the most immediate severe concern is the burning of corneal tissue. UVA light rays can burn corneal tissue by penetrating the eyelids even when they are shut.[10] For people who insist on using tanning booths, protective goggles must be worn at all times and exposure limits must not be exceeded.

Tanning booth customers should be aware that certain cosmetics (especially deodorant soaps and perfumes) and medicines do not interact well with light rays and can cause allergic responses and rashes. A tanning booth UVA tan offers little protection from an outdoor sunburn caused mainly by UVB rays. Persons who are warned by physicians to stay out of the sun should also avoid use of tanning booths and beds.[10]

of the uterus include abnormal bleeding between menstrual periods or other discharges. Risk factors associated with this form of cancer include age of first intercourse, number of sex partners, and a history of infertility. A lower incidence of cervical cancer in women who have used barrier contraceptives (condoms, diaphragms, and spermicides) suggests that this form of cancer may have a sexually transmitted component.[11] A higher incidence of endometrial cancer in women who were given estrogen following the onset of menopause is also reported. This, however, must be balanced against the risk of osteoporosis, which is discussed further on pp. 312-314.

Testicle

Cancer of the testicles is among the least common forms of cancer, however, it represents the most common solid tumor in males between the ages of 20 and 34 years. Cancer of the testicles shows a familial tendency and is more common in males whose testicles were undescended during childhood. The incidence of this cancer has been increasing in recent years.

Symptoms of cancer of the testicles include a small, painless lump on the side of the testicle, a swollen or enlarged testicle, or heaviness or a dragging sensation

Testicle Self-Examination

HOW TO EXAMINE YOUR TESTICLES

Your best hope for early detection of testicular cancer is a simple 3-minute monthly self-examination. The best time is after a warm bath or shower, when the scrotal skin is most relaxed.

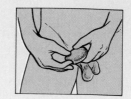

Roll each testicle gently between the thumb and fingers of both hands. If you find any hard lumps or nodules, you should see your doctor promptly. They may not be malignant, but only your doctor can make the diagnosis.

Following a thorough physical examination, your doctor may perform certain x-ray studies to make the most accurate diagnosis possible.

Testicular self-examinations are as important for men as breast self-examinations are for women.

in the groin or scrotum. Risk factors include confirmed injury, mumps, and hormonal treatments given to the mother before the child's birth.

The importance of testicle self-examinatin cannot be overemphasized for males in the at risk age group of 20 to 34 years. The box above describes this procedure.

The diagnosis of cancer

Is cancer survivable? The answer is, of course, yes. The chances for survival (living 5 years after diagnosis) depend greatly on the promptness of identification, diagnosis, and treatment.

In addition to the three factors affecting survival from cancer mentioned above, survival is also dependent on the type of cancer and the stage of its development. Without exception, a person's chances for surviving cancer are highest when treatment is undertaken while the disease is localized, and lowest when the disease is more generalized (spread).

Thus the chances for recovery from cancer are best when cancer is detected early. The familiar "cancer's seven warning signals" can serve as a basis for early detection (see the box on p. 303). As widely discussed and familiar as these signals are, they are frequently disregarded. Many people may recognize a cancer warning sign but prefer to attribute it to other (noncancer) causes. An awareness of these seven warning signals, nevertheless, remains the first line in the process of early cancer identification. Also, unexplained weight loss can be a signal for the presence of a malignancy. Weight loss, however, is not usually an early indicator of cancer. Persistent headaches and visual changes should be evaluated by a physician.

In addition to the recognition of danger signals, undergoing regularly scheduled *screening* for malignancy-related changes is important. Note that breast self-examination for all women over the age of 20 is recommended. Further, we would strongly recommend testicular self-examination for men. Step-by-step procedures for both of these self-examinations are provided in the boxes on p. 298 and above. The remaining screening procedures require the services of a medical practitioner.

Treatment

In today's approach to cancer treatment, proven therapies and promising new experimental approaches are often combined. The traditional therapies are surgery, radiation, and chemotherapy. Used independently or in combination, they form the backbone of our increasingly successful efforts in treating cancer. Newer, more experimental therapies are also being employed on a limited basis. One or more of these experimental approaches may join surgery, radiation, and chemotherapy as a basis for treatment.

Beyond the technical aspects of cancer treatment that will be described, the treatment of cancer also involves a variety of factors that are understandable on the basis of human emotions. These include pain, discomfort, fear, confidence, trust, and a willingness to be compliant. Treatment for cancer and recovery, regardless of the particular therapy used, is demanding. Patients must accept the need for therapy as being in their best interest. They must participate fully in their own treatment. And, for some, eventual death will need to be faced. (See Chapter 20 for a discussion of hospice program.)

In the section that follows, a brief description of each treatment scheme is described.

Surgery Surgical removal of tissue suspected to contain cancerous cells is the oldest approach to cancer therapy. When undertaken early in the course of the disease, surgery is particularly suited for tumors of the gastrointestinal tract, breast, uterus, and cervix. Minimal procedures are undertaken whenever possible, and radiation or chemotherapy is often used with surgery to assure maximum effectiveness.

Radiation The treatment of malignancies through the use of radiation or high-energy particles is both an old and a new approach. The implantation of radioactive materials into organs and the use of supervoltage x-ray and cobalt are well established therapies. More recent use of radiation and high-energy sources include the injection of tumor-specific sources of radioactive material, linear accelerators for the production of photons and electrons, and cyclotrons capable of producing high-energy particles.

Cancer's Seven Warning Signals

1 Change in bowel or bladder habits
2 A sore that does not heal
3 Unusual bleeding or discharge
4 Thickening or lump in breast or elsewhere
5 Indigestion or difficulty in swallowing
6 Obvious change in wart or mole
7 Nagging cough or hoarseness

If YOU have a warning signal that persists for more than 5 days, see your doctor!

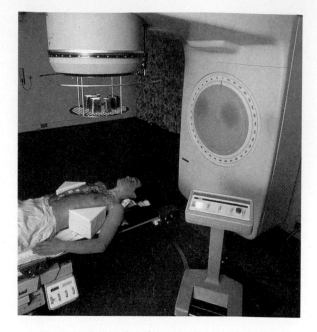

Radiation therapy for cancer patient.

Regardless of the procedure employed, the intent is to destroy cancer cells through disruption of their reproductive process. In doing so the therapist must balance loss of healthy tissue against the radiation's destructive influence on malignant cells. Radiation may be used in an attempt to achieve cure or as a **palliative** measure against pain and suffering. For some tumors, radiation will be the primary therapy, while others combine radiation and surgery.

palliative
measure taken to reduce pain and discomfort but not to cure a disease.

Chemotherapy The major advances in successful treatment of cancer can be attributed to advances in chemotherapy, both in terms of new drugs and the more effective combination of familiar chemotherapeutic agents. Four major classifications of chemotherapy agents are currently employed[11a]:

- *Alkalizing agents.* Injectable agents such as nitrogen mustard, which damages the cells' DNA
- *Antimetabolites.* Agents that alter the cell's ability to successfully synthesize several important chemical constituents
- *Antibiotics.* Drugs derived from lower life forms that are capable of interfering with the cancer cell's synthesis of RNA
- *Vinca alkaloids.* Drugs derived from the periwinkle plant that function as agents capable of controlling the mitotic activities of the cancerous cells

Immunotherapy In the belief that cancer cells have the ability to inactivate the body's immune system, researchers are pursuing ways in which to reactivate the system. *Monoclonal antibodies* to substances produced by cancer cells are currently being used in an attempt to aid the immune system in recognizing its own malignant cells and to stimulate the production of "killer" cells. Interleukin-2, a drug that can boost the activity level of the immune system, also shows promise in enhancing the production of killer cells.[12] Advances in genetic engineering make immunotherapy the most promising new approach to the treatment of cancer. Nevertheless, an immunization for cancer is still in the distant future.

Hyperthermia Through the use of *ultrasound* or microwaves the internal temperatures of cancer cells can be raised, thus subjecting critical protein-synthesizing processes to the destructive effects of heat.

Hyperbaric therapy For radiation therapy to have its maximal effect, the tissue being treated must possess an adequate level of oxygen. Because the central portions of solid tumors have little oxygen, radiation is less than maximally effective in these areas. Treatment delivered in a hyperbaric chamber, therefore, increases the effectiveness of the radiation therapy.

As cancer research progresses, the prognosis for survival will certainly increase. The box on p. 307 lists resources offering support for cancer victims. Since quackery is prevalent in cancer treatment, we recommend that you consult Chapter 17 for additional information about potentially fraudulent treatments.

Risk reduction

Because cancer will probably continue to be the second most common disease among adults, it is important that you explore ways to reduce your risk of developing some form of cancer. The following factors, which could make you vulnerable to cancer, can be controlled, or at least recognized.

- *Select your parents carefully.* This statement seems absurd, but its intent is constructive: you are the recipient of the genetic strengths and weaknesses of your biological parents. If cancer is prevalent in your family medical history, you cannot afford to disregard this fact. Individuals with a familial predisposition to breast cancer, for instance, must faithfully carry out monthly self-examinations, which are already recommended, of course, for all women.
- *Select your occupation carefully.* Because of recently discovered relationships between cancer and occupations that bring employees into contact with carcinogenic agents, you must be aware of risks with certain job selections and assignments. Gainful employment is an important facet of modern life, but to risk that life in a carcinogenic work environment is hardly prudent.
- *Do not use tobacco products* You may want to review the discussion on the overwhelming evidence linking all forms of tobacco use (including nonsmokeless) to the development of cancer. Smoking cigarettes will increase your risk of developing lung cancer by a factor of nine or ten. So detrimental is smoking to health that it is considered the number one preventable cause of death.
- *Follow a prudent diet* By returning to Chapter 5, you can review the relationships that exist between certain dietary practices and the incidence of various diseases, including cancer. Current preliminary research is focusing on the role of nutrients in preventing cancer. Vitamin A family compounds, calcium, vitamins B_6, B_{12}, and E, folic acid, and selenium are currently being studied. Should research demonstrate a clear role for these nutrients, "chemoprevention" may become a widely practiced component of cancer prevention. In planning meals and preparing food, increase consumption of foods high in fiber, avoid burning or overgrilling meat, and limit food that is high in nitrates. Certainly by reducing saturated fats in your diet and increasing the fiber, you may be able to decrease your risk of developing certain cancers.

Dietary Precautions for Cancer

The American Cancer Society recommends the following dietary precautions to help reduce the risk of getting cancer:
- Avoid obesity
- Reduce total fat intake
- Eat more high fiber foods
- Include foods rich in Vitamins A and C in your daily diet
- Include cruciferous vegetables in your diet
- Avoid smoked, salt-cured, and nitrate-cured foods
- Moderate alcohol consumption

How much sun is enough?

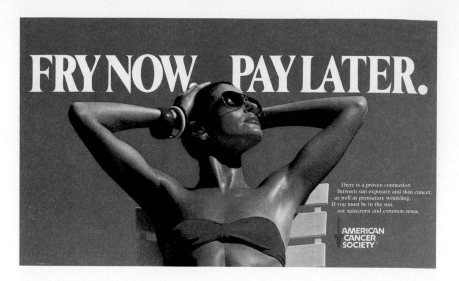

- *Control your body weight.* Particularly for women, obesity is related to a higher incidence of cancer of the uterus, ovary, and breast. Maintaining a desirable body weight could improve overall health and lead to more successful management of cancer should it develop.
- *Limit your exposure to sun.* It is important to heed this message, even if you enjoy many outdoor activities. Particularly for people with light complexions, the radiation received through chronic exposure to the sun may foster the development of skin cancers. Although most skin cancers are readily treatable, one form, malignant melanoma, can be life threatening.
- *Consume alcohol in moderation.* Although the evidence linking alcohol use and an increased rate of cancer is at best circumstantial, heavier users of alcohol do experience an increased prevalence of cancer of the oral cavity, larynx, and esophagus. Whether this results directly from the presence of carcinogens in alcohol or is more closely related to the alcohol user's tendency to smoke is not yet established. It is known, however, that people who have developed alcohol-related sclerotic changes of the liver are more likely to develop a malignancy at that site.

All risk factor reduction is, in the final analysis, relative in nature. Our observation and experiences lead us to believe that life cannot be totally structured around the desire to achieve maximum longevity or reduce morbidity at all costs. Most people need a balance between life that is emotionally, socially, and spiritually satisfying and life that is structured solely for the purpose of living a long time and minimizing exposure to illness.

Cerebral Palsy

Cerebral palsy (CP) is manifested as a loss of voluntary control over motor function resulting from a brain disorder or accident either before or after birth. The most probable cause of cerebral palsy is a lack of proper oxygenation at birth.[13] Other common causes are thought to be accidental poisoning, brain infections in childhood, and severe head injuries. Heredity is not considered a significant factor.

Resources Offering Support for Cancer Victims

For cancer victims and their families, many resource lines have been set up offering information and referrals:

- **American Cancer Society National Hotline:** (800) ACS-2345. Also, ACS recommends calling local ACS chapters for support group information.
- **National Cancer Institute Cancer Information Service:** (800) 4-CANCER.
- **National Coalition for Cancer Survivorship** (umbrella group for cancer survivor units nationwide): (505) 764-9956.
- **Candlelighters Foundation:** Information on support groups for children with cancer and their families: (202) 659-5136.
- *Cope* **magazine hotline:** Some referrals. Publishes national magazine for cancer survivors: (800) 343-2673.
- **Surviving:** Support group. Publishes newsletter for Hodgkin's survivors. Stanford University Medical center, Radiology Dept, Room C050, 300 Pasteur Dr, Stanford, CA 94305.
- **Vital Options:** Support group for young adults, 17 to 40, who are cancer survivors: (818) 508-5657.

The loss of motor function in cerebral palsy can express itself over a wide continuum. Impaired function can range from near complete paralysis to minor uncontrolled movements. Difficulties with speech may also be apparent. Some persons may have seizures. Although some people with cerebral palsy have concurrent mental retardation, many persons with cerebral palsy are not mentally retarded.

With the possible exception of the use of muscle relaxant drugs, physical therapy, and braces, treatment for cerebral palsy is focused on integrating the person into society. When provided with appropriate opportunities in a stimulating academic and social setting, persons with cerebral palsy are often able to show the world that a neurological accident does not imply a life that is less than successful, enjoyable, or contributive.

Premenstrual Syndrome (PMS)

Premenstrual syndrome has been described as follows[14]: "The premenstrual syndrome is characterized by psychological (depression, lethargy, irritability, aggressiveness, etc.) or somatic (headache, backache, asthma, acne, epilepsy, etc.) symptoms that recur in the same phase of each menstrual cycle, followed by a symptom-free phase in each cycle."

In the margin is a list (based on a compilation by the National Center for Premenstrual Syndrome and Menstrual Distress) that identifies some of the more frequently reported symptoms of PMS. Symptoms and severity may vary from month to month. A woman with PMS will experience the symptoms on a predictable cyclic basis during the *secretory phase* of the menstrual cycle. The condition's recurring nature is normally interrupted by only three events—pregnancy, *menopause*, and treatment with ovarian hormones.

The cause of PMS appears, most likely, to be hormonal. Perhaps a woman's

Some Common PMS Symptoms

Tension
Depression
Irritability
Headache
Tender breasts
Bloated abdomen
Backache
Dizziness
Fainting
Abdominal cramps
Weight gain
Fatigue

Personal
Assessment

Are You at Risk for Skin, Breast, and Cervical Cancer?

Some people may have more than an average risk of developing certain cancers. These people will be identified by certain risk factors.

This simple self-testing method is designed by the American Cancer Society to help you assess your risk factors for three common types of cancer. These are the major risk factors and by no means represent the only ones that might be involved.

Check your response to each risk factor. Add the numbers in the parentheses to arrive at a total score for each cancer type. Find out what your score means by reading the information in the right column. You are advised to discuss this information with your physician if you are at higher risk.

Skin Cancer

1 Frequent work or play in the sun
  a Yes (10)   **b** No (1)

2 Work in mines, around coal tars or around radio-activity.
  a Yes (10)   **b** No (1)

3 Complexion—fair skin and/or light skin.
  a Yes (10)   **b** No (1)

Your total points _____

EXPLANATION

1 Excessive ultraviolet light causes skin cancer. Protect yourself with a sun screen medication.

2 These materials can cause skin cancer.

3 Light complexions need more protection than others.

Interpretation

Numerical risks for skin cancer are difficult to state. For instance, a person with dark complexion can work longer in the sun and be less likely to develop cancer than a light complected person. Furthermore, a person wearing a long sleeve shirt and a wide brimmed hat may work in the sun and be less at risk than a person who wears a bathing suit for only a short period. The risk goes up greatly with age.

The key here is if you answered "yes" to any question, you need to realize that you have above-average risk.

Breast Cancer

1 Age groups
  a 20-34 (10)   **c** 50 and over (90)
  b 35-49 (40)

2 Race group
  a Oriental (5)   **c** White (25)
  b Black (20)   **d** Mexican American (10)

3 Family history
  a Mother, sister, aunt or grandmother with breast cancer (30)
  b None (10)

Your total points _____

4 Your history
  a No breast disease (10)
  b Previous noncancerous lumps or cysts (25)
  c Previous breast cancer (100)

5 Maternity
  a First Pregnancy before 25 (10)
  b First pregnancy after 25 (15)
  c No pregnancies (2)

Interpretation

Under 100   Low-risk women should practice monthly breast self-examination (BSE) and have their breasts examined by a doctor as part of a cancer-related checkup.

100-199   Moderate-risk women should practice monthly BSE and have their breasts examined by a doctor as part of a cancer-related checkup. Periodic breast x-rays should be included as your doctor may advise.

200 or higher   High-risk women should practice monthly BSE and have the above examinations and mammograms related to you.

Cervical Cancer*

1 Age group
   a Less than 25 (10)   c 40-54 (30)
   b 25-39 (20)   d 55 & over (30)

2 Race
   a Oriental (10)   d White (10)
   b Puerto Rican (20)   e Mexican American
   c Black (20)   (20)

3 Number of pregnancies
   a 0 (10)   c 4 and over (30)
   b 1 to 3 (20)

4 Viral infections
   a Herpes and other viral infections or ulcer formations on the vagina (10)
   b Never (1)

5 Age at first intercourse
   a Before 15 (40)   c 20-24 (20)
   b 15-19 (30)   d 25 and over (10)

6 Bleeding between periods or after intercourse
   a Yes (40)   b No (1)

Your total points _____

EXPLANATION

1 The highest occurrence is in the 40 and over age group. The numbers represent the relative rates of cancer for different age groups. A 45 year old woman has a risk three times higher than a 20 year old.

2 Puerto Ricans, Blacks, and Mexican Americans have higher rates of cervical cancer.

3 Women who have delivered more children have a higher occurrence.

4 Viral infections of the cervix and vagina are associated with cervical cancer.

5 Women with earlier intercourse and with more sexual partners are at a higher risk.

6 Irregular bleeding may be a sign of uterine cancer.

Interpretation

40-69   This is a low risk group. Ask your doctor for a pap test. You will be advised how often you should be tested after your first test.

70-99   In this moderate risk group, more frequent pap tests may be required.

100 or higher   You are in a high risk group and should have a pap test (and pelvic exam) as advised by your doctor.

*Lower portion of uterus. These questions would not apply to a woman who has had a complete hysterectomy.

body is insensitive to a normal level of progesterone, or her ovaries fail to produce a normal amount of progesterone. These reasons seem plausible, because PMS-type symptoms do not occur during pregnancy, a time during which natural progesterone levels are very high, and because women with PMS seem to feel much better after taking high doses of natural progesterone in suppository form. When using oral contraceptives that supply synthetic progesterone at normal levels, many women report relief from some symptoms of PMS.[15]

At this writing, two factors make the treatment of PMS with large doses of progesterone a speculative issue. The first is, of course, a lack of long-term data on the effects of high levels of progesterone on the body. The second factor is research bias, when the treatment method is known to both the physician and the patient.[16] Until both of these issues are carefully researched, it is unlikely that the medical community will deal with PMS through any approach other than a relatively conservative treatment of symptoms through the use of *analgesic drugs* (including *prostaglandin inhibitors*), *diuretic drugs*, dietary modifications (including restriction of caffeine and salt), vitamin B_6 therapy, exercise, and stress reduction exercises.

In addition to the role of progesterone in PMS, other causes have been considered. Aldosterone, a hormone associated with fluid retention,[17] and serotonin, a neurotransmitter have been identified by some as playing a role in the development of PMS. The exact nature of PMS has been further complicated by the classification of severe PMS as a mental disturbance by some segments of the American Psychiatric Association.

Type 2 (Non-Insulin-Dependent) Diabetes Mellitus

My father is diabetic. In fact, his condition was diagnosed just last year. He's lost a lot of weight since then and he seems to be doing pretty well.

This statement is typical of those shared with us whenever diabetes mellitus is discussed in our personal health classes. Students routinely report that a parent's diabetes was discovered when routine tests were conducted for another medical problem. Most students also indicate that their parent was overweight when the diagnosis of *type 2 diabetes* was made.

Some of your friends may have *type 1 (insulin-dependent) diabetes mellitus, or juvenile diabetes mellitus.* For these people diabetes has probably been a part of their lives for years. These students have taken **insulin** from the time their condition was diagnosed, have followed strict dietary practices, and have carefully controlled their exercise—all in an attempt to keep the diabetes under the best management possible. These students have diabetes in its most serious form in that they have lost all insulin production.

In persons who do not have diabetes mellitus, the body's need for energy is met through the "burning" of glucose within the cells. Glucose is absorbed from the digestive tract and carried to the cells by the circulatory system. Passage of glucose into the cell is achieved through a transport system that moves the glucose molecule across the cell's membrane. Activation of this glucose transport mechanism in insulin-sensitive cells requires the presence of the hormone insulin, and specific receptor sites for insulin can be found on the cell membrane.[18] The movement of glucose into the insulin-insensitive cells of nerve, kidney, and liver tissue does not require insulin.

insulin
pancreatic hormone required by the body for the effective metabolism of carbohydrates.

In addition to its role in the transport of glucose into sensitive cells, insulin is also required for the conversion of glucose into glycogen in liver cells and the formation of fatty acids in adipose cells. Alteration of glucose in preparation for eventual conversion to carbon dioxide, water, and energy also requires insulin.

Insulin is produced in the cells of the islets of Langerhans within the pancreas. The release of insulin from the pancreas corresponds to the changing levels of glucose within the blood.

In adults with a **genetic predisposition** for developing type 2 diabetes mellitus, a trigger mechanism (most likely obesity) begins a process through which the body cells become increasingly less sensitive to the presence of insulin, although a normal amount of insulin is produced by the pancreas. The growing ineffectiveness of insulin in facilitating glucose transport into glucose-sensitive body cells, and the breakdown of glycogen and mobilization of fatty acids, result in the buildup of glucose in the blood. Elevated levels of glucose give rise to *hyperglycemia*, a hallmark symptom of type 2 diabetes mellitus.[19]

> **genetic predisposition** inherited tendency to develop a disease process if necessary environmental factors exist.

In response to the hyperglycemic state, the kidneys begin the process of filtering glucose from the blood. Excess glucose then spills over into the urine. This removal of glucose in the urine demands large amounts of water. *Diuresis*, a second important symptom of the adult onset diabetes, is experienced as the diabetic person feels the urge to drink large amounts of water. (One early method of diabetes diagnosis included tasting a drop of urine for its relatively sweet taste!)

The current treatment of type 2 diabetes mellitus is undergoing constant refinement as more is learned about insulin insensitivity. For many adults with diabetes, dietary restriction is the only treatment required to maintain an acceptable level of glucose utilization. Weight loss will improve the condition by "releasing" more insulin receptors, and, as a consequence, the person can return to a more normal state of functioning.[20]

For people whose condition is more advanced, dietary restriction and weight loss alone will not accomplish the level of management required, and oral drugs may be necessary. Currently four *sulfonylureas* (oral hypoglycemic agents) seem to be effective in stimulating the release of additional insulin from the pancreas.[20] This additional insulin "push" helps the advanced diabetic maintain normal metabolic functioning. Type 2 diabetes mellitus, unlike its juvenile (type 1) counterpart, is not insulin dependent, and as a consequence, the direct administration of insulin is not generally required, although when insulin is used it can be effective in lowering blood glucose levels.[21]

In addition to genetic predisposition and obesity as important factors in type 2 diabetes mellitus, unresolved stress appears to play a role in the development of hyperglycemic states. Although stress alone probably cannot produce a diabetic condition, it is likely that stress, through the presence of epinephrine, can create a series of endocrine changes that can lead to a state of hyperglycemia. Misdiagnosis of diabetes mellitus has occurred as the result of this stress-induced hyperglycemia.[22]

Diabetes can cause serious damage to several important structures within the body. The rate and extent to which persons with diabetes develop these pathological changes can be markedly influenced by the nature of their particular condition and the type of management to which they comply. For those who already have diabetes, understanding of the condition and a commitment to the management scheme are important elements in living with diabetes mellitus.

Common Complications of Diabetes

Cataract formation
Glaucoma
Blindness
Dental caries
Stillbirths/miscarriages
Neonatal deaths
Congenital defects

Identifying the changes caused by osteoporosis.

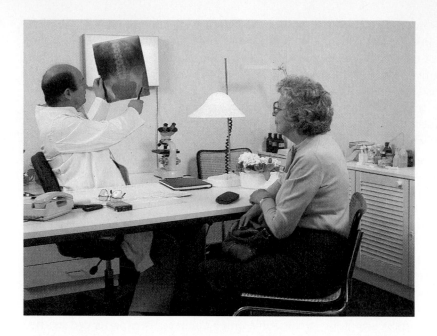

Osteoporosis

ON BEING PARENTS TO YOUR OWN PARENTS

One of the developmental undertakings that your parents are perhaps facing is that of becoming the "parents" of your grandparents. As your grandparents age, it may become increasingly necessary for your parents to begin making decisions, setting limits, and arranging care for their parents. Nothing forces midlife parents into this faster than, for example, when a grandmother fractures a hip and never totally returns to healthful independence she enjoyed before her fall.

As familiar as the broken-hip scenario is, the underlying cause of this accident is often misunderstood by both the elderly victim and the family who must respond to her needs. It is generally reported that the grandmother was doing little more than taking a calm walk or standing at the kitchen sink when she fractured her hip. In actuality, however, this sequence was probably reversed. The hip fractured first and then the fall occurred. All of this probably stemmed from osteoporosis, a condition resulting in a markedly weakened skeleton caused by calcium **resorption** from the bone.

It is not fully understood why white menopausal women are so susceptible to the increase in calcium loss that leads to fracture of the hip, wrist, and vertebral column. Well over 90% of all persons with osteoporosis are white women. From an anatomical point of view, the bones of an aging woman are not smaller in diameter than those of young women, nor do they have a different ratio of organic to mineral material. Rather, they lack the mass that is associated with the strong, healthy skeleton of a younger person.

As with premenstrual syndrome, the endocrine system may play a large role in the development of osteoporosis. At the time of menopause, a woman's ovaries begin a rapid decrease in the production of *estrogen,* one of the two hormones associated with the menstrual cycle. This lower level of estrogen may decrease the conversion of the precursors of vitamin D into the active form of vitamin D, the form necessary for absorbing calcium from the digestive tract. As

resorption
withdrawal of a chemical substance from a site in which it had been initially deposited.

a result, calcium may be drawn from the bones for use elsewhere in the body. To date, however, this mechanism has not been demonstrated as the sole basis of osteoporosis.[13] Fortunately, most dairy products and other food such as cereal, are fortified with vitamin D thus making the vitamin available.

Additional explanations of osteoporosis focus on two other possibilities— *hyperparathyroidism*[23] (another endocrine dysfunction) and the below-average degree of muscle development seen in osteoporotic women. In this latter explanation, the reduced muscle mass is associated with decreased activity that in turn deprives the body of the mechanical stimulation needed to facilitate bone growth. In the margin is a list that identifies some factors that may contribute to excess bone loss.

Premenopausal women have the opportunity to build and maintain a healthy skeleton through an appropriate intake of calcium. Current recommendations are for an intake of 1,000 mg of calcium per day. This amount can be obtained by some women completely through dietary intake, particularly from dairy products. Three to four daily servings of low-fat dairy products should provide sufficient calcium. Adequate vitamin D must also be in the diet because it aids in the absorption of calcium.

Many women do not intake an adequate amount of calcium. Calcium supplements, again in combination with vitamin D, can be used in achieving recommended calcium. Dairy products are a rich source of calcium. Current studies suggest that many of the more heavily advertised calcium supplements are relatively ineffective in supplying needed calcium because of their failure to dissolve. It is now known that calcium carbonate, a highly advertised form of calcium, is no more easily absorbed by the body than are other forms of calcium salts. Consumers of calcium supplements should compare brands to determine which, if any, they will buy.

In premenopausal women, calcium deposition in bone is facilitated by exercise, particularly exercise that involves movement of the extremities. Our stu-

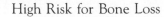

High Risk for Bone Loss

Women at highest risk for excess bone loss are those who:
- Are not physically active
- Have a low dietary calcium intake
- Smoke
- Drink excessive amounts of alcohol, coffee, tea, or soft drinks
- Have never been pregnant
- Have fair complexions
- Are thin and have small bones
- Have experienced an early menopause, either naturally or by surgical removal of the ovaries
- Have a family history of osteoporosis
- Regularly use steroid drugs, antiseizure medications, or anticoagulants

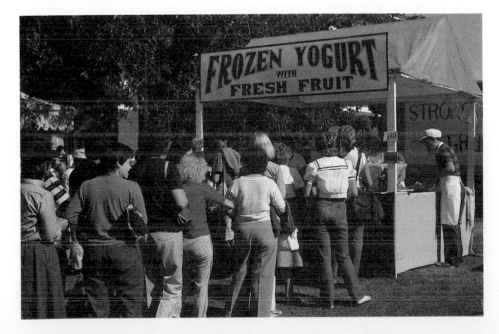

Yogurt is an excellent source of calcium.

dents are encouraged to consume at least the recommended servings from the milk group and engage in regular physical activity that involves the weight-bearing muscles of the legs, such as aerobics, jogging, or walking.

Postmenopausal women who are not elderly can markedly slow the resorption of calcium from their bones through the use of estrogen replacement therapy. When combined with a daily intake of 1,500 mg of calcium, vitamin D, and regular exercise, estrogen therapy almost eliminates calcium loss. A postmenopausal prevention program that does not include estrogen will have considerably less ability to protect against serious calcium loss.[24] Of course, women will need to work closely with their physicians in monitoring the use of estrogen.

The exact mechanism underlying osteoporosis is not clearly understood. Nevertheless, it is apparent that calcium consumption and regular physical activity should be maintained by women throughout the life cycle. Physicians can treat osteoporosis with hormonal and nutritional therapy, but good preventive health practices should minimize the need for these.

Allergic Disorders

antigens
disease-producing microorganisms or foreign substances that on entering the body trigger an immune response; foreign proteins stimulate the body's immune system to produce antigens.

allergens
environmental substances to which persons may be hypersensitive; allergens function as antigens.

People who have allergies have abnormal body reactions to certain substances called **antigens,** or **allergens.** These antigens might include certain molds, foods, plant pollens, drugs, dust, animal hair, and insect stings. When exposed to the antigens, people display allergic reactions, including nasal congestion, red, swollen, watery eyes, and sneezing. Itching of the ears, nose, throat, and mouth are often reported. Some people develop characteristic *hives.* Others occasionally indicate asthmalike symptoms that make breathing quite difficult.

Allergies tend to run in families. In fact, you may know families in which all the members have hay fever, ragweed allergies, or poison ivy sensitivity. Allergies may be seasonal difficulties that present themselves only when the antigen is prevalent. People who are sensitive to one antigen are likely to be sensitive to other antigens in the same general group. For example, those who are sensitive to dog hair may also be sensitive to most kinds of animal fur.

The cause of allergies lies in a disturbance in one's immune system. For unknown reasons, after an initial exposure to a particular antigen, some peoples' bodies prepare an overly elaborate defense system to counter subsequent exposures to that antigen. These people are said to have developed a *hypersensitivity* to the antigen. When they come into contact with the antigen, their body tissues release large amounts of histamines. These chemical substances constrict smooth muscle, such as that in the air passages, and alter normal circulatory activity.[25] In certain extreme cases, a person's body may overwhelmingly react to an antigen and produce such congestion that *anaphylactic shock,* asphyxiation, and death may result.

Allergies are often diagnosed by a health history, reported symptoms, and an allergy skin test. During an allergy skin test, small amounts of common antigens are either injected or "scratched" just beneath the skin of the patient's back, arm, or legs. Antigens that produce abnormal redness and swelling are easily identified.

Once the antigens are identified, people can attempt to avoid exposure to them, control the symptoms if an allergic response occurs, and undergo a preventive treatment called *desensitization* or immunotherapy.[22] In desensitization treatment a small amount of the offending antigen is injected so that the immune system can gradually develop an appropriate, normal defensive reaction to that antigen. The success of such therapy is variable.

Other treatment methods include the use of drugs to treat the symptoms of the allergic response. This is done generally by the use of *antihistamines* (to block the release of histamines), *antiinflammatory agents* (to reduce the inflammation response), and *decongestants* (to relieve nasal and chest congestion).

Fibrocystic Breast Condition

In reproductively mature females the menstrual cycle is accompanied by a corresponding cyclic process within the breast tissue. There, during the **proliferative phase** of the menstrual cycle, rising levels of estrogen initiate a rapid development of the tubular duct system of the breast. The proliferation of the **secretory cells** lining these ducts and the saclike tissue at the end of each duct is dependent upon progesterone and occurs during the latter half of the cycle. Should pregnancy occur, the breast tissue that was "primed" by estrogen and progesterone during that particular menstrual cycle would be maintained by the progesterone released by the *placenta* until the latter weeks of pregnancy, when pituitary and placental hormones take control of milk development.[26]

In some women, particularly those who have yet to experience pregnancy (nulliparous women), stimulation of the breast tissue by estrogen and progesterone results in an unusually high degree of secretory activity by the cells lining the ducts. The copious fluid released by the secretory lining finds its way into the fibrous connective tissue areas in the lower quadrants of the breast, where in pocketlike cysts this fluid distends neighboring tissue. Excessive secretory activity produces in many women a fibrocystic breast condition characterized by swollen, nodular, tender breast tissue before menstruation. Controversy has surrounded the possible link between caffeine intake and fibrocystic breast condition, but the present consensus is that caffeine consumption is not significantly related to fibrocystic breast condition.[27]

Women who experience a more extensive fibrocystic condition can be treated with drugs that have a "calming" effect on progesterone production. Additionally, occasional aspiration of the fluid-filled cysts can bring relief. Cysts that yield up to 5 milliliters of fluid are not uncommon and certainly explain the patient's complaints about tenderness and fullness of the breasts.[28]

Endogenous (Primary) Depression

A sizable number of persons experience a type of depression that is attributable to clearly defined life situations. This depression is called *exogenous* (or *reactive, secondary*) depression (see Chapter 19). However, a number of adults also experience a different form of depression. They report to their physician or counselor that they feel blue, unhappy, or even overwhelmed. They say that most activities are no longer pleasurable and may feel fatigued, unmotivated, and pessimistic about the future. The ability of these persons to function efficiently is markedly reduced. Their outward appearance reflects their depressed mode, and their speech may be labored and lacking in vitality. Some people experience hypochondriasis and frequently think of suicide. This form of depression may last for months.

proliferative phase
first half of the menstrual cycle.

secretory cells
specialized cells within the breast that will, on stimulation, produce milk.

Exogenous, or secondary, depression occurs in reaction to a particular life situation. *Endogenous,* or primary, depression is genetic and biochemical in origin.

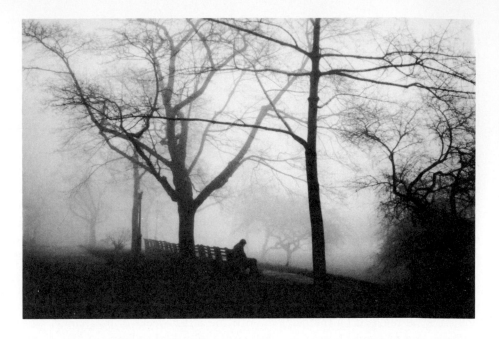

The difference between exogenous depression and this latter type is that in the second instance no event, situation, or set of circumstances is responsible for the person's depressed outlook. The physician identifies this form of depression as *endogenous,* because it is centered in the brain's biochemical function.[29] Endogenous depression, therefore, is primary in origin, while exogenous depression is secondary to factors that lie outside the person. Occasionally both types of depression may be operating. More commonly, however, one type clearly predominates and is the basis for a medical diagnosis.

The cause of endogenous depression is, most likely, genetic in origin and involves an alteration in the normal functioning of two neurotransmitters. (See Chapter 7 for related information.) Depending on the specific types of endogenous depression involved, the action of either serotonin or norepinephrine is altered. More than likely, the neurotransmitter is absorbed too quickly after its release by the synaptic terminal, thus making it less than fully capable of exerting its maximum effect on the transmission of nerve impulses.

The current approach to the treatment of endogenous depression involves two markedly different methods. The first and most immediate in terms of results involves the use of **electroconvulsive therapy (ECT).** In some cases improvements in the patient's outlook following shock therapy may be seen within a matter of a few hours. In other cases no improvement is reported. Much controversy surrounds this treatment method.[28]

electroconvulsive therapy (ECT)

use of electrical shock to alter the neurotransmitter activity within the brain.

The second method of management is drug therapy. The use of antidepressant drugs has ebbed and flowed over the course of the last 30 years. A family of drugs, the tricyclics, can be used in treatment. These drugs have the ability to block the rapid reabsorption of norepinephrine and serotonin on the presynaptic side of the synapse. However, because of the presence of a natural **homeostatic mechanism** that initially offsets the effect of the drug, a 2- or 3-week period is necessary before the level of neurotransmitter is sufficient to cause an elevation in mood. This time lag, in combination with unpredictable side effects, dictates the tricyclics be used with caution.

homeostatic mechanism

complex biological mechanism that attempts to moderate processes within the body so that a balance or equilibrium is maintained.

A new group of drugs, the *tetracyclics*, are now available. The tetracyclics possess the same properties of the tricyclics in slowing the rapid uptake of the neurotransmitter, but tetracyclics also possess the ability to counter the homeostatic mechanism mentioned in conjunction with tricyclics. Because of this quality, the tetracyclics reduce the time lag between the initial administration of the drug and the first sign of its effect and thus allow for safer uses of drug therapy in treating endogenous depression.[23]

Although we could have selected conditions other than depression to reflect the influence of neurochemistry on illness, endogenous depression is so subtle and pervasive that some experts believe it to be the most underdiagnosed condition seen by internists and family physicians.

Epilepsy

Epilepsy is characterized by sudden changes in mental function, state of consciousness, sensory activity, or movements of the body caused by misfiring of cerebral nerve cells. Epilepsy is the most common organic disorder of the nervous system, with about 1 in every 200 persons exhibiting some form. Epilepsy should not be considered a specific disease, but rather an umbrella term for a variety of symptoms that can originate from a number of causes, including brain injuries, brain infections, and brain tumors.

Epilepsy produces temporary disruptions in normal brain function, resulting in a variety of types of seizures. A number of persons with epilepsy report that an aura precedes their seizures. The aura is an advanced warning or sensation that alerts the person that a seizure may follow.

The Epilepsy Foundation of America has recategorized the types of seizures noted in persons with epilepsy (see Appendix 2). Note the great variation in the physical presentation of seizures, as well as the current nomenclature.

If you are with someone who appears to be having a seizure, the most important points to remember are (1) do not restrain the person, and (2) protect the person from accidentally hurting himself or herself. Appendix 2 describes the most appropriate first aid measures in seizure-related situations. You may note that the assistance of emergency first aid personnel is usually not needed.

In the treatment of epilepsy, surgery for the removal of brain tissue is not frequently indicated. For many persons with epilepsy, drug therapy, which includes the use of *anticonvulsant drugs*, has been effective in controlling the frequency and severity of seizures.[29] (As with the antihypertensive drugs, these drugs are only able to control a condition—they do not cure epilepsy.) Unfortunately the social stigma attached to epilepsy causes some persons to avoid regular compliance with drug therapy, since this behavior confirms the fact that they are, in some way, "different."

Multiple Sclerosis

For proper nerve conduction to occur within portions of the brain and spinal cord, an insulating sheath of *myelin* must surround *neurons*. In the progressive disease multiple sclerosis (MS) and other sheath-destroying diseases, the cells that produce myelin (oligodendrocytes) are altered, and myelin production ceases. With the cessation of myelin production, the neuron's sheath is replaced with nonfunctioning scarlike tissue. *Demyelination*, and its resultant disruption to normal neurological functioning, eventually reaches an extent to which vital functions of the body can no longer be carried out.[21] The condition is fatal.

Multiple sclerosis is a disease that most often appears for the first time during the young adult years—the traditional college years. Following its onset, the disease progresses episodically over the next 20 to 25 years. Symptoms vary from time to time, and periods of remission, with accompanying periods of euphoria, are common. The initial symptoms of the condition are often visual impairment, prickling and burning in the extremities, or an altered **gait.**[21] Degeneration of neurological function occurs in various forms during the course of MS. In the disease's most advanced stages, movement is greatly impaired and mental deterioration may be present.

Treatment for MS involves attempts to reduce the incapacitating nature of the symptoms and extend the periods of remission. Today a variety of therapies are employed, including steroid drugs, drugs to relieve muscle spasms, injections of **nerve blockers,** and physical therapy. In addition, psychotherapy is an important adjunct to the treatment of MS. Profound periods of depression, often accompany the initial diagnosis of this condition. Emotional support is helpful in dealing with the progressive impairment associated with the condition. Support by the family members of the victim is of great importance in the victim's attempt to adjust to the disease. Likewise support for the victim's family may be required during particularly difficult periods.

The cause of MS is not fully understood. Research continues to focus on virus-induced **autoimmune** mechanisms and on the role of genetic alterations in myelin production.

The genetic nature of MS is interesting, in light of the unusual demographic distribution of the condition. Anthropologists and epidemiologists now believe that genetic susceptibility of MS arose in one area of northern Europe. The prevalence of the disease in certain European countries and in particular areas of the United States and its absence in African black populations contribute to the belief that the genetic abnormality may have been introduced into the gene pool—possibly by an isolated strain of virus.

Low Back Pain

A common experience for adults is the sudden painful onset of lower back pain. Each year 10 million adults develop this condition to the point that they miss work, lose sleep, and generally feel incapable of engaging in day-to-day activities. Eighty percent of all adults who have experienced this condition will in fact do so two to three times per year.[21]

Although lower back pain can in some cases reflect potentially serious health problems, most lower back pain results from *mechanical* (postural) causes. Specifically, the *lordotic curvature* that normally exists in the lumbar portion of the spinal column may be lost because of prolonged straightening of the lower back during bending, lifting, or sitting. Once this curvature is lost, sharp pain is felt in the lower back slightly below the belt line, in the buttocks, or in the thigh and upper leg. As uncomfortable as lower back pain is, the problem is usually self-correcting within a week or two.[30] The services of a physician, physical therapist, or chiropractor are not generally required after an initial visit. However, surgery must be performed when lower back pain is caused by structural

gait
one's pattern of walking.

nerve blockers
drugs that can stop the flow of electrical impulses through the nerves into which they have been injected.

autoimmune
immune response against the cells of a person's own body.

changes in the vertebral column—such as in the case of a **herniated disk.** Annually only about 250,000 persons of the 10 million who experience lower back pain will require back surgery. Even this number may fall in the future as alternatives to surgery are developed. The approval of *chymopapain,* an enzyme that can destroy a portion of a herniated disk and thus allow it to shrink, offers an alternative to surgery for some.

After one experiences the onset of mechanical back pain, exercises can be begun that will restore the lordodic curvature to the back. As the lower back returns to its normal curvature, tissues near the spinal column are no longer stretched, the intervertebral disks are no longer compressed, and the spinal nerves return to their normal position. Reduction of pain follows quickly thereafter.

Prevention of mechanical back pain can be achieved by implementing a relatively few ostural practices during day-to-day activity. The following modifications in the way you might normally bend, pick up objects, and sit are suggested by a leading international authority in the field of mechanical back pain.

Sitting

When sitting for prolonged periods, the maintenance of the lordotic curvature is essential. It does not matter if you maintain this with your own muscles or with the help of a supportive roll placed in the small of the back.

In addition to sitting correctly with a lumbar support, you should interrupt prolonged sitting at regular intervals. On extended car journeys you should stop, walk around for a few minutes, and slowly bend backward five or six times.

Bending forward

When engaged in activities that entail prolonged forward bending or stooping—for example, gardening, vacuuming, and concreting—you must regularly stand upright, restore the lordotic curvature, and bend backward five or six times before pain commences.

Frequent interruption of prolonged forward bending by straightening up and bending backward to restore and accenutate the lordotic curvature should enable you to continue with most of the activities you are used to doing.

Lifting

If a load to be lifted weighs more than 30 pounds, the strain must be taken with the lower back in lordosis and your knees bent. You must lift by straigtening your legs.

If the object weighs less than 30 pounds, less care is required, unless you have been in a bent or sitting position for some time before lifting. If this has happened, you must lift as though the weight exceeds 30 pounds.

In addition to correct lifting technique, you must stand upright and bend backward five or six times before and after lifting.

An orthopedist at Harvard Medical School further advises exercise to strengthen the abdominal muscles as a sound preventive practice. Dr. Augustus White recommends swimming, walking, jogging, and bicycling as good forms of exercise for your back. However, golf, bowling, baseball, diving, and gymnastics all increase your chances of developing back problems.[29] The box on p. 320 shows exercises that strengthen the back and prevent lower back problems.

herniated disk
protrusion of an intervertebral disk from its normal position between adjoining vertebra.

Preventing Back Pain

To prevent back pain, you should alter the ways in which you:
- Sit
- Bend
- Lift
- Exercise

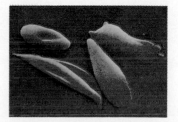
Sickled red blood cells.

The Williams Exercise Schedule

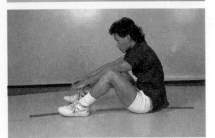

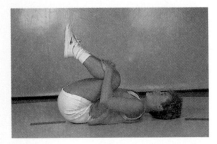

1

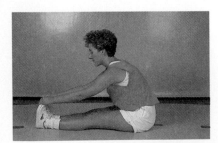

2

1 *Abdominal muscles.* A, To strengthen the abdominal muscles, raise your trunk off the floor as far as possible. Keep arms folded. Repeat 5 to 20 times. B, This is a less strenuous version of 1, as the arms are always extended.

2 *Gluteus maximus.* To strengthen the gluteus maximus muscle, place your feet about 9 inches from your buttocks. Place your hands just above your navel to make sure that the lumbar spine is not lifted. Contract the buttock muscles to rotate the pelvis backwards. The buttocks are lifted while the base of the spine remains on the floor. Repeat 10 to 20 times.

3 *Lumbar curve.* To obliterate the lumbar curve, place your arms around your knees and pull them towards your chest. Keep head relaxed on the floor. Lift the very base of the spine only. Repeat 10 times.

4 *Lumbar spine, hamstrings.* To improve flexion of the lumbar spine and stretch contraction of the hamstring muscles, bend your trunk forward while trying to touch your toes. Lower your head close to your knees. Relax. Repeat 10 times. (CAUTION: Do not perform this exercise if you experience pain radiating down your legs.)

5 *Pelvic area.* To relieve stiffness in the pelvic area, bend one leg and extend the other straight behind you. Arms are extended so that hands are on the floor 12 inches apart and in front of the bent leg. Press your pelvis down so that a definite stretch is felt in the front of the thigh of the extended leg. Repeat 10 times on each leg.

6 *Lumbar spine.* A, To flex the lumbar spine, stand with your feet about 12 inches apart. B, Bend the trunk and sink into a deep squat with your feet firmly planted on the floor. Hold. Resume standing position. (CAUTION: Do not perform this exercise if you experience knee problems.)

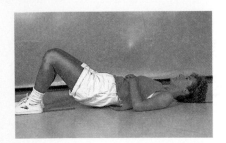

3

5

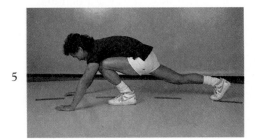

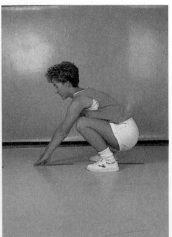

4

6

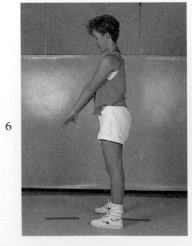

By paying a bit more attention to your back, particularly during bending, lifting, and sitting, you can minimize the occurrence of this uncomfortable and incapacitating condition.

Sickle Cell Trait and Sickle Cell Disease

Of all the chemical compounds found within the human body, few occur in as many forms as hemoglobin, the iron-based pigment that binds oxygen to the red blood cell. It is estimated that approximately 300 structurally different forms of hemoglobin exist. Two forms of hemoglobin, those with the genotypes HbAS and HbSS, are associated with the sickle cell trait and sickle cell disease, respectively. Black Americans can be the recipients of either form of the abnormal hemoglobin. Those who inherit the HbAS (heterozygous) hemoglobin do not develop sickle cell disease, but are capable of transmitting the gene for abnormal hemoglobin to their offspring. Persons inheriting the HbSS (homozygous) hemoglobin experience sickle cell disease and will face a shortened life characterized by periods of pain and impairment.[13]

Approximately 8% of all black Americans have sickle cell trait.[13] These people experience relatively little impairment. However, when they are in an environment with a reduced level of oxygen, clinical manifestation of the sickle cell condition can occur. However, the primary concern for people with sickle cell trait is the possibility of transmitting this trait.

For approximately 0.15% of black American children, sickle cell disease (HbSS) is a painful, incapacitating, and life-shortening disease.[13] The disease expresses itself in the form of red blood cells that undergo a chemical reorganization, in the presence of reduced oxygen. This reorganization results in an elongated, crescent-shaped cell—thus the term "sickle cell." Once having assumed this abnormal form, the sickled cells become rigid and are unable to pass through the body's most minute capillaries. Capillary blockage leads to reduced oxygen-

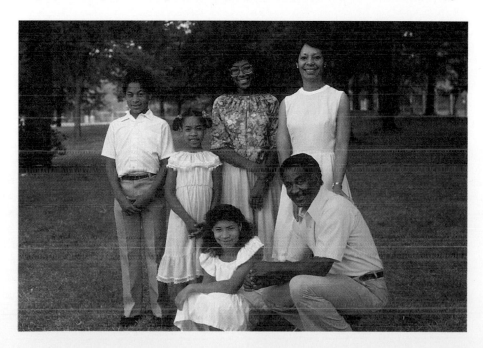

Could members of this family carry the sickle cell trait?

ation in distal tissue and increased sickling of red blood cells in that area. The body responds to the presence of these abnormal red blood cells by removing them in much less than the usual 120 days for normal red blood cells. This sets the stage for **anemia** in some people with sickle cell disease.

anemia
condition reflecting abnormally low levels of hemoglobin.

The clinical manifestations of sickle cell disease begin to appear as early as the sixth month of life. Throughout the remainder of the person's life (death usually occurs before the young adult years), the victim experiences numerous infections, reflecting damage to the spleen and other components of the immune system. Periods of significant pain centered in the abdomen, chest, and joints, as well as **pleurisy,** are also characteristic of the disease's progression.

pleurisy
inflammation of the lining of the chest cavity and outer surface of the lung.

In adults with sickle cell disease, the later years are characterized by an extensive array of serious medical problems, including impaired pulmonary function, congestive heart failure, gallbladder infections, altered urine production, bone changes, including scoliosis and osteomyelitis, and possible abnormalities of the eye and skin. For those who reach the young adult years, the prognosis for an extended life is not encouraging.

Although research for a drug that stimulates hemoglobin production is under way, a cure is not available.[31] Management of the disease is focused on preventing infections and minimizing the pain that can accompany the disease. For persons with sickle cell disease who must undergo surgery, red blood cell transfusions are required.

If a key exists to preventing the occurrence of sickle cell trait and disease, it lies in the area of *genetic counseling.*[13] Persons who have the condition in either of its forms must make careful decisions concerning reproduction, including pregnancy termination. Genetic counseling may provide help for many concerned couples. The decision to have children and perhaps risk passing on the gene for defective hemoglobin to the next generation is a matter that must be made by the persons involved. This is the case for all couples who may be at risk for transmitting diseases.

Arthritis

Arthritis is an umbrella term for over 100 forms of joint inflammation. The most common forms are **osteoarthritis** and **rheumatoid arthritis.** It is likely that as we age, all of us will develop osteoarthritis to some degree. Often called "wear and tear" arthritis, osteoarthritis occurs primarily in the weight-bearing joints of the knee, hip, and spine. In this form of arthritis, joint damage can occur to bone ends, cartilaginous cushions, and related structures as the years of constant friction and stress take their toll.

osteoarthritis
arthritis that develops with age; largely caused by weight and deterioration of the joints.

rheumatoid arthritis
the result of autoimmune deterioration of the joint.

The other commonly recognized form of arthritis is rheumatoid arthritis. Like allergic disorders, rheumatoid arthritis is considered an autoimmune disease process. For unknown reasons, in some persons the body's immune system attacks perfectly good cells in virtually all of the joints in the body. Approximately 2% of the population above the age of 15 have some degree of rheumatoid arthritis.[12] For those whose condition is recent in its onset, stiffness and joint pain are relatively common characteristics. In persons whose condition is more advanced, swelling, redness, throbbing pain, muscle atrophy, joint deformity, and limited mobility are often reported. Significantly greater numbers of women than men develop this form of arthritis.

Interestingly, a traumatic or stressful event often appears to serve as a triggering event in bringing a person's rheumatoid arthritis to a clinical level of expression. In many cases an individual's first indication of the condition follows an accident or a period of unusual stress. It is currently thought that there may be a genetic predisposition for developing rheumatoid arthritis.[13]

The destructive, painful effects of rheumatoid arthritis are noticed when the body's own specialized white blood cells, *phagocytic leukocytes,* begin to attack and destroy the *synovial cells* that line the joint capsules. Thus the production of synovial fluid from these cells diminishes. Additionally, a layer of granular tissue, the *pannus,* forms. The pannus attacks joint cartilage and eventually erodes the bone ends. Both synovial fluid reduction and bone erosion form the basis for the increasing degree of joint destruction seen in rheumatoid arthritis.

The objective of current management of arthritic conditions is not to cure the disease; rather, the practitioner attempts to aid the patient by reducing discomfort, limiting joint destruction, and maximizing joint mobility. Aspirin products, prostaglandin inhibitors, gold salts, and *immunosuppressive drugs,* are all employed in the management of arthritis.[13] In addition to drugs, physical therapy is routinely employed. In recent years surgery has also played an increasingly important role in the management of arthritis. Today surgery may involve tendon repair, joint replacement, and synovectomy. Unfortunately, arthritis is another condition often exploited by fraudulent practitioners and purveyors of useless products.

Cirrhosis of the Liver

Cirrhosis is a general term used to describe the replacement of normally functioning tissue within an organ with tissue composed of nonfunctioning cells. Cirrhosis of the liver as a major source of adult mortality may not be fully appreciated by the general population. Many illnesses are capable of initiating cirrhosis of the liver, including viral hepatitis, cardiovascular disease, bile duct obstruction and the most familiar of causes, chronic heavy alcohol use.[25] See Chapter 8 for a discussion of heavy alcohol use.

When normal liver tissue is replaced with nonfunctioning scarlike tissue, a gradual loss of liver function will be observed. Fatigue, **jaundice,** mental changes, and bleeding disorders occur and one's health declines. Most importantly, cirrhosis of the liver is associated with serious changes in the ability of the blood to reach the liver through the normal *hepatic-portal* route. This gradually developing obstruction of the portal vein results in the development of hypertension within the vessel and the rerouting of blood within the body. Eventually, because of these circulatory changes, spleen enlargement and internal hemorrhage will occur. In advanced cirrhosis of the liver, internal bleeding is the most frequent cause of death.[13]

In cases of cirrhosis of the liver attributed to chronic heavy alcohol use, the gradual development of the condition requires an extended period (10 years or more) and will progress through stages.[13] Initially, changes in the liver involve the gradual deposition of fat within the organ. Later, but before the development of actual cirrhosis, the liver will become chronically inflamed and liver cells will be destroyed. Last, actual replacement of liver cells with nonfunctioning fibrous tissue will occur.[13]

jaundice
yellowing of the skin as a result of the abnormal accumulation of bile pigment within the body.

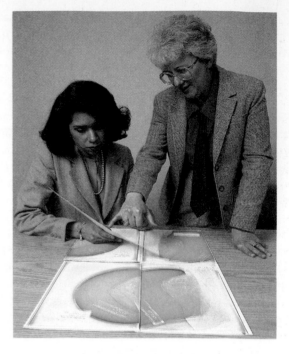

Preventing serious health problems requires periodic evaluations.

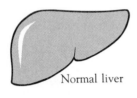

Normal liver

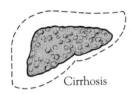

Cirrhosis

During the period of alcohol use that leads to cirrhosis of the liver, the user will exhibit observable changes in health. The effects of anemia, vitamin deficiencies, pancreatic inflammation, chronic inflammation of the gastric lining, vomiting, loss of appetite, and unpleasant changes in peripheral nervous sensation will eventually be seen. Securing medical attention for these symptoms may, in fact, begin the care needed to discontinue alcohol use and stop further liver damage.

SUMMARY

Numerous health problems that influence young adults were presented in this chapter. Cancer is a condition reflecting cellular dysfunction in its most extreme form. Since cancer is the second leading cause of death among adults, extensive ongoing research is being conducted. Much of the current cancer research focuses on oncogenesis—the development of cancer-causing genes.

Although cancer claims many lives, it is still survivable. The chances for recovery from cancer are best enhanced when a person is fully aware of cancer's seven warning signals and performs either breast self-examination or testicular self-examinations. Regular medical examinations also contribute to early diagnosis. Treatment for cancer generally combines proven therapies and experimental approaches. This chapter presented a brief description of many of these therapies.

In addition to cancer, 13 other health problems were identified and discussed in this chapter. For each condition, the suspected cause, diagnosis, treatment, and prognosis were presented. These conditions were selected for discussion because of their significance in young adults. The likelihood that we could develop one or more of these conditions is real. Certainly most of us have contact with a friend or relative with one or more of these health problems.

REVIEW QUESTIONS

1 Explain what cancer is. What major problem results from the fact that clinical identification of a malignant mass may not be possible until 5 years or more after tumor
activity has begun?
2 Define protooncogene and oncogene. Explain how carcinogens relate to the formation of oncogenes. What other areas of cancer research look promising? How likely
is it that there will soon be a cure for cancer? Why?
3 What are the most helpful activities people can do to enhance their chances for the
eary detection of cancer? What are the seven warning signals of cancer?
4 What are some of the treatments for cancer? Describe each one.
5 How do osteoarthritis and rheumatoid arthritis differ? Which form will most of us
eventually develop to some degree?
6 What is the physiological mechanism that causes some people to be allergic to a
specific antigen and others not to be allergic?
7 How do sickle cell trait and sickle cell disease differ? What is the prognosis of each
condition?
8 What are some of the primary causes of epilepsy? For cerebral palsy?
9 Can you explain how type 1 (insulin-dependent) diabetes mellitus and type 2 (noninsulin-dependent) diabetes mellitus differ with regard to causes and treatments?
10 Discuss the two general categories of depression.

QUESTIONS FOR PERSONAL CONTEMPLATION

1 Do you feel you could cope with a significant health problem at this time in your
life? If not, what steps might you take to prepare yourself for dealing with such a
condition in yourself or a loved one?
2 Do you know anyone who has or has had cancer? How did cancer affect that person's
life? In what ways? Do you feel that person dealt effectively with most aspects of the
disease? Why or why not?
3 How regularly do you perform either breast or testicular self-examinations? If you do
not do these on a regular basis, why not? Will you tell your close friends about these
important self-tests? Why or why not?
4 If you were diagnosed as having a terminal illness, how willing would you be to serve
as a subject in a research project that tested a potentially toxic experimental drug?
5 Which conditions in this chapter are you likely to develop and which are you not
likely to develop? Which ones might you conceivably "pass one" to your offspring?

REFERENCES

1 US Bureau of the Census: Statistical abstract of the United States: 1987, ed 107, Washington,
DC, 1987, US Department of Commerce.
2 Fisher, W: Oncologist, Personal interview, September 1987.
3 Bishop, JM: Cancer genes come of age, Cell 32:1010-1020, 1983.
4 Asok, A, and Hoffman, R: Oncogenes and the molecular biology revolution in cancer research,
Indiana Medicine 78:1081-1085, 1985.
5 Mertens, T: Geneticist, Personal interview, September 1987.
6 Friend, S, et al: A human DNA segment with properties of a gene that predisposes to retino-
blastoma and osteosarcoma, Nature 323:643-650, 1986.
7 American Cancer Association: Cancer Facts and Figures: 1987, Dallas, 1987, The Association.
8 Public Health Service Task Force on Women's Health Issues, Women's Health Report 100:87-
88, 1985.
9 Fisher, B: Ten-year results of a randomized clinical trial comparing radical mastectomy and total
mastectomy with or without radiation, The New England Journal of Medicine 312:674-686,
1985.

10   Health club tanning booths: risky business, The Physician and Sports Medicine 15:7, 59, 1987.

11   Songer, J: Oncologist, Personal interview, September 1987.

11a   Josey, W, Nahmias, A, and Naib, Z: Viruses and cancer of the lower genital tract, Proceedings of the American Cancer Society's National Conference on Gynecologic Cancer, Philadelphia, September, 1975, The Society, pp. 526-533.

12   Rosenberg, S, et al: A progress report on the treatment of 157 patients with advanced cancer using lymphokine-activated killer cells and interleukin-2 or high-dose interleukin alone, The New England Journal of Medicine 312:674-686, 1985.

13   Braunwald, E, et al: Harrison's Principles of Internal Medicine, ed 11, New York, 1987, McGraw-Hill Inc.

14   The National Center for Premenstural Syndrome and Menstrual Distress: Does PMS exist?, Boston, 1982, The Center.

15   Rubinow, D, and Stegge, J (discussants) and Kase, N, (moderator): Premenstrual Syndrome, 1983, The American College of Obstetricians and Gynecologists.

16   Egan, A: The selling of premenstrual syndrome, Ms. 10:26-31, 1983.

17   Benson, R, editor: Current obstetric and gynecologic diagnosis and treatment, ed 5, Los Altos, Calif, 1982, Lange Medical Books.

18   Kozak, G: Clinical diabetes mellitus, Philadelphia, 1982, WB Saunders Co.

19   The disease called "sugar diabetes," part 1 The Harvard Medical School Health Letter 10:1-7, 1985.

20   Ellenberg, M, and Rifkin, H: Diabetes mellitus: theory and practice, ed 3, New Hyde Park, New York, 1983, Medical Examination Publishing Co. Inc.

21   Firth, R, Bell, P, and Rizza, R: Effects of tolazamide and exogenous insulin on insulin action in patients with noninsulin-dependent diabetes mellitus, The New England Journal of Medicine, 314:20, 1280-1286, 1986.

22   Bogdonoff, M, Bressler, R, and Subak-Sharpe, G, editors: The physicians manual for patients, New York, 1984, Time Books.

23   Stein, J, editor: Internal Medicine, ed 2, Boston, 1986, Little, Brown & Co, Inc.

24   Riis, B, Thomsen, K, and Christiansen, C: Does calcium supplementation prevent postmenopausal bone loss? The New England Journal of Medicine 316:4, 173-177, 1987.

25   Groer, MW, and Shekleton, ME: Basic pathophysiology: a conceptual approach, St Louis, 1983, The CV Mosby Co.

26   Thibodeau, GA: Anatomy and physiology, St Louis, 1987, Times Mirror/Mosby College Publishing.

27   Schairer, C, Brinton, L, and Hoover, R: Methylxanthines and benign breast disease, American Journal of Epidemiology 124:4, 603-611, 1986.

28   Hunter, R: MD, personal interview, September 1987.

29   Ray, O, and Ksir, C: Drugs, society, and human behavior, ed 4, St Louis, 1987, Times Mirror/Mosby College Publishing.

30   Your aching back—what doctors can do about it: interview with Augustus White, MD, authority on back problems, US News & World Report 10:85-86, 1983.

31   Al-khatti, A, et al: Stimulation of fetal hemoglobin synthesis by erythropoietin in baboons, The New England Journal of Medicine 317:7, 415-420, 1987.

ANNOTATED READINGS

Bright, M: Living with your allergy, Englewood Cliffs, NJ, 1983, Prentice-Hall, Inc.
   The nature of allergies is described; numerous categories of allergies, including food, drug, pet, insect, and occupation-related allergies are reviewed.

Gach, M: The bum back book, Berkeley, Calif, 1983, CelestiaArts.
   A self-help book describing the role of acupressure in relieving back pain and problems generated by back tension. Includes illustrations and photographs depicting how acupressure is applied.

Gershwin, E, and Klingelhofer, E: Asthma—stop suffering start living, Reading, Mass, 1986, Addison-Wesley Publishing Co, Inc.
   A comprehensive look at the many types of asthma and their relationship to specific aspects of living such as exercise, pregnancy, diet, and occupational settings. Treatments, both conventional and unconventional, are discussed.

Jovanovic, J, Bierman, J, and Toohey, B: The diabetic woman, New York, 1987, Jermey P Tarcher, Inc.
   A broadly based account of the impact of diabetes on the lives of women. Pregnancy, fertility control, breastfeeding, weight loss, and medical care are discussed.

Lark, S: Dr. Susan Lark's premenstrual syndrome self-help book, Los Angeles, 1984, Forman Publishing, Inc.
   A very practical master plan for relieving over 150 symptoms of PMS. A woman's guide to feeling good all month.

Rosenbaum, EH: Can you prevent cancer? St Louis, 1983, The CV Mosby Co.
   Gives realistic guidelines for developing cancer-preventive life habits. Includes discussions on genetic counseling, diet, environment, smoking, and other life-style habits.

Smedley, H, and Stepney, R: Cancer what it is and how it's treated, New York, 1985, Basil Blackwell, Inc.
   Explains what cancer is, how it alters the body functions, and how it is treated. Risk factors are discussed. Both conventional and unconventional treatments are described.

CHAPTER 12

Infectious Diseases
A Shared Concern

Key Concepts

Infectious diseases continue to pose a threat to our society.

▪

Most common infectious diseases are caused by one of six types of pathogens.

▪

A pathogenic agent can be transmitted through the chain of infection.

▪

Within a new host, an infectious disease progresses through four distinct stages.

▪

The body protects itself from disease by using both its mechanical and biochemical defense systems.

▪

College students are susceptible to a variety of common infectious diseases.

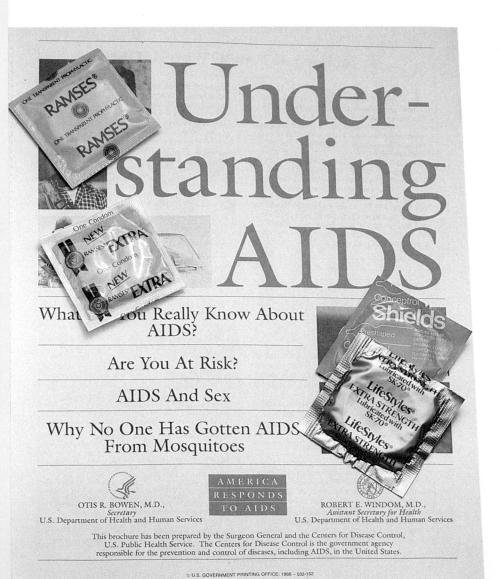

T*he information sticker we sometimes see attached to the door of restroom stalls succeeds in identifying the important concept underlying the study of infectious diseases:*

GONORRHEA: THE GIFT THAT KEEPS ON GIVING

We can see how this message can extend to other infectious diseases. Infectious diseases are, in a sense, "gifts" from people that we may pass on to other people. In this chapter we will explore the basic processes underlying the **etiological factors** and management of several of today's important infectious diseases.

INFECTIOUS DISEASES IN THE 1980s

Before the turn of the twentieth century, infectious diseases were the leading cause of death. These deaths came after exposure to the organisms that produced such diseases as smallpox, tuberculosis, influenza, whooping cough, typhoid, diphtheria, and tetanus. However, since the early 1900s the widespread use of antibiotic drugs as a treatment method and vaccinations as preventive therapy considerably reduced the numbers of persons dying from infectious diseases. People now die from chronic, long-term disease processes. We die from complications of cardiovascular disease, cancer, diabetes, liver damage, kidney disease, or other conditions.

Perhaps because of this shift in the causes of death, we have become rather complacent about infectious diseases. Many people cannot imagine that an infectious disease might ever really jeopardize their health or threaten their lives. Who ever heard of someone these days dying from whooping cough? Few people can say they know someone who is debilitated after having had measles, mumps, or even a sexually transmitted disease. We just do not believe that these can happen to us in this "high-tech, quick-cure" world we live in.

But as we shall see, such tragic consequences can happen. As a collective society, we have not fully realized that most harmful infectious diseases have not been eradicated. Today all too many parents are neglecting to have their children properly immunized against a wide variety of infectious diseases. Many young adults fail to realize the possible seriousness of such common diseases as influenza, measles, and the wide variety of sexually transmitted diseases. And, of course, AIDS and related conditions threaten millions of persons in many areas of the world. This chapter can make you more aware of some of the potentially serious infectious diseases, their causes, treatments, and methods of prevention. As a college-educated adult, you can use this information to keep yourself healthier and consequently happier and more productive throughout the rest of your life.

INFECTIOUS DISEASE TRANSMISSION

Infectious diseases can generally be transferred from person to person, although this is not always a direct transfer from one person to another. Infectious diseases can be especially dangerous because of their ability to spread to large numbers of people, producing **epidemics** or **pandemics.**

329

Pathogens

For a disease to be transferred, a person must come into contact with the disease-producing agent, or **pathogen.** When pathogens enter our bodies, they are sometimes able to resist our body defense systems, flourish, and produce a morbid (ill) state. We commonly call this morbid state an *infection.* Because of their small size, pathogens are sometimes referred to as microorganisms, microbes, or germs. As Table 12-1 indicates, many common infectious diseases are caused by *viruses, bacteria, fungi, protozoa, rickettsia,* and *parasitic worms.* The table also identifies some representative disease processes.

Table 12-1   Pathogens and Common Communicable Diseases

Pathogen	Description	Representative Disease Processes
Viruses	Smallest common pathogens; nonliving particles of DNA surrounded by a protein coat	Red measles, mumps, chickenpox, rubella, influenza, warts, colds, oral and genital herpes, shingles, AIDS, genital warts
Bacteria	One-celled microorganisms with sturdy, well-defined cell walls; three distinctive forms are spherical (cocci), rod-shaped (bacilli), and spiral-shaped (spirilla)	Tetanus, strep throat, scarlet fever, gonorrhea, syphilis, chlamydia, toxic shock syndrome, Legionnaires' disease, bacterial pneumonia, meningitis, diphtheria, food poisoning
Fungi	Plantlike microorganisms; molds and yeasts	Athlete's foot, ringworm, histoplasmosis, San Joaquin Valley fever, candidosis
Protozoa	Simplest animal form; generally one-celled organisms	Malaria, amebic dysentery, trichomoniasis vaginitis
Rickettsia	Viruslike organisms that require a host's living cells for growth and replication	Typhus, Rocky Mountain spotted fever, rickettsialpox
Parasitic worms	Multicellular organisms; represented by tapeworms, leeches, and roundworms	Abdominal pain, anemia, lymphatic vessel blockage, lowered antibody response, respiratory and circulatory complications

DNA

Cocci   Bacilli   Spirilla

Mold   Yeast

Amoeba

Rickettsia

Parasitic worms

Chain of Infection

The transmission of a pathogenic agent through the various links in the chain of infection forms the basis for an understanding of how diseases spread. Not every pathogenic agent will move all of the way through the chain of infection, because various links in the chain can be broken. Therefore the presence of a pathogen creates only the potential for a disease.

The first link in the chain of infection is the agent—the causal pathogen of a particular disease. This agent resides in a *reservoir*—the natural habitat of the pathogen. Reservoirs include such habitats as humans, animals, plants, soils, or discharges from humans and animals. Nonliving reservoirs (fingernails, dirty sheets, filthy restroom facilities) are sometimes called **fomites.** For an agent to be transferred, it must depart the reservoir from a *portal of exit.* Such departure points in humans include the mouth, nose, anus, open sores, and wounds. Blood (as in a transfusion) can also be considered a portal of exit.

Once having left the reservoir, the agent enters some route of transmission. Four common routes exist: (1) *direct transmission,* by kissing, touching, blood transfusions, sexual intercourse, or inhaling the fine droplets that are carried only a few feet by sneezing, talking, or coughing; (2) *indirect transmission,* by coming into contact with a pathogen by touching objects or fomites (towels, sheets, eating utensils, food products) already infected with the pathogen; (3) *airborne transmission,* by the transfer of agents through the air—suspended droplets can be transferred great distances in air or dust before coming into contact with a new host; and (4) *vector-borne transmission,* by the transfer of a pathogen by insects or animals. Flies, mosquitoes, and fleas are common vectors.

Once the agent is transferred, it must continue through the chain to the next link—the *portal of entry* into the new host. The new host's portals of entry are the points of invasion where the agent can enter the body—mouth, nose, ears, open sores, mucous membranes, or the urogenital system. The skin is also an entry point for many biting creatures (fleas, animals, flies) or blood-sucking insects (mosquitoes, leeches, ticks, chiggers).

The last link in the chain of infection is the establishment and proliferation of the agent in the *new host.* If the agent can overcome the host's resistance, it can produce an infection. The onset of the infectious process produces the signs and symptoms that in turn form a basis for the clinical diagnosis of a disease.

fomite
nonliving reservoir of a disease.

Stages of Infection

When a new host is assaulted by a pathogenic agent, a reasonably predictable sequence of events takes place. That is, the disease moves through four rather distinctive stages. You may be able to recognize these four stages of infection each time you catch a cold.

1 *The incubation stage.* This stage lasts from the time a pathogen enters your body until it multiplies significantly enough to produce recognizable characteristics (signs and symptoms) of the disease. The length of this stage can vary from a few hours to a month or more, depending on the agent and the host's resistance. This stage has been called a silent stage. Transmission of the pathogen to a new host is possible but not probable during this stage. Thus a host may be infected during this stage, but not infectious. AIDS is an exception to this rule.

The Four Stages
of Infection

1 Incubation
2 Prodromal
3 Peak
4 Recovery

2 *The prodromal stage.* The stage of incubation is followed by a short period during which the host may experience a variety of general signs and symptoms. Watery eyes, runny nose, slight fever, and overall tiredness (malaise, apathy) are indicative of this stage. These symptoms are nonspecific in nature and may not be so overwhelming that the host is forced to rest. During this stage, the pathogenic agent continues to multiply. Now the host is capable of transferring this pathogen to a new host should the appropriate links in the chain of infection be connected.

3 *The peak stage.* This stage, also called the *acme* or *acute stage,* is often the most unpleasant stage for the host. At this time, the disease reaches its highest point of manifestation. All of the clinical signs and symptoms for the particular disease can be seen or analyzed by appropriate laboratory tests. Communicability is most probable during this stage.

This stage can be likened to a pivotal military battle. During this peak stage, all of our available defense mechanisms are in the process of resisting further damage from the pathogen. For most of us, our body defense systems are sufficient to provide over 70 years of victories over invading microorganisms. We may harbor some infections throughout our lives, but never totally lose a battle.

4 *The recovery stage.* Also called the *convalescence stage,* this stage is characterized by victory over the invading agent. The pathogenic agent dies (or is reduced to an impotent level) and the host's signs and symptoms gradually disappear. Disease transmission during this stage is possible but not probable. Until the host's overall health has been strengthened, he or she may be especially susceptible to another (perhaps different) disease pathogen. Fortunately, after the recovery stage, further susceptibility to the causative agent should be reduced because of the body's buildup of immunity to that particular pathogen. This buildup of immunity is not certain, however. For example, many sexually transmitted diseases can be contracted repeatedly.

Identifying an infectious disease agent.

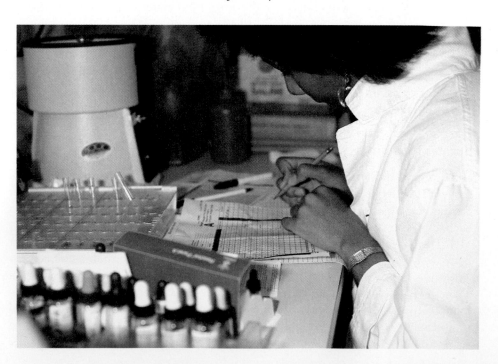

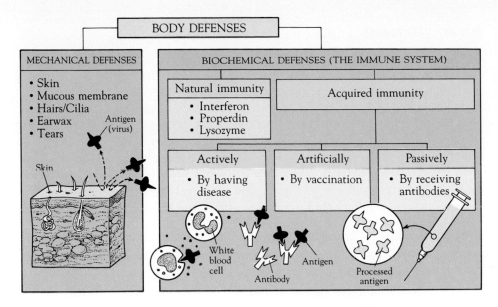

Figure 12-1
The body has a variety of defenses against invading organisms. Mechanical defenses are the body's first line of defense. Biochemical defenses include chemicals and antibodies that provide immunity against subsequent infections.

YOUR BODY'S RESPONSE TO PATHOGENIC AGENTS: DEFENSES

Much as a military installation is protected by a series of defensive alignments, so too is the body. These defenses can be initially classified as being either mechanical or biochemical (Figure 12-1). *Mechanical defenses* are "first line" defenses, since they physically separate the internal body from the external environment. Included among these are the skin, the mucous membranes, the respiratory and gastrointestinal tracts, the tiny hairs and cilia that filter incoming air, ear wax, and even tears. These perimeter defenses are more general than the biochemical defenses and serve primarily as a shield against foreign materials, which may contain pathogenic agents.

The second major classification of the body's defense resources is a *biochemical defense* system. This biochemical system is, in comparison to the mechanical system, far more specific, having as its primary mission the elimination of specific bacterial, viral, and fungal invaders. This biochemical system, usually referred to as the **immune system,** is subdivided into natural immunity and acquired immunity components.

immune system
system of biochemical and cellular elements that protect the body from invading pathogens and foreign materials.

Natural Immunity

The **natural immunity** component of the immune system incorporates specific white blood cells and a series of chemicals produced by the body that are capable of destroying or inactivating microorganisms or their toxins. Granulocytes and macrophages are specific white blood cells that attack and break down bacteria and other invading pathogens. Natural immunity also utilizes biochemical substances such as *interferon,* a protein that inactivates viruses; *properdin,* a large protein that destroys gram-negative bacteria; *polypeptides,* which also destroy gram-negative bacteria; and *lysozyme,* a polysaccharide capable of killing bacteria. Collectively, these chemicals provide the body with an important defense against a variety of pathogenic invaders.[1]

natural immunity
component of the immune system that uses specialized blood cells and chemicals produced by the body to destroy pathogens.

acquired immunity
major component of the immune system associated with the formation of antibodies and specialized blood cells that are capable of destroying pathogens.

actively acquired immunity
type of acquired immunity resulting from the body's response to naturally occurring pathogens.

artificially acquired immunity
type of acquired immunity resulting from the body's response to pathogens introduced into the body through immunizations.

passively acquired immunity
temporary immunity achieved by providing antibodies to a person exposed to a particular pathogen.

antibodies
chemical compounds produced by the body's immune system to destroy antigens and their toxins.

vaccination
medical procedure through which specially prepared antigens are introduced into the body for the purpose of activating the immune system.

antigens
disease-producing microorganism or foreign substance that, on entering the body, triggers an immune response.

sensitized lymphocytes
specialized white blood cells that produce lymphokine, a chemical that inactivates fungi, viruses, and cancer cells.

Acquired Immunity

Acquired immunity, a second major component of the body's immune system, involves a number of blood cells that have acquired the ability to recognize specific microorganisms and respond to them in a destructive fashion. This ability to recognize and respond, once initially developed, remains intact and will be activated should a subsequent invasion occur. Acquired immunity can be obtained in one of three ways. **Actively acquired immunity** develops when you have had a particular infectious disease. **Artificially acquired immunity** results when laboratory preparations containing weakened or killed pathogens are introduced into the body through *immunization.* **Passively acquired immunity** is a temporary form of immunity a person develops after receiving **antibodies** from another source.

The process of **vaccination** (also called immunization or inoculation) has been used for a hundred years to produce a state of acquired immunity in persons who have not yet experienced a particular disease. The **antigens** necessary for stimulating the body's immune system to produce the antibodies or **sensitized lymphocytes** are derived from dead microorganisms, toxins, or attenuated (weakened) microorganisms. The artificially acquired immunity resulting from vaccination is identical to that obtained from having contracted the disease. The advantage of vaccination over the actively acquired immunity you get from having survived the disease is that you will not experience the full effects of the disease.

If a person has been exposed to an antigen and he or she has no actively or artificially acquired immunity, it is possible for that person to receive short-term protection by receiving an injection of antibodies or sensitized lymphocytes. This passively acquired immunity lasts for 2 to 3 weeks if the antibodies are taken from another human. Antibodies or sensitized lymphocytes taken from an animal provide protection for a few days. Passive immunization is obviously a short-term solution, providing protection until such a time when the person can develop actively acquired immunity for that disease.

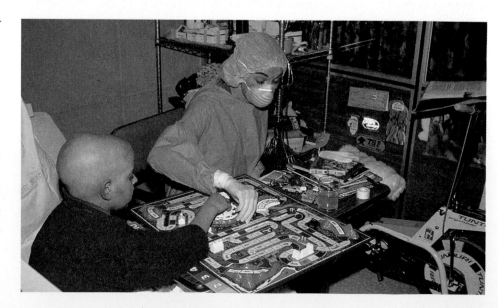

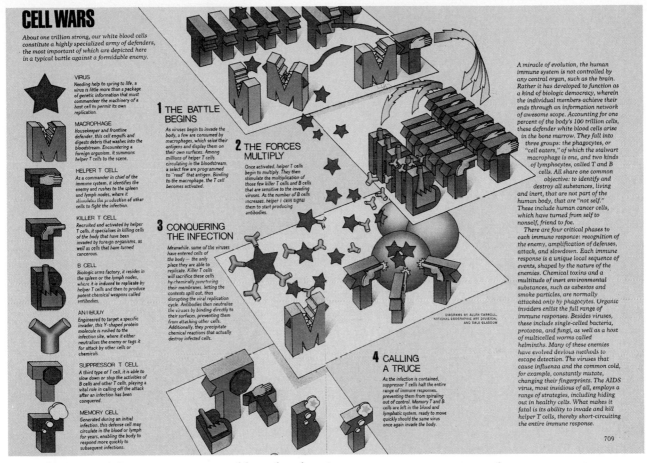

The four phases of the immune system and how they function.

All three forms of acquired immunity use two systems for attacking invading pathogens. The first system, *humoral immunity*, is primarily directed against bacterial invaders and reinvading viruses. The principal factors in humoral immunity are circulating white blood cells called *B-lymphocytes*. B-lymphocytes are capable of being converted into specialized cells called *plasma cells*. After making contact with bacterial or viral *antigens*, these plasma cells then are able to produce specific antibodies. It is currently thought that an activated plasma cell can produce approximately 2,000 identical antibodies per second over several days.[2]

Once produced by the plasma cells, the antibodies inactivate the viral or bacterial antigens in one of several specific ways. Antibodies produced by this initial contact with the antigen remain available to fight subsequent infections. Thus a host has developed actively acquired immunity to a specific antigen.

The second system, *cellular immunity*, occurs primarily in response to viruses, fungi, cancer cells, and foreign tissue (as in organ transplants).[2] Circulating white blood cells called *T-lymphocytes* form the basis for this form of immunity. Circulating T-lymphocytes are attracted by invading antigens. Four specialized forms of T-lymphocytes respond to an invading antigen: helper T-cells, killer T-cells, suppressor T-cells, and memory T-cells. (See figure above.) Each T-cell performs a specific role in protecting the body in response to the antigen.

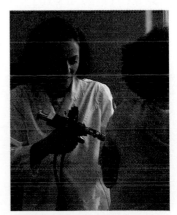

Vaccination provides artificially acquired immunity.

ETIOLOGICAL FACTORS AND MANAGEMENT OF SELECTED INFECTIOUS DISEASES OF THE YOUNG ADULT PERIOD

This section will focus on some of the common infectious diseases that are contracted or developed by college students, including some diseases that, although not especially common, have received much media attention in the past couple of years. We hope this information will provide some reference points you can use to judge your own disease susceptibility.

The Common Cold

The common cold, an acute, upper respiratory tract infection, must reign as mankind's supreme infectious disease. Also known as **acute rhinitis,** this highly contagious viral infection is caused by one of over 100 known rhinoviruses.[3] College students are easily at risk because they expose themselves to large numbers of people in crowded classrooms, residence halls, and social groups.

The signs and symptoms of a cold are fairly predictable. Runny nasal passages, watery eyes, general aches and pains, a listless feeling, and a slight fever may all accompany your cold in its early stages. Eventually your nasal passages swell and the inflammation may spread to the throat. Stuffy nose, sore throat, and coughing may follow. Since your senses of taste and smell are blocked, you probably will not feel like eating very much. Your body is telling you to rest.

And rest you should. After a few days, most of the cold's symptoms subside. In the meantime, isolate yourself from others, drink plenty of fluids, eat moderately, and rest. Please keep in mind that antibiotics are only effective against bacterial infections—not viral infections.

Your management of a cold can be aided by using some of the many over-the-counter cold remedies. These remedies will not cure your cold but may lessen the impact of the infection. Nasal decongestants, **expectorants,** cough syrups, and aspirin (or acetaminophen) can all provide some temporary relief. Use of some of these products for more than a few days is not recommended, however, since a **rebound effect** may occur.

If your cold appears to become more involved, as evidenced by prolonged chills, noticeable fever above 103° F, chest heaviness or aches, shortness of breath, coughing up a rust-colored mucus, or persistent sore throat or hoarseness, you should contact a physician. Always remember to blow your nose gently so as not to spread the infection to the *sinus cavities* or middle ear. Since colds are now thought to be transmitted most readily by hand contact, frequent handwashing and the use of tissues are recommended.

Influenza

Influenza is also an acute, contagious disease caused by a virus. Some influenza outbreaks have produced widespread death, as seen in the influenza pandemics of 1889-1890, 1918-1919, and 1957. The viral strains that produce this infectious disease (for example, Hong Kong, Asian, Victorian, swine, and influenza A, B, and C strains) have the potential for more severe complications than the viral strains that produce the common cold. The viral strain for a particular form of influenza enters the body through the respiratory tract. After brief incubation

---

acute rhinitis
the common cold; the sudden onset of nasal inflammation.

expectorants
drugs that help bring mucus and phlegm up from the respiratory system.

rebound effect
excessive congestion that results from the overuse of nosedrops and sprays.

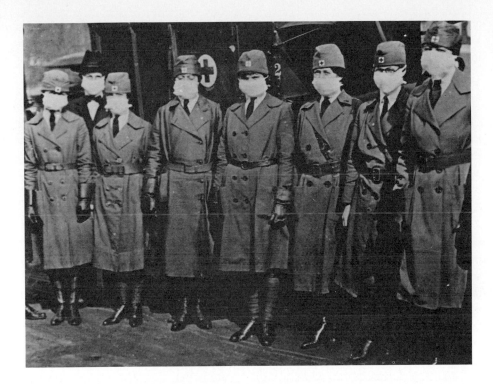

Members of the St. Louis Red Cross Motor Corps during the 1918 influenza epidemic.

and prodromal stages, the host develops signs and symptoms not just in the upper respiratory tract but throughout the entire body. These symptoms include fever, chills, cough, sore throat, headache, gastrointestinal disturbances, muscular pain, and **neuralgia.**

Except for possible *secondary bacterial infections,* antibiotics are not generally prescribed for people with influenza. For this reason you should not feel slighted if your physician recommends only aspirin, fluids, and rest. Some antiviral drugs, including amantadine hydrochloride for influenza A, hold promise for those persons who have developed a serious infection.[4]

Most young adults can cope with most of the milder strains of influenza that are prevalent each winter or spring season. Although we may be very uncomfortable for a while, most of us can return to our normal activities in about a week. However, pregnant women and older people—especially older people with additional health complications (heart disease, kidney disease, emphysema, chronic bronchitis)—are not so capable of handling this viral attack. They may quickly develop secondary bacterial complications (especially pneumonia), which can prove fatal. Each year in the United States, about 10,000 people die from flu and its resultant complications. In severe seasons, the death toll has reached 40,000.[5] Susceptible people must attempt to prevent an influenza infection from ever reaching them in the first place. Therefore flu vaccinations are routinely recommended for older people.

For strains that appear to be especially dangerous, most health authorities recommend that all of us receive a flu vaccination. This preventive approach attempts to confer artificially acquired immunity by inoculating us with the specific (though noninfectious) viral antigen. Some inoculations may include antigens for more than one strain of virus. These are the *polyvalent vaccines.* Two serious but extremely rare complications from flu vaccinations have been re-

neuralgia
painful inflammation of a nerve.

ported: allergic reactions and *Guillain-Barré syndrome*. Fortunately, flu vaccines subsequent to the swine flu vaccine in 1976 have not been associated with an increased frequency of Guillain-Barré syndrome.[5]

Mononucleosis

mononucleosis ("mono") viral infection characterized by weakness, fatigue, swollen glands, and low-grade fever.

Of all the common infectious diseases that a college student can contract, **mononucleosis ("mono")** can force a lengthy period of bed rest on you during a semester or quarter when you can least afford it. Other common diseases that can attack you can be managed with minimal amounts of disruption. However, the overall weakness and fatigue seen in many people with mono sometimes require a month or two of rest and recuperation.

Mono is a viral infection in which the body produces an excess number of *mononuclear leukocytes*. After uncertain, perhaps lengthy, incubation and prodromal stages, the acute symptoms of mono can appear, including weakness, headache, low-grade fever, swollen lymph glands (especially in the neck), and sore throat. Mental fatigue and depression are sometimes reported as side effects of mononucleosis. Usually after the acute symptoms disappear the weakness and fatigue remain—perhaps for a few months. Mono is clinically diagnosed by a *Monospot test*, a blood test that determines the percentage of white blood cells that are mononuclear leukocytes.

Since this disease is caused by a virus (Epstein-Barr virus), antibiotic therapy is not recommended. Treatment most often includes bed rest and the use of over-the-counter remedies for fever (aspirin or acetaminophen) and sore throat (lozenges).[3] Appropriate fluid intake and a well-balanced diet are also important in the recovery stages of mono. Fortunately, the body tends to develop actively acquired immunity to the mono virus, so subsequent infections of mono are unusual.

For years mono has been labeled the "kissing disease," perhaps by authoritarian adults who understood that mono tends to be relatively common among young people. Although it is true that the disease is seen most frequently in persons aged 15 to 24, mono is not highly contagious and is known to be spread by direct transmission in ways other than kissing. At this time, no vaccine has been developed to confer artificially acquired immunity to mononucleosis. The best preventive measures include the steps that you can take to increase your resistance to most infectious diseases: (1) eat a well-balanced diet, (2) exercise regularly, (3) sleep sufficiently, (4) use health care services appropriately, and (5) live in a reasonably healthy environment.

Chronic Epstein-Barr Virus Syndrome

Recently, a new illness has been reported in the medical literature that seems to strike mostly women in their thirties and forties. This illness produces severe exhaustion, fatigue, headaches, muscle aches, fever, inability to concentrate, and depression. The symptoms can last indefinitely and resemble those seen in mononucleosis.

First identified in 1985 during a possible outbreak in Nevada, chronic Epstein-Barr virus syndrome (CEBV) continues to be investigated as a valid disease.[6]

However, CEBV has been difficult to study. It has been called a mystery disease, since many factors are thought to be related to its development (for example, stress, weakened immune system, presence of other viruses, depression, and anxiety). Some skeptics argue that CEBV has become a generic, catch-all illness created for hypochondriacs who like to attribute their problems to a physical illness. Some have called this the "malaise of the '80s" or the "yuppie flu."[7] Until medical experts agree that this is truly a disease with identifiable causes, the debate about CEBV will probably continue.

Red Measles

Thought to be only a childhood disease, red measles (also called **rubeola** or common measles) has recently been seen in large numbers on some American college campuses. Red measles is the highly contagious type of measles characterized by a short-lived, relatively high fever (103° to 104° F) and a whole-body red spotty rash that lasts about a week. The other type of measles, *German measles* (**rubella** or 3-day measles), is a much milder form of measles that has serious implications for newborn babies of mothers who contracted this disease during pregnancy (see Chapter 10). Highly successful vaccines are now available for both varieties of measles and are usually given in the same injection. Women should receive these vaccinations *before* they become pregnant.

The outbreak of red measles among college students in the spring of 1983 again points to the fact that our society mistakenly believes that all infectious diseases have now been eliminated. In the spring of 1983, many college students contracted red measles. Public health experts realized that those who were contracting the disease either had never been vaccinated or had been vaccinated with a "killed" variety vaccine used before 1969. Only students who had already had red measles as children or who had been vaccinated with a "live" virus were guaranteed full immunity against the red measles virus. Since most of the students had not received this type of vaccine, nearly 50,000 immunizations were provided to students in Indiana alone.[8]

Unfortunately, 5% to 20% of today's college students still do not have documented immunity to measles and/or rubella and remain susceptible to these diseases.[9] Red measles should be avoided, because serious complications are known to take place in about 1 out of every 15 measles victims. These complications include pneumonia, deafness, and **encephalitis**. In unusual cases, brain damage and death can occur. Measles lowers one's resistance to other infections and, as some college students in 1983 realized, can severely jeopardize an academic quarter or semester. At this writing, only about half of American colleges require proof of vaccination when students enroll.[9] Have you been vaccinated? If not, we advise you to do so.

The method of rounding up children in a neighborhood and exposing them to a child who has an active case of measles is truly old-fashioned and dangerous. Rather, children should receive the recommended series of vaccinations from their health clinic or family physician. Many public school systems are requiring documented proof of immunization from a physician or clinic before children can attend classes. As an educated future parent, you should be conscientious about adhering to immunization schedules for your children.

rubeola
red or common measles.

rubella
German or 3-day measles.

encephalitis
inflammation of the brain.

toxic shock syndrome
potentially fatal condition
resulting from the proliferation of certain bacteria in
the vagina that enter the
general blood circulation.

Could You Have Toxic Shock Syndrome? Recognize Its Symptoms

Fever (102° F or above)
Headache
Vomiting
Sore throat
Diarrhea
Muscle aches
Sunburnlike rash
Low blood pressure
Bloodshot eyes
Disorientation
Reduced urination
Peeling of skin on the palms
    and soles of the feet

Toxic Shock Syndrome

Toxic shock syndrome (TSS), first reported in 1978,[10] made front-page head-lines in 1980, when it was reported by the Centers for Disease Control (CDC) that there was a connection between toxic shock syndrome and the presence of a specific bacterial agent (*Staphylococcus aureus*) in the vagina associated with the use of tampons. A 1980 CDC epidemiological study indicated that 98% of 928 women who developed TSS did so during a menstrual period. The highest incidence of TSS was in females in the 15 to 19 age group.[11]

TSS presents signs and symptoms as listed in the margin. Superabsorbent varieties of tampons apparently can irritate the vaginal lining three times more quickly than regular tampons.[12] This vaginal irritation is enhanced when the tampons remain in the vagina for long periods of time (over 5 hours). Once this irritation has begun, the staphylococcal bacteria (which are commonly present in the vagina) have relatively easy access to the victim's bloodstream. Prolifera-tion of these bacteria in the circulatory system produces the toxic shock syn-drome. Left untreated, the victim can die—usually as a result of cardiovascular failure. Fortunately, less than 10% of women diagnosed as having TSS actually die.

Although the extent of this disease is still quite limited (only about 3 to 6 cases per 100,000 women per year) and the mortality figures are low (comparable to those in women who use oral contraceptives), each woman should still exer-cise reasonable caution in the use of tampons during her period. Recommenda-tions are that (1) women should not use only tampons during their menstrual periods, and (2) women should not leave tampons in place for too long at a time.[12] Women should change tampons every few hours and intermittently use sanitary napkins. Tampons should not be used during sleep. Because the use of highly absorbent tampons increases the risk of TSS by 10 times over the use of regular tampons, medical experts now recommend that women use the least absorbent tampon that fits their needs.[13] Some physicians recommend that all tampon use be curtailed if a woman wants to be extraordinarily safe from TSS.

The incidence of TSS has dropped significantly since the early 1980s. Possible reasons for this decrease are the removal of certain superabsorbent tampons from the market, clearer warnings written on the tampon package inserts, and wom-en's overall increased knowledge of and concern about TSS.

Acquired Immune Deficiency Syndrome (AIDS)

Acquired immune deficiency syndrome (AIDS) is rapidly becoming the most devastating infectious disease to have occurred in modern times. AIDS was first identified in 1980. The Surgeon General has predicted that by the end of 1991 an estimated 270,000 cases of AIDS will have occurred, with 179,000 deaths. Fur-thermore, by 1991 between $8 and $16 billion will be required annually to care for people who have AIDS.[14] The toll in human lives and the financial burden AIDS will place on our health care system make AIDS a frightening disease.

Cause of AIDS

AIDS is caused by a virus that attacks the T-helper lymphocytes of the immune system (see p. 335). This virus has been called HTLV-III (human T-lympho-

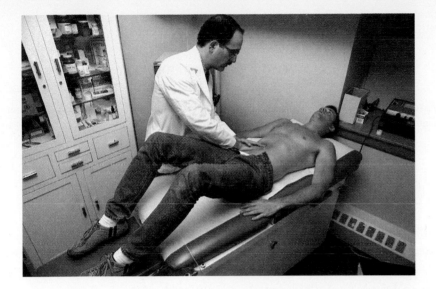

Examination of an AIDS patient.

tropic virus, type III), but HIV (human immune deficiency virus), is now the more commonly recognized name. For simplicity, we will call it the "AIDS virus" in this discussion.

When the AIDS virus attacks T-helper cells, the victim loses the ability to fight off a variety of infections that a person with a normal immune system could destroy. AIDS victims become vulnerable to infection by bacteria, protozoa, fungi, and a number of viruses and malignancies. Such infections are called "opportunistic infections," since they develop when the immune system is weakened.

Two diseases that commonly develop in AIDS patients are a lung infection, *Pneumocystis carinii* pneumonia, and a skin cancer called Kaposi's sarcoma. These diseases are rare in people with intact immune systems; however, about 78% of AIDS patients have had one or both of these diseases.[15] The AIDS virus can also invade the nervous system and cause brain damage. More than 50% of all persons diagnosed with AIDS have died. The breakdown of AIDS cases is given in the margin.

How is AIDS spread?

AIDS cannot be contracted easily. The chances of contracting AIDS through casual contact with AIDS patients at work, school, or at home are extremely rare or nonexistent.[14] AIDS is known only to be spread by direct sexual contact involving the exchange of body fluids (including blood, semen, vaginal secretions, and saliva), the sharing of intravenous drug needles, transfusion or infected blood or blood products, and perinatal transmission (from an infected mother to a fetus or newborn baby). For the AIDS virus to be transmitted, it must enter the bloodstream of the noninfected person. The AIDS virus enters the bloodstream of noninfected persons through contaminated blood or needles and tears in body tissues lining the rectum, mouth, and reproductive system. Current research also indicates that AIDS is not transmitted by insects.[16] Although the AIDS virus has been found in tears and saliva, the concentration has been too little to support transmission.

The Scope of the Problem

According to the Centers for Disease Control, the persons most likely to develop AIDS are homosexual or bisexual males and intravenous drug users. As of July 1987, the breakdown of AIDS cases was as follows[15]:

Homosexual or bisexual males	66%
Intravenous drug users	17%
Homosexual and bisexual males who also are intravenous drug users	8%
Heterosexuals	4%
Undetermined	3%
Blood transfusion recipients	2%
Hemophiliacs	1%
TOTAL	101%

*The sum of cases is 101% because an individual may be counted in more than one category.

Table 12-2   **Spectrum of HIV Infection**

	Asymptomatic	ARC (AIDS-related complex)	AIDS
External signs	No symptoms Looks well	Fever Night sweats Swollen lymph glands Weight loss Diarrhea Minor infections Fatigue	Kaposi's sarcoma Pneumocystis carinii pneumonia and other opportunistic infections Neurological disorders
Incubation	Invasion of virus to 3 months	Several months to 10 years	Several months to 10 years
Internal level of infection	Antibodies are produced Immune system remains intact Positive antibody test	Antibodies are produced Immune system weakened Positive antibody test	Immune system deficient Positive antibody test
Possible to transmit HIV?	Yes	Yes	Yes

What are the signs and symptoms of AIDS?

Most persons infected with the AIDS virus initially feel well and have no symptoms. The incubation period for AIDS is generally considered to be from 6 months to 10 years or more, with the current average being 7 years. Infected persons who are asymptomatic are still able to transmit the virus.

Eventually, many persons infected with the AIDS virus develop signs and symptoms that may include tiredness, fever, loss of appetite and weight, diarrhea, night sweats, and swollen lymph glands (lymph nodes)—usually in the neck, armpits, or groin. Anyone who has these symptoms for 2 weeks should see a physician.

These infected patients seem to develop only these signs and symptoms without actually developing the classic disease we know as AIDS. These patients are said to have developed AIDS-related complex (ARC). ARC patients remain infected with the AIDS virus and are capable of transmitting the virus to others. The precise percentage of ARC patients who eventually will develop classic AIDS is not known, although the percentage is expected to be high (see Table 12-2).

How is AIDS diagnosed?

The Centers for Disease Control has established specific criteria that physicians and researchers use to define AIDS.[17] In addition to a clinical examination and laboratory tests for accompanying infections, AIDS is diagnosed by a simple blood test that detects the presence of antibodies to the AIDS virus. Within a few weeks after exposure to the AIDS virus, a person's body will develop antibodies. The presence of these antibodies indicates that a person has been exposed to the AIDS virus—not that a person has AIDS or will develop AIDS for certain. It is estimated that up to 1.5 million persons in the United States have been infected with the AIDS virus.

This antibody test is now used to screen donated blood and plasma to help prevent cases of AIDS that come from blood transfusions or the use of blood products (such as factor VIII used by hemophilia patients). *A person cannot contract AIDS by donating blood or plasma.*

Treatment for AIDS

Presently there is no cure for AIDS. Physicians are limited to treating a patient's opportunistic infections on a case-by-case basis. Even the most optimistic estimates indicate that a vaccine to prevent AIDS may not be developed for a number of years. Because the AIDS virus mutates rather easily, a vaccine will be extremely difficult to develop.

The search for an antiviral drug to kill the AIDS virus continues. For some patients, one drug that seems helpful in inhibiting the replication of the AIDS virus is azidothymidine (AZT). AZT does not restore normal immune function and is not considered a cure for AIDS. Two principal drawbacks to this drug are its toxicity (it suppresses bone marrow function) and its expense (a single year of full-dose therapy costs over $10,000). At this time, AZT is administered only to AIDS patients who are likely to benefit from the therapy and whose physicians first enroll them with the Burroughs Wellcome Pharmaceutical Company (the current manufacturer of AZT).[18]

Prevention of AIDS

Can AIDS be prevented? The answer is a definite "yes." There are a number of steps an individual can take to reduce the risk of contracting and transmitting the AIDS virus. All of these steps involve understanding one's behavior and the methods by which the AIDS virus can be transmitted. The U.S. Public Health Service has provided recommendations (1) for the general public, (2) for persons

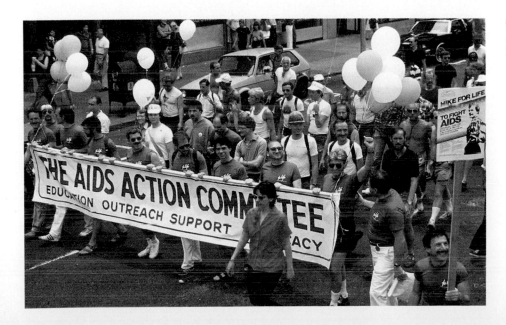

Community support for AIDS education is increasing.

at increased risk of infection, and (3) for persons with a positive result to an AIDS antibody test. The Public Health Service has a toll-free AIDS telephone hotline (1-800-342-AIDS) and local or state hotlines may exist in your area. Keep informed about AIDS!

The best preventive action is sound public education about AIDS. As college-educated persons, you are in one of the best positions to be fully aware of this epidemic. You should have easy access to library materials and resource persons to help you answer any questions you have about AIDS. The box below lists safe sex practices that will reduce your risk of contracting AIDS.

Concern and hysteria about AIDS

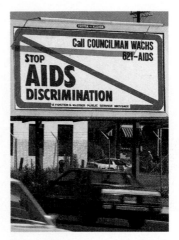

Strong feelings are associated with AIDS.

Not surprisingly, concern about AIDS has caused many young people to change their sexual behavior. In a recent Gallup poll three of four unmarried people over age 18 said that they have changed their sexual habits because they feared contracting AIDS. Approximately one third of those polled reported more frequent use of condoms, one third said they had fewer sexual partners, and one third said that they question their partners more closely about their sexual histories.[19] Students in our classes also report that their concern about AIDS has affected both their dating practices and attitudes toward casual sex.

For many people concern about AIDS has developed into a near-hysterical fear of the disease. This fear increases the discrimination that will be felt by the gay community and people who test positive for the AIDS virus.[20] Despite overwhelming scientific evidence indicating that AIDS is not contracted through casual contact, some people remain terrified that they might "catch" the disease. These people seem to be searching for absolute answers concerning the transmission of AIDS.

As with all other medical questions, absolute 100% guarantees are impossible to provide. We live in a world in which medical experts can only supply us with statistical probabilities about the likelihood of developing serious illnesses, such

Safer Sex Practices: Reduce Your Risk

- Know the name and address of your sex partner.
- Limit your sex partners.
- Always use condoms correctly and consistently.
- Avoid contact with body fluids, feces, and semen.
- Curtail use of drugs that impair good judgment.
- Never share hypodermic needles.
- Refrain from sex with known IV drug abusers.*
- Avoid sex with AIDS patients, those with signs and symptoms of AIDS, and the partners of high risk individuals.*
- Get regular tests for STD infections.
- Do not insert any foreign objects into the rectum.
- Practice proper hygiene (shower before and after sex).

*Recent studies indicate that the elimination of high-risk persons as sexual partners is the single most effective "safe sex" practice that can be implemented.

The Latest AIDS Position

Controversy concerning the prevalence of HIV in the heterosexual population has been generated by Masters, Johnson, and Kolodny in a book entitled, *Crisis: Heterosexual Behavior in The Age of AIDS.* The authors contend that the federal government is understating the risk heterosexuals have of contracting AIDS.

Masters, Johnson, and Kolodny suggest that HIV can be contracted by heterosexuals not only through sexual relations and intravenous drug use, but also by contact with an open wound (such as a small cut) of an infected person. The authors also contend that the blood supply remains a source of transmission to a greater extent than that admitted by the government.

Masters, Johnson, and Kolodny's theories regarding the risk to heterosexuals remain to be proven. Until better data is available, their book is being perceived as "alarmist."

as cancer, pneumonia, Alzheimer's disease, or heart disease. However, when it comes to AIDS, some people are not satisfied with statistical assurances. They demand statistical absolutes. When these absolutes cannot be promised, they rebel—sometimes in ways that resemble lynch mobs at the turn of the century.

AIDS hysteria has developed in some communities that have allowed children infected with the AIDS virus (through no fault of their own) to attend public schools. Concerned parents have led boycotts, petitioned school boards, and picketed schools where children with AIDS have been admitted.[21] Families of these children have been physically threatened, and their houses have been fire-bombed.

It is statistically more likely that a child will die while being transported to school than from contracting AIDS through casual contact with a fellow student. Only through aggressive public health education can we hope to allay the insecurities some people have about AIDS. The box above gives recent theories concerning AIDS transmission.

SEXUALLY TRANSMITTED DISEASES

Sexually transmitted diseases (STDs) were once referred to as venereal diseases (for Venus, the Roman goddess of love). Today the term veneral disease has been superseded by the broader term sexually transmitted disease. The current emphasis is on the successful prevention and treatment of STDs rather than on the ethics of sexuality. Hence this material appears in this chapter on infectious diseases rather than in a chapter on sexual behavior. These diseases are, first and foremost, medical problems—problems that have the potential for causing infertility, birth defects, and long-term disability.

This section will focus on the most frequently diagnosed STDs among college students (chlamydia, gonorrhea, herpes genitalis, syphilis, and pubic lice). A short section follows covering common vaginal infections, some of which may occur without sexual contact.

sexually transmitted diseases (STDs)
infectious diseases that are spread primarily through intimate sexual contact.

Chlamydia (Nonspecific Urethritis)

chlamydia
the most prevalent sexually transmitted disease. Caused by a nongonococcal bacterium.

Chlamydia is considered the most prevalent STD in the United States today. Chlamydial infections occur an estimated 5 times more frequently than gonorrhea and up to 10 times more frequently than syphilis. Since physicians are not required to report cases of chlamydia to the Centers for Disease Control, the true extent of the disease is not known.

Chlamydia trachomatis is the bacterial agent that causes the chlamydial infection. Chlamydia is the most common cause of nonspecific urethritis (NSU).[22] NSU refers to infections of the **urethra** and surrounding tissues that are not caused by the bacterium responsible for gonorrhea. Only when a culture smear test for suspected gonorrhea proves negative do clinicians diagnose NSU, usually by calling it chlamydia. About 80% of men with chlamydia indicate gonorrhea-like signs and symptoms, including painful urination and a whitish pus discharge from the penis. As in gonorrheal infections, most women report no overt signs or symptoms. A few women might exhibit a mild urethral discharge, painful urination, and swelling of *vulval* tissues. Whereas oral forms of penicillin are used in the treatment of gonococcal infections, oral tetracycline or doxycycline is prescribed for chlamydia and other NSUs.[22]

urethra
passageway through which urine leaves the urinary bladder.

As with all STDs, both sexual partners should receive treatment to avoid the "ping-pong" effect. This effect refers to the back-and-forth reinfection that occurs among couples when only one partner receives treatment. Further, as with other STDs, having chlamydia does not effectively confer actively acquired immunity.

Unresolved chlamydia can lead to the same negative health consequences that result from untreated gonorrheal infections. Initially your body's immune system might contain the infection to a subclinical level, where you temporarily exhibit no ill effects. However, in men the pathogens can invade and damage the deeper reproductive structures (the prostate gland, the seminal vesicles, and the Cowper's glands). Sterility can result. The pathogens can spread further and produce joint problems (arthritis) and heart complications (damaged heart valves, blood vessels, and heart muscle tissue).

pelvic inflammatory disease (PID)
acute or chronic infection of the peritoneum or lining of the abdominopelvic cavity; associated with a variety of symptoms and a potential cause of sterility.

In women the initial invasion sites are the urethra or the cervical area. If not properly treated, the invasion can reach the deeper pelvic structures, producing a syndrome called **pelvic inflammatory disease (PID).** The inner uterine wall (endometrium), the fallopian tubes, and any contiguous structures may be attacked to produce this painful syndrome. A variety of further complications can result, including sterility and **peritonitis.** Infected women can transmit a chlamydial infection to the eyes and lungs of newborn children during a vaginal delivery.[22] For both men and women the early detection of chlamydia and other NSUs is of paramount concern.

peritonitis
inflammation of the peritoneum or lining of the abdominopelvic cavity.

Gonorrhea

Probably the second most common STD, gonorrhea is caused by a bacterial pathogen *(Neisseria gonorrhoeae).* In men this bacterial agent can produce a milky white discharge from the penis, accompanied by painful urination. About 80% of men who contract gonorrhea report varying degrees of these two symptoms. The other 20% of men with gonorrhea are *asymptomatics;* that is, they

Personal Assessment

What is Your Risk of Contracting a Sexually Transmitted Disease?

A variety of factors interact to determine your risk of contracting a sexually transmitted disease (STD). This inventory is intended to provide you with an estimate of your level of risk.

Circle the number in each row that best characterizes you. Enter that number on the line at the end of the row (score line). After assigning yourself a number in each row, total the number appearing in the score column. Your total score will allow you to interpret your risk in contracting an STD.

							Points
Age	1 0-9	3 10-14	4 15-19	5 20-29	3 30-34	2 35 +	_____
Sexual Practices	0 Never engage in sex	1 One sex partner	2 More than one sex partner but never more than one at a time	4 Two to five sex partners	6 Five to ten sex partners	8 Ten plus sex partners	_____
Sexual Attitudes	0 Will not engage in premartial sex	1 Premartial sex is okay if it is with future spouse	8 Any kind of premarital sex is okay	1 Extramarital sex is not for me	7 Extramarital sex is okay	8 Believe in complete sexual freedom	_____
Attitudes Toward Contraception	1 Would use condom to prevent pregnancy	1 Would use condom to prevent STDs	6 Would never use a condom	5 Would use the birth control pill	4 Would use other contraceptive measure	8 Would not use anything	_____
Attitudes Toward STD	3 Am not sexually active so I do not worry	3 Would be able to talk about STD with my partner	4 Would check an infection to be sure	6 Would be afraid to check out an infection	6 Can't even talk about an infection	6 STDs are no problem—easily cured	_____

Your total points _____

Interpretation

5-8   Your risk is well below average
9-13   Your risk is below average
14-17 Your risk is at or near to average
18-21 Your risk is moderately high
22 +   Your risk is high

show no overt signs of the disease. These figures are approximately reversed for women: only about 20% of women are *symptomatic* and thus report varying degrees of frequent, painful urination, with a slimy yellow-green discharge from the vagina or urethra. Oral sex with an infected partner can produce a gonorrheal infection of the throat (pharyngeal gonorrhea). Gonorrhea can also be transmitted to the rectal areas of both men and women.

Diagnosis of gonorrhea is made by a culture smear test in which a cotton swab transfers the discharge onto a culture medium. After being incubated for a couple of days, the specific bacterium can be identified through a microscope. Antibiotic treatment regimens include use of penicillin, tetracycline, ampicillin, or other drugs. The specific use of one or more of these drugs depends on physician preference, site of infection, concurrent STD infections, and one's allergic response to penicillin. Some strains of gonorrhea (penicillin-resistant strains) are much more difficult to treat than others.[23] Follow-up cultures should be obtained from the infected sites 4 to 7 days after completion of the treatment plan. It should be noted that the treatment methods for NSU and gonorrhea are overwhelmingly effective.

Transmission of gonorrhea to newborns is possible. Thus it is imperative that proper prenatal care includes *endocervical cultures* for gonococcal bacteria. This preventive care can prevent the bacterium from being present in the mother's vagina during childbirth. If gonorrhea is present in the vagina during childbirth, a newborn could easily contract the infection in the mucous membranes surrounding the eyes. The resultant infection, *gonococcal ophthalmia,* is highly contagious and can quickly lead to blindness.[22] Most states still require that silver nitrate or other appropriate antibiotic (in eyedrop form) be administered to all newborns to prevent this infection.

Herpes Simplex Infections

Public health officials think that the sexually transmitted genital herpes virus infection rivals NSU and gonorrhea as the most prevalent STD. In fact, some researchers estimate that 25% to 30% of the adult population is infected with the genital herpes virus. However, because most persons remain asymptomatic for genital herpes and physicians are not required to report cases of this disease, we may never fully realize the magnitude of this condition. Herpes is really a

shingles
viral infection affecting the
nerve endings of the skin.

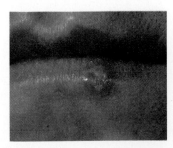

Oral herpes.

family of over 50 viruses, some of which produce recognized diseases in humans (chickenpox, **shingles,** mononucleosis, and others). One subgroup called herpes simplex 1 virus (HSV-1) produces an infection called *labial herpes* (oral or lip herpes). Labial herpes produces common fever blisters or cold sores seen around the lips and oral cavity. Herpes simplex 2 virus (HSV-2) is a different strain that produces similar clumps of blisterlike lesions in the genital region. Laypersons have referred to this second type of herpes as the STD type, although both types produce identical clinical pictures. (The structural differences in these strains are seen only through an electron microscope.) Both forms can exist at either site. Oral-genital sexual practices have resulted in from 10% to 50% of genital herpes cases now being caused by HSV-1.[22]

The herpes virus is a contact infectious agent; it is not an airborne agent. We contract this pathogen by physical contact with someone who has an active lesion present. Most of us initially contracted labial herpes in childhood when we were kissed by loving relatives—relatives with active fever blisters. People who today have the genital form of herpes probably contracted herpes by having intercourse with someone with an active lesion in his or her genital region. Of course, it is also possible to self-inoculate the genital region by touching an active labial blister and touching one's own genital region. Also, oral sex can transmit HSV-1 and HSV-2 strains to either site.

Herpes appears as a single sore or as a small cluster of blisterlike sores. These sores burn, itch, and (for some) become quite painful. The infected person might also report swollen lymph glands, muscular aches and pains, and fever. Some patients feel weak and sleepy when their blisters are present. The lesions may last from a few days to a few weeks. A week is the average time for active viral shedding. Then the blisters begin scabbing and new skin is formed.

Herpes is an interesting virus for several reasons. It can lie dormant for extended periods in the nerve clusters near the cheek-bone (the trigeminal nerve ganglia) or in the nerve cluster near the tailbone (the sacral ganglia). For reasons not well understood, but perhaps related to stress, diet, or overall health, the viral particles can be stimulated to travel along the nerve pathways to the skin and then create an active infection. Thus herpes can be considered a recurrent infection. Fortunately for most people recurrent infections are less severe than the initial episode and do not last as long.[22] Herpes is also interesting because, unlike most STDs, no treatment method has been successful at killing the virus. Acyclovir (Zovirax), in oral, ointment, and intravenous forms, has been used successfully in reducing the frequency, duration, and severity of genital herpes infections in certain groups of patients.[22] There are also some medications that may provide symptomatic relief.

Diagnosis of genital herpes is almost always made by a clinical examination. Currently used blood tests and tissue cultures can confirm the clinical diagnosis, but these are quite expensive and time consuming.

Herpes can also produce further complications:

1 Newborn babies are especially susceptible to the virus should they come into contact with an active lesion during the birth process. Newborns have not developed the defense capabilities to resist the invasion. They can quickly develop a systemic, general infection (neonatal herpes) that is often fatal, or local infections that produce permanent brain damage or blindness. Fortunately, most of these possible problems can be prevented through proper prenatal care. If there is any chance that the viral particles may be present at birth, a **cesarean section** delivery will be performed. This may reduce the likelihood of herpes transmission.

2 *Herpes keratitis* is a corneal infection of the eye that can occur if the viral particles are spread to the eye. This infection, if untreated with antiviral drugs, produces the second most common form of blindness caused by a disease process (next to glaucoma). Most cases are thought to be a result of self-inoculation—perhaps by touching a fever blister from the lip and rubbing the eye or by cleaning a contact lens in your mouth.

3 *Herpes encephalitis* is a rare form of brain infection that occurs when the herpes virus travels along nerve pathways to the brain. Early treatment with antiviral drugs may prevent this often fatal infection.

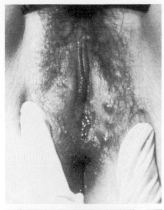
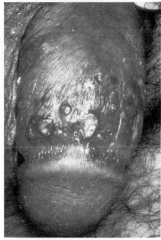

Genital herpes.

cesarean section
surgical removal of a fetus
through the abdominal wall.

Pap smear
cancer screening procedure in which cells removed from the cervix are examined.

4 An increased link with cervical cancer and herpes genitalis exists in women. A woman with herpes in the genital region is more likely to develop cervical cancer than a woman without the infection. Of course, this is only one of a few suggested correlates with cervical cancer (two others are intercourse at an early age and multiple sex partners). Fortunately, a **Pap smear** can detect cervical cancer in the early stages of development.

The best prevention against ever getting a herpes infection is to avoid all direct contact with a person who has an active infection. Do not kiss someone with a fever blister—or let them kiss you (or your children) if they have an active lesion. Do not share drinking glasses or eating utensils. Do not have intimate sexual contact with someone who displays the blisterlike clusters or rash. (Condoms are only marginally helpful and cannot protect against lesions on the female vulva or the lower abdominal area of the male.) Be careful not to self-inoculate yourself by touching a blister and then touching any other part of your body.

If you still manage to contract herpes, or if you already have some form of it, realize that it is not the end of the world. You will just have to be so meticulous that you do not further inoculate yourself or transmit the virus to others. Yes, you can still lead a normal life in all other respects. You can still have friends and lovers, and you can still bear children. Perhaps an antiviral drug will soon be developed that can effectively kill the virus completely. Until this time, try to keep a positive outlook and remember that you are not alone. At least as many adults have some form of herpes as those who do not have it.

Telling Your Partner About Herpes

Although herpes rarely has serious consequences, the lesions tend to reappear and are infectious. It is important to talk openly with your partner about this sexually transmitted disease. Here are some tips to make things easier:

Educate yourself.
  Be aware that herpes is rarely dangerous.
  Learn when the disease is most contagious (during the eruption and blister stage), and when sex is safest.

Choose the right time to talk.
  Discuss herpes with your partner only after you have gotten to know each other.

Listen to your partner.
  Be prepared to answer any questions that he or she may have.

Together, put things in perspective.
  Keep a positive outlook.
  Remember that you are not alone.
  Be aware that using a condom and abstaining from coitus during the most infectious period can prevent transmission of the disease.
  Although there is no known cure, research continues on an antiviral drug.
  Join a local support group together.

Genital Warts

Caused by a virus, genital warts are not considered especially serious. Found most commonly on the penis or scrotum, labia, or around the anus, genital warts can spread and should be reported to a physician. These pinkish-white lesions may be found in raised clusters that resemble tiny heads of cauliflower. Methods of treatment are often successful and include cryosurgery (freezing), electrocautery (burning), and surgical removal, and a topical agent (podophyllin).

Syphilis

Like gonorrhea, syphilis is caused by a bacterium (*Treponema pallidum*) and is transmitted almost exclusively by sexual intercourse. The incidence of syphilis, a CDC-reportable disease, is far lower than that of gonorrhea, however. For every 100 reported cases of gonorrhea, only about 3 cases of syphilis are reported.[24] Surely herpes and chlamydia are also much more common than syphilis. However, since the occurrence of syphilis seems to be increasing we have provided an overall summary of syphilis and its distinctive stages in the box on p. 352.

Pubic Lice

Three types of lice infect humans: the head louse, the body louse, and the pubic louse all feed on the blood of the host. Except for the relatively uncommon body louse, these tiny insects do not carry diseases. They are, however, quite annoying.

Pubic lice, also called *crabs*, attach themselves to the base of the pubic hairs, where they live and attach their eggs (nits). These eggs move into a larval stage after 1 week, and after 2 more weeks develop into mature adult crab lice.

People usually notice they have a pubic lice infestation when they are confronted with intense itching in the genital region. The lice and their tiny nits are sometimes visually evident. Fortunately, both prescription and over-the-counter creams lotions, and shampoos are extremely effective in killing both the lice and their eggs.

Lice are not transmitted exclusively through sexual contact, but also by contact with bedsheets and clothes that may be contaminated. You should be careful when you borrow a spare dormitory bed on a weekend when you visit friends at another college! Should you inadvertently develop a pubic lice infestation, you will have to treat yourself, your clothes, your sheets, and your furniture.

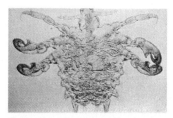

Pubic louse.

Vaginal Infections

A large number of bacteria and other microorganisms can cause vaginal discomfort and discharge.[25] Two common pathogens produce uncomfortable vaginal infections in women. The first is the yeast or fungus pathogen *Candida (Monilia) albicans*, which produces the classic yeast infection often called *thrush*. These organisms, commonly found in the vagina, seem to proliferate when some unusual stressor (pregnancy, use of birth control pills, diabetes, use of antibiotics) affects a woman's body. The yeast proliferation (candidosis) is easily noticed by

Syphilis: The On-Again Off-Again STD

Although we may think less often of syphilis than other sexually transmitted diseases, it remains a serious disease that if left untreated is capable of causing death. The course taken by syphilis is well established.

INFECTION

The bacterium of syphilis, *Treponema pallidum,* a spirochete, is transmitted from infected person to new host through intimate contact. Moist, warm tissue, such as that lining the reproductive, urinary, and digestive systems, offers an ideal environment for the agent.

INCUBATION

After infection, an asymptomatic period of from 10 to 90 days gives way to the characteristic first stage of the disease.

FIRST STAGE

Lasting 1 to 5 weeks, the first stage of syphilis is associated with the formation of a small, raised, painless sore called a *chancre.* In 90% of women and 50% of men this highly infectious lesion is not easily identified; thus treatment is generally not sought. Lymphatic enlargement in the groin may also be observed.

SECOND STAGE

The extremely contagious second stage of the disease is seen 2 to 6 months after initial infection. Because the infectious agents are now systemic, symptoms may include a generalized body rash, a sore throat, or a patchy loss of hair. A blood test (VDRL) will be positive, and treatment can be effectively administered. If untreated, the second stage will subside within 2 to 6 weeks. This is a stage during which syphilis can easily by transmitted by a pregnant woman to her fetus. Congenital syphilis often results in stillbirth or an infant born with a variety of life-threatening complications. Early treatment of an infected pregnant woman can prevent congenital syphilis.[22]

LATENT STAGE

After the second stage subsides, an extended period of noninfectiousness is seen. The infectious agents remain dormant within the body cells, and few clinical signs exist during this stage.

LATE STAGE

Syphilis can recur for a third time 15 to 25 years after initial contact. In late stage syphilis, tissue damage will be profound and irreversible. Damage to the cardiovascular system, central nervous system, eyes, and skin occurs, and death from the effects of the disease is likely.

TREATMENT

Syphilis is treated with pencillin, tetraycline, or erythromycin. Such treatment can kill the pathogen at any stage of the infection, but it cannot reverse the physical damage caused during the late stage of syphilis.

a white or cream-colored vaginal discharge that resembles cottage cheese. Vaginal itching and swelling are also commonly reported. Treatment often consists of an oral antibiotic or antibiotic douche to reduce the organisms to a normal level. (Men rarely report this monilial infection, although some may report mildly painful urination or a mild discharge at the urethral opening or beneath the foreskin of the penis.)

A second common agent that produces a vaginal infection is the protozoan *Trichomonas vaginalis*. This parasite can be transmitted through sexual intercourse or by contact with contaminated (often damp) objects, such as towels, clothing, or toilet seats that may contain some vaginal discharge. Men infrequently contract this infection (trichomoniasis) but may harbor the organism without realizing it. In women, this "trich" infection produces a foamy, yellow-green, foul-smelling discharge that may be accompanied by itching, swelling, and painful urination. Treatment consists of a 2-week course of oral medication that helps to kill the parasite.

Since the vagina is warm, dark, and moist, it is an ideal breeding environment for a variety of organisms. Normal hygienic measures seem to help keep vaginal infections at a minimum. Unfortunately, use of some highly promoted commercial products seems to lead to increased incidences of vaginal infections. Among these are tight pantyhose (without cotton panels), which tend to increase the vaginal temperature, and commercial vaginal douches, which can alter the acidic level of the vagina. Use of both of these products might promote infections. Women are advised to "wipe from front to back" after every bowel movement to reduce the opportunity for direct transmission of pathogenic agents from the rectum to the vagina. The avoidance of public bath facilities is also a good suggestion. Of course, if you notice any atypical discharge from the vagina, you should report this to your physician.

Cystitis and Urethritis

Cystitis, an infection of the urinary bladder, and *urethritis*, an infection of the urethrea, are conditions that can be caused by a sexually transmitted organism. Other modes of transmission are also associated with cystitis and urethritis, including infection with the organisms that cause vaginitis and organisms found in the intestinal tract. A laboratory culture is required to determine the specific pathogen associated with a particular case of cystitis or urethritis.

Cystitis and urethritis are most frequently found in women. The short and relatively straight urethra of the female and the closeness of the urethral opening to the vagina and rectum increase the likelihood of infection. Although the conditions are easily treated (with antibiotics) when discovered early, some women experience chronic cystitis and urethritis.

The symptoms include pain when urinating, the need to urinate frequently, a dull aching pain above the pubic bone, and the passing of blood-streaked urine. When the infection results from an organism associated with vaginitis, many women will report that the discomfort on urination seems to be "external." Infections associated with sexual transmission or self-contamination more often produce discomfort that is described as "internal."

Regardless of the focus of the discomfort, cystitis and urethritis can be easily treated when the specific organism has been identified. Few complications result from infections that are treated promptly. If cystitis and urethritis are left untreated, the possibility exists for the infectious agents to move upward in the urinary system and produce an infection of the ureters and kidneys. These upper urinary infections are more serious and require more extensive evaluation and aggressive treatment.

Prevention of cystitis and urethritis depends to some degree on the source of infectious agent. In a general sense, however, the incidence of infection can be lowered by urinating completely (to fully empty the urinary bladder) and by drinking ample quantities of fluids to flush the urinary tract. Whether the drinking of cranberry juice helps reduce urinary tract infections is a debatable issue.

SUMMARY

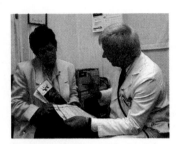

Responsible sexual behavior requires an understanding of STDs.

Infectious diseases are those diseases that have a specific pathogen as their cause. Although infectious diseases are no longer the major cause of death in our society, the risk of serious consequences from infectious diseases still poses a serious threat to those who are susceptible. Most of our common diseases are caused by one of six types of disease-producing agents, or pathogens. These pathogens are viruses, bacteria, fungi, protozoa, rickettsiae, and parasitic worms.

The transmission of a pathogenic agent through the links in the chain of infection forms the basis for an understanding of how diseases spread. The links in the chain include the agent, reservoir, portal of exit, route of transmission, portal of entry, new host, and proliferation of the agent in the new host. If the agent can overcome the host's resistance, it can produce an infection. Once the agent begins to produce infection, the disease moves through four distinctive stages: incubation, prodromal, peak, and recovery stage.

Your body responds to pathogenic agents with both mechanical and biochemical defense systems. Incorporated in your mechanical defenses are the skin, mucous membranes, cilia, earwax, and tears. The biochemical system is usually referred to as the immune system and is subdivided into natural and acquired components. The responses of these defense systems determine whether your body will be able to resist a specific infection.

In this chapter, information about common infections of the young adult period was presented to help you determine your own susceptibility to the common cold, influenza, mononucleosis, chronic Epstein-Barr virus syndrome, red measles, toxic shock syndrome, and AIDS. Also discussed were preventive measures college students can take to reduce the chances of contracting these diseases and infections. Sexually transmitted diseases were presented as medical conditions, and a review of the most common sexually transmitted diseases among college students was also included in this chapter.

REVIEW QUESTIONS

1 What category of disease (infectious or chronic) do most people today die from? Has this always been the case?
2 List the six most common types of pathogens. Describe each type of pathogen and give examples of the types of diseases or infections that each one can cause.
3 Explain the importance of the chain of infection in understanding how diseases are spread. What are the seven links in the chain of infection?

4 Identify and give examples of each of the four common routes of transmission of infectious agents.

5 Identify and describe the four distinctive stages that a disease moves through once a pathogenic agent has invaded a new host.

6 Give examples of mechanical defenses in your body. What is the primary function of the biochemical defense system in your body?

7 Define the following components of the immune system and explain how they differ from each other: natural immunity, actively acquired immunity, artificially acquired immunity, and passively acquired immunity.

8 Identify the pathogenic agent, signs and symptoms, treatment, serious consequences, and preventive measures for each of the following infectious diseases: the common cold, influenza, mononucleosis, red measles, toxic shock syndrome, and acquired immune deficiency syndrome.

9 Identify the causative agent, signs and symptoms, treatment, serious consequences, and preventive measures for each of the following sexually transmitted diseases: chlamydia, gonorrhea, herpes simplex, syphilis, and pubic lice.

10 Describe the most prevalent vaginal infections: candidosis and trichomoniasis. Are these considered sexually transmitted diseases? How can one reduce the possibility of developing vaginal infections?

QUESTIONS FOR PERSONAL CONTEMPLATION

1 How do you feel when a classmate or co-worker comes to class or work ill? Is it fair for this person to expose you to his or her illness? How can you deal with such a situation? Think about your own behavior with regard to this issue. Have you acted responsibly in similar situations?

2 Which infectious disease have you had in the recent past? What type of impact did this infection have on your day-to-day activities? What measures did you personally take to combat the infection? After having read this chapter, would you change your response to the next infectious disease you contract? In what ways?

3 Many of the once common infectious diseases of childhood are no longer a major threat because of immunizations. However, they still exist and pose the risk of serious consequences. How would you feel if you found out your child had become deaf after having measles because you neglected to have your child immunized? How can such tragic consequences be avoided?

4 What diseases have you been immunized against? If you are not certain, do you know where to get this information? Will you make an effort to locate this information?

5 Many infectious diseases (such as AIDS and sexually transmitted diseases) carry moral implications as well as medical risks. What would your initial reaction be if you found out that someone close to you had one of these diseases? What attitudes can you develop within yourself to avoid judgmental feelings about yourself and others who have contracted one of these diseases?

REFERENCES

1 Wistreich, GA, and Lechtman, MD: Microbiology, ed 4, New York, 1984, Macmillan Publishing Co.

2 Thibodeau, G: Anatomy and physiology, St. Louis, 1987, Times Mirror/Mosby College Publishing.

3 The physician's manual for patients, New York, 1984, Times Books.

4 Update on influenza activity in the US, availability of influenza vaccines, and recommendations for the use of vaccines and amantadine, Morbidity and Mortality Weekly Report 35:805-807, 1987.

5 Advisory Committee on Immunization Practices: prevention and control of influenza, Morbidity and Mortality Weekly Report 36:373–387, 1987.

6 Straus, SE: EB or not EB—that is the question, Journal of the American Medical Association 257:2335-2336, 1987.
7 Findlay, S: The 'yuppie flu' strikes—and stays, USA Today April 30, 1987, p 1.
8 Area physicians alerted about measles outbreak at Purdue, Muncie Star February 8, 1983, p 5.
9 Immunization practices in colleges—United States, Morbidity and Mortality Weekly Report 36:209-202, 1987.
10 Todd, J, et al: Toxic shock syndrome associated with phage-group-1 staphylococci, Lancet 2:1116-1122, 1978.
11 Toxic shock syndrome: Morbidity and Mortality Weekly Report 30:25-28, 33, 1981.
12 Price, JH: Update: toxic shock syndrome, The Journal of School Health 51:143-145, 1981.
13 Berkley, SF, et al: The relationship of tampon characteristics to menstrual toxic shock syndrome, Journal of the American Medical Association 258:917-920, 1987.
14 Surgeon General's report on acquired immune deficiency syndrome, Public Health Service, 1987, US Dept of Health and Human Services.
15 Facts about AIDS, Public Health Service, 1987, US Dept of Health and Human Services.
16 Booth, W: AIDS and insects, Science 237:355-356, 1987.
17 Revision of the CDC surveillance case definition for acquired immunodeficiency syndrome, Morbidity and Mortality Weekly Report Supplement No 1s 36:3s-15s, 1987.
18 FDA approves retrovir (AZT), Indiana State Board of Health, AIDS Update, 2:1-2, 1987.
19 New Yorkers shun homosexuals, Sexuality Today 10:1, 1987.
20 Chng, CL, and Roddy, WM: Ethical implications: screening for and treatment of AIDS, Health Education 18:4-7, 1987.
21 Monmaney, T: Kids with AIDS, Newsweek 110:50-59, 1987.
22 Braude, AI, Davis, CE, and Fierer, J, editors: Infectious diseases and medical microbiology, ed 2, Philadelphia, 1986, WB Saunders Co.
23 Penicillinase-producing Neisseria gonorrhoeae—Mortality Weekly Report 36:107-108, 1987.
24 Progress toward achieving the national 1990 objectives for sexually transmitted diseases, Morbidity and Mortality Weekly Report 36:173-176, 1987.
25 Haas, K, and Haas, A: Understanding sexuality, St. Louis, 1987, Times Mirror/Mosby College Publishing.

ANNOTATED READINGS

Berger, M: Dr. Berger's immune power diet, New York, 1985, Signet Books.
> A national bestseller, this book was written by a physician who feels that one's diet influences the effectiveness of the immune system. Using quizzes, case histories, menus, and recipes, Dr. Berger shows how proper eating can affect a person's overall health.

Brandt, A: No magic bullet: a social history of venereal disease in the United States since 1880, New York, 1987, Oxford University Press.
> A detailed history of the social and political factors related to sexually transmitted diseases. A chapter on AIDS updates the content of this book to the present time.

Jaffe, H, Rudin, J, and Rudin, M: Why me? Why anyone?, New York, 1986, St Martin's Press.
> The personal story of a 46-year-old rabbi who developed a rare form of leukemia. Using a spiritual focus, the authors describe this man's personal struggles with self-doubt, anger, and despair. The book supports the idea that we can learn to make every minute count.

Lauersen, N, and Whitney, S: It's your body: a woman's guide to gynecology, New York, 1985, Berkley Publishing.
> A comprehensive guide to the female body. Includes the latest research on estrogen, birth control, abortion, and toxic shock syndrome.

Weiner, A: Maximum immunity, New York, 1987, Pocket Books.
> A clear, comprehensive explanation of the human immune system. This book shows how to bolster the immune system so that it can function most effectively. Using extensive references, the author points out how to strengthen your natural resistance and reduce the likelihood of developing such diseases as cancer, AIDS, allergies, and colds.

Mastering Tasks

Illness and major health problems influence the progress we make with respect to the four developmental tasks: self-identity, independence, responsibility, and social interaction. The reverse is also true. The progress we make regarding these developmental tasks has some bearing on our susceptibility to illness and our ability to recover from illness. Let us look more closely at each task.

■ **Forming an Initial Adult Self-Identity** Most of us probably go through life without really believing that we might one day become seriously ill. We prefer to imagine ourselves as always being free from major health problems. Our identity is based upon a healthy view of ourselves.

However, we encourage you to think occasionally about how your self-identity might be changed if you were to contract or develop a serious illness. What would the impct be on your view of yourself, your interactions with others, and your dreams for the future? We believe that such introspection is healthy, because it serves two purposes: it prepares us for the future and it allows us to appreciate the good health we have today.

■ **Establishing a Sense of Relative Independence** As you move into and through adulthood, you will probably find yourself increasingly seeking ways of expressing your individualism, your freedom, your independence. In turn, the collective society expects you to temper this independence with some realism. You will be expected to manage your own finances, make academic and career decisions, and select friends according to your own criteria. Most college students relish these new opportunities.

Developing an independent lifestyle also means that you will be gradually moving away from those people you have regularly turned to for advice and support. With respect to the content in Unit IV, this emerging independence means that you may be forced to start experiencing illnesses all by yourself. The years of having others care for all of your health needs may nearly be over. Thus as an emerging independent adult you must become familiar with many techniques regarding self-care, prevention, and access to the health care system. Fortunately, you are the beneficiary of this growth process.

■ **Assuming Increasing Levels of Responsibility** Nearly every day, we are being encouraged by health professionals to be active participants in the promotion of our own health. We are asked to become more responsible for aspects of our health that we can control, such as our weight, our alcohol and other drug use, our fitness level, and our dietary practices. Indeed, the collective society is losing patience with people who blatantly disregard the necessity of living a healthy life.

Not only do irresponsible persons hurt themselves, but they also make a significant impact on the lives of others. Those who, by their own actions, are frequently ill and absent from work, overuse group health insurance protection, and place great burdens on family and friends reduce the quality of life for everyone. Practicing preventive health measures enables you to be responsible to the collective society.

■ **Developing the Skills for Social Interaction** The content in Chapters 10, 11, and 12 provides a large stage for the practice and rehearsal of your social skills. From the social involvement with friends who have a chronic health condition to the intimate discussions couples have concerning possible STD transmission, it is important to feel comfortable while communicating with others. Interacting with sick people, their families, and members of the health care delivery system sometimes takes persistence and a good deal of tact. For most persons, these social skills tend to develop with practice.

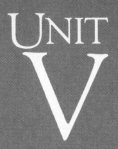

UNIT V

Our sexuality is an integral part of our being. It colors the way in which we interact with the world around us and affects how we will plan for our lives in terms of goals, relationships, reproductivity, and our role in society.

- **Physical Dimension of Health** Sexuality is closely related to the physical dimension of our health. Common physical changes related to sexuality include maturation at puberty, responses to sexual arousal, changes associated with contraception or pregnancy, and adaptations to increased age. How well we respond to these varied developmental processes may reflect our ability to feel comfortable about our sexuality.

Another point that connects sexuality and the physical dimension of health is that sexual experiences and relationships can be very demanding. Intense, pleasurable sexual experiences are fueled by energy and time. These experiences, and the relationships that accompany them, are certainly enhanced when the body is well maintained, energized, and relatively free from illness and pain.

- **Emotional Dimension of Health** As emerging adults, the gender schemas you are forming are, out of necessity, changing as your perceptions of being a woman or a man change. For example, few of you hold the same picture of femininity or masculinity today that you held when you were 14 years old. Your changing perceptions and priorities about being a man or a woman can be emotional stressors.

One of the most stressful aspects of living for many young adults concerns sexual intimacy. Your feelings about your own sexually intimate behavior can range from exhilaration to ambivalence to depression. Being comfortable with your sexuality comes from acting on the basis of your core values, recognizing when you are using someone or are being used by another, and being able to recover from disappointment.

- **Social Dimension of Health** As your adult sexuality emerges, your interest in other people develops rapidly. Because sexuality often involves interactions with other persons, the development of social skills is imperative. For many, dating provides an excellent arena in which to establish a base of social skills. As dating relationships become more serious, skills in communication can grow significantly. These skills are, of course, important factors in the process of mate selection and marriage.

- **Intellectual Dimension of Health** Within the context of a growing relationship, opportunities abound for individuals to contemplate, analyze, and interpret currently available information. Your intellectual resources may be challenged when you examine information concerning reproductive anatomy, fertility, sexual response, contraception, and the birth process.

Sexual relationships are also valuable in providing the opportunity for the growth of the intellect through the process of introspection. Sexual relationships quickly force individuals to sort through their feelings, values, and past experiences to find guidance in pursuing a relationship.

- **Spiritual Dimension of Health** Paired sexual experiences can provide you with an arena in which to serve others. In dating, courtship, and particularly in marriage, you are provided the opportunity to extend empathy, support, and love to another person. These responses exemplify the highest spiritual values to which most of us aspire.

The growth of a paired sexual relationship also presents an excellent opportunity for an individual to explore behavior and beliefs that relate to the spiritual dimension of health. Your sense of morality, the appropriateness of premarital sexual intimacy, and the value of fidelity within a marital relationship are specific touch points that you may wish to examine.

By carefully examining your core beliefs about sexuality, you will be better able to avoid situations in which your actions differ from your beliefs. You will also be better able to support your moral position when that position is being attacked by others. You may also gain a measure of tolerance for the feelings of other people.

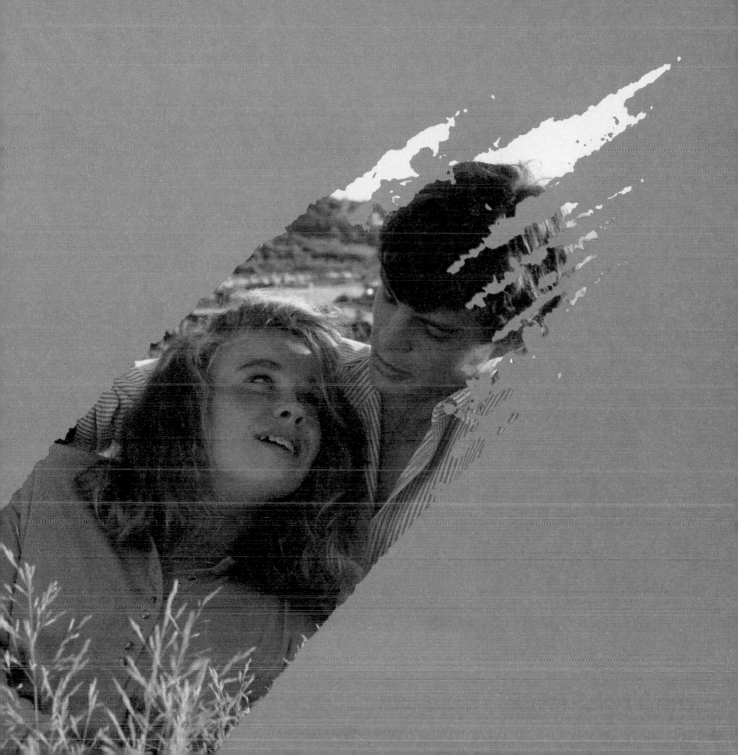

Sexuality
The Person, the Partner, the Parent

CHAPTER

13

Sexuality
Biological and Psychosocial Origins

Key Concepts

Both biological and psychosocial factors contribute to the complex expression of our sexuality.

The most basic level of biological sexuality begins at the moment of conception.

Psychosocial sexuality develops through the processes of gender identity, gender preference, and gender adoption.

The male and female reproductive systems are largely influenced by hormones.

Throughout a lifetime, each person will exhibit varying degrees of reproductive, genital, and expressionistic sexuality.

Increasingly, our society supports the most positive qualities of an androgynous lifestyle.

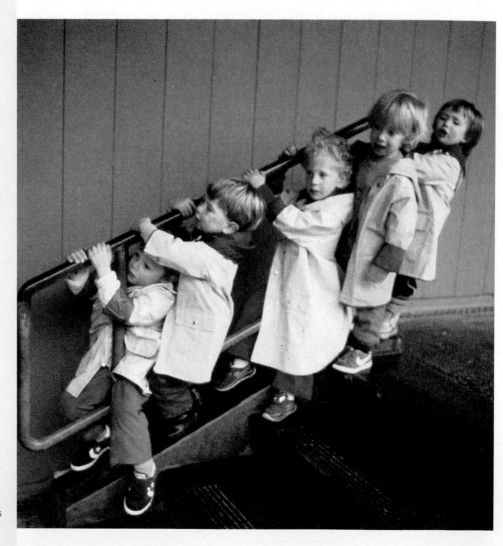

Beginning in the 1970s it appeared that a segment of the American public was in the process of discarding two old and familiar labels—male and female. Unisex fashions prevailed. Government agencies and private corporations rushed to de-gender position titles and to purge publications of sexist pronouns. As a collective society, we were strongly attracted to the idea that biology was an unacceptable basis on which to describe human behavior. Indeed, the nonsexist concept of "person" had emerged. Chairmen became chairpersons, mailmen became mail carriers, and the widespread use of the pronoun "he" was curtailed.

Today it appears that we have achieved a more even balance in our ability to realize that both biological and psychological factors contribute to the complex expression of our **sexuality.** As a society we are now inclined to view human behavior in terms of a complex script written on the basis of both biology and conditioning. Reflecting this understanding is the way in which we use the words "male or female" to refer to the biological roots of our sexuality and the words "man or woman" to refer to the psychosocial roots of our sexuality.

In this chapter we will explore human sexuality as it relates to the dynamic interplay of the biological base and the psychosocial base that form your **masculinity** or **femininity.** At points, the content related to the biological dimension of sexuality may seem complex, but the experiences that form the learned psychosocial portion should make the overall topic understandable.

THE BIOLOGICAL BASES OF HUMAN SEXUALITY

Observers in delivery rooms routinely report that within a few seconds following the birth of a baby, someone (a doctor, nurse, or parent) emphatically labels the child: "It's a boy," or It's a girl." For the parents, and the society as a whole, the child's **biological sexuality** is being displayed and identified. Another male or female enters the world.

Genetic Basis

For most students, the idea that biological sexuality begins at birth is recognized as being inaccurate. Rather, it is at the moment of conception that a Y-bearing or an X-bearing sperm cell joins with the X-bearing ovum to establish the true basis of biological sexuality. A fertilized ovum reflecting the chromosomal configuration of XX is a biological female, while the fertilized ovum bearing the XY configuration is a biological male. Genetics form the most basic level of an individual's biological sexuality.

Gonadal Basis

By the fifth or sixth week after conception the *embryo* is moving toward an additional level of biological sexuality—the establishment of a gonadal basis for its sexuality. Until this time, some people consider the embryo neither male nor female, because the reproductive structures are not evident. (Some even refer to all embryos as females, because the rudimentary *duct systems* appear to resemble female structures.) The seventh week begins true gonadal differentiation. Clearly defined testes can be identified at this time but it is not until the eleventh or twelfth week of fetal development that the ovaries are as clearly defined.[1]

sexuality
the quality of being sexual; can be viewed from many biological and psychosocial perspectives.

masculinity
behavioral expressions traditionally observed in males.

femininity
behavioral expressions traditionally observed in females.

biological sexuality
male and female aspects of sexuality.

361

Only recently has the control mechanism for the differentiation of the gonads been identified. It is now established that a testis-determining factor gene located on an "arm" of the Y chromosome controls the development of the undifferentiated gonad into the testis that is associated with the male.[2]

Internal Structural Development

mesonephric
duct system within the male embryo that gives rise to several internal reproductive structures.

paramesonephric
duct system within the female embryo that gives rise to several internal reproductive structures.

While gonadal differentiation is taking place within the embryo, two distinct duct systems are being influenced that will in turn help form the internal reproductive structures of the male and female. The development of these two duct systems (the **mesonephric** and **paramesonephric** systems) is controlled by the presence or absence of two hormones produced by the testes—*androgen* and the *inducer substance.*[3]

With both of these hormones present, the mesonephric duct system of the male embryo develops into the internal male reproductive structures. Since the female embryo possesses ovaries rather than testes, no androgen and inducer substances are produced. Thus the paramesonephric duct system of the female embryo develops into the internal female reproductive structures.[4]

External Structural Development

labia minora
small, liplike folds of skin immediately adjacent to the vaginal opening.

labia majora
larger, more external skin folds that surround the vaginal opening.

During the fourth through ninth weeks of intrauterine development, differentiation of the *genital tubercle, labioscrotal swellings,* and *urogenital folds* is found in both male and female embryos. In the male embryo, androgen exerts its masculine influences on certain tissues, resulting in the gradual development of the structures of the penis. The labioscrotal swellings fuse to form the scrotum, which during the twenty-eighth week is filled with the descended testes.[3]

Under the influence of *estrogen* from the placenta, the corresponding female embryonic tissues undergo differentiation to form the female external genitalia. The genital tubercle elongates to become the *clitoris,* while the urogenital folds are transformed into the **labia minora** and labioscrotal swellings remain unfused as the **labia majora.**[4]

Biological Sexuality and the Childhood Years

puberty
achievement of reproductive ability.

The growth and development of the child in terms of reproductive organs and physiological processes have traditionally been thought to be "latent" during the childhood years. However, a gradual degree of growth occurs in both the female and male child. The reproductive organs, however, will undergo more greatly accelerated growth at the onset of **puberty** and will achieve their adult size and capabilities shortly thereafter.

Puberty

menarche
time of a female's first menstrual cycle.

Entry into pubescence is a gradual maturing process for young females and males. In the young female, the typical transition into biological adulthood begins near the age of 11 with the budding of her breasts and the development of pubic hair. A spurt in skeletal growth is generally in synchrony with these initial indicators of sexual maturation. The onset of menstruation, the **menarche,** generally fol-

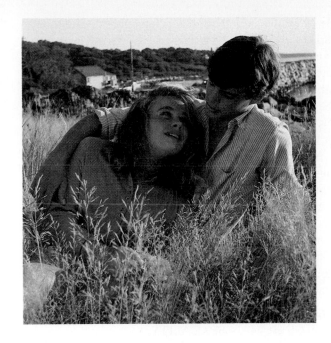

Puberty signals physical and emotional changes.

lows these changes by approximately 1 year. Thus menstruation is usually established by the age of 13.[1,5] A variation of plus or minus 2 years may characterize a particular girl's development in comparison to the group's average.

In the past century and a half, the average age of the menarche has been steadily falling. Data from the 1830s established the age of the menarche at 17 years, while today's average age is 13 years.[1] Improved nutrition and health care may be responsible for this change. Recent data suggest, however, that the movement toward an increasingly earlier menarche may have run its course.

It is not unusual for the first several menstrual cycles to be *anovulatory*.[6] This may be interpreted to mean that the young woman produces sufficient estrogen to stimulate uterine wall development, but not sufficient luteinizing hormone to move ova development to the point of ovulation.

The onset of biological maturation in the male follows a similar course. In the male, however, the process begins approximately 2 years later than it does in the female. The first indication that the young male's reproductive system is moving toward maturity is noted near the age of 12, when the testes and the scrotum begin to display rapid growth. Axillary (underarm) hair development may also be noted at this time. A growth spurt generally follows within 1 year, as does penile enlargement and the development of pubic hair. Growth of the larynx, with concomitant lowering of the voice, also occurs. The male's first ejaculation is generally experienced by the age of 14, most commonly through **nocturnal emission** or masturbation. Mustache and beard growth, at least to the point that shaving is deemed reasonable, is generally seen between the ages of 15 and 18.[1]

A question exists about the mechanism that signals the anterior pituitary gland to begin the production of **gonadotrophic hormones** required for the maturation of the reproductive system. For females the theory most frequently cited as to what starts the body's movement toward maturity is that of body weight or the percent of body fat. When evaluated on the basis of group data, children

nocturnal emission
ejaculation that occurs during sleep; "wet dream."

gonadotrophic hormones
hormones that influence the functioning of the testes and ovaries.

that are in the upper levels of height and weight development for their grade tend to experience the earliest expressions of puberty. Certainly in mature women who develop anorexia (see Chapter 6) or undertake a strenuous aerobic exercise program (see Chapter 4), weight loss can occur to the point that menstruation ceases. The often-heard contention that better nutrition underlies the earlier onset of the menarche is in keeping with the concept of a *threshold weight*.

Once obtained, reproductive capability only gradually declines over the course of the adult years. In the female, however, the relatively sudden onset of **menopause** signals a more pronounced turning off of the reproductive system than is the case for the adult male (see Chapter 19). By the early to mid-fifties, virtually all women have entered a postmenopausal period, whereas for males, relatively high level **spermatogenesis** may continue for a decade or two.[1]

The story of sexual maturation and reproductive maturity cannot, however, be solely focused on the changes that take place in the body. Clearly, the emotional, social, intellectual, and spiritual development of the individual must be considered as well. Now we will discuss the psychosocial processes that accompany the biological changes.

menopause
decline and eventual cessation of hormone production by the reproductive system.

spermatogenesis
process of sperm production.

THE PSYCHOSOCIAL BASES OF HUMAN SEXUALITY

If growth and development of our sexuality were to be visualized as a step ladder (see Figure 13-1), then one vertical rail of the ladder would represent our biological sexuality. Arising at various points along this rail would be rungs representing the sequential unfolding of the genetic, gonadal, and structural components.

Figure 13-1
Our sexuality develops through biological and psychosocial stages.

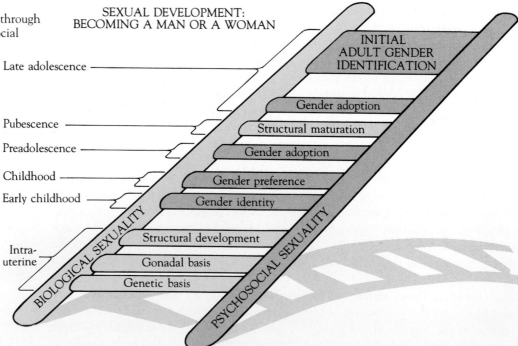

SEXUAL DEVELOPMENT:
BECOMING A MAN OR A WOMAN

INITIAL ADULT GENDER IDENTIFICATION

Late adolescence

Gender adoption

Pubescence — Structural maturation

Preadolescence — Gender adoption

Childhood — Gender preference

Early childhood — Gender identity

Structural development

Intra-uterine — Gonadal basis

Genetic basis

BIOLOGICAL SEXUALITY

PSYCHOSOCIAL SEXUALITY

Because humans, more so than any other life forms, have the ability to rise above a life centered on reproduction, a second dimension or rail to our sexuality exists—our **psychosocial sexuality.** As to why we possess the ability to be more than reproductive beings is a question to direct to the theologian or philosopher. The fact remains, however, that we are considerably more complex than functions determined by biology. The process that transforms male into man and female into woman begins at birth and continues to influence us through the course of our lives.

psychosocial sexuality
masculine and feminine aspects of sexuality.

Gender Identity

Although parents awaiting the birth of a baby may hold a preference for a baby of one **gender** over the other, they are frequently forced to wait until the birth of the baby to have their question answered. The answer, in the form of an emotionally charged statement, "It's a girl!" or "It's a boy!" occurs within seconds of the delivery. At that moment expectations and aspirations for the baby close or remain open on the basis of the child's gender. External genitals "cast the die," and femininity or masculinity begins to receive its traditional reinforcement.

gender
general term reflecting a biological basis of sexuality; the male gender or the female gender.

The process that leads to the child's recognition of his or her gender includes components so familiar that it is easy to overlook their importance. Hospitals routinely participate in the formalizing of gender by attaching a GIRL or BOY card to the nursery crib. In many hospitals, pink bows are still attached to the hair (or hands) of girl babies. Blue or pink blankets swaddle the new arrival, and within a few days a gender-identifying name is assigned by the parents. Within the first week of life the collective society has been served notice. You are what your genitals say that you are—a girl or a boy.

During the first year and a half, the effects of parenting practices begin to "inform" children of the gender to which they have been assigned. Toy selection, room decorations, clothing selection, language use, and the type of physical contact employed by the parents effectively educate a child's subconscious as to what gender he or she is. By the eighteenth month, typical children have both the language and the insight to correctly identify their gender. They have established a **gender identity.**[7] The first rung rising from the psychosocial rail of the ladder has been climbed.

gender identity
recognition of one's gender.

Gender Preference

During the preschool years children receive the second component of the *scripting* required for the full development of psychosocial sexuality—the desire to prefer the gender to which they have been assigned. The process whereby **gender preference** is transmitted to the child is more than likely a less subtle form of the practices observed during the gender identity period (the first 18 months). Parents begin to actively control the child's exposure to experiences traditionally reserved for children of the opposite sex. Particularly for boys, parents will stop play activities they perceive as being too feminine. In our society, the label "sissy" will be quickly assigned to the boy whose interests are too closely akin to those of his sister.

gender preference
emotional and intellectual acceptance for the gender that one is.

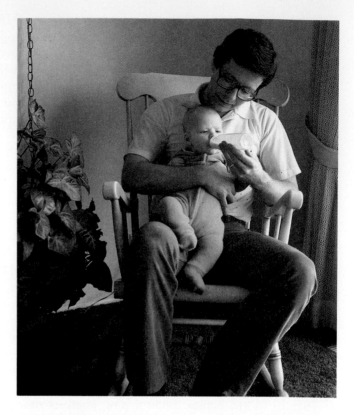

Is this baby a boy?

Although girls and boys are thought to arrive at an appropriate gender preference at about the same time, there exists a mechanism that allows some girls to delay selecting the appropriate preference as quickly as is expected for boys. This mechanism is, of course, "tomboyism." Traditionally, little girls are allowed to act like little boys much longer than little boys are allowed to act like little girls.[8]

With the recent acceleration in the importance of competitive sports for women, many of the skills and experiences once "reserved" for boys are now being fostered in young girls. What effect, if any, this movement will have on the speed at which gender preference is reached will be a topic of further research.*

Gender Adoption

The process of reaching an initial adult sexual identity requires a considerable period of time. The specific knowledge, attitudes, and behaviors characteristic of adults must be observed, analyzed, and practiced. The process of acquiring and personalizing these "insights" about how men and women think, feel, and act is reflected by the term **gender adoption,** the first and third rungs below the initial adult gender identification rail of the ladder in Figure 13-1.

For both the child and the adolescent, a personalized script of what he or she will be like as an adult is an undertaking of considerable importance. Parents, the parents of friends, teachers, neighbors, and the adults seen in the media are

gender adoption
lengthy process of learning the behaviors that are traditional for one's gender.

*If you want to test the existence of gender preference, ask a group of first or second grade boys or girls if they would be happier being a member of the opposite sex. Be prepared for some frank replies.

carefully studied. They become role models for the child. When the opportunity presents itself, the child puts these observations into practice. Play groups, adult-planned school and club activities, sports, early dating, and other peer group activities provide the stages on which the child's script can be rehearsed.

In addition to the construction of a personalized version of a sexual identity, it is important that the child and particularly the adolescent construct a *gender schema* for a member of the *opposite* sex.[9] Clearly, the world of adulthood, with its involvement with intimacy, parenting, and employment, will require that men know women and women know men. Gender adoption provides an opportunity to begin to assemble this equally valuable "picture" of what the other sex is like.

If the gender schemas of young persons could be studied, it would be interesting to see how well or how poorly they are being scripted. Human nature suggests that for some young people, the gender adoption would be undertaken with care and insightfulness, whereas for others the script will be haphazardly developed. For those young persons who have access to numerous physically, emotionally, socially, intellectually, and spiritually healthy adult role models, we would expect to see a gender schema capable of serving them well in the initial years of adulthood. These young people will have a good grasp of what it means to be a woman or a man. For those who do not have access to such clear role models, the traits found in their newly constructed schemas may limit their understanding of female and male adulthood. Interestingly, society seems comfortable in leaving this complex process to chance.

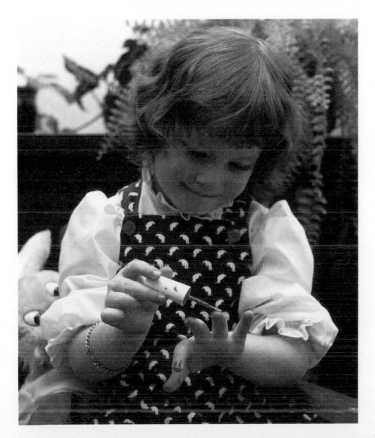

Practicing at being a woman.

Initial Adult Gender Identification

gender identification
achievement of a personally
satisfying interpretation of
one's masculinity or femininity.

By the time young people have climbed all of the rungs of the sexuality ladder, they have arrived at the chronological point in the life cycle when they are charged to construct an initial adult **gender identification.** If this label seems remarkably similar to the terminology used in identifying one of the developmental tasks being used in this textbook, your observation is accurate. In fact, the task of forming an initial adult self-identity is closely related to developing an initial adult self-image of oneself as a man or a woman. Although most of us currently support the concept of "person" in many gender-neutral contexts, (for some very valid reasons), we still must identify ourselves as either a man or a woman. The world is comprised of males and females thinking, feeling, and behaving as men and women, because our sexuality is an inseparable part of our life experience.

THE REPRODUCTIVE SYSTEMS

The most familiar aspects of biological sexuality are the structures that compose the reproductive systems. Each structure contributes in unique ways to the reproductive process. Thus with these structures males have the ability to impregnate. Females have the ability to become pregnant, give birth, and nourish infants through breastfeeding. Additionally, many of these structures are associated with nonreproductive sexual behaviors (see Chapter 14).

The Male Reproductive System

ICSH (interstitial cell stimulating hormone)
a gonadotrophic hormone of
the male required for the
production of testosterone.

The male reproductive system consists of external structures or genitals (the penis and scrotum), and internal structures (the testes, various passageways or ducts, seminal vesicles, the prostate gland, and the bulbourethral glands) (see Figure 13-2, A). The *testes* (also called *gonads* or *testicles*) are two egg-shaped bodies that lie within a saclike structure called the *scrotum*. During most of fetal development, the testes lie within the abdominal cavity. They descend into the scrotum during the last 2 months of fetal life. The testes are housed in the scrotum because a temperature lower than the body core temperature is required for adequate sperm development. The walls of the scrotum are composed of contractile tissue and have the ability to draw the testes closer to the body during cold temperatures (and sexual arousal) and to relax during warm temperatures. Scrotal contraction and relaxation allow a constant, productive temperature to be maintained in the testes.

A cross-sectional view of a single testis reveals an intricate network of structures called *seminiferous tubules* (see Figure 13-2, B). It is within these 300 or so seminiferous tubules that the process of sperm production (*spermatogenesis*) takes place. Sperm cell development starts at about age 11 in boys and is influenced by the release of the hormone **ICSH (interstitial cell stimulating hormone)** from the pituitary gland. ICSH does primarily what its name suggests: it stimulates specific cells (called *interstitial cells*) within the testes to begin producing the male sex hormone *testosterone.* Testosterone in turn is primarily responsible for the gradual development of the male secondary sex characteristics at the onset of puberty. By the time a boy is approximately 15 years old, sufficient levels of testosterone exist so that the testes become capable of full spermatogenesis.

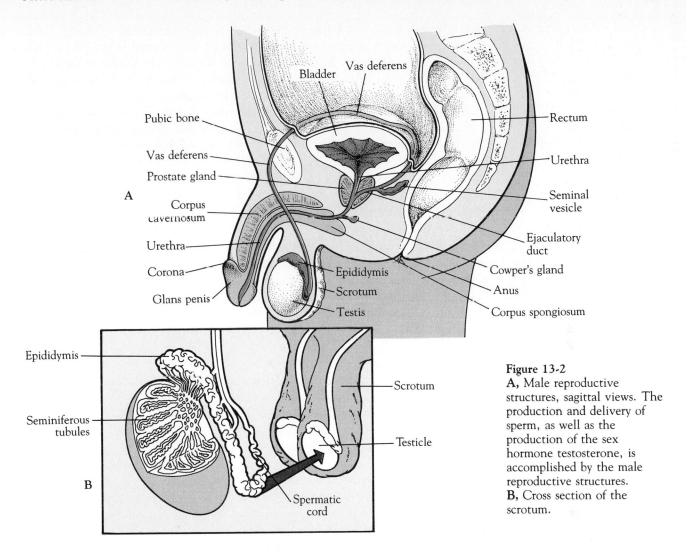

Figure 13-2
A, Male reproductive structures, sagittal views. The production and delivery of sperm, as well as the production of the sex hormone testosterone, is accomplished by the male reproductive structures. **B,** Cross section of the scrotum.

Before the age of about 15, most of the sperm cells produced in the testes are incapable of fertilization. The production of fully mature sperm (*spermatozoa*) is triggered by another hormone secreted by the brain's pituitary gland—**FSH (follicle stimulating hormone).** FSH influences the seminiferous tubules to begin to produce spermatozoa that are capable of fertilization.

Spermatogenesis takes place around the clock, with hundreds of millions of sperm cells produced daily. The sperm cells do not stay in the seminiferous tubules, but rather are transferred through a system of ducts that lead into the *epididymis*. The epididymis is a tubular coil that attaches to the back side of each testicle. These collecting structures house the maturing sperm cells for a period of 2 to 3 weeks. During this period, the sperm finally become capable of motion, but remain inactive until they mix with the secretions from the accessory glands (the seminal vesicles, prostate gland, and the Cowper's gland).

Each epididymis leads into an 18-inch passageway known as the *vas deferens*. Sperm, moved along by the action of hairlike projections called *cilia*, can also remain in the vas deferens for an extended time without losing their viability.

The two vas deferens extend into the abdominal cavity, where each meets

FSH (follicle stimulating hormone)
a gonadotrophic hormone required for initial development of ova (in the female) and sperm (in the male).

with a *seminal vesicle*—the first of the three accessory structures or glands. Each seminal vesicle contributes a clear, alkaline fluid that nourishes the sperm cells with fructose and permits the sperm cells to be suspended in a movable medium. The fusion of a vas deferens with the seminal vesicle results in the formation of a passageway called the *ejaculatory duct*. Each ejaculatory duct is only about 1 inch long and empties into the final passageway for the sperm—the urethra.

This juncture takes place in an area surrounded by the second accessory gland—the *prostate gland*. The prostate gland secretes a milky fluid containing a variety of substances, including proteins, cholesterol, citric acid, calcium, buffering salts, and various enzymes. The prostate secretions further nourish the sperm cells and also raise the pH level, making the mixture quite alkaline. This alkalinity permits the sperm greater longevity as they are transported during ejaculation through the urethra, out of the penis, and into the highly acidic vagina.

The third accessory glands, the *bulbourethral* or *Cowper's glands*, serve primarily to lubricate the urethra with a clear, viscous mucus. These paired glands empty their small amounts of preejaculatory fluid during the arousal stage of the sexual response cycle. Alkaline in nature, this fluid also neutralizes the acidic level of the urethra. It is hypothesized that viable sperm cells can be suspended in this fluid and can enter the female reproductive tract before full ejaculation by the male.[8] This may account for many of the failures that accrue to users of the "withdrawal" method of contraception.

The sperm cells, when combined with secretions from the seminal vesicles and the prostate gland, from a sticky substance called **semen**. Interestingly, the microscopic sperm actually make up less than 5% of the seminal fluid discharged at ejaculation. Contrary to popular belief, the paired seminal vesicles contribute up to 70% of the semen volume, while the prostate gland adds most of the remainder.[10] Thus the fear of some men that a **vasectomy** will destroy their ability to ejaculate is completely unfounded (see Chapter 15).

During *emission* (the gathering of semen in the upper part of the urethra), a sphincter muscle at the base of the bladder contracts and inhibits semen from being pushed into the bladder and urine from being deposited into the urethra.[8] Thus semen and urine rarely intermingle, even though they leave the body through the same passageway.

Ejaculation takes place when the semen is forced out of the penis through the urethral opening. The involuntary, rhythmic muscle contractions that control ejaculation result in a series of pleasurable sensations known as *orgasm*.

The urethra lies on the underside of the *penis* and extends through one of three cylindrical masses of erectile tissue. Each of these three spongy bodies provides the vascular space required for sufficient erection of the penis. When a male becomes sexually excited, these spongy areas become congested with blood (*vasocongestion*). After ejaculation, or when a male is no longer sexually stimulated, these spongy bodies release the blood into the general circulation and the penis returns to a **flaccid** state.

The *shaft* of the penis is covered by a thin layer of skin that is an extension of the skin that covers the scrotum. This loose layer of skin is sensitive to sexual stimulation and extends over the head of the penis, except in males who have been circumcised. The *glans* (or head) of the penis is the most sexually sensitive (to tactile stimulation) part of the male body. Nerve receptor sites are especially prominent along the *corona* (the ridge of the glans) and the *frenulum* (the thin tissue at the base of the glans).

---

semen

secretion containing sperm and other nutrients discharged from the urethra at ejaculation.

vasectomy

surgical procedure in which the vas deferens are cut to prevent the passage of sperm from the testicles; the most common form of male sterilization.

flaccid

nonerect; the state of erectile tissue when vasocongestion is not occurring.

The Female Reproductive System

The external structures (genitals) of the female reproductive system consist of the mons pubis, labia majora, labia minora, clitoris, and vestibule (see Figure 13-3). Collectively these structures form the *vulva* or vulval area. The *mons pubis* is the fatty covering over the pubic bone. The mons pubis (or mons veneris or mound of Venus) is covered by pubic hair and is quite sensitive to sexual stimulation. The *labia majora* are large longitudinal folds of skin that cover the entrance to the vagina, while the *labia minora* are the smaller longitudinal skin folds that lie within the labia majora. These hairless skin folds of the labia minora join at the top to form the *prepuce*. The prepuce covers the glans of the *clitoris*, which is the most sexually sensitive part of the female body.

A rather direct analogy can be made between the clitoris and the penis. In terms of tactile sensitivity, both structures are the most sensitive parts of the male and female genitals. Both contain a glans and a shaft (although the clitoral shaft is beneath the skin surface). Both organs are composed of erectile tissue that is capable of becoming engorged with blood. Both are covered by skin folds

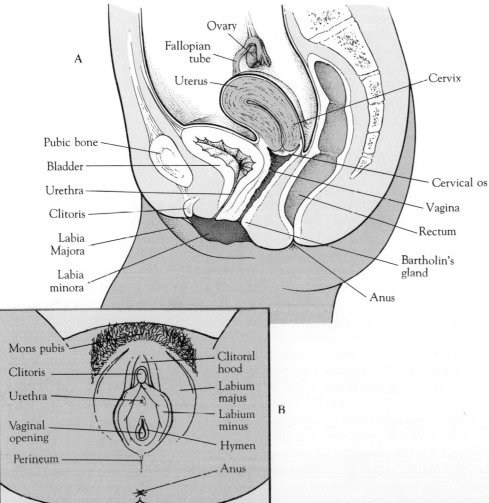

Figure 13-3
A, Female reproductive structures, sagittal view. The formation of ova, production of the sex hormones estrogen and progesterone, and support for the developing fetus are functions of the structures of the female reproductive system. **B,** External view of female genitals.

smegma
cellular discharge that can accumulate beneath the clitoral hood and the foreskin of an uncircumcised penis.

(the clitoral prepuce of the female and the foreskin of the male) and both structures can collect **smegma** beneath these tissue folds.[6]

The *vestibule* is the region enclosed by the labia minora. Evident here are the urethral opening and the entrance to the vagina (or vaginal orifice). Also located at the vaginal opening are the *Bartholin's glands,* which secrete a minute amount of lubricating fluid during sexual excitement.

The *hymen* is a thin layer of tissue that stretches across the opening of the vagina. Once thought to be the only indication of virginity, the intact hymen rarely covers the vaginal opening entirely. Openings in the hymen are necessary for the discharge of menstrual fluid and vaginal secretions. Many hymens are stretched or torn to full opening by adolescent physical activity or by the insertion of tampons. In women whose hymens are not fully ruptured, the first act of sexual intercourse will generally accomplish this purpose. Pain may accompany first intercourse in females with relatively intact hymens.

The internal reproductive structures of the female include the vagina, uterus, fallopian tubes, and ovaries. The *vagina* is the structure that accepts the penis during sexual intercourse. Normally the walls of the vagina are collapsed, except during sexual stimulation, when the vaginal walls widen and elongate to accommodate the erect penis. Only the outer third of the vagina is especially sensitive to sexual stimulation. In this location, vaginal tissues swell considerably to form the **orgasmic platform.** This platform constricts the vaginal opening and, in effect, "grips" the penis—regardless of its size.[6] Thus the belief that a woman receives considerably more sexual pleasure from men with large penises is not supported from an anatomical standpoint.

orgasmic platform
expanded outer third of the vagina that during the plateau phase of the sexual response pattern grips the penis.

The *uterus* (or *womb*) is approximately the size and shape of a small pear. This organ is a highly muscular organ capable of undergoing a wide range of physical changes, as evidenced by its enlargement during pregnancy, its contractions during menstruation and labor, and its movement during the orgasmic phase of the female sexual response cycle. The primary function of the uterus is to provide a suitable environment for the possible implantation of a fertilized ovum, or egg. This implantation, should it occur, will take place in the innermost lining of the uterus—the *endometrium.* In the mature female, the endometrium undergoes cyclic changes as it prepares a new lining on a near-monthly basis.

The lower third of the uterus is called the *cervix.* The cervix extends slightly into the vagina. Sperm can enter the uterus through the cervical opening, or *cervical os.* Mucous glands in the cervix secrete a fluid that is thin and watery near the time of ovulation. This viscosity apparently facilitates sperm passage into the uterus and deeper structures. However, this mucus is much thicker during portions of the menstrual cycle when pregnancy is improbable and during pregnancy, when bacterial agents and other substances are especially dangerous to the developing fetus.

The upper two thirds of the uterus is called the *corpus* or *body*. This is where implantation of the fertilized ovum generally takes place. The upper portion of the uterus opens into two *fallopian tubes* (or *oviducts*)—each about 4 inches long. The fallopian tubes are each directed toward an *ovary.* They serve as a passageway for the ovum in its week-long voyage toward the uterus. In most cases, conception takes place in the upper third of the fallopian tubes.

The ovaries are analogous to the testes in the male. Their function is to produce the *ova*, or eggs. Usually, one ovary produces and releases just one egg each month. Approximately the size and shape of an unshelled almond,[10] an ovary produces viable ova in the process known as *oogenesis*. The ovaries also produce the female sex hormones through the efforts of specific structures within the ovaries. These hormones play multiple roles in the development of female secondary sex characteristics, but their primary function is to prepare the endometrium of the uterus for possible implantation of a fertilized ovum. In the average healthy female, this preparation takes place about 13 times a year for a period of about 35 years.[11] At menopause, the ovaries shrink considerably and stop nearly all hormonal production.

The Menstrual Cycle

Each month or so, the inner wall of the uterus prepares for a possible pregnancy. When a pregnancy does not occur (as is the case throughout most months of a woman's fertile years), this lining must be released and a new one prepared. The breakdown of this endometrial wall and the resultant discharge of blood and endometrial tissue is known as *menstruation* (or *menses*) (see Figure 13-4). The cyclic timing of menstruation is governed by hormones released from two sources: the pituitary gland and the ovaries.

Girls generally have their first menstrual cycle (*menarche*) sometime between 12 and 14 years of age. Body weight, nutrition, heredity, and overall health are factors that are related to menarche. Interestingly, after a girl first menstruates, she may be **anovulatory** for a year or longer before she releases a viable ovum during her cycle. She will then continue this cyclic activity until about age 45 to 55.

anovulatory
not ovulating.

For purposes of explanation, this text will refer to a menstrual cycle that lasts 28 days. Be assured that few women display absolutely perfect 28-day cycles. Most women fluctuate by a few days to a week around this 28-day pattern. Some women vary extremely from this average cycle.

Your knowledge about the menstrual cycle is critical for your understanding of pregnancy, contraception, menopause, and issues related to the overall health and comfort of women. Although at first it may sound like a complicated process, each segment of the cycle can be studied separately for better understanding.

The menstrual cycle can be thought of as occurring in three segments or phases. The first is the menstrual phase (lasting about 1 week); the second is the proliferative phase (also lasting about 1 week); and the third is the secretory phase (lasting about 2 weeks). Day 1 of this cycle starts with the first day of bleeding, or menstrual flow.

The *menstrual phase* signals the woman that a pregnancy has not taken place and that her uterine lining is being sloughed off. During a 5- to 7-day period, a woman will discharge about one-fourth to one-half cup of blood and tissue. (Only about 1 ounce of the menstrual flow is actual blood.) The menstrual flow is heaviest during the first days of this phase. Since the muscular uterus must contract to accomplish this tissue removal, some women experience uncomfortable cramping during menstruation. Most women, however, report more pain and discomfort during the few days before the first day of bleeding. (See the discussion of premenstrual syndrome [PMS] in Chapter 11.)

MENSTRUAL CYCLE

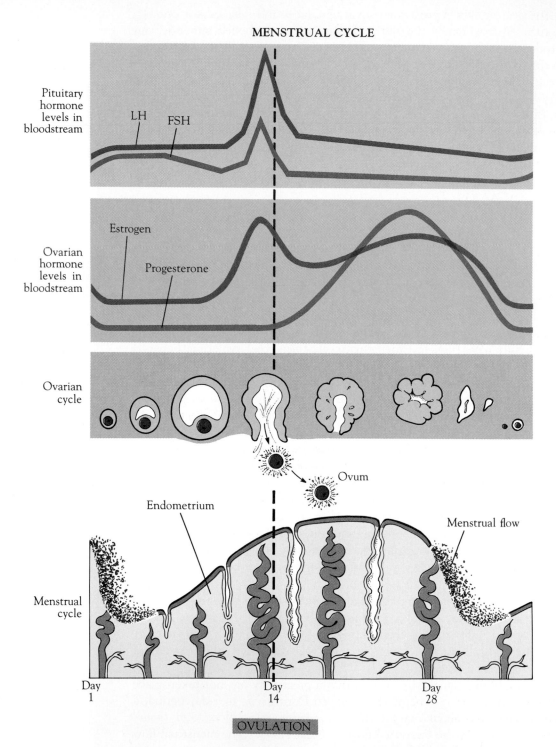

Pituitary hormone levels in bloodstream

LH   FSH

Ovarian hormone levels in bloodstream

Estrogen

Progesterone

Ovarian cycle

Ovum

Endometrium

Menstrual flow

Menstrual cycle

Day 1   Day 14   Day 28

OVULATION

Figure 13-4
The menstrual cycle involves the development and release of an ovum, supported by hormones from the pituitary, and the buildup of the endometrium, supported by hormones from the ovary, for the purpose of establishing a pregnancy.

Modern methods of absorbing menstrual flow include the use of tampons and sanitary napkins. Caution must be exercised by the users of tampons to prevent the possibility of toxic shock syndrome (TSS) (see Chapter 12). Since menstrual flow is a positive sign of good health, women are encouraged to be normally active during menstruation.

The *proliferative phase* of the menstrual cycle starts about the time menstruation stops. Lasting about 1 week, this phase is first influenced by the release of follicle stimulating hormone (FSH) from the pituitary gland. FSH circulates in the bloodstream and directs the ovaries to start the process of maturing approximately 20 primary ovarian *follicles*. Thousands of primary egg follicles are present in each ovary at birth. These follicles resemble shells that house immature ova. As these follicles ripen under FSH influence, they release the hormone *estrogen*. Estrogen's primary function is to direct the endometrium to start the development of a thick, highly vascular wall. As the estrogen levels increase, the pituitary gland's secretion of FSH is reduced. Now the pituitary gland prepares for the surge of the **luteinizing hormone (LH)** required to accomplish ovulation.[12]

In the days immediately preceding ovulation, one of the primary follicles (called the *graafian follicle*) matures fully. The other primary follicles degenerate and are absorbed by the body. The graafian follicle moves toward the surface of the ovary. When LH is released in massive quantities about day 14, the graafian follicle bursts to release the fully mature ovum. The release of the ovum is called **ovulation.**

The ovum is quickly captured by the fingerlike projections (*fimbriae*) of the fallopian tubes. In the upper third of the fallopian tubes, this ovum is capable of being fertilized for a period of 24 to 36 hours. If the ovum is not fertilized by a sperm cell, it will begin to degenerate and eventually be absorbed by the body.

After ovulation, the *secretory phase* of the menstrual cycle starts when the remnants of the graafian follicle restructure themselves into a **corpus luteum.** The corpus luteum remains inside the ovary secreting estrogen as well as a fourth hormone—*progesterone*. Progesterone (literally meaning "for pregnancy") continues to direct the endometrial buildup. If pregnancy occurs, the corpus luteum monitors progesterone and estrogen levels throughout the pregnancy. If pregnancy does not occur, high levels of progesterone signal the pituitary to stop the release of LH and the corpus luteum starts to degenerate on about day 24. When estrogen and progesterone levels diminish significantly by day 28, the endometrium is discharged from the uterus and out the vagina. The secretory phase ends and the menstrual phase begins. The cycle is complete.

luteinizing hormone (LH)
luteinizing hormone; a gonadotrophic hormone of the female required for fullest development and release of ova; ovulating hormone.

ovulation
the release of a mature egg from the ovary.

corpus luteum
cellular remnant of the graafian follicle after the release of an ovum.

ADDITIONAL ASPECTS OF HUMAN SEXUALITY

Earlier in this chapter we identified the biological and psychosocial bases of our sexuality. In this section we will explore three additional aspects of our sexuality—reproductive, genital, and expressionistic—around which many of our important decisions in life are made.* With these new perspectives in mind, you will be better able to see the complexity associated with our development as productive and satisfied beings.

---

*We cite no specific source for the terms *reproductive sexuality, genital sexuality,* and *expressionistic sexuality.* Rather, they are labels we and our colleagues use in instructional units associated with human sexuality.

Personal Assessment

Sexual Attitudes: A Matter of Feelings

Respond to each of the following statements by selecting a numbered response (1-5) that most accurately reflects your feelings. Circle the number of your selection. At the conclusion of the questionnaire, total these numbers for use in interpreting your responses.

1　Agree strongly
2　Agree moderately
3　Uncertain
4　Disagree moderately
5　Disagree strongly

1 Men and women have greater differences than they have similarities.	1	2	3	4	5
2 Homosexuality and bisexuality are immoral and unnatural.	1	2	3	4	5
3 Our society is too sexually oriented.	1	2	3	4	5
4 Pornography encourages sexual promiscuity.	1	2	3	4	5
5 Children know far too much about sex.	1	2	3	4	5
6 Education about sexuality is solely the responsibility of the family.	1	2	3	4	5
7 Dating begins far too early in our society.	1	2	3	4	5
8 Sexual intimacy before marriage leads to emotional stress and damage to one's reputation.	1	2	3	4	5
9 Sexual availability is far too frequently the reason that people marry.	1	2	3	4	5
10 Reproduction is the most important reason for sexual intimacy during marriage.	1	2	3	4	5
11 Modern families are too small.	1	2	3	4	5
12 Family planning clinics should not receive public funds.	1	2	3	4	5
13 Contraception is the woman's responsibility.	1	2	3	4	5
14 Abortion is the murder of an innocent child.	1	2	3	4	5
15 Marriage has been weakened by the changing role of women in society.	1	2	3	4	5
16 Divorce is an unacceptable means of resolving marital difficulties.	1	2	3	4	5
17 Extramarital sexual intimacy will destroy a marriage.	1	2	3	4	5
18 Sexual abuse of a child does not generally occur unless the child encourages the adult.	1	2	3	4	5
19 Provocative behavior by the woman is a factor in almost every case of rape.	1	2	3	4	5
20 Reproduction is not a right but a privilege.	1	3	3	4	5

Your total points _____

Interpretation

20-34 points　　A very traditional attitude toward sexuality
35-54 points　　A moderately traditional attitude toward sexuality
55-65 points　　A rather ambivalent attitude toward sexuality
66-85 points　　A moderately open attitude toward sexuality
86-100 points　A very open attitude toward sexuality

Reproductive Sexuality

Of these three aspects of sexuality, *reproductive sexuality* reflects the most basic level of sexuality over which the adult must exercise direction and display insight. Simply stated, reproductive sexuality is related to your knowledge of, desire for, and ability to participate in the act of *procreation.* Pregnancy, delivery, natural childbirth, breastfeeding, fertility control, and pregnancy termination are terms related to this dimension of sexuality. Demographic data indicate that most (but not all) of you will choose to be active in this dimension of your sexuality by becoming parents.

Genital Sexuality

Genital sexuality refers to the nonreproductive use of the reproductive organs. In comparison to the concept of reproductive sexuality, genital sexuality implies *recreation* and *communication* rather than procreation. The behaviors and meanings associated with the terms orgasm, having sex, making love, oral-genital sex, prostitution, and sexual responsiveness are genital in their orientation.

In the most positive sense, sexual experiences that are genitally oriented should be sensual, erotic, and stimulating, and should give the individual a sense of release. Genital sexuality reflects our gift to ourselves and to our partners as well. However, many forms of genital sexuality may not be condoned by certain groups of people or religions.

For some persons genital sexuality can be a volatile experience. We base this contention on the closeness of genital sexuality to reproduction. Far too frequently a genitally centered sexual experience results in an unanticipated and unwanted pregnancy. In such circumstances, the couple, or more often the female acting alone, is forced to make decisions that could significantly influence the future. An unexpected pregnancy, even for the relatively mature college person, may result in a series of necessary compromises. Also, the close association between genital sexuality and sexually transmitted diseases (including AIDS) makes some sexual activities potentially dangerous.

For some people genital sexuality becomes the mode of communication with which they feel most comfortable. In such cases, partners may be known only in a very limited way. Growth in sexual technique may readily occur within the context of a genitally centered relationship, but little in the way of a fully developed relationship will occur. Genitally based relationships are rarely elevated to a much higher level.

Expressionistic Sexuality

Expressionistic sexuality represents the most broadly based dimension of yourself as a man or woman. As its name implies, this is your "expression" of your current gender schema. Cognitively, **affectively,** and behaviorally, you are "playing out" your initial adult gender identification. The way you dress, the occupation you pursue, and the leisure activities you develop are all aspects of this dimension of your sexuality.

affective
pertaining to one's beliefs, values, and predispositions.

Expressionistic sexuality encompasses the reproductive and genital dimensions of your sexuality, but it is more. It is the sexuality that will serve you most fully

Ideas about traditional sex roles are changing.

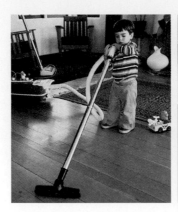 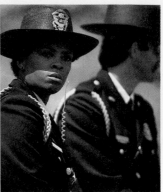

for the rest of your life. Most adults probably are conventional in their patterns of expressionistic sexuality, yet a variety of additional patterns also exist (see Chapter 14).

ANDROGYNY: SHARING THE PLUSES

Although there may still be some pocket of resistance, in the last 15 years our society has increasingly accepted an image of a person who possesses both masculine and feminine qualities. This accepted image has taken years to develop, because our society traditionally has reinforced only limited masculine roles for males and limited feminine roles for females.

In the past, from the time a child was born, we assigned and reinforced only those roles and traits that were thought to be directly related to his or her biological sex. Boys were not allowed to cry, play with dolls, or help in the kitchen. Girls were not encouraged to become involved in sports; they were told to learn to sew, cook, and babysit. Males were encouraged to be strong, expressive, dominant, aggressive, career oriented, while females were encouraged to be weak, shy, submissive, passive, and home oriented.

These traditional biases have resulted in some interesting phenomena related to career opportunities. Women were denied jobs requiring above-average physical strength, denied admittance into professional schools (law, medicine, and business) requiring high intellectual capacities, and denied entry into most levels of military participation. Likewise, men have not been encouraged to enter traditionally feminine careers, such as nursing, clerical work, and elementary school teaching. Such traditional biases started disappearing in the 1980s.

androgyny
the blending of both masculine and feminine qualities.

For a variety of reasons, the traditional picture has changed. **Androgyny,** or the blending of both feminine and masculine qualities, is more clearly evident in our society now than ever before. Today it is perfectly acceptable to see men involved in raising children (including changing diapers) and doing routine housework. On the other hand, it is also acceptable to see women entering the workplace in jobs traditionally managed by men and participating in sports traditionally played by men. Men are not scoffed at when seen crying after a touching movie. Women are not laughed at when they choose to assert themselves. The disposal of numerous sexual stereotypes has probably benefitted our society immensely by relieving persons of the quest to be 100% "womanly" or 100% "macho."

The fact that some research data suggest that androgynous people are better able to cope with many of life's stressors than those who fit rigid sex roles should encourage you to be unafraid to break the stereotypical sex role occasionally.[13] So, women: if you want to pump iron, repair your roof, tune up your car, or play rugby, by all means, DO IT. So, men: if you want to do aerobic exercise, make a quiche, learn to iron, or practice needlepoint, by all means, DO IT. You may find yourself much happier than you would be if you tried to repress these urges, and you may find yourself a much more flexible, talented person.

SUMMARY

In our society we have come to recognize that both biological and psychosocial factors contribute to the complex expression of our sexuality. Biological sexuality begins at the moment of conception and is determined on a genetic basis. The gonadal basis of sexuality begins to develop the fifth or sixth week after conception. The structural basis of sexuality is established as the internal and external reproductive structures develop in the fetus.

At birth, children are labeled female or male according to their external reproductive structures. During the childhood years, only a gradual degree of growth occurs in the reproductive systems. However, during puberty, greatly accelerated growth takes place until the reproductive systems achieve their adult structure and capabilities.

Virtually all individuals go through several processes that transform them into beings who are more complex than simply their biological makeups. These psychosocial processes include gender identity, gender preference, and gender adoption. By the time individuals move through these psychosocial stages, they are ready to construct an initial adult gender identification.

The male and female reproductive systems consist of external and internal structures. The menstrual cycle's primary functions are to produce a viable ovum and to develop a supportive environment in the uterus.

The complexity of our adult sexuality is reflected in three distinct facets of our sexuality; reproductive, genital, and expressionistic. Expressionistic sexuality is the type of sexuality that all of us display on a daily basis through our physical structure, dress, mannerisms, and lifestyle.

For many reasons, there is now an increasing acceptance of androgynous individuals—people who possess both masculine and feminine qualities. Androgynous people seem to be better able to cope with life's stressors. Additionally, the acceptance of androgyny is opening many career opportunities that were once closed to either men or women.

REVIEW QUESTIONS

1 Explain the following bases of our biological sexuality: genetic, gonadal, internal structural development, and external structural development.
2 Explain the role of the hormone androgen in the structural development in female and male embryos.
3 Describe the physical changes that take place in both males and females during puberty.

4 Define and explain the following terms: gender identity, gender preference, gender adoption, gender schema, and initial adult gender identification.

5 Identify the major components of the male and female reproductive systems. Explain the structure of each component and its function in the reproductive process.

6 Trace the passageways for sperm and ova.

7 Explain the menstrual cycle. Identify and describe the three stages of the menstrual cycle.

8 Differentiate among reproductive, genital, and expressionistic aspects of sexuality.

9 Define androgyny. What are the advantages of an androgynous lifestyle? What are the disadvantages?

QUESTIONS FOR PERSONAL CONTEMPLATION

1 Think about the years when you were growing up. What kinds of activities were you involved in, or encouraged to be involved in? Were they activities typically thought of as male or female? Are your current activities traditional ones for your gender? Why do you think you selected these activities?

2 Do you have positive or negative feelings about the gender you are? What do you think causes these feelings? How can you deal with them if they are negative feelings?

3 Do you agree or disagree with the contention that biological processes may influence sexuality more strongly than was once believed?

4 Do you feel your character is mostly masculine, mostly feminine, or androgynous? What behaviors could you change in your own life that would make you more androgynous? Do you see any value in making these changes?

REFERENCES

1 Hyde, JS: Understanding human sexuality, ed 3, New York, 1986, McGraw-Hill Book Co.

2 Mosher, D, et al: The sex-determining region of the human Y chromosome encodes a finger protein, Cell 51:1091-1104, 1987.

3 Moore, K: The developing human, ed 3, Philadelphia, 1982, WB Saunders Co.

4 Spence, AS: Basic human anatomy, ed 2, Menlo Park, Calif, 1986, The Benjamin-Cummings Publishing Co.

5 Masters, W, Johnson, V, and Kolodny, R: Human sexuality, ed 2, Boston, 1985, Little, Brown & Co, Inc.

6 Crooks, R, and Baur, K: Our sexuality, ed 3, Menlo Park, Calif, 1987, The Benjamin-Cummings Publishing Co.

7 Money, J, and Tucker, P: Sexual signatures: on being a man or a woman, Boston, 1975, Little, Brown & Co.

8 Haas, K, and Haas, A: Understanding sexuality, St. Louis, 1987, Times Mirror/Mosby College Publishing.

9 Money, J, and Ehrhardt, A: Man and woman, boy and girl: differentiation and gender identity from conception to maturity, Baltimore, 1972, The Johns Hopkins University Press.

10 Tortora, GJ, and Anagnostakos, NP: Principles of anatomy and physiology, ed 5, New York, 1987, Harper & Row Publishers, Inc.

11 Lein, A: The cycling female: her menstrual rhythm, San Francisco, 1979, WH Freeman & Co, Publishers.

12 Hatcher, RA, et al: Contraceptive technology 1986-1987, New York, 1986, Irvington Publishers, Inc.

13 Bem, SL: Beyond androgyny: some presumptuous prescriptions for a liberated sexual identity. In Sherman, J, and Denmark, F, editors: Psychology of women: future directions of research, New York, 1981, Psychological Dimensions, Inc.

ANNOTATED READINGS

Denney, NW, and Quadagno, D: Human sexuality, St. Louis, 1987, Times Mirror/Mosby College Publishing.

A college-level textbook suitable for an introductory human sexuality course. Presents a comprehensive overview of issues and scientific topics related to sexuality. The authors draw from the social, behavioral, biological, and health sciences.

Durden-Smith, J, and deSimone, D: Sex and the brain, New York, 1983, Warner Books, Inc.

Identifies the biological inheritance that separates males from females, and challenges all accepted social scientific teachings. Attempts to answer these questions: What is the real difference between man and woman? Is there something that makes the male brain qualitatively different from the female brain?

Field, E: The good girl syndrome: why women are programmed to fail in a man's world, New York, 1986, Macmillan Publishing Co.

Discusses the difficulties that confront women as they attempt to compete with men in areas traditionally in the sole domain of men. Provokes consideration of the behavioral patterns that could be used by women to succeed in "a man's world."

Hubbard, R, Henefin, M, and Fried, B: Biological woman—the convenient myth, Cambridge, Ma, 1982, Schenkman Books, Inc.

A collection of 12 scholarly feminist essays that counter the argument that biology is the most important determinant of our masculinity and feminity. Some of the essay titles are "Have Only Men Evolved?" "Taking the Men out of Menopause," and "Displaced—The Midwife by the Male Physician."

Money, J, and Tucker, P: Sexual signatures: on being a man or a woman, Boston, 1975, Little, Brown and Co, Inc.

A classic book for the nonprofessional that details in an understandable manner the pathways our sexuality takes in reaching its fullest expression. The interrelationship of the biological and psychosocial forces that make the behavior of males and females both alike and different is an important focus of the book.

Sarrel, LJ, and Sarrel, PM: Sexual turning points: the seven stages of adult sexuality, New York, 1984, Macmillan Publishing Co.

Presents the view that there is a direct connection between life events and sexuality. Presents seven stages, including sexual unfolding and childhood-adolescent sexual experiences and their effects.

Stechert, K: On your own terms: a woman's guide to working with men, New York, 1987, Vintage Books.

Intended to help women better understand the men with whom they work. Describes ways in which men use humor, aggressiveness, power, and money.

Sexuality
A Variety of Behaviors and Relationships

Key Concepts

The human sexual response pattern consists of four predictable stages.

Sexual behavior is enhanced through good communication and concern for yourself and your partner.

Couples can move through three distinct stages as they progress from dating to marriage.

Alternatives to marriage include divorce, singlehood, cohabitation, and single parenthood.

Variant sexual behavior is seen in a variety of forms.

The causes of homosexuality are not fully understood.

Sexual victimization is pervasive in our society.

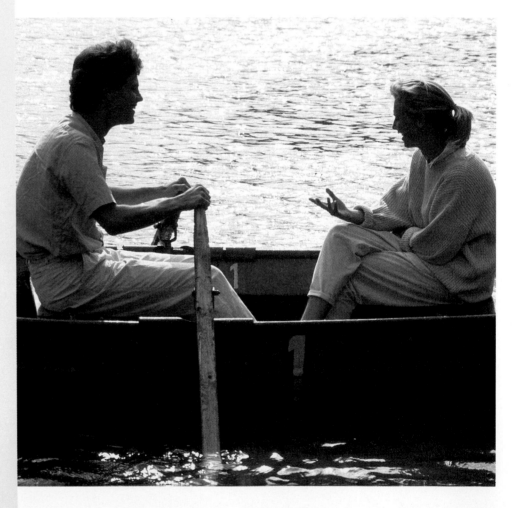

*I*n this chapter, the genital and expressionistic dimensions of sexuality discussed in Chapter 13 will be reexamined in more depth. However, rather than focusing on sexuality as it relates solely to you as an individual, the focus of this chapter will be on sexuality as it relates to your experiences in paired relationships. The specific topics of sexual responsiveness, patterns of sexual behavior, standards of sexual intimacy, dating, mate selection, marriage, alternatives to marriage, sexual preferences and variations, and sexual victimization will be explored.

THE HUMAN SEXUAL RESPONSE PATTERN

Genital sexuality—the sexuality of recreation, communication, and performance—exists because of the ability of the human body to respond to erotic stimuli. Rooted in biological function, sexual responsiveness links the biologically based reproductive sexuality with the psychosocially conditioned expressionistic sexuality. Genital sexuality can be an important component in human relationships. The healthy adult can take pleasure in the fact that there is an easily accessible pathway whereby arousal, release, and intense satisfaction can be gleaned from structures whose primary purpose is reproduction.

Although history is replete with written and visual accounts of the human's ability to be sexually aroused, it was not until the pioneering work of Masters and Johnson[1] that the events associated with arousal were clinically documented. Five questions posed by these researchers gave direction to a series of studies involving the scientific evaluation of human sexual response:

1 Is there a definitive pattern associated with the sexual response of males and females?
2 Is the sexual response pattern stimuli specific?
3 What variations occur in the sexual response patterns of males and females? What variations might be found among members of the same sex? Within a given individual?
4 What are the basic physiological mechanisms underlying a sexual response pattern?
5 What role is played by specific organs and organ systems within the sexual response pattern?

Question 1—A Predictable Response Pattern

The answer to the first question posed by the researchers was a definitive "yes." A predictable sexual response pattern was identified.[1] The sexual response pattern consists of an initial **excitement stage**, a **plateau stage**, the **orgasmic stage**, and a **resolution stage**. Each stage involves predictable changes in the structural characteristics and physiological function of reproductive and nonreproductive organs in both the male and female. A detailed description of sequentially occurring changes noted in each stage and depictions of the locations and changing size of anatomical structures is shown in the box on pp. 384-385.

Question 2—Stimuli Specificity

The research of Masters and Johnson[1] clearly established an answer to the second question concerning a stimuli specificity. Their findings demonstrated that

excitement stage
initial arousal stage of the sexual response pattern.

plateau stage
second stage of the sexual response pattern; a leveling off of arousal immediately before orgasm.

orgasmic stage
third stage of the sexual response pattern; the stage during which neuromuscular tension is released.

resolution stage
fourth stage of the sexual response pattern; the return of the body to a preexcitement state.

Sexual Response Pattern

UNAROUSED STAGE

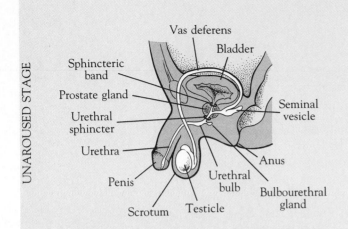
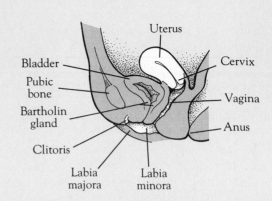

Vas deferens
Bladder
Sphincteric band
Prostate gland
Urethral sphincter
Urethra
Penis
Scrotum
Testicle
Urethral bulb
Anus
Seminal vesicle
Bulbourethral gland

Uterus
Bladder
Pubic bone
Bartholin gland
Clitoris
Labia majora
Labia minora
Cervix
Vagina
Anus

EXCITEMENT STAGE

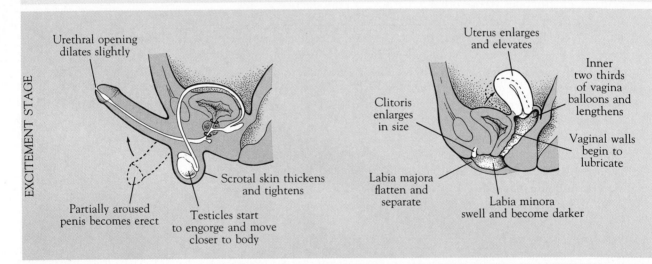

Urethral opening dilates slightly
Partially aroused penis becomes erect
Testicles start to engorge and move closer to body
Scrotal skin thickens and tightens

Uterus enlarges and elevates
Clitoris enlarges in size
Labia majora flatten and separate
Labia minora swell and become darker
Inner two thirds of vagina balloons and lengthens
Vaginal walls begin to lubricate

PLATEAU STAGE

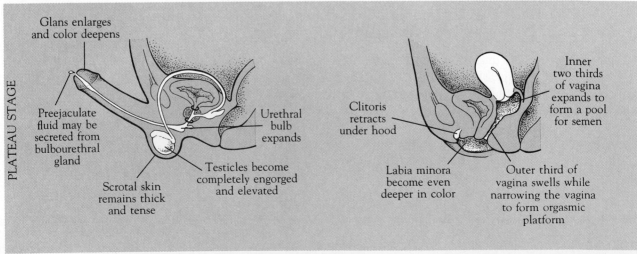

Glans enlarges and color deepens
Preejaculate fluid may be secreted from bulbourethral gland
Scrotal skin remains thick and tense
Testicles become completely engorged and elevated
Urethral bulb expands

Clitoris retracts under hood
Labia minora become even deeper in color
Inner two thirds of vagina expands to form a pool for semen
Outer third of vagina swells while narrowing the vagina to form orgasmic platform

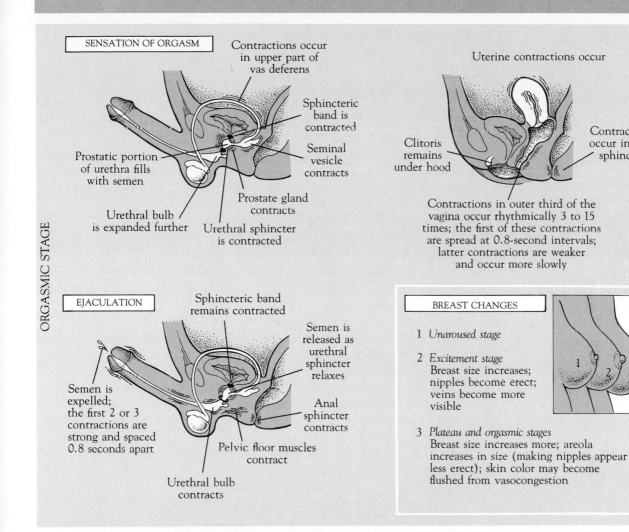

ORGASMIC STAGE

SENSATION OF ORGASM

Contractions occur in upper part of vas deferens

Sphincteric band is contracted

Seminal vesicle contracts

Prostatic portion of urethra fills with semen

Urethral bulb is expanded further

Prostate gland contracts

Urethral sphincter is contracted

Uterine contractions occur

Clitoris remains under hood

Contractions occur in anal sphincter

Contractions in outer third of the vagina occur rhythmically 3 to 15 times; the first of these contractions are spread at 0.8-second intervals; latter contractions are weaker and occur more slowly

EJACULATION

Sphincteric band remains contracted

Semen is released as urethral sphincter relaxes

Semen is expelled; the first 2 or 3 contractions are strong and spaced 0.8 seconds apart

Anal sphincter contracts

Urethral bulb contracts

Pelvic floor muscles contract

BREAST CHANGES

1 *Unaroused stage*

2 *Excitement stage*
   Breast size increases; nipples become erect; veins become more visible

3 *Plateau and orgasmic stages*
   Breast size increases more; areola increases in size (making nipples appear less erect); skin color may become flushed from vasocongestion

1 2 3

RESOLUTION STAGE

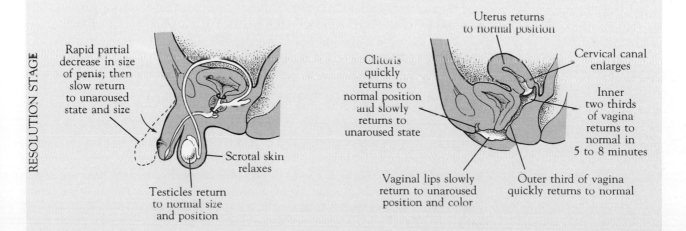

Rapid partial decrease in size of penis; then slow return to unaroused state and size

Scrotal skin relaxes

Testicles return to normal size and position

Uterus returns to normal position

Clitoris quickly returns to normal position and slowly returns to unaroused state

Cervical canal enlarges

Inner two thirds of vagina returns to normal in 5 to 8 minutes

Vaginal lips slowly return to unaroused position and color

Outer third of vagina quickly returns to normal

a wide variety of sensory modalities can supply the stimuli necessary for initiating the sexual response pattern. While tactile stimuli might initiate arousal in most persons and maximize it for the vast majority of persons, in both males and females, visual, olfactory, auditory, and *vicariously formed stimuli* can accomplish the same sexual arousal patterns.

Question 3A—Male Versus Female Response Pattern

In response to the third question, several variations are observable when comparing the sexual response patterns of males and females:

- With the exception of some late adolescent males, the vast majority of males are not multiorgasmic. The **refractory phase** of the resolution stage prevents most males from experiencing more than one orgasm in a short period of time, even though sufficient stimulation is available.
- Females possess a **multiorgasmic capacity.** As many as 10% to 30% of all adult females routinely experience multiple orgasms.[1]
- Although they possess multiorgasmic potential, some 10% of all adult females are *anorgasmic*—that is, they never experience an orgasm.[2] For some anorgasmic females, orgasms can be experienced when masturbation, rather than **coitus,** provides the stimulation.
- When measured during coitus, males reach orgasm far more quickly than do females. However, when masturbation is the source of stimulation, females reach orgasm as quickly as do males.[1]

More important than any of the differences pointed out is the finding that the sexual response patterns of males and females are far more alike than they are different. Not only do males and females experience the four basic stages of the response pattern, but they also have similar responses in specific areas, including the **erection** and *tumescence* of sexual structures; the appearance of a **sex flush;** the increase in cardiac output, blood pressure and respiratory rate; and the occurrence of *rhythmic pelvic thrusting.*[1]

Question 3B—Variation: Within a Same-Sex Group

When a group of subjects of the same sex was studied in an attempt to answer questions about similarities and differences in the sexual response pattern, Masters and Johnson noted considerable variation. Even when variables such as age, race, education, and general health were held constant, the extent and duration of virtually every stage of the response pattern varied.

Question 3C—Variation: Within the Same Individual

For a given person, the nature of the sexual response pattern does not remain constant, even when observed over a relatively short period of time. A variety of internal and external factors can alter this pattern. The aging process, changes in general health status, levels of stress, altered environmental settings, use of alcohol and other drugs, and behavioral changes in a sexual partner can cause one's own sexual response pattern to change from one sexual experience to another.[3]

---

refractory phase
that portion of the male's resolution stage during which sexual arousal cannot occur.

multiorgasmic capacity
potential to have several orgasms within a single period of sexual arousal.

coitus
penile-vaginal intercourse.

erection
the engorgement of erectile tissue with blood; characteristic of the penis, clitoris, nipples, labia minora, and scrotum

sex flush
the reddish skin response that results from increasing sexual arousal

Question 4—Physiological Mechanisms Underlying the Sexual Response Pattern

The basic mechanisms in the fourth question posed by Masters and Johnson are now well recognized. One factor, *vasocongestion,* or the retention of blood or fluid within a particular tissue, is of major importance in the development of physiological changes that promote the sexual response pattern.[1] The presence of erectile tissue underlies the changes that can be noted in the penis, breast, and scrotum of the male, and the clitoris, breast, and labia majora of the female.

A second mechanism now recognized as necessary for the development of the sexual response pattern is that of *myotonia,* or the buildup of *neuromuscular tonus* within a variety of body structures.[1] At the end of the plateau stage of the response pattern, a sudden release of the accumulated neuromuscular tension gives rise to the rhythmic muscular contractions and muscular spasms that constitute orgasm as well as ejaculation in the male. In both sexes, however, the subjective interpretations of this release of neuromuscular tension are important in shaping the feelings of satisfaction associated with orgasm.

Question 5—Role of Specific Organs in the Sexual Response Pattern

The fifth question posed by Masters and Johnson concerning the role played by specific organs and organ systems during each stage of the response pattern can be readily answered by referring to the material presented in the box on pp. 384-385. As you study this box, remember that direct stimulation of the penis and either direct or indirect stimulation of the clitoris are the principal avenues toward orgasm. Also, intercourse represents only one activity that can lead to orgasmic pleasure.

A recent development in the study of sexual response patterns centers on a presumed erogenous zone in the upper anterior portion of the vaginal wall, the *Grafenberg spot.*[4] First reported in 1940 by Ernst Grafenberg, this spot is believed to be the female counterpart of the male prostate gland. Proponents of the "G spot" theory contend that when deeply stimulated, this small area of erectile tissue on the anterior wall of the vagina becomes erect and upon orgasm, releases a moderate quantity of alkaline fluid. Many gynecologists, pathologists, and anatomists dispute the existence of the Grafenberg spot.

PATTERNS OF SEXUAL BEHAVIOR

While sex researchers may see sexual behavior in terms of the human sexual response pattern just described, most people are more interested in the observable dimensions of sexual behavior. From the definitions of sexuality developed for use in this textbook, we will now direct your attention to the blending of your genital sexuality and your expressionistic sexuality. We will begin by discussing celibacy and end with heterosexual coital behavior.

Celibacy

Celibacy, or secondary virginity, may be defined as self-selected abstinence from sexual intimacy.[5] Usually thought of in conjunction with religious orders, this behavioral choice is sometimes chosen by persons not affiliated with such orders. There are many reasons why a man or woman would choose not to establish a sexually intimate relationship with another person. Some physical handicaps might preclude sexual activity. The threat of AIDS transmission may discourage some people from sexual intimacy. Others who are celibate may include those who find partners unavailable or unappealing. Some may be protecting their virginity until marriage.

Still others, perhaps the vast majority, prefer celibacy simply because it seems most appropriate for them. Celibacy does not preclude deep, intimate relationships with others—just sexual relations with others. Perhaps celibacy simplifies life, allows for greater emphasis on work or creative efforts, allows for cerebral focus on the self, or fosters experimentation in asceticism. Celibacy may be short-term or may last a lifetime, and no identified physical or psychological complications appear to result from a celibate lifestyle.

Masturbation

The following passage, taken from a 1901 medical school textbook entitled *Perfect Womanhood,* reflects a negative view of masturbation, which was held in the early decades of this century.

> On going to his bed, after he had gone to sleep, she found his hands still upon the organ, just as they were when he fell asleep. She watched this carefully for a few days, then took him in her confidence and told him of the dreadful evil effects. Finding the habit so firmly fixed, she feared that telling him, at his age, what effect it would have upon his future would not eradicate the evil as soon as she hoped. So after studying the case for a time, she hit upon the following remedy. Although unscientific, literally speaking, it had the desired effect. Feeling that something must be done to stop, and to stop at once, the awful habit, she said, "Did you know, Charlie, that if you keep up this habit of 'self-abuse' that a brown spot will come on your abdomen, light brown at first, and grow darker each week, until it eats a sore right into your system, and if it keeps on, will eventually kill you?"[6]

Whether the rationale underlying this negative view of masturbation arose out of Judeo-Christian beliefs concerning coitus as the only legitimate sexual behavior, or whether this view was centered in a misguided concern for health, is primarily of historical importance. The point that is relevant today is that masturbation is very widely practiced.

For those who are interested in the variety of procedures that are applicable to the act of masturbation, we would recommend some of the books currently used in human sexuality courses. (These may be found in many university bookstores and libraries.) What is more important to us, however, is the fact that the near universal practice of masturbation among college-age men and women suggests the value of dealing with sexual needs. The following can be easily seen as positive dimensions of masturbation.

- For some individuals masturbation is the only form of sexual behavior that is available and, at the same time, acceptable and safe to engage in.
- Masturbation provides a means for exploring the sexual response pattern and thus experiencing a dimension of one's sexuality.
- Masturbation provides an outlet for tension and the reduction of stress. Some contend that masturbation is the most useful facilitator for sleep that they have discovered.

For some, masturbation is the only source of tactile and vicarious stimulation that will produce an orgasm. As mentioned previously, females who
are anorgasmic during coitus are often orgasmic during masturbation.
A study conducted by Hunt,[7] which found that approximately 70% of married
men and women continue to masturbate well into the first decade of marriage,
reflects the staying power of this form of sexual behavior.

Fantasy and Erotic Dreams

The brain is the most sensual organ in the body. In fact, many sexuality experts
classify **sexual fantasies** and **erotic dreams** as forms of sexual behavior. Particularly for people whose verbal ability is highly developed, the ability to create
rich vicarious scenes enriches other forms of sexual behavior.

Various types of sexual fantasies are forms of sexual behavior generally found
in association with some second type of sexual behavior. When occurring before
coitus or masturbation, fantasies prepare a person for the behavior that will follow. As an example, fantasies experienced during a course lecture may focus
your attention on sexual activity that will occur later in the day.

When fantasies occur in conjunction with another form of sexual behavior,
the second behavior may be greatly enhanced by the supportive fantasy. Both
females and males fantasize during foreplay and coitus. Masturbation and fantas-
izing are inseparable activities.[5]

Erotic dreams occur during sleep in both men and women. The association
between these dreams and ejaculation resulting in a nocturnal emission (wet
dream) is readily recognized in males. In females, erotic dreams can lead not
only to vaginal lubrication, but to orgasm as well.[4]

Shared Touching

Virtually the entire body can be an erogenous zone when sensual contact between partners is involved. A soft, light touch, a slight application of pressure,
the brushing back of a partner's hair, and gentle massage are all forms of communication that heighten sexual arousal.

Genital Contact

Your grandparents' generation called it "heavy petting." A generation later it
was referred to as "feeling up." You too no doubt have a term to describe the
act of stimulating a partner's genitals. Regardless of the words used, genital contact has long been a popular form of sexual behavior for couples of all ages.

Two important uses can be identified for the practice of stimulating a partner's
genitals. The first is that of being the tactile component of **foreplay.** Genital
contact, in the form of holding, rubbing, stroking, or caressing heightens arousal
to a level that allows for progression into coitus.

The second role of genital contact is that of *mutual masturbation to orgasm.*[8]
Stimulation of the genitals so that both partners experience orgasm is a form of
sexual behavior practiced by many adolescents as well as couples during the
late stage of a pregnancy. For couples not wishing a pregnancy, the risk of pregnancy is virtually eliminated when this becomes the form of sexual intimacy
practiced.

sexual fantasies
fantasies with sexual themes;
sexual daydreams or imaginary events.

erotic dreams
dreams whose content elicits
a sexual response.

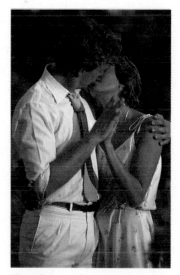
Touching enhances intimacy.

foreplay
activities, often involving
touching and caressing, that
prepare individuals for sexual intercourse.

In terms of specific techniques, rubbing of the vulva, including indirect contact with the clitoris, and insertion of one or more fingers into the vagina are commonly employed techniques for stimulating the female. For males, rubbing, pulling, and caressing the penis and the scrotum are effective forms of genital contact. Finger penetration of the anus can be erotically stimulating for both sexes. Care must be taken, however, not to contaminate other structures with bacteria from the anus. Vibrators can be used in stimulating the genitals of both the male and female.

As is the case of other aspects of intimacy, genital stimulation is best enhanced when partners can talk about their needs, expectations, and reservations. Practice and communication can shape this form of contact into a pleasure-giving approach to sexual intimacy.

Oral-Genital Stimulation

Sexual behaviors, like other human behaviors, are not static but change over the course of time. The practice of oral-genital sex is no exception. In the 1950s, according to Kinsey's data, slightly over 55% of college-educated married couples had experienced oral sex. Research in the 1970s by Hunt revealed a significant increase in the incidence of reported oral sex. Ninety percent of all married couples had experienced oral-genital stimulation, while 70% of unmarried adolescents reported the same.[7]

Oral-genital stimulation brings together two of the body's most erogenous areas: the genitalia and the mouth. Couples who engage in oral sex consistently report that this form of intimacy is highly satisfactory. Some persons have experimented with oral sex and found it unacceptable, and some have never experienced this form of sexual intimacy. Some couples prefer not to participate in oral sex because they consider it immoral (according to religious doctrine), illegal (which it is in some states), or unhygienic (because of a partner's unclean genitals). Some couples may refrain because of the mistaken belief that oral sex is a homosexual practice. Regardless of the reason, a person who does not consider oral sex to be pleasurable should not be coerced into this behavior.

fellatio
oral stimulation of the penis.

cunnilingus
oral stimulation of the vulva or clitoris.

Three basic forms of oral-genital stimulation are practiced by both heterosexual and homosexual couples. **Fellatio,** in which the penis is sucked, licked, or kissed by the partner, is the most common of the three. Knox[4] reports three current studies that indicate that between 60% and 95% of women and men claim that their petting sometimes includes fellatio. **Cunnilingus,** in which the vulva of the female is kissed, licked, or penetrated by the partner's tongue, is only slightly less frequently practiced. Among married couples, Petersen's 1983 study[9] indicated that nine out of ten husbands enjoy performing cunnilingus with their wives.

Mutual oral-genital stimulation, the third form of oral-genital stimulation, combines both fellatio and cunnilingus. When practiced by a heterosexual couple, the female partner performs fellatio on her partner, while her male partner performs cunnilingus on her. Obviously, the partners must be lying in opposite directions. Since this positioning resembles the figure "69," mutual oral-genital stimulation is frequently referred to as "69." Homosexual couples can practice mutual fellatio or cunnilingus.

Couples considering oral-genital stimulation as an adjunct to their sexual

Sexual Performance Difficulties and Therapies

For all of the predictability of the human sexual response pattern, many people find that at some point in their lives, they are no longer capable of responding sexually. The inability of a person to perform adequately is identified as a sexual difficulty or dysfunction. Sexual difficulties can have a corrosive influence on a person's sense of sexual satisfaction and on a partner's satisfaction. Fortunately, most sexual difficulties can be resolved through strategies that use individual, couple, or group counseling. Most sexual performance difficulties stem from psychogenic factors.

Difficulty	Possible Causes	Therapeutic Approaches
WOMEN **ORGASMIC DIFFICULTIES**		
Inability to experience orgasm	Anxiety, fear, guilt, anger, poor self-concept; lack of knowledge about female responsiveness; inadequate sexual arousal; interpersonal problems with partner	Counseling to improve a couple's communication; educating a woman and her partner about female responsiveness; teaching a woman how to experience orgasm through masturbation
VAGINISMUS		
Painful, involuntary contractions of the vaginal muscles	Previous traumatic experiences with intercourse (rape, incest, uncaring partners); fear of pregnancy; religious prohibitions; anxiety about vaginal penetration of any kind (including tampons)	Counseling to alleviate psychogenic causes; gradual dilation of the vagina with woman's fingers or dilators; systematic desensitization exercises; relaxation training
DYSPAREUNIA		
Painful intercourse	Insufficient sexual arousal; communication problems with partner; infections, inflammations; structural abnormalities; insufficient lubrication	Individual and couple counseling with a focus on relaxation and communication; medical strategies to reduce infections and structural abnormalities
MEN **IMPOTENCE**		
Inability to achieve an erection	Chronic diseases (including diabetes, vascular problems, and chemical dependencies); trauma; numerous psychogenic factors (including anxiety, guilt, fear, poor self-concept)	Medical intervention (including possible vascular surgery or the use of penile implants); couple counseling using sensate focusing, pleasuring, and relaxation strategies
RAPID EJACULATION		
Ejaculating too quickly after penile penetration; premature ejaculation	Predominately psychogenic in origin; a male's need to prove his sexual prowess; anxiety associated with previous sexual experiences	Counseling to free the man from the anxiety associated with rapid ejaculation; altering coital position; masturbation prior to intimacy; use of the squeeze technique as orgasm approaches
DYSPAREUNIA		
Painful intercourse	Primarily physical in origin; inability of the penile foreskin to retract fully; urogenital tract infections; scar tissue in seminal passageways; insufficient lubrication	Medical care to reduce infection or repair damaged or abnormal tissue; additional lubrication

practices might wish to discuss any initial reservations they might have. Clearly, participation in oral sex should not be forced on one partner by another. Couples engaging in oral sex should probably reach a prior agreement on such issues as how to dispose of the ejaculate and whether cunnilingus will be practiced during the menses. For relatively few, oral-anal stimulation will become a logical extension of their oral-genital practices.

Coitus

Although various words and phrases are used to describe the act of penile-vaginal intercourse, technically the term *coitus* is preferred. Of all the groups of sexual behaviors described thus far, coitus (or *coition*) is the only practice that is limited to heterosexual couples. Thus penile-anal intercourse (*sodomy*)—practiced by some heterosexual and male homosexual couples—is not encompassed by the term coitus. Furthermore, no other sexual practice is as directly associated with **procreation** as is coitus. For many, coitus is considered the only natural and appropriate form of sexual intimacy.

procreation
reproduction.

    The incidence and frequency of coital behavior is a much-studied topic. Information concerning the percentages of married and unmarried persons who have experienced sexual intercourse is readily available in textbooks used in human sexuality courses. In making personal interpretations of these data, however, you are reminded that the collection of this information relies on people reporting their own intimate behaviors. Interviews and questionnaires do not always reflect behavior as closely as researchers would like. Furthermore, the AIDS epidemic has had a major impact on the sexual practices of many people, including young adults.

    Despite limitations associated with the collection of data about the sexual behavior of unmarried young adults, we can generalize about three areas of change in coital behavior that have occurred in the past 20 years.

1 Significantly higher percentages of women now report experiencing sexual intercourse than did 20 years ago.
2 Slightly higher percentages of men now report experiencing sexual intercourse than did 20 years ago.
3 Men still report overall higher frequencies of premarital coitus than do women, but this gap is quickly narrowing.[3]

As is true for other forms of sexual behavior described in this chapter, a mature approach to coitus requires concern for yourself and your partner as well as a commitment to communicate. Particularly for coitus, the "wham, bam, thank you, ma'am" attitude that has traditionally been the male mindset is rapidly becoming a thing of the past. Couples need to share their expectations concerning coital techniques and the desired frequency of intercourse. Even the "performance" factors, such as depth of penetration, nature of body movements, tempo of activity, and timing of orgasm are of increasing importance to many couples. These factors also need to be revealed through open communication.

    Because this textbook is not intended to be a performance manual in the area of intimate sexual behavior, we would again refer you to a variety of books (including textbooks) which provide written as well as visually explicit information on coital positions. We will simply suggest that four basic positions for coitus—*male above, female above, side by side,* and *rear entry*—each offer relative advantages and disadvantages. Personal preferences based on such criteria as body size, physical limitations, pregnancy, and the need for variation and heightened eroticism will dictate the coital techniques you and your partner use.

NONMARITAL AND EXTRAMARITAL SEXUAL INTIMACY

In spite of all its ability to provide pleasure and release, the sexual response capacity described earlier has been tightly scrutinized by society—particularly for young unmarried adults and adolescents. Sanctions against nonmarital **intimacy** have a rich and interesting history in Western society. **Normative standards** controlling nonmarital sexual intimacy are not, however, only of historical interest; they exist today.

Traditionally, an individual was expected to be emotionally, socially, intellectually, and spiritually intimate so that the mate selection process could function effectively. Physical intimacy, however, was to be delayed until marriage. This standard still exists today. Other standards, however, also seem to exist.

You have probably already made your decision concerning nonmarital sex. In making this decision, did you entertain all of the possible choices and understand fully the rationale associated with each choice?

In our opinion, perhaps the most useful set of terms through which to identify the various normative standards is that offered by Isadore Rubin.[10] These standards, in modified form, appear below. Study each standard. Next, try to identify the standard that best reflects your belief about the appropriateness of nonmarital intimacy. Certainly not everyone reading this textbook will choose the standard you have identified. What is important, however, is that you recognize that all of these standards coexist and that you should spend time attempting to understand and feel comfortable with the standard you have chosen.

- *Traditional repressive asceticism.* Regardless of what your body is trying to tell you, disregard its message. Nonmarital sexual intimacy is wrong because it offends God. Even sexual intimacy in marriage should be engaged in only for its intended purpose—to have children.
- *Enlightened asceticism.* Again, disregard messages received from your body regarding sexual stimulation and intimacy. It is definitely not in your best interest to give in to something as unfulfilling as nonmarital sexual intimacy. Your strength of character will be realized when you can control your desires to do what you know is not in your best interest. You will become a better, stronger person by having mustered this inner strength.
- *Humanistic liberalism.* Nonmarital sexual intimacy could be acceptable for you so long as you and your partner love each other. A sense of commitment and permanence must exist. In addition, should pregnancy occur, you will marry. Even more desirably, you and your partner should be responsible users of contraceptives to avoid a pregnancy.
- *Humanistic radicalism.* Sexual intimacy before marriage is acceptable so long as you and your partner have established a set of mutually agreed upon ground rules. No one is to be purposefully hurt because of the decision to be sexually active. Love and commitment are not necessary, because sexual intimacy is yet another medium for communication between mature people.

intimacy
any close, mutual verbal or nonverbal behavior within a relationship.

normative standards
statements of societal expectations concerning behavioral conduct.

Couples need to arrive at a mutually agreeable sexual standard.

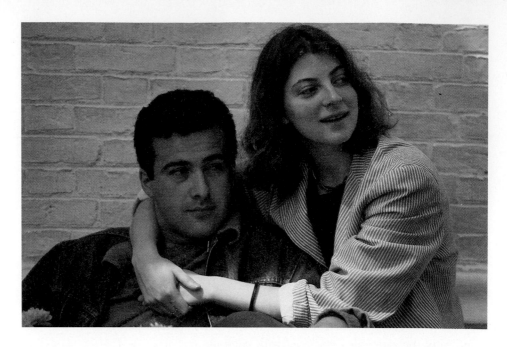

Fun morality. Like many other activities that hold the potential for pleasure and release, sexual intimacy is such a fun activity. A sexual partner is there for the purpose of allowing you to feel pleasure, stimulation, and release. Enjoy yourself, life is there for the taking.

Did you find your sexual standard among those appearing above? Is it likely that each of the five standards has representatives among the students taking this personal health course with you? If you are involved in a paired relationship, would your partner agree that his or her standard is the same as yours?

Although these normative standards are presented within the context of premarital sexual intimacy, the same basic standards exist for married persons considering a nonmarital (extramarital) relationship. In light of the statistical probability that extramarital sexual intimacy will be a part of many marriages, you should consider these standards whether you are married or engaged.

In a recent survey of 240 married couples, 60% of the men responding said they had had an extramarital relationship, compared with slightly less than 50% of the women surveyed. Researchers said these results were comparable to those of other recent studies.[11] With increasing concern over the transmission of sexually transmitted diseases, these percentages are likely to drop. Interestingly, while many of our own traditional-age students find these figures surprisingly high, our nontraditional students report that these figures do not surprise them.

Intimacy, before and outside of marriage, is a reality of today's world. Thoughtful insights, such as those provided by Rubin, can help you gain a sense of understanding about the decisions you make concerning sexual intimacy.

DATING AND MATE SELECTION

Rubin's standards presented in the previous section are not standards made by society solely for the purpose of depriving persons of the stimulation of sexual intimacy. Traditionally, they have been used in an attempt to help couples understand the role sexual intimacy will play in their relationship before marriage, particularly during the mate selection process.

In this section we will examine the process that brings young adults together so that they will eventually marry. Dating, the first phase of this process, facilitates initial contact with others. Mate selection, the second and more substantive phase, establishes the paired relationship. Of course, dating is also a process entered into for purposes other than beginning the search for a marital partner. For the vast majority of you, however, on at least one occasion, the process will move from initial dating to marriage.

Dating: Beginning a Paired Relationship

From the hundreds of persons that you have had contact with through school, employment, and leisure activities, how does it happen that you will choose one person, or at most a few people, to seriously consider as a mate? What makes a particular person that much different from all the others? We do not have the answers to these questions, and doubt seriously whether specific answers could be obtained. We can, however, suggest to you a few of the more familiar factors that seem to narrow the field of eligibles for most people.

The most powerful process in operation that moves you toward certain persons and away from others is **homogamy.** Similarities in age, racial and familial background, educational aspirations, and, to a degree, religious preference not only place you in a college environment but also narrow the field of persons with whom you will feel comfortable as a friend, a dating partner, and, eventually, a spouse. People usually seek intimacy (and ultimately marriage) with a person who is similar in these regards.

A second important factor that narrows the field of eligibles is that of **physical proximity.** Individuals who are or will be physically accessible to you are much more "affordable" as friends and dating partners. From a pragmatic point of view, the costs of carrying on relationships that are separated by great distance are much higher than those undertaken locally. Time, money, and difficulty in communicating are all expenses that can seriously detract from the continuation of these relationships. Absence usually does not make the heart grow fonder. Physical proximity also tends to reflect the existence of homogamy, because persons who share similar backgrounds and interests tend to live, study, work, and play together.

The factors of **complementary needs, compatible needs,** and **parental image** also help explain the chemistry that brings two persons together and helps keep them together. The meeting of complementary needs applies to dating situations in which two people have complementing voids in their own personalities that need to be filled. As an example, the overly quiet man sometimes seeks as a partner a woman whose outgoing nature can be used to make him more sociable. The outgoing woman, at the same time, seeks him as a partner because of his ability to curtail or refine her gregariousness. Thus the adequacy of one person's personality becomes a resource for the partner.

As the name implies, compatible needs are similar needs. According to this interpretation, two persons who have the same needs will probably choose each other as partners. In so doing they "pool" their resources for meeting those needs. Although we may often hear that "opposites attract," it is much more

homogamy
existence of similar or shared traits among members of a group.

physical proximity
physical closeness of individuals in terms of their places of residence, employment, and recreation.

complementary needs
needs of a potential mate that are different than those possessed by the partner.

compatible needs
needs of a potential mate that are the same as the needs possessed by the partner.

parental image
characteristics of a potential mate that remind a person of traits of his or her parent of the opposite sex.

Personal Assessment

How Compatible Are You?

This quiz will help test how compatible you and your mate's personalities are. You should each rate the truth of these 20 statements based on the following scale. Circle the number that reflects your feelings. Total your scores and check the interpretation following the quiz.

1 Never true
2 Sometimes true
3 Frequently true
4 Always true

We can communicate our innermost thoughts effectively.	1 2 3 4
We trust each other.	1 2 3 4
We agree on whose needs come first.	1 2 3 4
We have realistic expectations of each other and of ourselves.	1 2 3 4
Individual growth is recognized as important within our relationship.	1 2 3 4
We will go on as a couple even if our partner doesn't change.	1 2 3 4
Our personal problems are discussed with each other first.	1 2 3 4
We both do our best to compromise.	1 2 3 4
We usually fight fairly.	1 2 3 4
We try not to be rigid or unyielding.	1 2 3 4
We keep any needs to be "perfect" in proper perspective.	1 2 3 4
We can balance desires to be sociable and the need to be alone.	1 2 3 4
We both make friends and keep them.	1 2 3 4
Neither of us stays down or up for long periods.	1 2 3 4
We can tolerate the other's mood without being affected by it.	1 2 3 4
We can deal with disappointment and disillusionment.	1 2 3 4
Both of us can tolerate failure.	1 2 3 4
We can both express anger appropriately.	1 2 3 4
We are both assertive when necessary.	1 2 3 4
We agree on how our personal surroundings are kept.	1 2 3 4

Your total points _____

Interpretation

20-35 points   You and your partner seem quite incompatible. Professional help may open your lines of communication.

36-55 points   You probably need more awareness and compromise.

56-70 points   You are highly compatible. But be aware of the areas where you can still improve.

71-80 points   Your relationship is very fulfilling. Ask your mate to take this test, too. You may have a one-sided view of a "perfect" relationship.

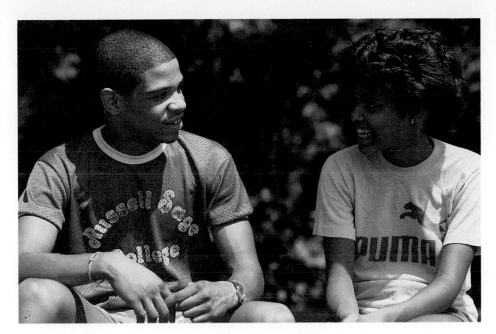

Through dating we begin to define what qualities a potential mate will have.

likely that those with compatible needs will be strongly attracted to each other.

The parental image explanation of why two persons are attracted suggests that to one person the partner displays traits he or she values in a parent. Proponents of this explanation contend, for example, that a young woman seeks in a male partner the traits she admires in her father, while the young man seeks the strengths of his mother in the personality of a young woman.

Regardless of how two persons are initially attracted as dating partners, the fact remains that they are attracted. In so doing, the opportunity exists for the process of moving from casual dating through engagement to marriage.

THREE-STAGE DATING–MATE SELECTION MODEL

Although a dating–mate selection sequence involving casual dating, steady dating, and engagement is very familiar to you, the process that propels two persons along this continuum may be unfamiliar. Therefore we will present a three-stage model to account for this movement. A greatly modified version of a courtship model initially proposed by Murstein[12] serves as the basis for this model. We recognize, of course, that a model can be nothing more than a word picture to describe how a process might occur. Your experiences will be the criteria on which you can validate its content.

Stage 1—The Marketing Stage

The earliest stage of dating begins when, after meeting a new person, you construct an "ideal" image of yourself that you want to transmit to this person. The very same process is, of course, being undertaken by the new partner. You become the recipient of a carefully constructed facade. You both are "putting your best foot forward." **Infatuation** with your partner may be strong during this stage.

Characteristics of
Stage 1 Dating

Putting your best foot forward
Relatively short-lasting stage

infatuation
an often shallow, intense attraction to another person.

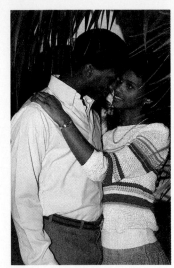

Infatuation initiates many relationships.

Characteristics of
Stage 2 Dating

Mutual exploration of beliefs
  and feelings
"Steady" dating
Movement toward permanence

In this initial stage of dating, and at each of two remaining stages, both you and your partner are operating on the basis of personal gains and losses. Relationships continue at one level so long as gains at that level are deemed sufficient. Relationships progress when both partners wish to experience new and more highly valued gains and are willing to risk greater losses. Difficulties begin when partners progress at different rates in their desire for greater gains.

For most young adults, dating at this marketing stage may last only a relatively short time as both partners quickly tire of dealing with shallow "perfection" and begin to want to know what exists beyond the partner's titles, affiliations, wardrobe, or physical appearance. For these individuals, dating will progress to the second level of our dating–mate selection model.

Stage 2—The Sharing Stage

The second stage in the progression from casual dating to marriage is made possible by a desire of the partners to explore the underlying belief systems that account for the compatibility found during the latter portion of the marketing stage. The fact that two persons appear to have things in common and appear to enjoy each other is no longer sufficient justification for continuing a relationship. Maturity and self-awareness whet the appetite for discovering why the relationship seems to be headed in the direction of increased commitment and permanence. Infatuation declines as the relationship deepens.

The sharing stage of the dating–mate selection model can only occur when the two partners are willing to act on their interest in knowing more about each other. A commitment to engaging in the verbal exchange of ideas and information is critically important. Open and honest discussions about aspirations, priorities, beliefs, and concerns must occur regularly.

This stage of the dating–mate selection process will more than likely be labeled by the observer as steady dating. As the relationship grows in its depth of understanding, the movement toward permanence becomes more evident. Time alone cannot, however, sustain the growth of a relationship if the exchange of value-centered information by both partners does not take place. And certainly an enjoyable sexual relationship cannot alone suffice for the absence of communication.

As was the case in the cautious stage of the dating–mate selection process, both partners must feel they are making sufficient gains to justify their continued participation. Particularly because of the need to be increasingly open and honest with yourself and your partner, feelings of vulnerability are common during this stage.

Indeed, the sharing stage of the dating–mate selection process is critically important. If you marry after moving through only the marketing stage of the process, the marriage's stability will be extremely questionable. A marriage after you move through the second stage of the process should be much better equipped to handle the demands of marriage.

Stage 3—The Behavior Stage

As you might well have determined by now, the third stage of the dating–mate selection process centers around the ability of you and your partner to transfer values into consistently observable behaviors. For you or your partner to have verbalized these values during the sharing stage is, of course, important to the maturing of your relationship. In the third stage, however, you must now determine whether your behaviors are consistent with the values you shared in the second stage. The mate selection process will not be fully completed until this stage has been undertaken.

Characteristics of Stage 3 Dating

Transferring beliefs into behaviors
Relationship matures

LOVE

Love may be one of the most elusive, yet widely recognized, concepts that describe some level of emotional attachment to another. Haas and Haas[2] describe five forms of love, including erotic, friendship, devotional, parental, and altruistic love. Other behavioral scientists[3] have focused primarily on two types of love most closely associated with dating and mate selection: *passionate love* and *companionate love*.

Passionate love, also described as romantic love or infatuation, is a "state of extreme absorption in another. It is characterized by intense feelings of tenderness, elation, anxiety, sexual desire, and ecstasy."[3] Often appearing early in a relationship, passionate love typically does not last very long. Passionate love is driven by the excitement of being closely involved in a relationship with a person whose character is not fully known.

If a relationship progresses into the sharing stage of the dating and mate selection model, passionate love is gradually replaced by companionate love. This type of love is "a less intense emotion than passionate love. It is characterized by friendly affection and a deep attachment that is based on extensive familiarity with the loved one."[3] This is a love that is enduring and capable of sustaining long-term, mutual growth. Central to companionate love are feelings of empathy, support, and tolerance of the partner.

MARRIAGE

Just as there is no single way for two persons to move through dating and mate selection, marriage is an equally variable undertaking. In marriage, two persons join their lives in a way that affirms each as an individual and both as a legally constituted pair. However, for a large percentage of couples, the demands of marriage are too rigorous, confining, and demanding. They will find resolution for their dissatisfaction through divorce or extramarital affairs. However, for the majority, marriage will be an experience that alternates periods of happiness, productivity, and admiration with periods of frustration, unhappiness, and disillusionment with the partner. Each of you who marries will find the experience unique in every regard.

As we enter the 1990s, certain trends regarding marriage are evident. The most obvious of these is the age at first marriage. Today men are waiting longer than ever to marry. Now the average age at first marriage for men is 25.8 years.[14] Additionally, these new husbands are better educated than in the past and are more likely to be established in their careers.

Women are also waiting longer to get married and tend to be more educated and career oriented. Recent statistics indicate that the average age at first marriage is 23.6 years.[13]

Some Tips for Partners

Take the time and make the effort to show you care for your partner.
Share plans, activities, and friendships.
Listen to your partner; find out what is important to him or her.
Tell your partner what is important to you.
Don't expect your partner to fulfill all your needs.
Try to accept your partner's shortcomings.
Don't blame your partner for all your problems; learn to see when you are at fault.
Learn to compromise.
Handle conflicts at the earliest opportunity; find a solution that benefits both of you.
Keep a sense of humor; have fun together.

Marriage still appeals to the majority of adults. Currently, approximately 80% of adults age 18 and older are either married, widowed, or divorced.[14] Thus only about one fifth of today's adults have not married. Within the last decade, the percentage of adults who have decided not to marry has nearly doubled. Single-hood and other alternatives to marriage will be discussed later in this chapter.

FORMS OF MARRIAGE

To describe the nature of marital relationships, we will use the familiar categories of marital relationships advanced by Cuber and Harroff.[15] The marriage types described should not be viewed as being either "good" or "bad." Rather, you should recognize one simple reality: these marriages are routinely found and apparently meet the needs of the individuals involved. Some of the types of marriages we will present began in the form in which they are being described. Others, however, evolved into their present form, having once been a very different type of marital relationship.

Conflict-Habituated Marriage

"We fought on our first date, our honeymoon was a disaster, and we've disagreed on everything of importance ever since." This frank description of a marital relationship characterized by confrontation, disagreement, and perhaps physical abuse reflects a *conflict-habituated marriage*. The central theme of this type of marital relationship is conflict, and its continuous presence suggests that no attempt at resolution is actively sought. Couples in conflict-habituated marriages agree to disagree and, on this basis, the relationship takes its form.

Devitalized Marriage

In the same way a dying person is said to possess failing signs, a *devitalized marriage* has lost its signs of life. Unlike the conflict-habituated marriage, which since its beginning was chronically impaired, the devitalized marriage was once a more active and satisfying marital relationship. For some reason, however, one or both partners have lost their desire to maintain the marriage in its original, dynamic state.

The future of a devitalized marriage is difficult to predict. Some marriages of this type can be revitalized. Effective marriage counseling, a new job, or moving to a new community can rekindle a relationship. Other devitalized marriages are able to remain intact because one or both partners find vitality through an extramarital relationship. Some devitalized marriages persist at low levels of involvement and commitment with little hope for improvement. We would not be surprised that for those of you who have witnessed the dissolution of your parents' marriage, devitalization was an important factor in its ending.

Passive-Congenial Marriage

"Passive" refers to a low level of commitment or involvement, while the word "congenial" suggests warmth and friendliness. When these two familiar words are combined as they are in *passive-congenial marriage*, they describe perfectly the type of marital relationship sought by some couples.

Ending Conflict

Psychologist and author Don Dinkmeyer suggests the following for resolving conflicts:

Show mutual respect.

Identify and resolve the real issue.

Seek areas of agreement.

Mutually participate in decision-making.

Be cooperative and specific.

Focus on the present and future—not the past.

Don't try to assign blame.

Say what you are thinking and feeling.

Set a time limit for discussing problems.

Accept responsibility.

Schedule time together.

For some of today's young professionals, the passive-congenial marriage offers a safe harbor from the rigors encountered in the world of corporate positions and professional practices. Children may not be valued "commodities" in the passive-congenial marriage. The added financial and personal stressors that are related to child rearing could compromise an already established lifestyle. You may be able to construct an image of a passive-congenial couple if you can picture two people meeting after work for a quiet dinner at a small restaurant, talking in muffled tones about their corporate battles, and planning their winter cruise.

Maintaining a passive-congenial marriage requires less time and energy than other forms of marriage. For two persons who feel certain that their major contributions to society will be made principally through their efforts in the workplace, this marriage may be ideal. Certainly you may know many couples who are choosing this increasingly popular form of marriage.

Total Marriage

In the *total marriage* little remains of the unique identities that existed between two people before their marriage took place. For reasons that are probably lost to the subconscious mind, two persons possessing individual personalities use marriage to fuse their identities into one identity—the total pair.

The total marriage requires that the individual partners set aside all aspirations for individual growth and development. Decisions are not made with "me" or even "you" as the focus of attention. Rather, energies are directed to what is best for "us." Life outside of the marital relationship and partner's presence does not exist, at least figuratively speaking. Eventually outsiders, when talking about these individuals, can no longer truly speak about the man or the woman, but are limited to speaking about the couple.

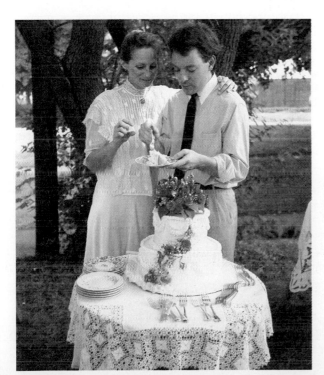

What form of marriage will evolve for this couple?

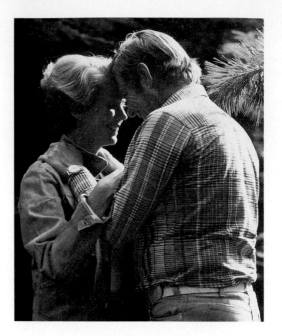

A vital marriage.

Vital Marriage

The *vital marriage* is undertaken with the intent that it will serve as an arena for the growth of both the individuals and of the pair. The concepts of "my growth," "your growth," and "our growth" prevail. In a vital marriage, personal goals may at times be subordinated for the good of the partner or the paired relationship. Yet both the man and woman (and the children) know that when it is possible and desirable, those once-subordinated goals will assume top priority. Equality of opportunity exists.

In describing the vital marriage, we must point out that this type of marital relationship is not perfect, nor is it appropriate for all couples. In today's complex society, the vital marriage may be especially difficult to maintain.

ALTERNATIVES TO MARRIAGE

Although the great majority of you have experienced or will experience marriage, viable alternatives certainly exist. This section will briefly explore divorce, singlehood, cohabitation, and single parenthood.

Divorce

Marriage relationships, like many other kinds of interpersonal relationships, can terminate. Today, marriages—relationships begun with the intent of permanence "until death do us part"—end nearly as frequently as not through divorce. Interestingly four years is the median length of marriages that end in divorce.[16] Four years appears to be the length of time needed for many couples to experience the initial demands of child rearing.

In the past two decades the rate at which divorces occur has been climbing steadily. As recently as 1982 this rate continued to climb. In 1983, however, the first sign of a downward trend was observed. When viewed again in 1987,

Improving Marriage

Few marital relationships are "perfect." All marriages are faced with occasional periods of strain or turmoil. Even marriages that do not exhibit major signs of distress can be improved, mostly through better communication. Marriage experts suggest that implementing some of these patterns can strengthen marriages:

- Problems that exist within the marriage should be brought into the open so that both partners are aware of the difficulties.
- Balance should exist between the needs and expectations of each partner. Decisions should be made jointly. Partners should support each other as best they can. When a partner's goals cannot be actively supported, they should at least receive moral support and encouragement.
- Realistic expectations should be established. Partners should negotiate areas in which disagreement exists. They should work together to determine the manner in which resources should be shared.

Beyond the patterns listed above, a sense of permanence helps sustain a marriage over the course of time. If the partners are convinced that their relationship can withstand difficult times, then they are more likely to take the time to make needed changes. Couples can develop a sense of permanence by implementing some of the patterns described above.

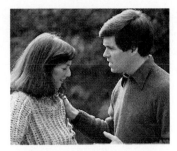

Conflicts will surface in any marriage.

this downward trend was again seen.[17] Probable factors influencing this include the later age of first marriage, a changing societal attitude toward divorce, and the growing tendency toward singlehood.

Regardless of the exact direction that divorce statistics take in the immediate future, the fact that nearly as many marriages end in divorce as continue should give us cause for reflection. Why should approximately 40% to 45% of marital relationships be so likely to end within a relatively few years? Unfortunately, marriage experts cannot provide one clear answer to this question. Rather, they suggest that divorce is a reflection of unfulfilled expectations for marriage on the part of one or both partners, including:

- The belief that marriage will ease your need to deal with your own faults and that your failures can be transferred to the shoulders of your partner
- The belief that marriage will change faults that you know exist in your partner
- The belief that the high level of romance of your dating and courtship period will be continued through marriage
- The belief that marriage can provide you with an arena for the development of your personal power, and that once married you will not need to compromise with your partner
- The belief that your marital partner will be successful in meeting all of your needs

If these expectations seem to approximate what you anticipate through marriage, then you may find that disappointments will abound. To varying degrees, marriage is a partnership that requires postponement and subordination of personal

Coping with Breakup

The end of a relationship is always a wrenching and painful experience. The following tips suggest both alternatives to breakup and ways to cope with it.

- *Talk first.* Try to deal effectively and directly with the conflicts. The old notion had it that it was good for a couple to fight. But anger can beget anger and even lead to violence. Freely venting anger is as likely to damage a relationship as to improve it. Therefore, cool off first, then talk and discuss fully and freely.
- *Trial separation.* Sometimes only a few weeks apart can convince a couple that it is far better to work together than to go it totally alone. It is generally better to plant the rules of such a trial quite firmly. Will the individuals see others? What are the responsibilities if children are involved? There should also be a time limit, perhaps a month or two, after which the partners reunite and discuss their situation again.
- *Obtain help.* The services of a *qualified* counselor, psychologist, or psychiatrist may help a couple resolve their problems. Notice the emphasis on the word qualified. Some people who have little training or competence represent themselves as counselors. For this reason a couple should insist on verifying the counselor's training and licensing.
- *Allow time for grief and healing.* When a relationship ends, people are often tempted to immediately become as socially and sexually active as possible. This can be a way to express anger and relieve pain. But it can also cause frustration and despair. A better solution for many is to acknowledge the grief the dissolution has caused and give oneself time for healing. Six months to a year of continuing one's life and solidifying friendships typically helps the rejected partner establish a new equilibrium.

expectations. Marriage can be a complicated proposition. Because of the high expectations that many people hold for marriage, the termination of marriage can be an emotionally difficult process to undertake.

When divorce occurs among people with children, concern is frequently voiced over the well-being of the children. Different factors, however, influence the extent to which divorce affects children. Included among these factors are the sex of the children, the age of the children, custodial arrangements, financial support, and the remarriage of one or both parents. For many children, adjustments must be made to accept their new status as a member of a blended family.

Singlehood

An alternative to marriage for adults is *singlehood*. For many people, being single is a lifestyle that affords the potential for pursuing intimacy, if desired, and provides an uncluttered path for independence and self-directedness. Other persons, however, are single because of divorce, separation, death, or the absence of an opportunity to establish a partnership.

Many different living arrangements are seen among singles. Some single persons maintain separate residences and choose not to share a household. Other habitation styles for singles include cohabitation, periodic cohabitations, single-hood during the week and cohabitation on the weekends or during vacations, or the *platonic* sharing of a household with others. Perhaps for some persons, singlehood is only a frame of reference that guides the way in which they pursue their marital relationships.

Like habitation arrangements, the sexual intimacy patterns of singles are individually tailored. Some singles practice celibacy, others pursue heterosexual or homosexual intimate relationships in a **monogamous** pattern, while others may have multiple partners. As in all interpersonal relationships, including marriage, the levels of commitment are as variable as the persons involved.

monogamous
paired relationship with one partner.

Because singlehood has not yet been as thoroughly studied as marriage, it is somewhat more difficult to address its effects on the level of satisfaction it provides for those who pursue it. Initial studies do suggest, however, that on a group basis it is a more positive lifestyle for women than for men.[4] For those single persons who later decide to marry, research suggests that they are more likely to marry a partner who has been once married, are less likely to pool resources in marriage, have either no children or have them quickly, and marry more quickly than younger couples once the decision to marry has been reached.

The key ingredients to satisfaction in singlehood may not be markedly different from those associated with happiness in marriage. Harayda[18] identifies some of the characteristics of single people that tend to make them satisfied and happy. Single people enjoy:

- Putting down roots
- Feeling economically secure
- Working without becoming workaholics
- Being supportive to the next generation
- Being committed to their chosen single lifestyle

Regardless of the exact form that singlehood takes in terms of habitation patterns, sexual intimacy practices, and the subsequent marriage roles, it is an extremely viable lifestyle that provides an attractive alternative to marriage for many of today's young and midlife adults.

Cohabitation

Cohabitation, or the sharing of living quarters by unmarried persons, represents yet another alternative to marriage. For adults of all ages, but for younger adults in particular, the practice is somewhat common but difficult to quantify with any exactness.

cohabitation
sharing of a residence by two unrelated, unmarried people; living together.

A current study suggests that approximately 50% of couples live together before marriage.[19] Additionally, the data suggest that cohabitation is evident in all age groups and accounts for some of the delay seen in the age of first marriage.

Although cohabitation may seem to imply a vision of sexual intimacy between male and female roommates, several forms of shared living arrangements can also be viewed as cohabitation. For some couples, cohabitation is only a part-time arrangement for weekends, during summer vacation, or on a variable schedule. Additionally, **platonic** cohabitation can exist when a couple shares living quarters but does so without establishing an intimate relationship. Close friends, persons of retirement age, and homosexuals might all be included in a group called "cohabitants."

platonic
close association between two people that does not include a sexual relationship.

The archetype of a cohabitation arrangement is the couple who has drifted into cohabitation as the result of a dating relationship in which sexual intimacy and occasional "overnighting" have already occurred. In the living arrangement that follows, both material possessions and emotional support are generally shared. Only occasionally is a contractual relationship established. Monogamy will predominate. Approximately 50% of cohabitation relationships will disband, and the persons involved will depart with the feeling that they would cohabit again if it appears desirable. Finally, cohabitation is neither more nor less likely to lead to marriage than is a more traditional dating relationship. It is, in fact, only an alternative to marriage.

Forms of Single Parenthood

The situation in which an unmarried young woman becomes pregnant and becomes a single parent is a continuing reality in this country. A new and significantly different form of single parenthood is, however, also a reality in this country. It is the planned entry into a single parenthood by older, better educated people, the vast majority of whom are women.

In contrast to the teenage girl who becomes a single parent through an unwed pregnancy, the more mature woman who desires single parenting has usually planned carefully for the experience. She has explored several important concerns, including questions regarding how she will become pregnant (with or without the knowledge of a male partner or through artificial insemination), the need for a father figure for the child, the effect of single parenting on her social life, and, of course, its effect on her career development. Once these questions have been resolved, no legal barriers stand in the way of her becoming a single parent.

Single parenthood can be rewarding and satisfying.

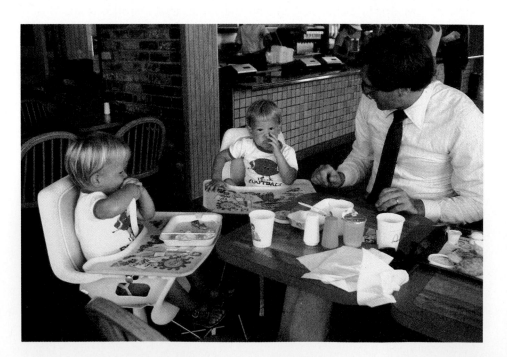

If You Are Single

Is your life on hold just because you are single? Are you living in limbo instead of making a real home for yourself?

To see if you're taking good care of yourself as a single "nester," try this quiz from Janice Harayda, adapted from her new book, *The Joy of Being Single*. Total your yes responses and check the interpretation following the quiz.

	Yes	No
1 Do you sleep on a real bed rather than a convertible sofa or a mattress on the floor?	____	____
2 Would you feel comfortable buying such items as monogrammed towels or antiques if you liked them and could afford them?	____	____
3 Do you have at least one specialty that you can cook with pride for friends?	____	____
4 Do you already own a condo, co-op, or house? If not, are you saving up for one?	____	____
5 Do you have family pictures displayed in your home?	____	____
6 Do you participate in at least one community or neighborhood group, such as a block association, a tennis committee, or the Jaycees?	____	____
7 Could you invite your boss to your home without feeling embarrassed?	____	____
8 Do you put up decorations on important holidays?	____	____
9 Do you occasionally give sit-down dinner parties instead of having the gang over for pizza and beer?	____	____
10 Do you look forward to coming home from work each night?	____	____

Interpretation

1-2   Your place probably feels more like a sensory deprivation chamber than a real home.

3-7   You are well on the way to creating a real home and a real life for yourself.

7+   Congratulations. You have a strong sense of who you are, and aren't afraid to let your place show it.

A very large number of women, and a growing number of men, are actively participating in single parenthood in conjunction with a divorce settlement involving sole or joint custody of children. On the basis of current statistical data, 23.4% of all families with children under age 18 are headed by a single parent. This represents 14.4 million children.[20] Studies are ongoing concerning the effect that being reared by a single parent has on the school performance and social adjustment of these children.

A few single parents have been awarded children through adoption. Given the limited pool of adoptable children, the likelihood of a single person's receiving a child is small, but more persons have been successful recently in single-parent adoptions.

For all groups of single parents, the process of rearing a child in the absence of a partner is a potentially satisfying—but certainly demanding—undertaking. Regardless of the liberalization in sexual standards that have occurred in the last two decades, we believe that the prevailing feeling remains that most children do best when reared within the context of a caring, nurturing partnership. As a consequence of this feeling, less support and understanding may be forthcoming from the general public than might be initially anticipated by some single parents.

SEXUAL PREFERENCES AND VARIATIONS

People express their sexuality in many ways. Some of the more familiar variations in sexual behavior are described in this section.

Homosexuality

In our society we have a tendency to label people by their overt behaviors. We call people either "shy" or "congenial," based on how we see them interact with others. After observing people, we may identify them as runners or nonrunners, academics or nonacademics, careful drivers or careless drivers. Sometimes we are accurate judges—often we are wrong.

So too it is with sexual behaviors. We tend to categorize others by only a few observations. We assume that a man and woman who are dating steadily are *heterosexual*. We assume that our friends who choose friends of the same sex might have *homosexual* tendencies. Occasionally, we may even make judgments about our own sexual inclinations. As a society, this judgmental thinking has led us to believe a variety of myths and to accept a number of stereotypes about *sexual object preferences*. We hope this section can clear the air about some of our misunderstandings.

Sexual object preference and sexual orientation apply to "the gender to whom an individual is attracted."[3] Homosexual orientation (or homosexuality) refers to an attraction toward same-sex partners. Heterosexual orientation (or heterosexuality) refers to an attraction to opposite-sex partners. *Bisexual* orientation (or bisexuality) refers to an attraction to both same-sex and opposite-sex partners.

The term "homosexuality" comes from the Greek word *homos*, meaning "same." The word homosexuality may be used with regard to males or females. Thus we use the terms "homosexual males" and "homosexual females." Frequently the word "gay" is used to refer to homosexual orientation in both males and females. *Lesbianism* is also commonly used to refer to the sexual attraction between females. This word stems from the Island of Lesbos, which the Greek poet Sappho described as an island for women in love.

The distinctions among the categories of sexual object preference are much less clear than their definitions might suggest. Most people probably fall somewhere along a continuum between exclusive heterosexuality and exclusive homosexuality. Kinsey in 1948 presented just such a continuum.[21] Any distinctions

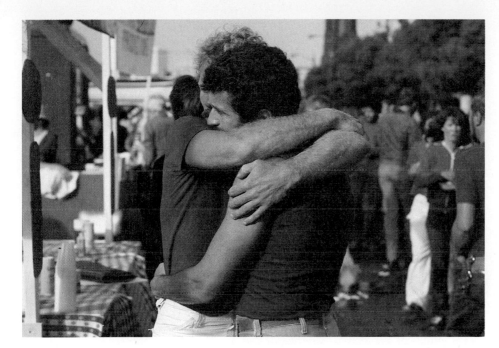

One expression of intimacy.

become further clouded when one considers that the definitions refer to sex object preference, not just to sexual behavior. Thus males who are sexually attracted to other males but never pursue a relationship with a male might be considered homosexual.

Why does a given individual have a homosexual orientation? Theories regarding the cause of homosexuality have focused on psychoanalytic factors, family environment factors, genetic factors, hormonal factors, and behavioral (social learning) factors. In the 1960s and 1970s, the behavioral theory (positive homosexual experiences reinforce continued homosexual behavior) and the family environment theory (dominant mother and detached father) received much support. In the late 1980s, a biological theory based on a genetic/hormonal predisposition has been more widely suggested to account for exclusive homosexuality.[3] However, for sexual orientation in general, no one theory has emerged that fully explains this developmental process. Regardless of cause, however, reversal to heterosexuality generally does not occur.

The extent of homosexuality in our society is a debatable issue. Undoubtedly, gathering valid information of this kind is difficult. The extent of homosexual orientation is probably much greater than many heterosexuals realize. Furthermore, many persons refuse to reveal their homosexuality and thus prefer to remain "in the closet."

Although operational definitions of homosexuality may vary from researcher to researcher, in 1948 Kinsey estimated that about 2% of American females and 4% of American males were exclusively homosexual.[21,22] More recent estimates place the overall combined figure of homosexuals at about 10% of the population.[3] Clearly the expression of same-sex attraction is not uncommon in our society.

Bisexuality

People whose preference for sexual partners includes both sexes are referred to as bisexuals. Bisexuals may fall into one of three groups: those who are (1) genuinely attracted to both sexes, (2) homosexual but also feel the need to behave heterosexually, (3) aroused physically by the same sex but attracted emotionally to the opposite sex.[23] Some persons participate in a bisexual lifestyle for extended periods, whereas others move quickly to a more exclusive orientation. Little research has been conducted on bisexuality, and thus the size of the bisexual population is not accurately known.

A particularly pressing reason for learning more about the bisexual lifestyle is its relationship to the transmission of AIDS. Currently in the United States "homosexual and bisexual males" represent the most cases of this deadly disease. By definition, bisexuals hold the greatest potential for extending the AIDS virus into the heterosexual population. Since the prevalence of bisexuality is unknown, the importance of safe sex practices becomes more important than ever.

Transsexualism

Transsexualism is a sexual variance of the most profound nature, because it represents a complete rejection by an individual of his or her biological sexuality. The transsexual male believes that he is a female and desires to be the woman that he knows he is. The female transsexual believes that she is a male and thus desires to become the man that she knows she should be.

sex reassignment operations surgical procedures designed to remove the external genitalia and replace them with genitalia appropriate to the opposite sex.

For transsexuals, the period of gender adoption is perplexing as they attempt, with limited success, to resolve the dissonance between what their mind tells them is true and what their body displays. Adolescent and young adult transsexuals often cross-dress, undertake homosexual relationships (which they view as being heterosexual relationships), experiment with hormone replacement therapy, and in some cases actively pursue a **sex reassignment operation.** Several thousand of these operations have been performed.

An interesting point that emerges from the study of transsexualism is that

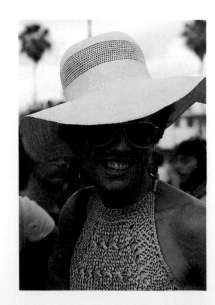

Is this person expressing a sexual variation?

concerning the most basic indicator of gender. Does a deeply held belief of being a male or female constitute the basis of gender? Does removal of external genitalia and the construction of new genitals change a person from one gender to another? Can a court of law accomplish this conversion?

Biologically the answers to these questions must be "no." Regardless of what can be accomplished through surgical, psychiatric, or legal intervention, the fact remains that the transsexual still possesses the XY or XX chromosomal benchmarks of his or her original gender.

Other Sexual Variations

It seems fairly simple to suggest that any sexual behavior not engaged in by a majority of people could be labeled a **variant** behavior. However, since the culture we live in is dynamic and thus changes constantly, getting a handle on what is "normal" and what is "variant" is difficult at best. For example, such behaviors as *masturbation* and *oral-genital stimulation,* which were considered variant a few decades ago, are now practiced by a majority of sexually active people. As we move closer to the twenty-first century, some behaviors that today appear to be variant may be considered socially or culturally acceptable behaviors in the future. Other variant behaviors, such as incest and pedophilia, are not likely to ever be considered culturally or socially acceptable.

Rathus[21] categorizes variations from normal sexual behaviors according to a person's (1) sex object preference or (2) choice of sexual activity. Fetishism, transvestism, and zoophilia involve choices of nonhuman sexual objects, while pedophilia and incest involve choices of human sexual objects. Variant choices of sexual activity include exhibitionism, voyeurism, sadism, and masochism.[24]

Fetishism refers to "a variation in choice of sexual object in which a bodily part or inanimate object elicits sexual arousal and is preferred repeatedly to a person."[24] Although it is normal for people to be stimulated by a partner's breasts, hands, buttocks, or revealing clothing, when these body parts or nonhuman objects become the sole stimuli for sexual arousal and preference, they can be considered fetishes.

Transvestism is a sexual variation in which a person participates in "recurrent, persistent cross-dressing for the purposes of sexual excitement."[24] Such a behavioral pattern is most commonly seen among males—males who prefer to dress, in part or completely, as females. Such behaviors are usually not openly displayed. The large proportion of such males are not homosexual, as many seem to believe. Rather, most transvestites are heterosexuals who lead otherwise normal lives. They have full-time careers, raise families, and become involved in community services.

Zoophilia refers to "sexual contact with animals as a repeatedly preferred source of sexual excitement; also called *bestiality.*"[24] Such a variation is quite unusual, although Kinsey[22] in 1953 reported about 8% of male subjects and 0.75% of female subjects as having had sexual contact with animals, primarily farm animals and house pets. Kinsey reported most of these contacts as having come during adolescence.

Pedophilia refers to a sexual variance with a human object. This variance can be defined as "sexual contact with children as the repeatedly preferred source of sexual excitement."[24] A person displaying this variant behavior would be called a *pedophiliac,* or in a legal sense, a child molester. Most pedophiliacs are male

variant
different from the statistical average.

fetishism
choice of a body part or inanimate object as a source of sexual excitement.

transvestism
recurrent, persistent cross-dressing as a source of sexual excitement.

zoophilia
sexual contact with animals as a preferred source of sexual excitement.

pedophilia
sexual contact with children as a source of sexual excitement.

incest
marriage or coitus (sexual intercourse) between closely related individuals.

exhibitionism
exposure of one's genitals for the purpose of shocking another person.

voyeurism
watching others undressing or engaging in sexual activity.

masochism
sexual excitement while being injured or humiliated.

sadism
sexual excitement achieved while inflicting injury or humiliation on another person.

sadomasochism
combination of sadism and masochism into one sexual activity; "S and M."

heterosexuals. The most common types of child molesting appear to be genital fondling and exhibitionism.

Incest is a second type of sexual variance with a human object. In this case, the behavior refers to "marriage or coitus between people so closely related that sexual activity is prohibited by virtue of their kinship tie."[24] Incest between brother and sister or father and daughter is probably the most common form of this variant behavior. Besides being illegal, incest can prove to be psychologically damaging to children who are coerced to participate in this behavior.

One variant choice, not of sexual object but of sexual activity, is **exhibitionism,** represented by the "repeated exposure of the genitals for the purpose of shocking the victim rather than sexually exciting her."[24] Exhibitionists are almost always males—the victims are female children and adult women. The exhibitionist's sexual stimulation comes through the element of risk, as well as the surprise or disgust shown by the victim. (Thus strippers are not generally thought of as exhibitionists). Most exhibitionists prefer exposure to strangers. Individuals who engage in exhibitionism tend to be quite passive and do not seek sexual contact with their victims. They usually flee quickly after exposing themselves.

Voyeurism is another variant sexual activity that includes "repetitive watching of unsuspecting people disrobing or engaging in sexual activity."[24] The sexual excitement gained by the viewer comes from observing an unsuspecting person or people. The element of risk may also be involved. For this reason, voyeuristic people (or "Peeping Toms") do not generally receive satisfaction from viewing pornographic magazines or watching adult-rated movies, since the models or actors in these forms of entertainment clearly expect to be seen.

A third variant sexual activity is **masochism.** Masochism refers to "experiencing enhanced sexual arousal as a result of pain, humiliation, or danger."[24] Women tend to be masochists more often than men. Preferred forms of masochism include being restrained with ropes (bondage), psychologically humiliated, beaten, or pinched by the sexual partner. The partner is commonly labeled a sadist.

The sexual activity of **sadism** is "the enhancing of one's sexual excitement by inflicting pain or humiliation on another."[24] Men tend to be sadists more often than women. The sadists' cooperative sexual partners are, of course masochists. The interacting behavior that occurs between sadists and masochists is known as **sadomasochism.** Sadomasochism is frequently referred to as "S and M." For most practicing couples, sadomasochistic behavior is relatively mild as far as actual injury to the participants. The sexual excitement appears to result from the fantasy that the activity could be real.

SEXUAL VICTIMIZATION

Ideally, sexual intimacy is a mutual, enjoyable form of communication between two people. Far too often, however, relationships are approached in an aggressive, hostile manner. These sexual aggressors always have a victim—someone who is physically or psychologically traumatized. *Sexual victimization* occurs in many forms and in a variety of settings. In this section we will briefly look at sexual victimization as it occurs in rape and sexual assault, sexual abuse of children, sexual harassment, and the commercialization of sex.

Rape Prevention Guidelines

- Never assume that you are an unlikely candidate for personal assault.
- Think carefully about your patterns of movement to and from class or work. Alter your routes frequently.
- Walk briskly with a sense of purpose. Try not to walk alone at night.
- Dress so that the clothes you wear do not unnecessarily restrict your movement or make you more vulnerable.
- Always be aware of your surroundings. Look over your shoulder occasionally. Know where you are so you won't get lost.
- If you think you are being followed, look for a safe retreat. This might be a store, a fire or police station, or a group of people.
- Be especially cautious of first dates, blind dates, or people you meet at a party or bar who push to be alone with you.
- Let trusted friends know where you are and when you plan to return.
- Keep your car in good working order. Think beforehand how you would handle the situation should your car break down.
- Trust your best instincts if you are assaulted. Each situation is different. Do what you can to protect your life.

Rape and Sexual Assault

As violence in our society increases, the incidence of rape and *sexual assault* correspondingly rises. The victims of these crimes fall into no single category. Victims of rape and sexual assault include young and old, male and female. Victims include the mentally retarded, prisoners, hospital patients, and college students. We all are potential victims and self-protection is critically important. (See the box on rape prevention above and the box on p. 414 for help for the rape victim.)

Despite the fact that we are potential victims, many of us do not fully understand how vulnerable we are. Rape in particular has associated with it a number of myths (false assumptions). Among these are:

- *Women are raped by strangers.* In approximately half of all reported rapes, the victim had some prior acquaintance with the rapist. Increasingly, women are being raped by husbands, dating partners, and relatives. The incidence of child molestation and sexual violence, including rape, is also on the rise.
- *Rapes almost always occur in dark alleys or deserted places.* The opposite is true. Most rapes occur in or very near the victim's residence.
- *Rapists are easily identified by their demeanor or psychological profile.* Most experts indicate that rapists generally do not differ significantly from their nonrapist counterparts.
- *Incidence of rape is overreported.* Estimates are that only one in five rapes is reported. Rape continues to be among the fastest rising of all major crimes, according to the FBI's Uniform Crime Report. One rape is committed in the United States every 7 minutes.[25]

Help for the Rape Victim

If you have been raped, seek help as soon as possible. The following procedures may be helpful.

1 *Call the police immediately to report the assault.* Police can take you to the hospital and start gathering information that may help them apprehend the rapist. Fortunately, many police departments now use specially trained officers (many of whom are female) to work closely with rape victims during all stages of the investigation.

2 If you would rather not contact the police immediately, *call a local rape crisis center.* Operated generally on a 24-hour hotline basis, these centers have trained counselors to help you evaluate your options, contact the police, escort you to the hospital, and provide aftercare counseling.[26]

3 *Do not alter any potential evidence related to the rape.* Do not change your clothes, douche, take a bath, or rearrange the scene of the crime. Wait until all the evidence has been gathered.

4 *Report all bruises, cuts, and scratches, even if they seem insignificant.* Report any information about the attack as completely and accurately as possible.

5 *You will probably be given a thorough pelvic examination.* You may have to ask for *STD* tests and pregnancy tests.

6 Although it is unusual for a rape victim's name to appear in the media, you might *request that the police withhold your name* as long as is legally possible.

- *Rape happens only to people in low socioeconomic classes.* Rape cuts across all socioeconomic classes. Each person, male or female, young or old, is a potential victim.
- *There is a standard way to escape from a potential rape situation.* Each rape situation is different. No one method to avoid rape can work in every potential rape situation. Because of this, we encourage personal health classes to invite speakers from a local rape prevention services bureau to discuss approaches to rape prevention.

Sometimes a personal assault begins as a physical assault that may turn into a rape situation. Rape is generally considered a crime of sexual aggression in which the victim is forced to have sexual intercourse. Current thought concerning rape characterizes this behavior as a violent act that happens to be carried out through sexual contact.

Date Rape

In recent years closer attention has been paid to the sexual victimization that occurs during dating relationships. Referred to as *date rape* or *acquaintance rape,* this form of violence involves forced sexual intercourse by a dating partner. Studies on a number of campuses suggest that about 20% of college women report having experienced date rape. An even higher percentage of women report being kissed and touched against their will. Some men have reported being psychologically coerced into intercourse by their female dating partners. In many cases, the aggressive partner will display certain behaviors that can be categorized (see the list in the margin).

Psychologists believe that aside from the physical harm of date rape, a greater amount of emotional damage may occur.[27] Nearly all victims of date rape seem to suffer from *posttraumatic stress syndrome*. They suffer from anxiety, sleeplessness, and nightmares. Guilt concerning their own behavior, self-esteem, and judgment of other people can be overwhelming and the individual may require professional counseling. Because of the seriousness of these consequences, all students should be aware of the existence of date rape.

Sexual Abuse of Children

One of the most tragic forms of sexual victimization is the sexual abuse of children. Children are especially vulnerable to sexual abuse because of their dependent relationships with parents, relatives, and caregivers (such as babysitters, teachers, and neighbors). Often children are unable to readily understand the difference between appropriate and inappropriate physical contact. Abuse may range from psychological trauma to blatant physical manipulation, including fondling, oral sex, and intercourse.

Because of the subordinate role of children in relationships involving adults, sexually abusive practices often go unreported. Sexual abuse can leave emotional scars that make it difficult to establish meaningful relationships later in life. For this reason, it is especially important for people to pay close attention to any information shared by children that could indicate a potentially abusive situation.

Sexual Harassment

Sexual harassment consists of "unwanted attention of a sexual nature that creates embarrassment or stress."[2] Examples of sexual harassment include unwanted physical contact, excessive pressure for dates, sexually explicit humor, sexual innuendos or remarks, job advancement based on sexual favors, and overt sexual assault. Unlike more overt forms of sexual victimization, sexual harassment may be applied in a subtle manner and can, in some cases, go unnoticed by coworkers and fellow students. Nevertheless, sexual harassment produces stress that cannot be resolved until the harasser is identified and forced to stop. Both males and females can be victims of sexual harassment.

Sexual harassment can occur in many settings, including employment and academic settings. On the college campus, harassment may be primarily in terms of "sex for grades." When this occurs, it is important that the student think carefully about the situation and document the specific times, events, and places where the harassment took place. Consult your college's policy concerning harassment. Next, you could report these events to the appropriate administrative officer (perhaps the Affirmative Action Officer, Dean of Academic Affairs, or Dean of Students). You may also want to discuss the situation with a staff member of the university counseling center.

If harassment occurs in the work environment, the victim should document the occurrences and report them to the appropriate management or personnel

Date Rape

To avoid date rape be cautious of the following behaviors:
Disrespectful attitude towards you and others
Lack of concern for your feelings
Violence and hostility
Obsessive jealousy
Extreme competitiveness
A desire to dominate
Unnecessary physical roughness

official. Reporting procedures will vary from setting to setting. Sexual harassment is a form of illegal sex discrimination and violates Title VII of the Civil Rights Law of 1964.

Commercialization of Sex

We live in a society that places a great deal of importance on sexuality. We are expected to be interesting, alluring, and provocative, particularly with regard to interpersonal relationships. It is not surprising, therefore, that a commercial side to sexuality has emerged over the course of time. To some extent, this commercialization of sex affects everyone.

As a direct consequence of certain forms of sexual commercialization, many people have become victimized, such as the prostitute and his or her client, the runaway teenager, the aspiring actress or actor, and the victim of child pornography. In a less detrimental way, few of us can make a consumer decision that is not in some way influenced by a sexual message. The car, the alcoholic beverage, the perfume, and the clothes we purchase are sold to us through sexually alluring commercials. Do you envision any change in our collective consciousness that will diminish the emphasis on the commercialization of sex?

SUMMARY

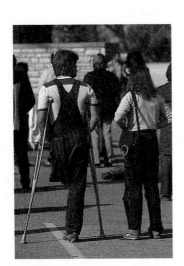

Relationships foster growth and development.

The focus of this chapter was on sexuality as it relates to your experiences in paired relationships. Five core questions were presented about the physiology of the human sexual response pattern. The predictable sexual response pattern consists of four stages: excitement, plateau, orgasmic, and resolution. Also presented were the similarities and variations in sexual response that exist between the sexes.

A discussion of sexual behavior patterns included information about celibacy, masturbation, sexual fantasy, erotic dreams, shared touching, genital contact, oral-genital stimulation, and coitus. A mature approach to these behaviors requires concern for yourself and your partner, as well as a commitment to communicate.

Many standards exist for sexual behaviors in our society, especially when premarital and extramarital sexual intimacy are concerned. A listing of some of these standards was presented. You were encouraged to study the standards and to try to identify, understand, and feel comfortable with the standard that best reflects your belief.

The process of dating and mate selection was examined. A three-stage model was presented to account for the process that propels two persons along the continuum from dating to marriage. The three stages are the marketing stage, sharing stage, and the behavior stage. The mate selection process provides an excellent opportunity to discuss the important issues that must be dealt with before a commitment to marriage is made.

Marriage experts identify various types of marital relationships. Regardless of their form, they exist because they seem to meet the needs of the individuals involved. The forms of marriage include conflict-habituated marriage, devitalized marriage, passive-congenial marriage, total marriage, and vital marriage.

Although at some point in their lives most people marry, there are a number of alternatives to traditional marriage. This chapter discussed some of the issues involving divorce, singlehood, cohabitation, and single parenthood.

Describing a number of sexual preferences as either "normal" or "variant" is not a simple task. To a large degree, the way in which people categorize sexual behavior depends on their personal perspectives and moral beliefs. Many variant sexual behaviors were discussed in this chapter, including homosexuality, bisexuality, and transexualism.

Sexual victimization practices produce physically or psychologically traumatized persons. Many forms of sexual victimization were discussed in this chapter. Among these are rape and sexual assault, date rape, the sexual abuse of children, and sexual harassment. The commercialization of sex was identified, especially as it pertains to the ways in which people can be victimized.

REVIEW QUESTIONS

1 Identify the four stages of the human sexual response pattern. Describe the changes that occur during each stage.
2 What variations exist between the sexual response patterns of males and females?
3 Define celibacy, masturbation, sexual fantasies, erotic dreams, shared touching, genital contact, oral-genital stimulation, and coitus.
4 Identify the three areas of change concerning coital behaviors of unmarried young adults in the past 20 years.
5 What are the three stages that couples generally move through from dating to marriage? Describe what takes place during each stage.
6 Identify and describe the five forms of marriage presented in this chapter. What advantages and disadvantages might there be in each type of marriage?
7 How would you explain the differences between homosexuality and bisexuality? How common are these sexual preferences in our society?
8 Explain what is meant by "variant sexual behaviors." What are some of the variant sexual behaviors discussed in this chapter?
9 Explain some of the myths associated with rape? What is date rape?
10 In what ways can the "commercialization of sex" produce victims?

QUESTIONS FOR PERSONAL CONTEMPLATION

1 Carefully examine the sexual behaviors mentioned in this chapter. Identify your own feelings about each of these behaviors in terms of acceptability, involvement, responsibility, and communication. Are your feelings about these behaviors in line with your actions? If not, what changes should you make in either your feelings or your actions?
2 Which of the following issues should be considered *and* discussed by couples who choose to be sexually active? Why or why not?
   a Partner's feelings
   b Your own feelings
   c What your friends think
   d Parents' feelings
   e Parents' rules regarding nonmarital sex
   f Contraception

   g   Risk of AIDS or other STDs

   h   Ability to communicate with partner

   i   Possible pregnancy

   j   Abortion

   k   Adoption

   l   Single parenthood

   m   Future career or school plans

   n   Your level of maturity

   o   Partner's level of maturity

   p   How you will feel after sexual involvement

   q   How much information you will share with others about your sexual activities

   r   Whether or not you've ever had sexual intimacy

   s   Religious teachings

   t   Moral values

   u   Legal statutes

3 How many of the items that you checked in question 2 do you think are usually discussed by a couple *before* they become sexually active? Why do you think this is true?

4 If you are currently involved in a paired relationship, examine this relationship in terms of the three-stage model presented in this chapter. What stage do you consider your relationship to be in? Do you see your current relationship eventually moving through all three stages to marriage? Why or why not?

5 Review the five forms of marriage presented in the chapter. If you are married, which form relates best to your own marriage? If you are not married, which form will you most likely have if you do choose to get married?

6 To what degree are the variant behaviors presented in this chapter acceptable to you? Which behaviors do you feel are unacceptable?

REFERENCES

1   Masters, W, and Johnson, V: Human sexual response, Boston, 1966, Little, Brown & Co, Inc.

2   Haas K, and Haas, A: Understanding sexuality, St. Louis, 1987, Times Mirror/Mosby College Publishing.

3   Crooks, R, and Baur, K: Our sexuality, ed 3, Menlo Park, Calif, 1987, The Benjamin-Cummings Publishing Co.

4   Knox, D: Human sexuality: the search for understanding, St. Paul, 1984, West Publishing Co.

5   Nass, G, Libby, R, and Fisher, M: Sexual choices, ed 2, Monterey, Calif, 1984, Wadsworth Publishing Co.

6   Melendy, M: Perfect womanhood: for maidens-wives-mothers, Chicago, 1901, Monarch Book Co.

7   Hunt, M: Sexual behavior in the 1970s, Chicago, 1974, Playboy Press.

8   Hyde, JS: Understanding human sexuality, ed 3, New York, 1986, McGraw-Hill Book Co.

9   Petersen, JR, et al: The *Playboy* readers' sex survey, part 2 Playboy March, 1983, pp 90-92, 178-184.

10   Rubin, I: Transition in sexual values–implications for the education of adolescents, Journal of Marriage and the Family 27:185-189, 1965.

11   Springer, B: Women think twice before affair, study shows, Associated Press, Muncie Evening Press, April 22, 1985, p 9.

12 Murstein, B, editor: Theories of attraction and love, New York, 1971, Springer Publishing Co, Inc.

13 Profile of the American husband, Statistical Bulletin 68:2-7, 1987.

14 US Bureau of the Census: Current population reports: Marital status and living arrangements, Series P-20, No 418, Washington, DC, 1987, US Government Printing Office.

15 Cuber, J and Harroff, P: Sex and the significant Americans, Baltimore, 1965, Penguin Books.

16 Hellmich, N: Divorce rears its head in 4th year, USA Today, December 8, 1986, p 1d.

17 Norton, A and Morrman, J: Current trends in marriage and divorce among American women, Journal of Marriage and the Family, 49:3-14, 1987.

18 Harayda, J: The joy of being single, New York, 1986, Doubleday & Co, Inc.

19 Gwartney-Gibbs, P: The institutionalization of premarital cohabitation: estimates from marriage license applications, 1970 and 1980, Journal of Marriage and the Family, 48:423-434, 1986.

20 US Bureau of the Census, Current population reports, Marital status and living arrangements: March 1985, Series P-20, No 410, Washington, DC, 1986, US Government Printing Office.

21 Kinsey, A, Pomeroy, W, and Martin, C: Sexual behavior in the human male, Philadelphia, 1948, WB Saunders, Co.

22 Kinsey, A, et al: Sexual behavior in the human female, Philadelphia, 1953, WB Saunders Co.

23 Gelman, D, et al: A perilous double love life, Newsweek, July 13, 1987, pp 44-46.

24 Rathus, SA: Human sexuality, New York, 1983, Holt, Rinehart & Winston.

25 Equal Opportunity/Affirmative Action Programs Office: Personal physical violence and rape: guide to awareness and prevention, ed 4, Muncie, Ind, 1982, Ball State University.

26 Bever, DL: Safety: a personal focus, ed 2, St. Louis, 1988, Times Mirror/Mosby College Publishing.

27 Brothers, J: Date rape, Parade, September 27, 1987, pp 4-6.

ANNOTATED READINGS

Davitz, LL, and Davitz, J: Living in sync: men and women in love, New York, 1986, The Bergh Publishing Group, Inc.

Men and women have different needs and expectations at different stages of marriage. The authors describe several stages of marriage in detail. Suggestions for enhancing the vitality of marriage are provided.

DeAngelis, B: How to make love all the time: secrets for making love work, New York, 1987, Rawson Associates.

Inadequacies in the bedroom that can carry over into other aspects of life are discussed. Many "bedroom roles" that can be used to a person's benefit are described.

Meshorer, M, and Meshorer, J: Ultimate pleasure: the secrets of easily orgasmic women, New York, 1986, St Martin's Press, Inc.

Easily orgasmic women are defined as those who reach orgasm in 75% of their sexual encounters. The authors studied sixty of these women who were between the ages 21 and 59. These women report being delighted in their sexuality and willing to share knowledge about their sexual success.

Rock, M: The marriage map: understanding and surviving the stages of marriage, Atlanta, 1986, Peachtree Publishers, Ltd.

Working, parenting demands, and the rigor of day-to-day living can devitalize a marriage. The author describes the critical stages in the evolution of modern marital relationships and ways they can be revitalized.

Vaughn, D: Uncoupling: turning points in intimate relationships, New York, 1986, Oxford University Press, Inc.

Vaughn examined 103 separated or divorced individuals to discover the steps that couples go through as they move toward ending their marriages. Armed with this information, couples may be better able to spot early warning signs of difficulty in a marriage.

CHAPTER 15

Fertility Control
An Exercise of Responsible Choice

Key Concepts

Birth control and contraception are related but not synonymous terms

People choose to use birth control methods for a variety of reasons.

Contraceptive methods can be evaluated by their theoretical and use effectiveness rates.

Control over the male and female reproductive systems can be achieved through any of four means.

Each method of birth control has advantages, disadvantages, and contraindications.

Decisions regarding abortion are highly personal and require serious consideration.

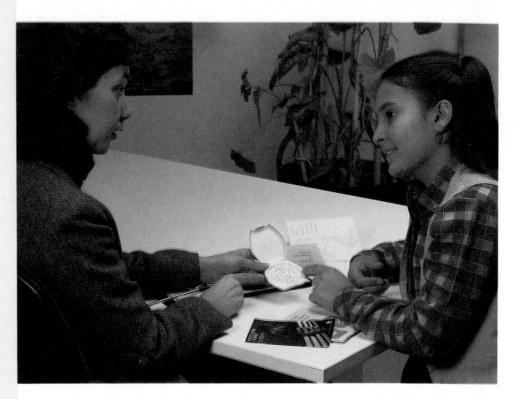

It has been said that the future belongs to the efficient. In a similar way, your own efficiency in controlling your **fertility** will have a significant impact on your future. Your understanding of information and the various issues related to fertility control will help you make responsible decisions in this complex, intriguing area.

Today's young adults form the first generation of people who have near-total control over their fertility. Most couples can now decide when (or if) they want to have children and at what intervals they want their children to be born. Understandably these decisions will require significant contributions from each of the five dimensions of health.

BIRTH CONTROL VERSUS CONTRACEPTION

Any discussion about the control of your fertility should start with an explanation of the subtle differences between the terms **birth control** and **contraception.** While many persons use the words interchangeably, they reflect different perspectives about fertility control. "Birth control" is an umbrella term that refers to all of the procedures you might use to prevent the birth of a child. Birth control includes all available contraceptive measures, as well as sterilization, use of the intrauterine device (IUD), and abortion procedures.

"Contraception" is a much more specific term for any procedure you or your partner might use to prevent the fertilization of an ovum. Contraceptive measures vary widely in the mechanisms they use to accomplish this task. They also vary considerably in their method of use and their rate of success in preventing conception. A few examples of contraceptive methods are the use of condoms, oral contraceptives, spermicides, and diaphragms.

Beyond the numerous methods mentioned above, could it also be possible that certain forms of sexual behavior not involving intercourse be considered forms of contraception? For example, mutual masturbation by couples substantially reduces the likelihood of pregnancy. This practice, as well as additional forms of sexual expression other than intercourse (such as kissing, touching, and massage), have been given the generic term **outercourse.**[1] Not only does outercourse protect against unplanned pregnancy, but it also may significantly reduce the transmission of sexually transmitted diseases, including AIDS.

REASONS FOR CHOOSING TO USE BIRTH CONTROL

People choose to use birth control for a variety of reasons. Many career-minded individuals carefully plan the time and spacing of children so that they can best provide for the children's financial support without sacrificing their own job status. Others choose methods of birth control to ensure that they will never have children. Some use birth control methods to permit safe participation in a wide variety of sexual behaviors. Fear of contracting a sexually transmitted disease prompts some people to use specific forms of birth control.

Financial and legal considerations can be significant factors in the use of certain birth control methods. Many people must, by necessity, take the cost of a method into account when selecting an appropriate birth control. The cost of sterilization and abortion can prohibit some low-income persons from choosing these alternatives, especially since federal funds do not support such procedures.

421

Family planning services are readily available.

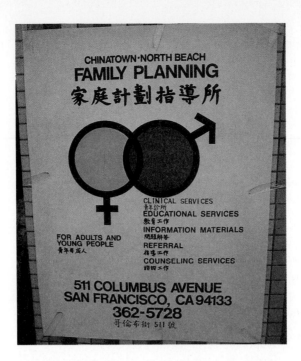

A number of states have established statutes and policies that make contraceptive information and medical services relatively difficult to obtain.

Another important consideration in the use of birth control methods is the availability of professional services. An example of the impact of this factor may be the selection of birth control methods by college students. Some colleges and universities provide contraceptive services through their student health centers. Students enrolled in these schools have easy access to low-cost, comprehensive contraceptive services. Students enrolled in colleges that do not provide such complete services may find that access to accurate information and clinical services is difficult and that private professional services are expensive.

For many persons religious doctrine will be a factor in their selection of a birth control method. This influence can be seen in the Roman Catholic Church's ban on the use of all forms of contraception other than natural family planning and in the condemnation of abortion by certain religious groups.

THEORETICAL EFFECTIVENESS VERSUS USE EFFECTIVENESS

Persons considering the use of a contraceptive method need to understand the difference between the two effectiveness rates given for each form of contraception. *Theoretical effectiveness* is a measure of a contraceptive method's ability to prevent a pregnancy when the method is used precisely as directed during every act of intercourse. *Use effectiveness,* however, refers to the effectiveness of a method in preventing conception when used in the way it is used by the general public. Use effectiveness rates take into account factors that lower effectiveness below that based on "perfect" use. Failure to follow proper instructions, illness of the user, forgetfulness, and a subconscious desire to experience risk or even pregnancy are but a few of the factors that can lower the effectiveness of even the most theoretically effective contraceptive technique.

Effectiveness rates are often expressed in terms of the percentage of women users of childbearing age who do not become pregnant while using the method for 1 year. For some methods the theoretical and use effectiveness rates are vastly different; the theoretical rate is always higher than the use rate. Table 15-1 presents data concerning effectiveness rates, advantages, and disadvantages of many birth control methods.

SELECTING YOUR CONTRACEPTIVE METHOD

In this section we will discuss some of the many factors that should be important to you as you consider selecting a contraceptive method. Remember that no method possesses equally high marks in all of the following areas. It is important that you and your partner select a contraceptive method that is both acceptable and effective, as determined by your unique needs and expectations.

For a contraceptive method to be acceptable to those who wish to exercise a large measure of control over their reproductive potential, the following should be given careful consideration.

It should be safe. The possibility that either you or your partner may face an unacceptable health risk from the use of a particular form of contraceptive should be minimized. A skilled clinician, provided with a complete medical history, can direct you to the contraceptive method best suited to your needs and limitations. You must also consider the possibility that a fetus might be put at risk should you become pregnant and continue to use certain forms of contraception.

It should be effective. Your use of a particular type of contraceptive is, in a sense, a game of odds. Even the most theoretically effective forms occasionally result in unwanted pregnancies. Since your objective is to prevent a pregnancy, you will probably select a method that has a high level of effectiveness.

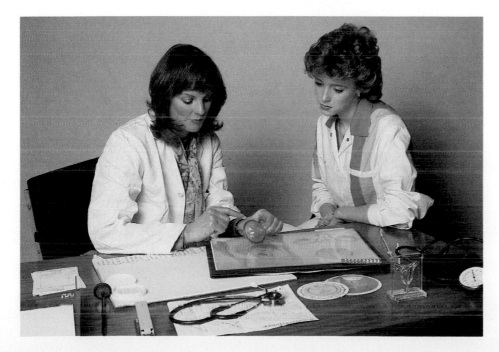

Reproductive counseling is part of family planning services.

Table 15-1 Effectiveness Rates of Birth Control for 100 Women During 1 Year of Use

Method	Effectiveness Best Observed	Typical Users	Advantages	Disadvantages
Withdrawal	85%	75% to 80%	No supplies or advance preparation needed; no side effects; men share responsibility for family planning	Interferes with coitus; may be difficult to use effectively
Fertility awareness techniques	94% to 98%	75% to 85%	No supplies needed; no side effects Men share responsibility for family planning; women learn about their bodies	Difficult to use, especially if menstrual cycles are irregular, as is common in young women; abstinence may be necessary for long periods; lengthy instruction and ongoing counseling may be needed
Spermicide	97% to 98%	80% to 90%	No health risks; helps protect against some STDs	Must be inserted 5 to 30 minutes before coitus; effective for only 30 to 60 minutes; some women may find them awkward or embarrassing to use
Condoms	98%	80% to 90%	Easy to use; inexpensive and easy to obtain; no health risks; very effective protection against some STDs; men share responsibility for family planning	Must be put on just before coitus; some men and women complain of decreased sensation
Diaphragm with spermicide	97% to 98%	80% to 90%	No health risks; helps protect against some STDs and cervical cancer	Must be inserted with jelly or foam before every coitus and left in place for at least 6 hours after coitus; must be fitted by health care personnel; some women may find it awkward or embarrassing to use; may be inconvenient to clean, store, and carry
Contraceptive sponge	90%	75% to 90%	Continuous protection for 24 hours; effective immediately after insertion; may help protect against some STDs	Must be moistened before insertion; some women may find it awkward or embarrassing to use; may cause vaginal irritation in some users; sometimes difficult to insert and remove; relatively expensive

Method	Effectiveness		Advantages	Disadvantages
	Best Observed	Typical Users		
Cervical cap	Effectiveness is estimated to be similar to the diaphragm, but no large-scale American studies to provide proof			Limited availability
IUD	99%	95% to 98%	Easy to use; highly effective in preventing pregnancy; does not interfere with coitus; repeated action not needed	Increases risk of pelvic inflammatory disease (PID) and infertility in women with more than one sexual partner; not usually recommended for women who have never had a child; must be inserted by health care personnel; may cause heavy bleeding and pain in some women; limited availability
Combined pill (estrogen-progestin):	99%	97% to 98%	Easy to use; highly effective in preventing pregnancy; does not interfere with coitus; regulates menstural cycle; reduces heavy bleeding and menstrual pain; helps protect against ovarian and endometrial cancer	Must be taken every day, requires medical examination and prescription; minor side effects such as nausea or menstrual spotting; possibility of circulatory problems such as blood clotting, strokes, and hypertension in a small percentage of users
Minipill (progestin only):	99%	96% to 97%		
Tubal ligation	99.96%	99.96%	Permanent; removes fear of pregnancy	Surgery-related risks; irreversible
Vasectomy	99.85%	99.85%	Permanent; removes fear of pregnancy	Irreversible
Calendar method (when used alone)	85%	70% to 80%	No supplies needed; no side effects; men share responsibility for family planning	Difficult to use, especially if menstrual cycles are irregular as is common in young women; abstinence may be necessary for long periods

It should be reliable. *Reliability* is a measure of the method's ability to be consistently effective, particularly when used in an appropriate manner. Should your method prove ineffective, even when used correctly and when the method has a high theoretical effectiveness, then you may be a unique user (in terms of your own body chemistry), or your particular device may be defective.

It should be reversible. You may want to have children at some point in your life. Should this be the case, it is important that you recognize that some forms of birth control are, for all practical purposes, irreversible. Male and female sterilization should be viewed as techniques best suited for those who are certain that they wish to be child free or those who have completed their families.

It should be affordable. Cost should not be a major factor in your decision to select a suitable contraceptive method. Expensive forms of contraception may force some people to neglect adequate protection, but for the typical college student, effective forms ar usually affordable. Furthermore, most family planning agencies and many college health centers provide effective methods at reduced prices to college students.

It should be easy to use. Any method of contraceptive protection that has complicated instructions has the potential for low effectiveness. Successful methods are those whose use can be easily understood. Do not make a rigid commitment about your contraceptive selection until you understand the nature of its use. Misuse is easy—even for those who have sufficient knowledge about contraceptives and high levels of motivation.

It should not interfere with sexual expression. An ideal contraceptive is one that should not serve as a "turn off" for you or your partner. It should not compromise your sense of esthetics, or be uncomfortable, or interfere with the overall enjoyment of your intimacy. For example, if you are a person who needs to protect the spontaneity of your sexual activity, then do not select a method that must be applied shortly before intercourse. A contraceptive that interferes too often with the quality of your sexual intimacy is a contraceptive that will not be consistently used in its most effective manner.

HOW BIRTH CONTROL METHODS FUNCTION

The intact reproductive systems are biologically designed to provide both the genetic material and support systems for new life. Because scientists adequately understand the male and female systems, control over these systems is possible. Birth control can be accomplished through the following four means.

1 Control achieved through preventing sperm from entering the female reproductive system. Methods include abstinence, coitus interruptus (withdrawal), condom, and male sterilization.

2 Control achieved through preventing sperm from contacting an ovum once sperm have entered the female reproductive system. Methods include rhythm, the diaphragm, vaginal spermicides, douching, the cervical cap, and the contraceptive sponge.

3 Control achieved through preventing the ovum from reaching sperm. Methods include the combined oral contraceptive and female sterilization.

4 Control achieved through disrupting a pregnancy. Methods include the IUD, the minipill, menstrual extraction, and abortion.

Developing Your Personal Life Plan

Your decisions concerning children and birth control must be made within the broad context of your reproductive life plan. To help you develop this plan, ask yourself each of the following questions. To further develop your reproductive life plan, discuss these questions with your partner or trusted friend.

1 Do I wish to marry?
2 At what age would I like to marry?
3 How many years of formal education would I like to complete?
4 When during or after my education would I like to marry?
5 Would I like to wait until I'm married to start having intercourse?
6 Would I like to have children one day?
7 How old would I like to be when I have my first child?
8 How concerned would I be if I (or my partner) were to become pregnant before we were married?
9 If I (or my partner) were to become pregnant when we did not want to be pregnant, what would I do? Raise the child? Adoption? Abortion?
10 How many children would I like to have?
11 Will I be able to support this family emotionally and financially?
12 How would I feel if I were not able to have *any* children?
13 Would I consider adoption an option were I unable to become pregnant?
14 What kind of obligation, if any, do I feel toward limiting the size of my family to help limit the pressure of overpopulation?
15 Would I like to work when my children are toddlers? When my children are in their childhood years? When my children are no longer in the home?
16 How do I expect my partner to participate in child rearing?
17 Of all the things I could do in my life, probably the most important thing would be . . .?
18 This life goal would be affected by marriage in the following ways: . . . By child rearing the the following ways: . . .
19 What would it mean to me if my marriage were to end in divorce?
20 Would I like to have sexual intercourse with the person I marry before that marriage occurs?
21 How would I feel if my spouse were to have an intimate sexual relationship outside of our marriage?
22 How would my spouse feel if I were to have an intimate sexual relationship outside of our marriage?
23 How would I feel if I were to have an intimate sexual relationship outside my marriage?
24 How does my life plan thus far fit in with my spiritual beliefs, with the beliefs of the family and society in which I live, and with my personal code of ethics? How does it fit in with what I feel is spiritually or ethically right or wrong *for me?* If my actions are in conflict with what I feel is right for me to be doing, how can I eliminate this potential conflict that may lead to loss of self-respect?

Although some of the specific methods can be placed under more than one category, today's management of the reproductive system focuses on these four means. It is possible that control mechanisms other than these may exist and eventually become the focus of birth control technology in the future.

CURRENT BIRTH CONTROL METHODS

Withdrawal

coitus interruptus (withdrawal)
a contraceptive practice in which the erect penis is removed from the vagina before ejaculation.

Withdrawal or **coitus interruptus,** is the contraceptive practice in which the erect penis is removed from the vagina just before ejaculation of semen. Theoretically this procedure prevents sperm from entering the deeper structures of the female reproductive system. The use effectiveness of this method, however, reflects how unsuccessful this method is in actual practice (see Table 15-1).

To be more effective this method requires a considerable amount of discipline on the part of the users. Withdrawing the penis before ejaculation is a physical maneuver quite contrary to most couples' intercourse behavior. Most men prefer deep penetration at the moment of ejaculation. Women generally prefer consistent thrusting movements, which tend to trigger their orgasms. Withdrawal tends to inhibit complete sexual enjoyment—especially for the woman.

There is strong evidence to suggest that the clear, preejaculate fluid that helps to neutralize and lubricate the male urethra can contain *viable* (capable of fertilizing) sperm.[3,4] This sperm can be deposited near the cervical opening before withdrawal of the penis. This phenomenon may in part explain the relatively low effectiveness of this method.

Understandably, the use of this method requires considerable trust by the woman. She trusts that her partner will recognize the signs of imminent ejaculation, and that he will "pull out" just in the nick of time. Such trust may not be fully warranted. Tucker[5] writes on this issue:

> Since it is women, not men, who get pregnant, it's not surprising that few women trust and few men deserve trust enough to use this method. . . The only good things about the technique are that it is free, available without a prescription and offers no health hazards other than pregnancy and mental frustration.

Despite the drawbacks of this method, its worldwide use by many couples may be much more extensive than one might expect.[1] The use of withdrawal by sexually active adolescents is reported to be rather high. Unfortunately, use of this method is quite common in teens who think they cannot get pregnant the first time they have intercourse.

Fertility Awareness Techniques

fertility awareness techniques
combined use of all three rhythm techniques of contraception.

There are three approaches included in the birth control strategy called **fertility awareness techniques:** (1) the calendar method, (2) the basal body temperature (BBT) method, and (3) the Billings cervical mucus method. All three methods attempt to determine the time a woman ovulates. Figure 15-1 shows a day-to-day fertility calendar used to calculate fertile periods. Most research indicates that an ovum is viable for only about 24 to 36 hours after its release from the ovary. Once a woman can accurately determine when she ovulates, she must

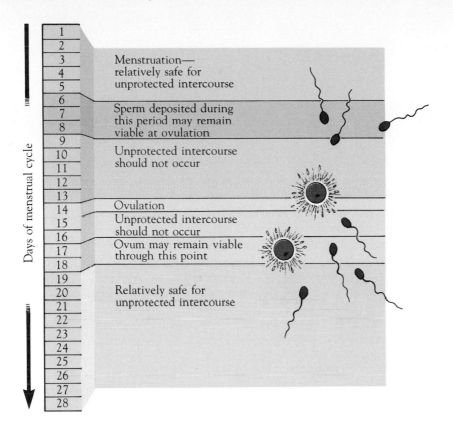

Figure 15-1
Fertility awareness techniques (natural family planning) combines use of the calendar, basal temperature, and Billings mucus techniques to identify the fertile period.

refrain from intercourse long enough for the ovum to begin to disintegrate. Periodic abstinence, rhythm, natural birth control, and natural family planning are terms synonymous with fertility awareness.

Fertility awareness techniques are the only acceptable methods endorsed by the Roman Catholic Church. Interestingly, only about 30% of all Roman Catholic women of childbearing age rely solely on fertility awareness techniques. For some persons who have deep concerns for the spiritual dimensions of their health, the selection of a contraceptive method other than fertility awareness technique may indicate a major compromise on their part.

The effectiveness of the various fertility awareness techniques depends on a woman's careful monitoring of her menstrual cycle. High motivation is a requisite for success. Some sources cite rhythm methods as being 80% to 98% effective when used correctly.[6] Of course, using combinations of these three techniques increases the effectiveness of the rhythm method.

The **calendar method** requires close examination of a woman's menstrual cycle for at least eight cycles. Records are kept of the length (in days) of each cycle. A *cycle* is defined as the number of days from the first day of bleeding of one cycle to the first day of bleeding of the next cycle.

To determine the days she should abstain from intercourse, a woman should subtract 18 from her shortest cycle of the past year. This is the first day she should abstain from intercourse. Now she should subtract 11 from her longest cycle: this is the last day she must abstain from intercourse.[1]

Perhaps the biggest drawback for the calendar method is that couples must

calendar method
form of natural family planning in which the variable lengths of a woman's menstrual cycle are used to calculate her fertile period.

Historical Perspective

Was it magic? Or demons? Or the sun? Was it something she ate? Why does a women initially feel tired and nauseated, then swell, and finally give birth to a child? Can you imagine not knowing the answers to these simple questions about pregnancy? Primitive people did not. Even today in some remote areas of the world people still do not clearly understand reproduction. Nevertheless, primitive people have tried to prevent the birth of babies—most with only limited success. Birth control may be as old as humanity.

Because women carry and deliver babies, the responsibility for controlling fertility was initially relegated to females. Even today almost all of the effective contraceptive technologies are designed to be used by women for their own reproductive systems. History has its own versions of our current oral contraceptive, intrauterine device, diaphragm, and vaginal spermicides.

ORAL CONTRACEPTIVES

Probably the first oral contraceptives were teas made from a variety of materials believed to prevent or terminate a pregnancy.

Others, over the centuries, have included many such "teas" made from various kinds of roots, weeds, and tree leaves; infusions of gunpowder; pills made of quicksilver; even drafts of such death poisons as arsenic . . . The women of Japan at one time ate honey containing the bodies of dead bees. Froth from a camel's mouth was swallowed hopefully by the women of North Africa, who at one time stoically and secretly drank water that had been used to wash the dead.[2]

INTRAUTERINE DEVICE (IUD)

The discovery of the role played by a foreign body placed within the uterus is nearly as old as recorded history. For centuries the leaders of camel caravans crossing the desert protected their female camels from pregnancy; the small stones placed in the uterus of the camels proved to be a relatively effective version of today's IUD.[3] Over the course of history, women have inserted foreign objects composed of various materials into the uterus.

DIAPHRAGM

The female barrier method of contraception has its own unusual history. The Egyptians practiced interesting approaches to stop sperm from entering the female reproductive system. One use was a pluglike device made from the droppings of a crocodile.[2]

Women from other cultures and eras have inserted plugs made of grass, seaweed, dried fruit, seeds, leaves, and cloth into the vagina. Chunks of rock salt and half of a lemon also have their place in the historical collection of diaphragms.

VAGINAL SPERMICIDE

Substances designed to kill sperm were used as early as any of the methods already mentioned.[2] In some cases, the acidity or alkalinity of these substances could have imparted some functional value to these early methods. E. Havemann says, "Aristotle recommended the use of oil of cedar or frankincense mixed with olive oil, and other Greek writers prescribed a mixture of peppermint juice and honey, gum of cedar, or ground pomegranate rind. Also used in this way have been lemon juice, alcohol, opium, and vinegar."[2]

In addition to these forms of female contraception, historical accounts of rhythm, douching, and vaginal swabs support the active pursuit of fertility control that our ancestors undertook.

The realization that vaginal penetration and ejaculation were associated with pregnancy led humans to explore male birth control.

COITUS INTERRUPTUS

Perhaps the oldest version of male-centered contraception is that of withdrawing the penis from the vagina just before ejaculation takes place. Even today, for many sexually active adolescents, this historical method may be the first (and least effective) form of contraception they use.

CONDOM

Although use of the condom is now common throughout the world, it is one of the more recent additions to the male's attempt to control the reproductive process. In a 1564 treatise, the Italian anatomist Gabriello Fallopio recommended the use of a linen sheath. Some early condoms were made of animal gut or leather.[2]

By today's standards most of the techniques mentioned are relatively ineffective, if not dangerous. Perhaps our currently adopted procedures may seem equally primitive by the family planning experts of the future. Regardless, like our forebears, we continue our efforts to counteract the uncanny effectiveness of our own reproductive systems.

stop intercourse for fairly lengthy periods of time. For sexually active couples whose primary sexual behavior includes penile/vaginal intercourse, this abstinence can be distracting, if not unbearable. Women with cycles that vary in length from 26 to 32 days, for example, would be required not to have intercourse from day 8 to day 21 of their subsequent cycles. Because many couples refrain from intercourse during the menstrual flow (day 1 to about day 6), there remain only about 10 days in the entire cycle for such couples to have intercourse. No wonder so many children have been born to couples exclusively practicing this method!

The *basal body temperature method* requires a woman (for about 3 or 4 successive months) to take her rectal temperature every morning before she rises from bed. A finely calibrated thermometer, available in many drugstores, is used for this purpose. The theory behind this method is that a distinct correlation exists between body temperature and the process of ovulation. Just before ovulation, the body temperature supposedly dips and then rises about 0.5° to 1.0° F for the rest of the cycle. The woman is instructed to refrain from intercourse during the interval when the temperature change takes place.

Drawbacks of this procedure include the need for consistent, accurate readings and the realization that all women's bodies are different. Some women may not fit the temperature pattern projection because of biochemical differences in their bodies. Also, body temperatures can fluctuate because of a wide variety of illnesses and physical stressors.

The *Billings cervical mucus method* is the most recently developed fertility awareness technique. Generally used as an adjunct to other fertility awareness techniques, this method requires a woman to evaluate the daily mucous discharge from her cervix. Users of this method become familiar with the changes in both appearance (from clear to cloudy) and consistency (from water to thick) of their cervical mucous throughout their cycles. Women are taught that the unsafe days are when the mucus becomes clear and is the consistency of raw egg whites. Such a technique of ovulation determination must be learned from a physician or family planning professional. For esthetic reasons, this method might not be suitable for all women.

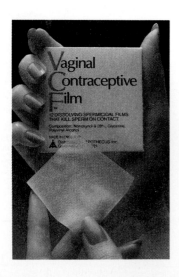

Vaginal Contraceptive Film (VCF)

A recently introduced spermicide developed in England is vaginal contraceptive film (VCF). Vaginal contraceptive film is a nonoxynol-9 impregnated sheet that is inserted over the cervical opening. Shortly after insertion of the VCF, it dissolves into a gel-like material that clings to the cervical opening. The VCF can be inserted up to an hour before intercourse. Over the course of several hours, the material will be washed from the vagina in the normal vaginal secretions.

This new spermicide is a nonprescription form of contraception that is as effective as other spermicidal foams and jellies. A box of 12 sheets costs about $7. Like other spermicidal agents, VCF may also help in minimizing the risk of STDs and PID.

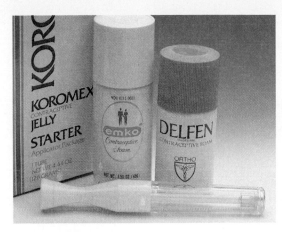

Vaginal spermicide.

Vaginal Spermicides

Although they are not recommended as your primary form of fertility control, spermicidal agents are often recommended to be used with other forms of birth control. Alone, **spermicides** offer a reasonable amount of protection for the woman who is sexually active on an *infrequent* basis. For the oral contraceptive user who has missed taking two or more birth control pills, spermicides are an excellent backup method of protection. For women who are experiencing menopause, spermicides provide protection from a pregnancy as well as lubrication for a vagina that has become drier as a result of estrogen depletion.

Modern spermicides are safe, reasonably effective, reversible forms of contraception that can be obtained without a physician's prescription; they can be purchased in most drugstores and in many supermarkets. Like condoms, spermicides are relatively inexpensive.

Spermicides, which are available in foam, cream, paste, or film form are made of water-soluble bases with a spermicidal chemical incorporated in the base. The base material is designed to liquefy at body temperature and distribute the spermicidal component in an even layer over the tissues of the upper vagina. The box on p. 432 describes a newly developed film-type spermicide.

Effervescent vaginal suppositories are composed of spermicides suspended in water-soluble bases. On insertion into the vagina, they dissolve and release their spermicides in a thin film covering the area around the cervix. Research has revealed that some suppositories do not adequately melt by the time their spermicidal protection is needed.[1]

Spermicidal foams, packaged in the form of aerosols, are placed in the vagina where they quickly become a foam. As the foam spreads over the region of the cervix, the spermicide it contains is available to attack sperm. While present, the foam will provide a degree of mechanical blockage to the passage of sperm. Foams, in comparison to other spermicidal products, are thought to offer the most protection.

Depending on the spermicide used, the spermicide will either attack the sperm cell's membrane or alter the metabolic activity within the sperm cell. Spermicides are not specific to sperm cells; they also attack certain bacterial cells, and thus may provide the woman with some additional protection against many sexually transmitted diseases and **pelvic inflammatory disease (PID)**.[7] In

spermicides
chemicals capable of killing sperm.

pelvic inflammatory disease (PID)
generalized infection of the pelvic cavity that results from the spread of an infection through a woman's reproductive structures.

Figure 15-2
Spermicidal foams and suppositories are placed deep into the vagina in the region of the cervix no longer than 30 minutes before intercourse.

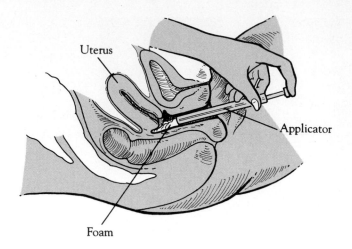

Uterus

Applicator

Foam

very few cases, spermicides have caused skin irritations to users. Some couples may find the smell or taste of certain spermicides either offensive or pleasing.

For women using vaginal spermicides, either as their sole form of fertility control or as an adjunct to their partner's use of the condom, the directions supplied by the manufacturer should be carefully followed (see Figure 15-2). Many family planning agencies advocate a more cautious set of directions than do most manufacturers. On the basis of these more conservative directions, users of vaginal spermicides are advised to take the following steps:

1 Insert the spermicide no longer than 30 minutes before intercourse.
2 Double the amount of spermicide to be applied over that recommended by the manufacturer.
3 Once the foam is inserted, do not walk around unnecessarily. Movement can, in some cases, cause the mechanical protection provided by the inert base to be lost too quickly.
4 For each act of intercourse following the first, insert an applicator full of spermicide into the vagina.
5 Do not douche or bathe for at least 8 hours after the last act of intercourse. The spermicidal action of the product's active ingredient could be removed before all sperm are incapacitated.

On the basis of these reservations, vaginal spermicides offer some measure of contraceptive protection for those females who are motivated to use them correctly. However, when combined with another form of contraception, these products can be considered effective forms of fertility control.

Condom

Colored or natural, smooth or textured, straight or shaped, plain or reservoir-tipped, dry or lubricated—the condom is approaching an art form. Exaggerated? Perhaps. Nevertheless, the familiar **condom** remains a safe, effective, reversible contraceptive device.

For couples who are highly motivated in their desire to prevent a pregnancy, the effectiveness of a condom can approach that of the oral contraceptive—especially if condom use is combined with a spermicide. (Some lubricated con-

condom
latex shield designed to cover the erect penis and retain semen upon ejaculation; "rubber."

doms now also contain a spermicide.) For couples who are less motivated or who use condoms on an irregular basis, the condom can be considerably less effective. This readily available and inexpensive method of contraception requires responsible use if it is to achieve a high level of effectiveness.

Why should couples consider the condom as a primary form of contraception when other forms are equally available and, in some cases, more effective? The following should be considered:

- The condom is readily available. Its use is not based on an examination or a prescription. It is sold openly in drugstores. At many universities, condoms are marketed in the health center at cost.
- It is safe. The condom is a barrier method of contraception that involves nothing more than a latex rubber material and a water-soluble lubricant. No chemicals are ingested, and only limited contact is made between the device and the bodies of the partners.
- It is one of the few effective forms of contraception that affords the man an active opportunity to assume responsibility for fertility control. Granted, the male partner could pay for birth control pills, wash or powder a diaphragm after use, or promise to withdraw before ejaculation, but these are limited opportunities for responsibility. The condom can be a shared form of contraceptive protection for the partners.
- The condom offers a measure of protection against sexually transmitted diseases. For both the man and the woman, chlamydial infections, gonorrhea, and AIDS and other sexually transmitted diseases are less likely to be acquired when the condom is used. When combined with a spermicide condoms may become even more effective against the spread of sexually transmitted diseases. See Chapter 12 for a more detailed description of the condom's role in safe sex practice. Although advertisements suggest that condoms provide protection against the transmission of genital herpes, users of condoms must remember that this protection is limited to the penis and vagina—not to the surrounding genital region, where most lesions are found.

Condoms.

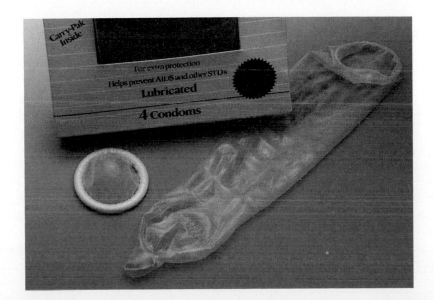

We believe that there are legitimate roles for the condom as a contraceptive agent. How can the condom be used to maximize its effectiveness? These simple directions, in combination with your motivation and commitment to regular use, should provide you with reasonable protection:

- Keep a supply of condoms at hand. Condoms should be stored in a cool, dry place so that they are readily available at the time of intercourse. Condoms that are stored in wallets or automobile glove compartments may not be in satisfactory condition when they are used. Temperature extremes are to be avoided. The shelf life of condoms is about 2 years.
- Do not test a condom by inflating or stretching it. Handle it gently and keep it away from sharp fingernails.
- For maximum effectiveness, put the condom on before genital contact. Either the man or the woman can put the condom in place. Early application is particularly important in the prevention of sexually transmitted diseases. Early application also lessens the possibility of the release of preejaculate fluid.
- Unroll the condom on the erect penis. For those using a condom without a reservoir tip, a small amount of space should be left to catch the ejaculate.
- Lubricate the condom if this has not already been done by the manufacturer. When doing this, be certain to use a water-soluble lubricant and not a petroleum-based product, such as petroleum jelly. Petroleum can deteriorate the latex material.
- After ejaculation, be certain that the condom does not become dislodged from the penis. Hold the rim of the condom firmly against the base of the penis during withdrawal. Do not allow the penis to become flaccid (soft) while still in the vagina.
- Inspect the condom for tears before throwing it away. If the condom is damaged in some way, immediately insert a spermicidal agent into the vagina.

Like other barrier methods of contraception, the condom is a reasonable choice for couples who are motivated in their desire to prevent a pregnancy and who are willing to assume the level of responsibility required.

Diaphragm

What form of birth control would you select if you were a woman faced with one or more of the following situations?

- Your partner wants no responsibility in preventing your pregnancy. He will not use a condom, practice withdrawal, or have a vasectomy.
- You have been informed that the oral contraceptive pill and the IUD are not especially "safe" for you.
- You are breastfeeding.
- You are sexually active, but on an infrequent basis.

diaphragm
soft, rubber cup designed to cover the cervix.

If you find yourself in one or more of the above situations, then a barrier method, particularly the **diaphragm,** could be an excellent choice for you. A growing body of evidence suggests that among women who are concerned about the potential risks associated with oral contraceptive or IUD use, the diaphragm is gaining popularity. In fact, some women are selecting the diaphragm for other

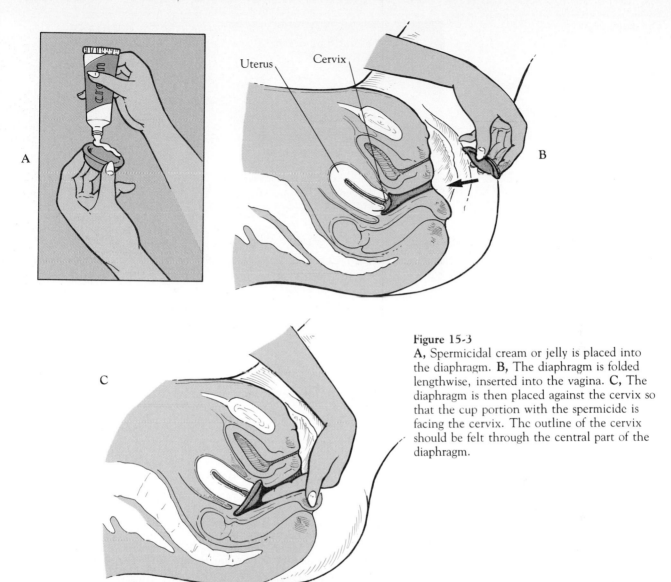

Figure 15-3
A, Spermicidal cream or jelly is placed into the diaphragm. **B,** The diaphragm is folded lengthwise, inserted into the vagina. **C,** The diaphragm is then placed against the cervix so that the cup portion with the spermicide is facing the cervix. The outline of the cervix should be felt through the central part of the diaphragm.

reasons—reasons associated with its ability to provide some protection against STDs and PID[1] and to provide additional lubrication during intercourse. The diaphragm does, however, require a high level of motivation and a commitment to careful use. When used incorrectly, its use effectiveness falls far below that of the pill, IUD, or combined spermicide-condom use.

The diaphragm is a soft, rubber cup with a springlike metal rim that when properly fitted and properly inserted by the user, rests in the top of the vagina. In its proper position, the diaphragm covers the cervical os (see Figure 15-3). During intercourse, the diaphragm stays in place quite well and cannot usually be felt by either the man or the woman.

The diaphragm is always used in conjunction with a spermicidal cream or jelly. The diaphragm should be covered with an adequate amount of spermicide

The diaphragm.

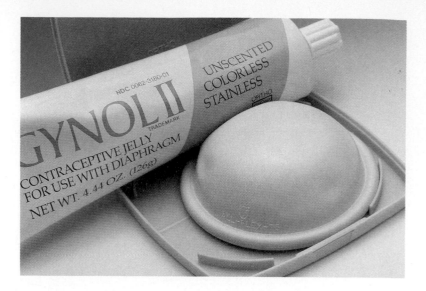

inside the cup and around the rim. When used properly with a spermicide, the diaphragm is an effective contraceptive, and when combined with the man's use of a condom, its effectiveness is even greater.

For some women, the diaphragm is not an acceptable form of contraception because of characteristics that are unacceptable for them. One or more of the following could be an important reason for you to select another method of birth control:

- A high level of motivation is required with the diaphragm.
- It is necessary for the user to handle her genitalia.
- To minimize the possibility of toxic shock syndrome, the diaphragm should not be used during the menses and it should not remain in place for more than 24 hours.[1]
- The diaphragm must be fitted and prescribed by a physician.
- The initial cost of the device may be relatively high. The continuing cost of spermicides also adds to this expense.
- The diaphragm must be inserted no longer than 6 hours before intercourse, it must remain in place for at least 6 hours following intercourse, and should additional episodes of intercourse take place, additional spermicide must be applied. Diaphragm use is considered "messy" by some people.
- Even when used correctly, the diaphragm is less effective than both the pill and the IUD.
- The diaphragm needs to be refitted once a year, after a weight gain or loss of 10 pounds, and after childbirth. The diaphragm should be replaced every 2 years because of the stress on the rubber material.

Cervical Cap

cervical cap
small, thimble-shaped device designed to fit over the cervix; limited availability.

The **cervical cap** is a small, thimble-shaped device that fits over the entire cervix. Resembling a small diaphragm, the cervical cap is placed deeper than the diaphragm. The cap is held in place by suction rather than by pushing against anatomical structures (see Figure 15-4). Like the diaphragm, a spermicide is used with the cervical cap. Thus it requires many of the same skills for insertion and care as the diaphragm. The use effectiveness of the cervical cap appears to be

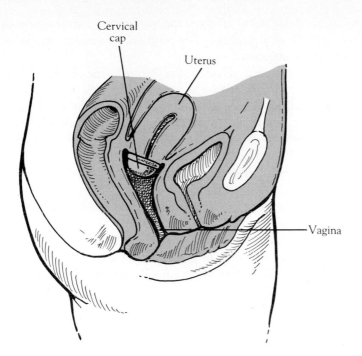

Cervical cap

Uterus

Vagina

Figure 15-4
After the spermicidal cream or jelly is placed in the cervical cap, the cap is inserted into the vagina and placed against the cervix.

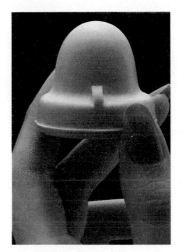

Cervical cap.

approximately equal to that of the diaphragm, but to date so few are used in this country that its effectiveness is largely based on a few limited studies.[7] Cervical caps were approved by the FDA in June 1988. These devices are manufactured only in Europe and are distributed in the United States through prescription by a physician.

Contraceptive Sponge

In April 1983 the FDA approved one brand (Today) of a new contraceptive device called the **contraceptive sponge.**[7] This over-the-counter product consists of a soft, spongy, disklike object that is moistened and inserted over the cervical area. The contraceptive sponge contains an appropriate dose of a common spermicide (nonoxynol-9). Thus this device both blocks sperm from entering the uterus and kills sperm. Each sponge is effective for about 24 hours and is not reusable. The safety and use effectiveness of this product is approximately equal to that of the diaphragm. There is some indication that use of the sponge decreases the risk of contracting chlamydial and gonorrhea infections.[8]

A small percentage of women experience unpleasant side effects and complications from the use of the sponge. Among these are vaginal irritation or allergic reactions, difficulty in sponge removal, tearing of the sponge into fragments, and increased vaginal dryness.[1] The predicted risk of toxic shock syndrome (see Chapter 12) among sponge users is similar to that in tampon users.[9]

contraceptive sponge
soft, spongy disk that is moistened and inserted over the cervical area.

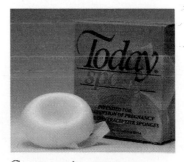

Contraceptive sponge.

Intrauterine Device

Recall that fertilization generally occurs in the upper third of a fallopian tube. The fertilized ovum begins the week-long journey down the tube to the uterus, which has already been prepared for its arrival. Once entering the uterus, the

intrauterine device (IUD)
small, plastic, medicated or
unmedicated device that
when inserted in the uterus
prevents continued preg-
nancy.

ovum's growing cellular mass initiates the process of implantation and subsequently the formation of a placenta. The pregnancy becomes established and the
gestational process is underway.

For the woman who has selected the **intrauterine device (IUD)** as her
method of birth control, the above scenario could well begin, but would not
continue, in all likelihood. IUD use seems to inhibit the implantation of the
fertlized ovum in the uterus. The pregnancy cannot continue. Birth control will
have been accomplished—contraception will not have been accomplished. In a
technical sense, the IUD is not a contraceptive device.

The mechanism underlying the functioning of the IUD is still being researched. The most currently accepted explanations include the following[10]:

■ *The IUD stimulates the production of a foreign-body response in the uterus.* Following insertion of the IUD, numerous phagocytic white blood cells appear
in the endometrium and the uterine fluids. These cells are followed by the
appearance of additional phagocytic cells, including giant cells, plasma
cells, and macrophages. Consumption of sperm or the fertilized ovum by
these cells is possible.

■ *The IUD causes changes in the normal cyclic nature of the uterine wall.* During
the menstrual cycle, the lining of the uterus moves through a growth stage
and into a secretory stage as it matures in anticipation of a fertilized ovum.
Should the normal course of this preparation be disrupted, as has been attributed to the IUD, the ovum could arrive in the uterus at a time when
the wall was too poorly prepared for implantation to be successful. The
ovum would be denied the support needed for continued growth.

The most widely used medicated IUD (Progestasert) is a T shaped, plastic
IUD that contains progesterone. This type of IUD helps to create a high progesterone concentration in the uterine wall tissue. The elevated level of progesterone prevents the uterine wall from reaching a state of development favorable
for implantation. The Progestasert must be replaced every 12 months.

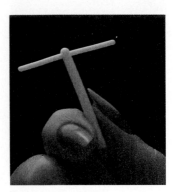

Progestasert IUD.

IUDs must be inserted by a skilled physician. Usually the IUD is inserted
during the time the woman is menstruating, because the cervical opening is
slightly dilated at this time, and the likelihood of being pregnant is quite remote.
A local anesthetic may be used.

IUDs are not recommended for all women. Troublesome side effects do occur
for some users of the IUD, including heavier and longer menstrual flow and
occasional mid-cycle spotting. Two potentially serious side effects of IUD use are
uterine perforation and the development of pelvic inflammatory disease. This disease is a generalized, life-threatening infection of the abdominal cavity. IUD
users, particularly young women with multiple sexual partners and a greater exposure to sexually transmitted diseases, are more likely to develop this infection
than are non-IUD users. Studies relating IUD use and PID are ongoing. Management of this dangerous infection appears to be possible with early diagnosis.

Women are becoming increasingly concerned about the use of the IUD. A
particular IUD, the Dalkon Shield, was linked to a number of deaths and
thousands of cases of infection and miscarriage (see Figure 15-5). Thousands
of liability lawsuits were filed against the manufacturer, the A.H. Robbins
Company, by women who claim to have been injured by the Dalkon Shield.
The Dalkon Shield is no longer manufactured and payments for injury are being
made.[11]

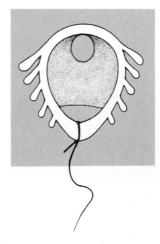

Figure 15-5
The Dalkon Shield.

In conjunction with the problems of the Dalkon Shield, the manufacturers of most other IUDs have ceased production. As of 1988 only two IUDs are marketed in the United States; one of these is the Progestasert.

The second IUD that is available in the United States is the recently introduced Copper-T 380A. This IUD is a refinement of earlier copper IUDs in which copper ions released by the IUD interfered with the normal function of endometrial tissue, thus preventing implantation of the fertilized ovum. The Copper-T 380A can be used for 4 years before it needs to be replaced.

Should a woman with an IUD become pregnant, the possible removal of it must be considered. If the IUD is in a position that does not interfere with the developing fetus, the IUD might be permitted to remain. However, if the location of the IUD poses a medical threat to the fetus or the mother, the device will most likely be removed. This minimizes the risk of *spontaneous abortion*.

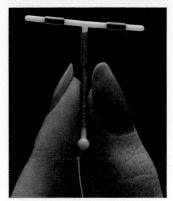

Copper-T 380A IUD.

Oral Contraceptives

Developed in the 1950s, the **oral contraceptive pill** provides the highest effectiveness rate of any single reversible contraceptive method used today. The pill is the method of choice for nearly 10 million users in the United States.[1]

Use of "the pill" requires a physician's examination and prescription. Since oral contraceptives are available in a wide range of formulas, follow-up examinations are important to ensure that a woman is receiving an effective dosage with as few side effects as possible. Matching the right prescription with the woman may require a few consultations.

All oral contraceptives contain synthetic (laboratory-made) hormones. The *combined pill* uses both synthetic estrogen and synthetic progesterone in each pill. The *sequential pill,* no longer used today, consisted of a series of estrogen-only pills followed by a series of progesterone-only pills.

Oral contraceptives function in several fascinating ways. The estrogen present in the pill tends to suppress the release of follicle-stimulating hormone (FSH) from the pituitary gland. Because of this action, no primary follicles in the ovaries are stimulated to begin maturation. The progesterone present in the pill serves to alter the usual menstrual sequence in three ways. First, progesterone suppresses the pituitary gland's release of luteinizing hormone (LH), reducing the chances of ovulation should a follicle have inadvertently matured. Second, the progesterone causes an inadequate development of the endometrial lining of the uterus. Finally, the progesterone helps to thicken the cervical mucus, thus making sperm penetration into the uterus difficult at best.

The physical changes produced by the oral contraceptive provide some beneficial side effects in women. Since the synthetic hormones are taken for 21 days and then are followed by **placebo pills** or no pills for 7 days, the menstrual cycle becomes regulated. Even women who have irregular cycles immediately become "regular." Since the uterine lining is not developed to the extent seen in a non-pill-taking woman, the uterus is not forced to contract with the same amount of vigor. Thus menstrual cramping is reduced and the resultant menstrual flow is diminished. The use of the pill increases the likelihood of contracting a chlamydial infection however, the pill does inhibit a number of other common STDs.[1] Recent research also suggests that oral contraceptive use may provide protection against noncancerous breast tumors, endometrial cancer, and cancer

oral contraceptive pill
pill taken orally, composed of synthetic female hormones that prevent ovulation or implantation; "the pill."

placebo pills
pills that contain no active ingredients.

Oral contraceptives.

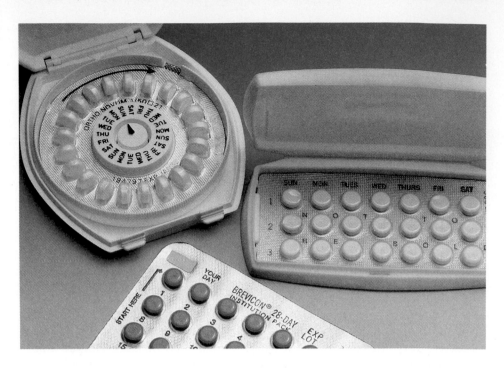

of the ovaries.[1,12,13] Some oral contraceptives have been found to lower LDL levels (see Chapter 10) thus fostering cardiovascular health. No evidence has been found linking breast cancer to long-term use.

The negative side effects of the oral contraceptive pill can be divided into two general categories: (1) unpleasant and (2) potentially dangerous. The unpleasant side effects generally subside within 2 or 3 months for most women. A number of women report some or many of the following symptoms:

- Tenderness in the breast tissue
- Nausea
- Mild headaches
- Slight, irregular spotting
- Weight gain
- Fluctuations in sex drive
- Mild depression
- Lowered resistance to vaginal infections

Interestingly, these reported symptoms closely approximate the symptoms some women report during the first few months of pregnancy. This should come as no surprise, because in a certain sense, the woman's body reponse to the pill mimics some of the body changes caused by hormonal fluctuations during the early stages of pregnancy. In both cases, FSH is suppressed and progesterone release is continued. Shouldn't the body reactions be rather similar? Of course, just as many pregnant women report no unusual side effects early in the pregnancy, many first users of oral contraceptives also report no unpleasant side effects.

The potentially dangerous side effects of the oral contraceptive pill are most often seen in the cardiovascular system. Blood clotting, strokes, hypertension, and myocardial infarction all seem to be associated with the estrogen component of the combined pill. When compared to nonusers, the risk of dying from cardiovascular complications is only slightly increased among healthy, young oral contraceptive users. *Migraine headaches* and gallbladder disease also are associated with oral contraceptive use. Nevertheless, the risks that are associated with pregnancy and childbirth are still much greater than those associated with oral contraceptive use.

It appears that there are some **contraindications** for the use of oral contraceptives. If you have a history of blood clotting, migraine headaches, liver disease, a heart condition, obesity, diabetes, epilepsy, anemia, or if you have not established regular menstrual cycles, the pill probably should not be your contraceptive choice.

Two additional contraindications are receiving considerable attention by the medical community. Cigarette smoking and advancing age are highly associated with an increased risk of potentially serious side effects. Increasing numbers of physicians are not prescribing oral contraceptives for their patients who smoke. The risk of cardiovascular-related deaths is greatly enhanced in women over age 35. The risk is even higher in female smokers over 35. The data are quite convincing.[1]

For the vast majority of women, however, the pill, when properly prescribed, is safe and effective. Careful scrutiny of one's health history and careful follow-up examinations when a problem is suspected are essential elements that can provide a margin of safety. The ease of administration, the relatively low cost, and the effectiveness of the pill make it a sound choice for many women.

However, some women prefer not to use the combined oral contraceptive pill. Thus to avoid some of the potentially serious side effects of the combined pill, some physicians are prescribing **minipills.** These oral contraceptives contain no estrogen—only low-dose progesterone. In a number of women, the minipill does not produce the cessation of ovulation seen in most users of the combined pill. The minipill seems to work by making an unsuitable environment for the transportation and implantation of the fertilized ovum. The effectiveness of the minipill is slightly lower than that of the combined pill.[1]

Breakthrough bleeding and **ectopic pregnancy** are more common in minipill users than in combined pill users. Long-term studies on the comparative safety of minipills over combined pills have not been completed.[1] However, it does seem plausible that the risks associated with only one hormone would be less than those from two hormones.

Oral contraceptives of the future

The future holds promise for better oral contraceptives. Both males and females may soon have access to contraceptive pills composed of "natural" hormones. Rather than replacing the natural hormones estrogen and progesterone, as birth control pills do, a new contraceptive pill will regulate egg production by enhancing the action of inhibitory hormones already produced by the female reproductive system. A similar contraceptive pill may be developed that regulates sperm production. A birth control pill for females that contains Inhibin, a recently identified nonsteroidal gonadal inhibitory factor, could appear in the early 1990s. The box on p. 444 describes another oral contraceptive that could be used in the future.

contraindications
factors that make the use of a drug inappropriate or dangerous for a particular person.

minipills
low-dose progesterone oral contraceptives.

ectopic pregnancy
a pregnancy wherein the fertilized ovum implants at a site other than the uterus, typically in the fallopian tubes.

Morning-After Pill

A "morning-after pill" is an oral contraceptive a woman can take to reduce the possibility of pregnancy following unprotected intercourse. The FDA has not officially approved any oral contraceptive that could be used in this fashion. Formerly, the drug DES (diethylstibesterol) was used as a type of morning-after pill, although it was primarily for women who were victims of rape. Because of its potentially dangerous side effects, DES was removed from the market. A relatively high dose progesterone-only oral contraceptive (Ovral) is now "unofficially" the drug of choice as a morning-after pill. Physicians, who have the right to prescribe drugs for purposes other than those specifically indicated by the FDA, are now prescribing Ovral for patients who have unprotected mid-cycle intercourse. Many physicians prefer not to use Ovral in this fashion. The use of Ovral initiates menstrual flow within a few weeks.[1]

The use of a morning-after pill in cases of rape or contraceptive failure is understandable. However use in cases of unprotected intercourse seems to many people to be a reflection of irresponsibility. Does this pill represent just another form of abortion? What do you think?

Sterilization

sterilization
generally permanent birth control techniques that surgically disrupt the normal passage of ova or sperm.

All of the contraceptive mechanisms or methods already discussed have one quality in common; they are reversible. Although microsurgical techniques are fast providing medical breakthroughs, **sterilization** should still be considered an irreversible procedure. When you decide to use sterilization, you no longer control you own fertility, because you no longer will be able to produce offspring.

For this reason, couples considering sterilization procedures usually must undergo extensive discussions with a physician or family planning counselor to identify their true feelings about this finality. People must be aware of the possible changes in self-concept they might have after sterilization. If you are a man who equates fertility with masculinity, you may have trouble accepting your new status as a sterile male. If you are a woman who equates motherhood with femininity, you might have adjustment problems after sterilization.

The male sterilization procedure is called a *vasectomy*. Accomplished under a local anesthetic in a physician's office, this 20- to 30-minute procedure consists of the surgical removal of a section of each vas deferens. After a small incision is made through the scrotum, the vas deferens is located and a small section removed. The remaining ends are either tied or *cauterized* (see Figure 15-6, A).

Most men report only mild to moderate discomfort for about 1 week after surgery. Use of an athletic supporter seems to provide comfortable support for some during the week following surgery. Follow-up physician's examinations are essential to determine the sperm count in the ejaculate. Within about 6 weeks, no sperm should be present in the ejaculate. Until the ejaculate is free of sperm, a backup method of contraception should be used.

Although most men report temporary mild anxiety about their sexual functioning after a vasectomy, the potential for normal functioning remains quite high. Men still produce male sex hormones, get erections, have orgasms, and

ejaculate. There should be no anticipated complications. (Recall that sperm accounts for only a small portion of the semen.) Some men even report increased
interest in sexual activity, since their chances of impregnating a woman are
virtually nonexistent.

What happens to the process of spermatogenesis within each testicle? Sperm
cells are still being produced, but they are destroyed by specialized white blood
cells called phagocytic leukocytes.

The most common method of female sterilization is *tubal ligation.* During this
procedure, the fallopian tubes are cut and the ends tied back. Some physicians
cauterize the tube ends to ensure complete sealing (see Figure 15-6, *B*).

The fallopian tubes are usually reached either through the abdominal wall or
the vaginal wall. In a *minilaparotomy,* a small incision is made through the abdominal wall just below the navel. The resultant scar is quite small and is the

Female Sterilization Methods

Tubal ligation
   Minilaparotomy
   Culpotomy
   Laparoscopy
   Culdoscopy
Ovariectomy
Hysterectomy

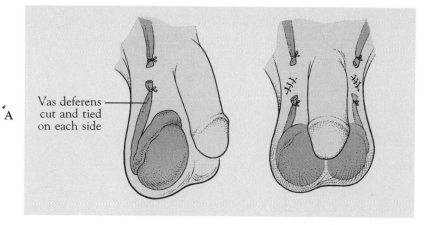

A

Vas deferens
cut and tied
on each side

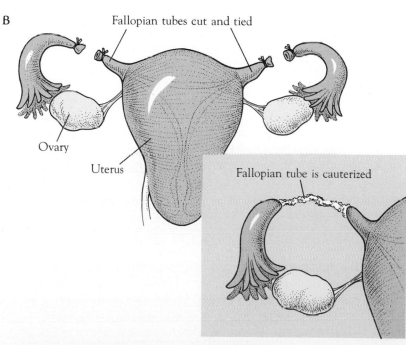

B

Fallopian tubes cut and tied

Ovary

Uterus

Fallopian tube is cauterized

Figure 15-6
The most frequently used
forms of male and female
sterilization. **A,** Vasectomy.
B, Tubal ligation.

basis for the term "band-aid surgery." In a *culpotomy,* the tubes are reached through an incision made in the vaginal wall. A culpotomy produces no external scarring, but since hemorrhage and infection rates are about twice as high as those for the minilaparotomy, this procedure is not routinely done.[2]

Female sterilization requires about 20 to 30 minutes, with the patient under a local or general anesthetic. The use of a *laparoscope* has made female sterilization much simpler than in the past. The laparoscope is a small tube equipped with mirrors and lights. Inserted through a single incision, the laparoscope locates the fallopian tubes before they are cut, tied, or cauterized. When an endoscope is used through an abdominal incision, the procedure is called a *laparoscopy.* If entry is made through the vaginal wall, the procedure is called a *culdoscopy.* Like the culpotomy, the culdoscopy is seldom performed.

Women who are sterilized still produce female hormones, ovulate, and menstruate. The ovum cannot move down the fallopian tube, however. Within a day of its release, the ovum will start to disintegrate and be absorbed by the body. Contrary to some beliefs, sterilization does not bring on menopause and it does not initiate male secondary sex characteristics in women. Freed of the possibility of becoming pregnant, many sterilized women report an increase in sex drive and activity.

Two other procedures produce sterilization in women. *Ovariectomy* (the surgical removal of the ovaries) and *hysterectomy* (the surgical removal of the uterus) accomplish sterlization. However, these procedures are used to remove diseased (cancerous, cystic, hemorrhaging) organs and are not primarily considered sterilization techniques.

A RANGE OF OPTIONS

Before discussing the technical procedures employed in terminating a pregnancy, let us first consider the options that are in theory available to all women:
- The pregnancy can be carried to term and the child kept*
- The pregnancy can be carried to term and the child placed for adoption*
- The pregnancy can be carried to term and the child placed into foster care, either to be taken later by the mother or placed for adoption*
- The pregnancy can be terminated†

These are the four options that exist for a woman who is pregnant and uncertain about whether or not to terminate her pregnancy. Reputable clinicians and family planning agencies will help clarify a woman's uncertainties by describing the full range of options available. The box on p. 448 further explains these options. For a particular woman, factors such as marital status, financial security, job security, interests of the father, religious beliefs, support of family and friends, and the availability of services are factors that personalizes the decision.

Abortion

Regardless of the circumstance under which pregnancy occurs, women may now choose to terminate their pregnancies. No longer must women who do not want to be pregnant seek potentially dangerous, illegal abortions. This formerly weak

*Assume the absence of a serious threat to the life or health of the woman.
†Contingent on the stage of the pregnancy and applicable state regulations.

Personal Assessment

Which Birth Control Method Is Best for You?

To assess which birth control method would be best for you, answer the following questions and check the interpretation below.

Do I: Yes   No

1 Need a contraceptive right away? _____ _____
2 Want a contraceptive that can be used completely independent of sexual relations? _____ _____
3 Need a contraceptive only once in a great while? _____ _____
4 Want something with no harmful side effects? _____ _____
5 Want to avoid going to the doctor? _____ _____
6 Want something that will help protect against sexually transmitted diseases? _____ _____
7 Have to be concerned about affordability? _____ _____
8 Need to be virtually certain that pregnancy will not result? _____ _____
9 Want to avoid pregnancy now but want to have a child sometime in the future? _____ _____
10 Have any medical condition or lifestyle that may rule out some form of contraception? _____ _____

Interpretation

If you have checked *Yes* to number:

1 Condoms, sponges, and spermicides may be easily purchased without prescription in any pharmacy.
2 Sterilization, oral contraceptives, cervical caps, and fertility awareness techniques do not require that anything be done just before sexual relations.
3 Diaphragms, condoms, sponges, or spermicides can be used by people who have coitus only once in a while. Fertility awareness techniques may also be appropriate, but require a high degree of skill and motivation.
4 IUDs should be avoided. Sometimes the use of oral contraceptives result in some minor discomfort and may have harmful side effects.
5 The sponge, condom, and spermicides do not require a prescription from a physician.
6 The condom and, to a lesser extent, spermicides and the sponge may help protect against some sexually transmitted diseases.
7 The cost of sterilization is high, but there is no additional expense for a lifetime. Those who have coitus daily or more often may find the diaphragm, oral contraceptives, or a cervical cap more economical than other methods.
8 Sterilization provides near certainty. Oral contraceptives or a diaphragm-condom-spermicide combination also gives a high measure of reliable protection. Fertility awareness, withdrawal, and douche methods should be avoided.
9 While it is sometimes possible to reverse sterilization, it requires surgery and is more complex than simply stopping use of any of the other other methods.
10 Smokers and people with a history of blood clots should not use oral contraceptives. Some people have an allergic reaction to a specific spermicide and should experiment with another brand. Some women cannot be fitted with a diaphragm or cervical cap because of the position of the uterus. The woman and her health care provider will then need to select another suitable means of contraception.

NOTE: There may be more than one method of birth control suitable for you. Study the methods suggested above and consult Table 15-1 to determine what techniques may be most appropriate.

Unwanted Pregnancy

A woman who is pregnant with an unwanted child faces a difficult decision. Available options for the pregnant woman include keeping the child, placing the child in foster care until it can be cared for by the mother or placed for adoption, placing the child for immediate adoption, or terminating the pregnancy. The decision between immediate adoption and terminating the pregnancy is, perhaps, the most difficult.

The decision to carry an unwanted pregnancy to term and then place the child for immediate adoption is appealing to many for two reasons: (1) it protects the life of the developing fetus, and (2) it provides a child for people who wish to adopt. Advocates of this choice would attempt to convince the pregnant woman that the short length of pregnancy, the low risk of delivery, the freedom from the guilt that may be associated with abortion, and the happiness of the adopting family outweigh the convenience of terminating the pregnancy.

In contrast to placing the child for adoption, women have the legal right to end an unwanted pregnancy—regardless of the reason. Once the decision to have an abortion is reached, women need only act within the time frame established by the Roe v. Wade decision. Advocates of this freedom of choice position remind women that they need not function as "baby factories" purely to meet the demands of the adoption market. Further, women who do not want to spend time being pregnant and face the risks of labor and delivery have the right to terminate the pregnancy. The integrity of the individual's body is the paramount concern.

Which position do you support? What is the basis of your choice?

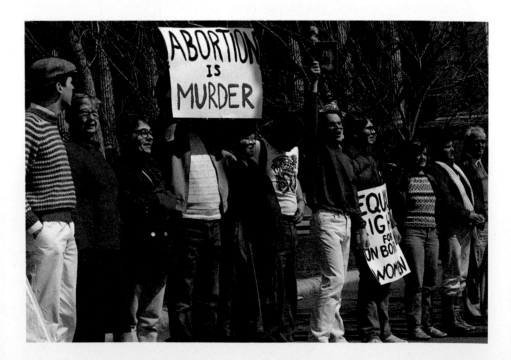

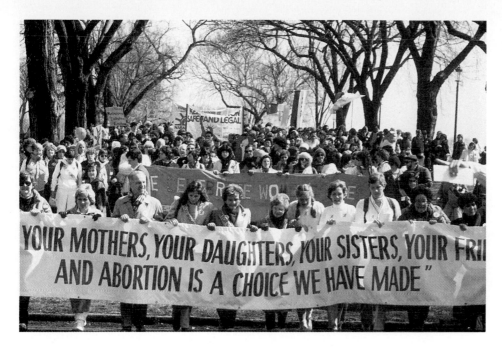

link in the fertility control chain has now been strengthened. On the basis of current technology and legality, women need never experience childbirth. The decision will be theirs to make.

We believe that **abortion** is not to be considered a first-line, preferred form of fertility control. Rather, abortion is a final, last-chance undertaking. It should be employed only when responsible control of one's fertility could not be achieved. The decision to abort a fetus is a highly controversial, personal one— one that needs serious consideration by each woman.

abortion
induced premature termination of a pregnancy.

On the basis of the landmark 1973 U.S. Supreme Court case *Roe v. Wade,* the United States joined many of the world's most populated countries in legalizing abortions within the following guidelines.

1 For the first 3 months of pregnancy (first trimester), the decision to abort lies with the woman and her doctor.
2 For the next 3 months of pregnancy (second trimester), state law may regulate the abortion procedure in ways that are reasonably related to maternal health.
3 For the last weeks of pregnancy (third trimester) when the fetus is judged capable of surviving if born, any state may regulate or even prohibit abortion except where abortion is necessary to preserve the life or health of the mother. If a pregnancy is terminated during the third trimester, a viable fetus would be considered a live birth and not be allowed to die.

Each year approximately 1,250,000 women make the decision to terminate a pregnancy in the United States.[14] Thousands of additional women probably consider abortion but elect to continue their pregnancies.

First trimester abortion procedures

Menstrual extraction Also referred to as menstrual regulation, menstrual induction, and preemptive abortion, menstrual extraction is a process carried out be-

First trimester abortion.

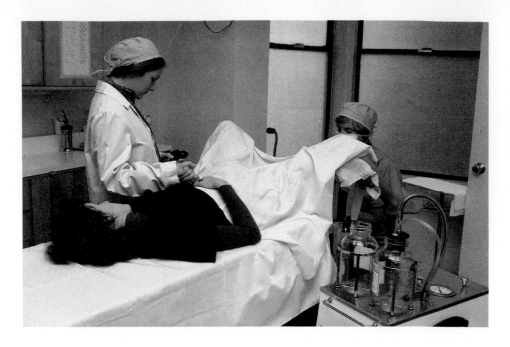

tween the fourth and sixth week after the last menstrual period (or in the days immediately after the first missed menstrual period). Generally performed in a physician's office under a local or *paracervical anesthetic,* a small plastic *cannula* is inserted through the undilated cervical canal into the cavity of the uterus. Once the cannula is in position, a small amount of suction is applied by a hand-held syringe. By rotating and moving the cannula across the uterine wall, the physician can withdraw the endometrial tissue.

When performed by an experienced clinician using the appropriate-sized cannula, menstrual extraction is a relatively safe procedure. Blood loss during aspiration of the endometrium is minimal, and a period comparable to a normal menstrual flow usually follows for the next few days. Although complications including cramping, spotting, infection, or retention of products of the conception are possible, chances of these are minimal.

Pregnancy tests are generally not done before performing the procedure, because menstrual extraction occurs so early in the gestational period. For some women, and perhaps for some clinicians, the necessity of not confirming a pregnancy may be a positive aspect of this procedure. Both will never really know if the woman was pregnant.

Vacuum aspiration Induced abortions undertaken during the sixth through ninth week of pregnancy are generally done through a procedure of *vacuum aspiration* of the uterine contents. Vacuum aspiration is a procedure similar in nature to menstrual extraction. Unlike menstrual extraction, however, vacuum aspiration may require **dilation** of the cervical canal and the use of a local anesthetic. In this more advanced stage of pregnancy, a larger cannula must be inserted into the uterine cavity. This process can be accomplished by using metal dilators of increasingly larger sizes to open the canal. After aspiration, the uterine wall may also be scraped to confirm complete removal of the uterine contents. Vacuum aspiration is the most commonly performed abortion procedure.

dilation
gradual expansion of an opening or passageway.

Dilation and curettage (D & C) When a pregnancy is to be terminated during the ninth through fourteenth weeks, vacuum aspiration gives way to a somewhat similar procedure labeled **dilation and curettage,** or more familiarly, D & C.

Like vacuum aspiration, the D & C involves the gradual enlargement of the cervical canal through the insertion of increasingly larger metal dilators. When the cervix has been dilated to a size sufficient to allow for the passage of a *curette,* the removal of the endometrial tissue can begin. Unlike the cannula, which attaches to a small mechanical pump, the currette is a metal instrument resembling a spoon, with a cup-shaped cutting surface on its end. As the curette is drawn across the uterine wall, the soft endometrial tissue and fetal parts are scraped from the wall of the uterus. (The D & C is also used in the medical management of certain health conditions of the uterine wall, such as irregular bleeding or the buildup of endometrial tissue.)

In both the vacuum aspiration and the D & C procedures, the tissues removed from the uterus are examined histologically to confirm the complete removal of the endometrium and fetal parts.

As in the case of menstrual extraction, both of these latter procedures are quite safe procedures for the woman. The need to dilate the cervix increases the risk of cervical trauma and the possibility of perforation, but these risks are low. Bleeding, cramping, spotting, and infections present minimal controllable risks when procedures are done by experienced clinicians under clinical conditions.

dilation and curettage (D & C)
surgical procedure in which the cervical canal is dilated to allow the uterine wall to be scraped.

Second trimester abortion procedures

When a woman's pregnancy continues beyond the fourteenth week of gestation, termination becomes a more difficult matter. The procedures at this stage become more complicated, take longer to be completed, and the complications become more common.

Dilation and evacuation Vacuum aspiration and D & C can be combined in a procedure called *dilation and evacuation (D & E)* during the earliest weeks of the second trimester (see Figure 15-7). The use of D & E increases the likeli-

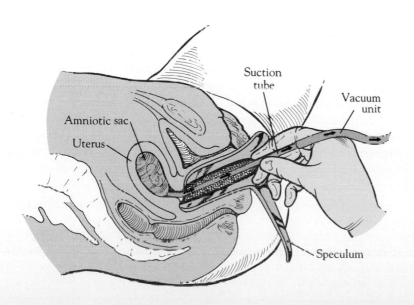

Suction tube

Vacuum unit

Amniotic sac

Uterus

Speculum

Figure 15-7
During dilation and evacuation the cervix is dilated and the contents of the uterus are aspirated out. This procedure is used to perform abortions up to 16 weeks of gestation.

hood of trauma and postprocedural complications. By the end of the six-teenth week this procedure will have reached the limits of its usefulness, and more intensive procedures will be required to terminate the late second trimester pregnancy.

Hypertonic saline procedure From the sixteenth week of gestation to the end of the second trimester, intrauterine injection of a strong salt solution into the amniotic sac is the procedure frequently used. The administration of intrauterine **hypertonic saline solution** requires a skilled operator so that the needle used to introduce the salt solution does in fact enter the amniotic sac. Once in place, amniotic fluid is withdrawn, allowing the saline solution to be injected.

hypertonic saline solution salt solution with a concentration higher than that found in human fluids.

In the place of the withdrawn amniotic fluid, 150 to 250 milliliters of a 20% to 25% saline solution is returned to the amniotic sac.[1] The saline solution is introduced slowly to avoid too much pressure, which might rupture the sac. Some physicians support the procedure by dilating the cervix with *laminaria* or another dilatory product and administering the hormone oxytocin to stimulate uterine contractions. The onset of uterine contractions will expel the dehydrated uterine contents with 24 to 36 hours.

Prostaglandin injection procedure *Prostaglandin intrauterine injections* are the second type of abortion procedure used during the second trimester. Prostaglandins are hormone-like chemicals that have a variety of useful effects on human tissue. Produced naturally within the body, these substances influence the contractility of smooth muscle. Since the uterine wall is composed entirely of smooth muscle, it is particulary sensitive to the presence of prostaglandins. When prostaglandin is administered in sufficient quantity, uterine contractions become strong enough to expel the fetal contents.

When prostaglandin is injected into the amniotic fluid, the result is an induced abortion. The procedure, like the saline method, involves the introduction of a needle into the amniotic sac. Synthetic prostaglandin is injected and within about a day, uterine contractions will begin expelling the fetus from the uterus. Delivery of a live fetus is a possibility and has been reported in the literature.[1] Prostaglandin can also be administered through a vaginal suppository.

Third trimester abortion procedures

Should termination of a pregnancy be required in the latter weeks of the gestational period, a surgical procedure in which the fetus will be removed (*hysterotomy*) or a procedure in which the entire uterus is removed (*hysterectomy*) can be undertaken. As one can imagine, these procedures are more complicated and involve longer hospitalization, major abdominal surgery, and an extended period of recovery. Because of the complete removal of the uterus, the hysterectomy not only terminates the pregnancy, it also ends the woman's fertility. The complicated nature and legal limitations of a third trimester abortion speaks strongly in favor of making a decision about an unwanted pregnancy as early as possible.

SUMMARY

The ability to manage one's reproductive system in a responsible manner is a significant challenge. Each person is responsible for numerous choices and the consequences of those choices. One of the initial decisions might involve the choice of a birth control or contraceptive method.

While evaluating the effectiveness of a birth control method, it is important to be aware of the difference between theoretical and use effectiveness rates. Theoretical effectiveness rates involve the perfect use of a method, while use effectiveness rates take into consideration human error. Other factors that should be considered when choosing a birth control method include safety, reliability, reversibility, affordability, ease of use, and whether or not it will interfere with sexual expression.

Birth control methods function by exerting control over the male and female reproductive systems. Four means of control are identified in this chapter: preventing the sperm from entering the female reproductive system, preventing the sperm from reaching an ovum, preventing the ovum from reaching the sperm, and disrupting a pregnancy. Many of the current methods of birth control have evolved through the centuries. An examination of these outdated methods helps put our current methods into a clearer perspective.

In this chapter the current methods of birth control were examined: how they work, their advantages, their disadvantages, and any contraindications for their use. The methods include withdrawal, fertility awareness techniques, vaginal spermicides, condoms, diaphragms, cervical caps, contraceptive sponges, intrauterine devices, and oral contraceptives. Sterilization was also presented as an option—one that requires additional consideration, since it is generally considered to be an irreversible procedure.

Abortion was also presented as a method of birth control. However, abortion was not suggested as one of the first-line preferred methods. Though abortion remains a woman's personal choice, it is still highly controversial and may be totally unacceptable to some persons. Should a woman make the decision to undergo an abortion, she needs to be aware that specific abortion procedures are done during each trimester of pregnancy. Abortions performed in the first trimester are those with the least risk to a woman's health.

REVIEW QUESTIONS

1 Explain the difference between the terms *birth control* and *contraception.* Give examples of each.

2 List several reasons why people choose to control their fertility.

3 Explain the difference between theoretical effectiveness rates and use effectiveness rates. Which one is usually higher? Why is it important to know the difference between these two rates?

4 Identify some of the factors that should be given careful consideration when selecting a contraceptive method. Explain each factor.

5 Identify and explain the four means of control that can be exerted over the male or female reproductive systems. For each means of control, give an example of a birth control method that uses that approach.

6 List some historical examples of birth control methods.

7 For each of the methods of birth control, explain the advantages, disadvantages, and contraindications for its use.

8 How do minipills differ from the combined oral contraceptive pill? What is a morning-after pill?

9 What general guidelines stemmed from the 1973 Supreme Court decision regarding abortion? What are the four alternatives a pregnant woman has regarding the outcome of her pregnancy?

10 Identify and describe the different abortion procedures that are used during each trimester of pregnancy. When is the safest time for an abortion?

QUESTIONS FOR PERSONAL CONTEMPLATION

1 Considering your lifestyle, which contraceptive method would be best for you? If you are sexually active, are you using this "best method"?

2 Assess each method of birth control in light of the religious beliefs you hold.

3 Do you think a couple who chooses not to use contraception should discuss what they will do if a pregnancy occurs? Why or why not?

4 If you were to become pregnant unexpectedly, how would you feel about your pregnancy? Which of the many options would you choose? Take some time to consider what effects a pregnancy would have on your current lifestyle and your future plans.

5 What are your own feelings about abortion? Consider the following questions:

a Should abortion be legal?

b Should the government help pay for abortions for those who are unable to afford them?

c Are there circumstances when you feel abortion is acceptable?

d Are there circumstances when you feel abortion is not acceptable?

REFERENCES

1 Hatcher, RA, et al: Contraceptive technology: 1986-1987, ed 13, New York, 1986, Irvington Publishers, Inc.

2 Havemann, E: Birth control, New York, 1967, Time Books, Inc.

3 Crooks, R, and Baur, K: Our sexuality, ed 3, Menlo Park, Calif, 1987, The Benjamin-Cummings Publishing Co.

4 Hyde, JS: Understanding human sexuality, ed 3, New York, 1986, McGraw-Hill Book Co.

5 Tucker, T: Birth control, New Canaan, Conn, 1975, Tobey Publishing Co, Inc.

6 Population Information Program: Youth in the 1980s: social and health concerns, Population Reports, Series M, no 9, Baltimore, 1985, The Johns Hopkins University.

7 Population Information Program: New developments in vaginal contraception, Population Reports, Series H, no 7, Baltimore, 1984, The Johns Hopkins University.

8 Rosenberg, M, et al: Effect of the contraceptive sponge on chlamydial infection, gonorrhea, and candidiasis, The Journal of the American Medical Association 257:2308-2312, 1987.

9 Centers for Disease Control: Toxic shock syndrome and the vaginal contraceptive sponge, Morbidity and Mortality Weekly Report 33:43-48, 1984.

10 Population Information Program: IUDs: an appropriate contraceptive for many women, Population Reports, Series B, no 4, Baltimore, 1982, The Johns Hopkins University.

11 Johnson, P, and Kates, A: Dalkon shield victims win in buy out plan, USA Today February 5, 1987, p 11a.

12 The Cancer and Steroid Hormone Study of the Centers for Disease Control and the National Institute of Child Health and Human Development: Combination oral contraceptive use and the risk of endometrial cancer, The Journal of the American Medical Association 257:796-800, 1987.

13 The Cancer and Steroid Hormone Study of the Centers for Disease Control and the National Institute of Child Health and Human Development: The reduction in risk of ovarian cancer associated with oral contraceptive use, The New England Journal of Medicine 316:650-655, 1987.

14 Painter, K: Abortions down for the first time since '69, USA Today August 24, 1987, p 1d.

ANNOTATED READINGS

Benderly, BL: Thinking about abortion, Garden City, NY, 1984, Dial Press, Doubleday & Co, Inc.

  Covers the emotional, moral, social, and medical aspects of abortion. The author, an award-winning science journalist, uses the case study approach to support her contention that women can recover from abortion experiences to be stronger and more resilient.

Chalker, R: The complete cervical cap guide, New York, 1987, Harper & Row Publishers, Inc.

  Traces the history, modern development, fitting, and use of the cervical cap. Indicates the effectiveness and advantages of this contraceptive device.

Gregersen, E: Sexual practices: the story of human sexuality, New York, 1983, Franklin Watts, Inc.

  Studies a wide range of sexual practices from a cross-cultural perspective. Information on historical methods of contraception is covered in detail. Heavily illustrated, this book views sexual practices from an anthropologist's perspective.

Hatcher, RA, et al: Contraceptive technology: 1986-1987, ed 13, New York, 1986, Irvington Publishers, Inc.

  Perhaps the most comprehensive guide to contraception, birth control, population and family planning, legal considerations, and sexually transmissible infections. Used as a primary reference by physicians, educators, and family planning clinics. Contributors include many staff members from The Centers for Disease Control (CDC).

Silber, S: How not to get pregnant, New York, 1987, Charles Scribner's Sons.

  A guide to the selection and use of various reliable forms of contraception, including natural family planning, sterilization, and the IUD. Background information on the structure and function of the reproductive system is provided.

CHAPTER 16

Sexuality
The Parent as Foundation for the Future

Key Concepts

Becoming pregnant and bearing and rearing children can have a significant impact on the lives of young adults.

Pregnancy is generally determined by testing for the hormone HCG and observing the characteristics of pregnancy.

All products that a pregnant woman consumes may affect fetal development.

The birth of a child involves three stages of labor.

One in six couples has a fertility problem.

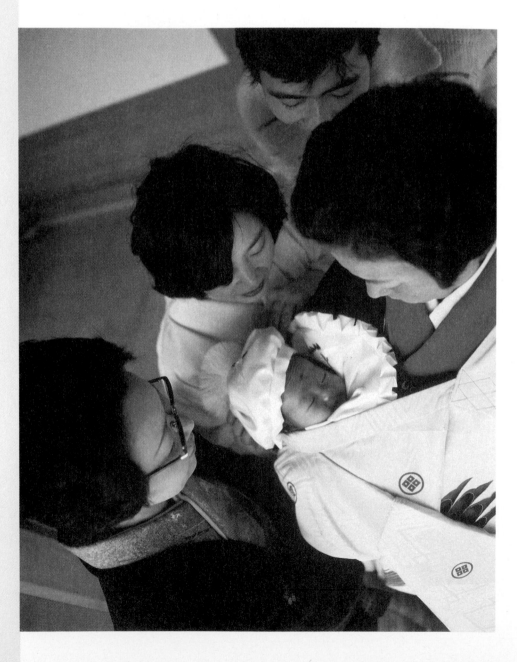

$\mathbf{Y}$ou may be surprised at the many diverse topics you will find in this chapter. Information ranges from parenthood, pregnancy, childbirth, and birth technology to infertility. The common thread throughout this chapter involves the choices you will make in terms of your reproductive sexuality.

Our students find these topics especially interesting. Most likely this is because the topics involve decisions nearly everyone must face. Many of our nontraditional students have already made parenting decisions. These students' experiences add insights that help our traditional students better see what lies ahead.

BASIC CONSIDERATIONS SHAPING PARENTHOOD

Within the last 2 or 3 decades, a major shift has taken place in the attitudes young adults have toward having children. These changed attitudes have been supported by actual changes in childbirth patterns. In the 1950s and early 1960s, marriage was the first in a series of predictable events that took place with nearly all recent college graduates. Within 2 years, couples routinely had their first of "3.2 children." Those who delayed having children until they were in their early thirties or couples who decided not to have children at all were clearly in the minority. Somehow, it just wasn't "right" not to have children. For a variety of reasons we will discuss, this attitude has softened. People are now waiting until a significantly later age to become parents, and an increasing number of couples have decided not to have children.

Why Have Children?

Perhaps before we examine some of the considerations that should be addressed by young adults as they consider parenthood, we should seek an answer to a more basic question: "Why do people wish to have children?" This question is especially meaningful because it is becoming increasingly clear that having children can be an exceedingly expensive proposition. Recent estimates indicate that its costs over $200,000 (in direct or indirect costs) to raise each child, in a middle-income family, from birth through college. Although children were real economic assets to parents when our society was more agrarian, children of today's parents must be seen as economic liabilities.

There must be other reasons why people wish to parent children. One comprehensive summary of the value that children have for parents has been presented by Thomas J. Espenshade,[1] who categorized eight reasons why parents have children:

1 *Adult status and social identity.* Having children is tangible evidence that one has reached adulthood, perhaps more so than completing school, taking a first job, or even getting married.

2 *Expansion of self, tie to a larger society, "immortality."* As a rule, children outlive their parents, and this may furnish parents with a sense of immortality, the realization that their characteristics, as reflected in their progeny, will survive after them.

3 *Morality.* This dimension refers to the subordination of self-interest to a higher goal. Children afford parents the opportunity to sacrifice for the good of someone else.

4 *Primary group ties, affiliation.* The family has historically been a stable and permanent institution, and affiliation with it may offer a sense of emotional security.

5 *Stimulation, novelty, fun.* A birth creates the sense that something new and different is happening, and in so doing may help to relieve the tedium of everyday life.

6 *Creativity, accomplishment, competence.* The challenges involved in raising children may fulfill these needs.

7 *Power, influence.* Having children enables parents to influence the course of others' lives.

8 *Social comparison, competition.* Where offspring are a sign of prestige or wealth, large numbers of children may elevate the parents' position in the community. They may also attest to the parents' sexuality. These motives are perhaps most commonly found in nonindustrialized societies.

You may be able to propose further reasons why some persons choose to have children. We would include such possibilities as the desire to (1) please your own parents, (2) extend a religious sect or follow the tenets of the church regarding procreation, (3) satisfy a couple's curiosity about what their child might be like, and (4) carry out a logical consequence of a loving relationship between the parents.

Additional Issues

Before deciding to have children, couples should have frank discussions about the impact that pregnancy and a newborn child will have on their lives. For those students contemplating single parenthood, we ask that you consider these issues as they relate to your particular situation and to excuse our consistent use of plural pronouns. In any event, some or all of the following basic considerations should be discussed:

- What impact will pregnancy have on us individually and collectively?
- Why do we want to have a child?
- What impact will a child have on the images we have constructed for ourselves as adults?
- Can we afford to have a child and provide for its needs?
- How will the responsibilities related to raising a child be divided?
- How will our professional careers be affected by the addition of a child?
- Are we ready now to accept the extended responsibilities that can come with a new child?
- How will we rear our child in terms of religious training, discipline, and participation in activities?
- Are we ready to part with much of the freedom associated with late adolescence and the early young adult years?
- How will we handle the possibility of being awakened by 6 AM each morning for the next couple of years?
- What plans have been made if we should discover that our baby (or fetus) is defective?
- Are we capable of handling the additional responsibilities associated with having a handicapped child?
- Are we comfortable with the thought of bringing another child into an already overcrowded, violent, bigoted, and polluted world?

If these questions seem strikingly negative in tone, there is indeed a reason for this. We believe that all too frequently the "nuts and bolts" issues related to childbearing and parenting are ignored, or at least are placed on the back burner. Although it is important for future parents to consider how cute and cuddly a new baby will be, how enhanced holidays will be with a new child, and how pleased the grandparents will be, we would consider that issues secondary to the major realities of having a child enter your lives.

Incidentally, many children are happily reared by parents who never considered all of the issues presented here. We are testimony to this fact. We are both in the process of rearing young children, and we honestly cannot say we analyzed the pros and cons of having children before we became parents. Perhaps we have been lucky. Our overall experiences of having and rearing children have been deeply rewarding, but the pathway has been rocky at times. Fortunately, sleepless nights, long waits in doctors' offices, slumber parties, cluttered houses, and depleted checkbooks are all forgotten when, after a long day, we get home to hear that daily roar: "Daddy's home!"

PREGNANCY: AN EXTENSION OF THE PARTNERSHIP

Pregnancy is a condition that requires a series of complex yet coordinated changes to occur in the female body. In this chapter pregnancy will be followed from its beginning with fertilization to its conclusion with labor of childbirth.

Personal Assessment

How Do You Feel About Parenting?

Respond to each of the following items based on your own opinions about parenting. Circle the letters that best match your response (see explanation of these abbreviations below). After completing this personal assessment, join three of your classmates in comparing and discussing your responses.

SA   Strong agree
A   Agree
U   Undecided
D   Disagree
SD   Strongly disagree

1 One cannot parent successfully without, at the same time, being a generally successful adult member of the community.	SA A U D SD	
2 It is inappropriate to view parenting as a method of achieving immortality.	SA A U D SD	
3 Parenting requires that one be willing to make major personal sacrifices for the benefit of the child.	SA A U D SD	
4 Parenting adds a large measure of vitality to an adult's life.	SA A U D SD	
5 Parenting demands greater creativity than any other adult pursuit.	SA A U D SD	
6 A person who cannot comfortably make decisions for others should not consider parenting.	SA A U D SD	
7 A family cannot exist in the absence of children.	SA A U D SD	

Physiological Obstacles and Aids to Fertilization

Many sexually active young people believe that they will only become pregnant (or impregnate someone) when they want to, despite their haphazard contraceptive practices. Because of this mistaken belief, many young people are not sold on the use of contraceptives. It is important for young adults to remember that from a species survival standpoint our bodies were designed to promote pregnancy. It is estimated that 90% of sexually active women of childbearing age will become pregnant within 1 year if they do not employ some form of contraception.[2]

With regard to pregnancy, each act of intercourse can be considered a game of physiological odds. There are obstacles that may reduce a couple's chance of pregnancy. The following is a list of some of these obstacles.

Obstacles to fertilization

1 *The acidic level of the vagina is destructive to sperm.* The low pH of the vagina will kill sperm that fail to enter the uterus quickly.
2 *The cervical mucus is thick during most of the menstrual cycle.* Sperm penetration is more difficult, except during the few days surrounding ovulation.
3 *The sperm must locate the cervical opening.* The cervical os is small in comparison to the rest of the surface area where sperm are deposited.
4 *Half of the sperm travel through the wrong fallopian tube.* Most commonly, only one ovum is released at ovulation. The two ovaries generally "take turns" each month. The sperm have no way of knowing which tube they should enter. Thus it is probable that half will travel through the wrong tube.
5 *The distance sperm must travel is relatively long compared to the tiny size of the sperm cells.* Microscopic sperm must travel about 7 or 8 inches once they are inside the female.
6 *The sperm's travel is relatively "upstream."* The anatomical positioning of the female reproductive structures necessitates an "uphill" movement by the sperm.
7 *The contoured folds of the tubal walls trap many sperm.* These folds make it difficult for sperm to locate the egg. Many sperm are trapped in this maze.

There are also a variety of aids that tend to help sperm and egg cells to join. Some of these are listed below.

Aids to fertilization

1 *An astounding number of sperm are deposited during ejaculation.* Each ejaculation contains about a teaspoon of semen. Within this quantity are between 200 and 500 million sperm cells. Even with large numbers of sperm killed in the vagina, millions are able to move to the deeper structures.
2 *Sperm are deposited near the cervical opening.* Penetration into the vagina by the penis allows for the sperm to be placed near the cervical os.
3 *The male accessory glands help make the semen nonacidic.* The seminal vesicles, prostate gland, and the Cowper's gland secrete fluids that provide an alkaline environment for the sperm. This environment helps the sperm be better protected in the vagina until they can manage to move into the deeper, more alkaline uterus and fallopian tubes.

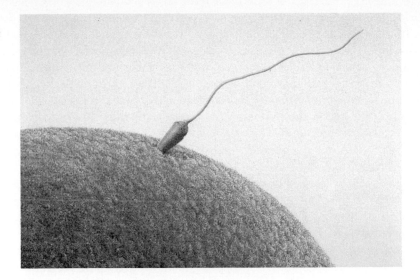

Ovum surrounded by sperm before fertilization.

4 *Uterine contractions aid sperm movement.* The rhythmic muscular contractions of the uterus tend to cause the sperm to move in the direction of the fallopian tubes.

5 *Sperm cells move rather quickly.* Despite their microscopic size, sperm cells can move relatively quickly—just under 1 inch an hour. Powered by sugar solutions from the male accessory glands and the whiplike movements of their tails, sperm can reach the distant third of the fallopian tubes in less than 8 hours as they swim in the direction of the descending ovum.

6 *Once inside the fallopian tubes, sperm can live for days.* Some sperm may be viable for up to a week after reaching the comfortable, nonacidic environment of the fallopian tubes. Most sperm, however, will survive an average of 48 to 72 hours. Thus they can "wait in the wings" for the moment an ovum is released from the ovary.

7 *The cervical mucus is thin and watery at the time of ovulation.* This mucus allows for better passage of sperm through the cervical opening when the ovum is most capable of being fertilized.

8 *Estrogen levels are at their highest point just before ovulation.* The term *estrogen* comes from the Greek word meaning "to make mad with desire." In lower female animals, high estrogen levels are associated with increased sex drive. In humans, however, this relationship is not as clear. Other psychosocial factors are probably more influential, yet from a biological and species survival standpoint, this phenomenon still remains plausible.

Pregnancy Determination

For centuries the only way to find out that a woman had become pregnant was to see if she stopped menstruating (because continued progesterone secretion helps keep the endometrial wall from deteriorating) and her abdomen began to enlarge. Within a couple of months, pregnancy could be determined rather reliably. Although this method would still work in this era, most couples want to find out more quickly.

Earlier in this century a newer way of determining pregnancy was routinely used. In this pregnancy test, urine from the woman was injected into laboratory animals, most often rabbits, mice, or frogs. If the woman was pregnant, the hormone *human chorionic gonadotropin (HCG)* in her urine would stimulate ovulation in female animals and stimulate ejaculation in male animals. Of course, the female animals had to be sacrificed and analyzed for ovluation. (Thus the phrase "the rabbit died" was coined to indicate that this test determined that a woman was pregnant.) Positive readings were only possible if the woman had been pregnant for 2 to 4 weeks and thereby had developed sufficiently high levels of HCG.[3]

HCG is initially released in large quantities by embryonic cells that later form the fetal part of the placenta. For the first 6 weeks of pregnancy, HCG's primary function is to maintain the corpus luteum's continued release of estrogen and progesterone. After the first 2 months, estrogen and progesterone are produced mainly by the placenta.[4]

immunoassay pregnancy test
pregnancy test that uses an antigen-antibody response to determine the presence of HCG in a urine sample.

A quicker, more accurate test is now available to determine pregnancy. This test, called the **immunoassay pregnancy test,** also determines whether HCG is present in a woman's urine. If the woman is pregnant, the embryo's HCG will combine with the anti-HCG antibody to form a brown ring. This takes about 2 hours to complete and is not 100% accurate. *False positive* readings occur in 3% of the tests, and *false negatives* are found in about 20% of the tests. It is thought that false negative readings result when the test is conducted within the first week after fertilization has occurred—too early for HCG to be circulating in amounts large enough to spill over into the urine. Various kinds of immunoassay pregnancy test kits can be purchased in drug stores and supermarkets in most communities. The box on p. 463 describes home pregnancy tests.

radioreceptor assay test
pregnancy test that uses a radioactive substance to determine the presence of HCG in a serum sample.

Most physicians and family clinics prefer to look for HCG through tests that analyze the blood rather than urine. These **radioreceptor assay tests** have higher degrees of accuracy than immunoassay tests. A newly developed pregnancy test for use by physicians employs *monoclonal antibodies* to detect HCG in a urine sample as quickly and accurately as the radioreceptor assay test.

The fetus at 14 weeks gestation within the amniotic sac.

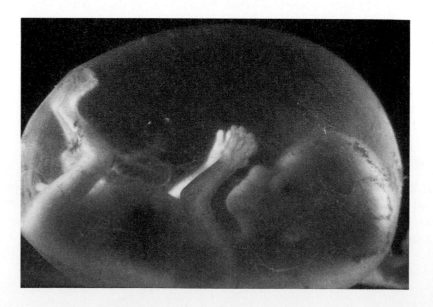

Home Pregnancy Tests

Home pregnancy tests have been available for several years. Using technology similar to that used by many laboratory-based pregnancy tests, home pregnancy tests give an accurate result in the privacy of the home, and are less costly than tests by physicians.

Home pregnancy tests identify the presence of HCG (human chorionic gonadotropin) in the urine of the pregnant woman. This hormone is produced by an implanted zygote to maintain ovarian support of the uterine wall through continuation of progesterone production. The presence of HCG in the urine is a highly reliable indicator of pregnancy. Home pregnancy tests have accuracy rates at or near 98%. Of course, a visit to a physician and subsequent prenatal care are important follow-up procedures.

Signs of Pregnancy

Aside from pregnancy tests done in a laboratory, a woman can sometimes recognize early signs and symptoms. The signs of pregnancy have been divided into three categories.[3]

Presumptive signs of pregnancy

Missed period after coitus the previous month
Nausea upon awakening (morning sickness)
Increase in size and tenderness of breasts
Darkening of the areolar tissue surrounding the nipples

Probable signs of pregnancy

Increase in the frequency of urination (the growing uterus presses against the bladder)
Increase in the size of the abdomen
Cervix becomes softer by the sixth week (detected by a pelvic exam by clinician)
Positive pregnancy test

Positive signs of pregnancy

Determination of a fetal heartbeat
Feeling of the fetus moving (quickening)
Observation of fetus by ultrasound or optical viewers

Fetal Life

After fertilization occurs, 5 to 8 days will pass before the cell mass implants into the endometrium of the uterus. Before entering the uterus, the cell mass is called a *morula* (Latin for "mulberry") (see Figure 16-1). Once it enters the uterus, the developing embryo is called a *blastocyst*. The blastocyst will implant 1 or 2 days after entering the uterus. After implantation, the cell mass is called an *embryo*. The embryonic stage lasts for 8 weeks before giving way to the **fetal stage**. Protected in its amniotic sac, the developing fetus is intimately connected to the

The Well-Managed Pregnancy

- Determine the time of ovulation and the time intercourse
- Assume that conception has occurred
- Avoid x-rays, unnecessary drugs, and exposure to infectious persons
- Eat wholesome foods from the basic food groups
- See your doctor as directed
- Exercise as prescribed
- Maintain approximate weight

fetal stage
stage of human development from the end of the eighth week of gestation until the time of birth.

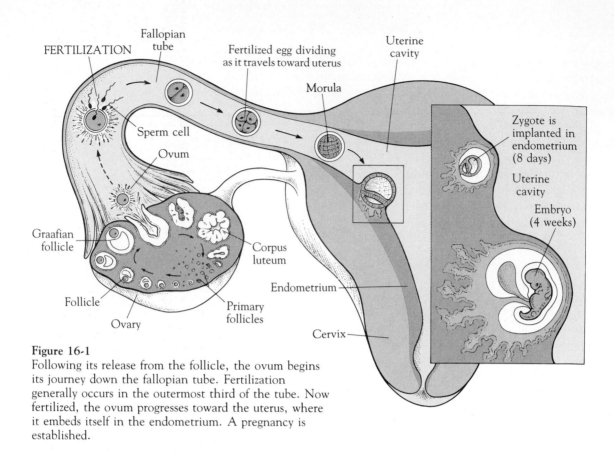

Figure 16-1
Following its release from the follicle, the ovum begins its journey down the fallopian tube. Fertilization generally occurs in the outermost third of the tube. Now fertilized, the ovum progresses toward the uterus, where it embeds itself in the endometrium. A pregnancy is established.

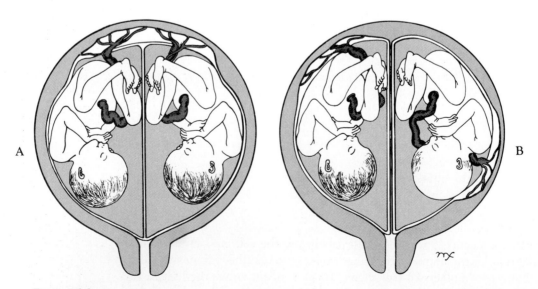

Figure 16-2
A, Identical twins.
B, Fraternal twins. Note differences in construction of amniotic sacs.

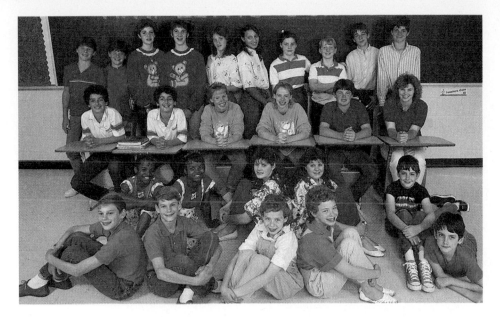

Can you identify which twins are identical and which are fraternal?

mother by the *placenta*. The placenta is the organ of exchange between the mother and her fetus. Through the placenta, the fetus receives oxygen and nourishment from the mother's bloodstream and disposes of carbon dioxide and other waste products. These exchanges take place through a *diffusion process* in the placenta, and the fetal and maternal blood never mix.

Multiple Births

The majority of pregnancies are single; however, some pregnancies lead to multiple births. The most common multiple birth is twins. On rare occasions, however, the birth of three, four, five, or more infants occurs. The use of fertility drugs has increased the occurrence of multiple births.

In one out of every 88 pregnancies, two babies will develop.[5] These twin-multiple births are of two types, depending on the numer of ova that have been fertilized.

Identical twins (monozygotic) result when only one ovum is fertilized but divides into two zygotes early in its development (see Figure 16-2, A). Identical twins possess the same genetic background and share the same placenta. These twins are always, of course, of the same sex.

Fraternal twins (dizygotic) result when two separate ova are fertilized by different sperm (see Figure 16-2, B). Fraternal twins can be of the same sex or opposite sex and are only slightly more similar in appearance than any two other siblings.[5] Each fetus has its own placenta.

In all multiple pregnancies, the developing infants must compete for space and, to some degree, share nutrients. As a result the incidence of prematurity is higher than in single pregnancies.[5] Prematurity is higher for identical twins than for fraternal twins, perhaps because of the need to share a single placenta.

In other types of multiple pregnancies, the likelihood of premature delivery is greater than that of pregnancies resulting in twins. In multiple pregnancies involving five infants (quintuplets) or more, the infant mortality rate is extremely high.

Natural Occurrence of Multiple Births

Twins	1 in 90
Triplets	1 in 9,000
Quadruplets	1 in 900,000
Quintuplets	1 in 85,000,000

Warning: Acne, Accutane, and Birth Defects

Accutane, manufactured by Roche Laboratories, may be the most effective prescription drug for severe cystic acne, a type of acne that often causes deep scarring. In the Spring of 1988, the FDA reissued an earlier warning that pregnant women should not use this drug since it is capable of causing severe birth defects such as brain, skull, facial, and cardiac abnormalities.[6] Women who use Accutane and are planning a pregnancy are encouraged to stop using the drug for two menstrual cycles before becoming pregnant. This gives the body time to clear Accutane from its system before conception. Some physicians recommend that women take a pregnancy test before beginning use of Accutane because of its severe affects on fetuses.

Agents That Can Damage a Fetus

A large number of agents that come into contact with a pregnant woman can affect fetal development. Many of these (rubella and herpes viruses, tobacco smoke, alcohol, and virtually all other drugs) have been discussed in other chapters of this text. The best advice for a pregnant woman is to maintain close contact with her obstetrician during pregnancy and to consider carefully the ingestion of any over-the-counter drug (including aspirin, caffeine, and antacids) that could adversely harm the fetus.

It is also important for any woman to avoid exposure to radiation during the pregnancy. Such exposure, most commonly through x-rays or radiation fallout from nuclear testing, can irreversibly damage fetal genetic structures. Epidemiological studies have shown that birth defects in the children of women exposed to radiation fallout are significantly higher than in the children of unexposed pregnant women.[3] Pregnant women are advised to avoid unnecessary x-ray exposure during pregnancy.

CHILDBIRTH: THE LABOR OF DELIVERY

Determination of the Due Date

The day at which a pregnancy will come to term is called the *due date*. Nine months, 40 weeks, or 280 days is the average length of a human pregnancy. With this in mind, the due date can be calculated in a simple fashion by adding 7 days to the first day of the last menstrual period and then counting back 3 months. For example, let us say that you think you are pregnant and the first day of your last period was September 1. Adding 7 days to this will result in September 8. By counting back three months from September 8, you can determine a due date of June 8. There is about a 50/50 chance that the actual birth will occur within 1 week of this calculated date.

Interestingly, female babies tend to be born a few days earlier than male babies. Women who exercise regularly also tend to deliver earlier than women who do not exercise, and women who have short menstrual cycles also tend to have shorter pregnancies.[3]

Parturition

Childbirth, or *parturition*, is one of the true peak experiences for both men and women. Most of the time childbirth is a wonderfully exciting venture into the unknown. For the parents, this intriguing experience can provide a stage for personal growth, maturity, and insight into a dynamic, complex world.

During the last few weeks of the third **trimester,** most fetuses will move deeper into the pelvic cavity in a process called *lightening*. During this movement, the fetus's body will rotate and the head will begin to engage more deeply into the mother's pelvic girdle. Many women will report that their babies have "dropped."

Another indication that parturition may be relatively near is the increased reporting of *Braxton-Hicks contractions*. These uterine contractions, which are of mild intensity and often occur at irregular intervals, may be felt throughout a pregnancy. During the last few weeks of pregnancy (*gestation*), these mild contractions can occur more frequently and cause a woman to feel as if she were going into labor **(false labor).**

Labor begins when uterine contractions become more intense and occur at regular intervals. The birth of a child can be divided into three stages: (1) *effacement* and dilation of the cervix, (2) expulsion of the fetus, and (3) expulsion of the placenta (see Figure 16-3). For a woman having her first child, the birth process lasts an average of 12 to 16 hours. The average length of labor for subsequent children is significantly shorter—from 4 to 10 hours on the average. Labor is very unpredictable: labors that last between 1 and 24 hours occur daily at most hospitals.

Stage one: effacement and dilation of the cervix

In the first stage of labor, the uterine contractions attempt to thin (*efface*) the normally thick cervical walls and to enlarge (*dilate*) the cervical opening. These contractions are directed by the release of *prostaglandins* and the hormone *oxytocin* into the circulating bloodstream. In women delivering first babies, effacement will occur before dilation. In subsequent deliveries, effacement and dilation usually occur at the same time.

The first stage of labor is often the longest of the three stages. The cervical opening must thin and dilate to a diameter of 10 centimeters before the first stage of labor is considered complete.[7] Often this stage begins with the dislodging of the cervical mucous plug. The subsequent *bloody show* (mucous plug and a small amount of blood) at the vaginal opening may indicate that effacement and dilation have begun. Another indication of labor's onset may be the bursting or tearing of the fetal amniotic sac. "Breaking the bag of waters" is a reference to this phenomenon, which happens in various measures in expectant women. Some amniotic sacs burst with a large gush of clear amniotic fluid; some merely have a slight tear that trickles a small amount of fluid. Some women may even continue through the delivery of the baby before the sac is torn by the attending clinician or physician.

trimester
three-month period of time; human pregnancies encompass three trimesters.

false labor
conditions that tend to resemble the start of true labor; may include irregular uterine contractions, pressure, and discomfort in the lower abdomen.

Figure 16-3
Labor, or childbirth, is a three-stage process. During effacement and dilation, the first stage, the cervical canal is gradually opened by contractions of the uterine wall. The second stage, birth of the baby, encompasses the actual expulsion of the baby from the uterus and through the birth canal. The expulsion of the placenta, the third stage, empties the uterus, thus completing the process of childbirth.

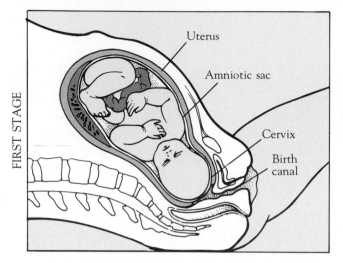

FIRST STAGE

Uterus

Amniotic sac

Cervix

Birth canal

Uterine contractions thin the cervix and enlarge the cervical opening

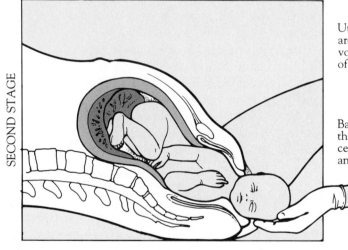

SECOND STAGE

Uterine contractions are aided by mother's voluntary contractions of abdominal muscles

Baby moves through dilated cervical opening and birth canal

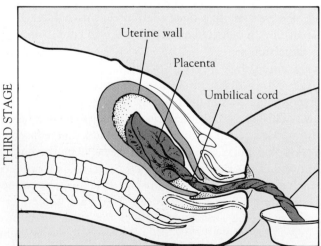

THIRD STAGE

Uterine wall

Placenta

Umbilical cord

Placenta detaches from uterine wall and is delivered through the vagina

The pain of the uterine contractions becomes more intense as the woman moves through this first stage of labor. As the cervical opening effaces and dilates from 0 to 3 centimeters, many women report feeling happy, exhilarated, and confident. In the early phase of the first stage of labor, the contractions are relatively short (lasting from 15 to 60 seconds) and the intervals between contractions range from 20 minutes to 5 minutes as labor progresses. However, these rest intervals will become shorter and the contractions more forceful when the woman's uterus contracts to dilate 4 to 7 centimeters.

In this second phase of the first stage of labor, the contractions usually last about 1 minute each, and the rest intervals drop from about 5 minutes to 1 minute over a period of 5 to 9 hours.

The third phase of the first stage of labor is called *transition*. During transition the uterus contracts to dilate the cervical opening to the full 10 centimeters required for safe passage of the fetus out of the uterus and into the vagina (birth canal). This period of labor is often the most painful part of the entire birth process. Fortunately, it is also the shortest phase of most labors. Lasting between 15 and 30 minutes, transition contractions often last 60 to 90 seconds each. The rest intervals between contractions are short and vary from 30 to 60 seconds.

An examination of the cervix by a nurse or physician will reveal whether full dilation of 10 centimeters has occurred. Until the full 10-centimeter dilation, women are cautioned not to "push" the fetus during the contractions (see Figure 16-4). Special breathing and concentration techniques help many women cope with the first stage of labor.

Stage two: expulsion of the fetus

Once the mother's cervix is fully dilated, she enters the second stage of labor, the expulsion of the fetus through the birth canal. Now the mother is encouraged to help push the baby out (with her abdominal muscles) during each contraction. In this second stage, the uterine contractions are less forceful than during the transition phase of the first stage of labor, and may last 60 seconds each with a 1- to 3-minute rest interval.

This second stage may last up to 2 hours in first births.[7] For subsequent babies, this stage will usually be much shorter. When the baby's head is first seen at the vaginal opening, *crowning* is said to have taken place. Generally the back of the baby's head appears first. (Infants whose feet or buttocks are presented first are said to be delivered in a *breech position*). Once the head is delivered, the baby's body rotates upward to let the shoulders come through. The rest of the body follows quite quickly. The second stage of labor ends when the fetus is fully expelled from the vagina.

Newly delivered babies often look far different from the babies seen on television commercials. Their heads are often cone-shaped as a result of the compression of cranial bones that occurs during the delivery of the baby through the birth canal. Within a few days following birth, the newborn's head will assume a much more normal shape. Most babies (of all races) appear bluish at first, until they begin regular breathing. All babies are covered with a coating of *vernix*, a white, cheeselike substance that protects the skin.

Stage three: expulsion of the placenta

Usually within 30 minutes after the fetus is delivered, the uterus will again initiate a series of contractions to expel the placenta (or *afterbirth*). The placenta

Figure 16-4
Cervical dilation during the three stages of labor.

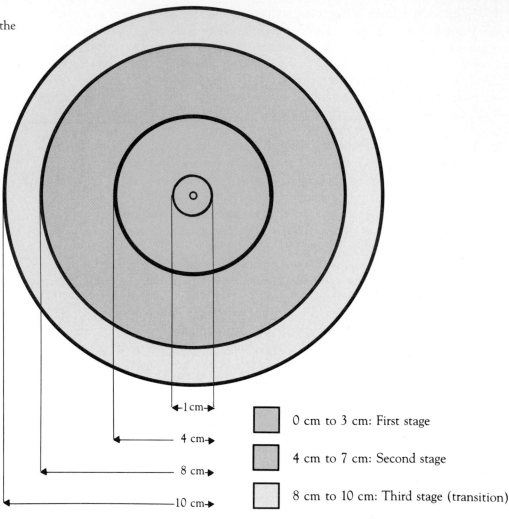

←1 cm→

4 cm→

8 cm→

10 cm→

0 cm to 3 cm: First stage

4 cm to 7 cm: Second stage

8 cm to 10 cm: Third stage (transition)

is examined by the attending physician to ensure that it was completely expelled. Torn remnants of the placenta could lead to dangerous *hemorrhaging* by the mother. Often the physician will perform a manual examination of the uterus after the placenta has been delivered.

Once the placenta has been expelled, the uterus will continue with mild contractions to help control bleeding and start the gradual reduction of the uterus to its normal, nonpregnant size. This final aspect of the birth process is called **postpartum.** External abdominal massage of the lower abdomen seems to help the uterus contract, as does an infant's nursing at the mother's breast.

postpartum
period of time after the birth of a baby during which the uterus returns to its prepregnancy size.

ADDITIONAL CONSIDERATIONS CONCERNING CHILDBIRTH

Medications

Despite the large movement toward prepared childbirth or natural childbirth methods of delivery, most women still receive some kind of medication during labor. The type of drug depends on the particular birth situation, physical preference, and pain tolerance of the mother. Since the use of any drug by the mother can potentially damage the fetus, the physician and mother need to discuss the use of any medications before the time of delivery.

Analgesics are drugs that are administered to reduce the mother's pain during labor. Analgesics are sometimes used with mild tranquilizers to reduce pain and encourage relaxation of the mother. *Anesthetics* are drugs that block off all sensations. *General anesthetics,* in the form of inhaled gases, were formerly used during the last 10 minutes or so of the second stage of labor. However, since it is now recognized that general anesthetics can damage a fetus and also do not allow the mother to participate actively in the final part of her delivery, general anesthetics are less commonly used now, except in some cesarean deliveries.

Most anesthetics used today are regional or local anesthetics. *Regional anes-thetics* are injected at specific points (near the spinal cord) and block off sensations in the body below the injection site. Some regional anesthetics can be injected that will allow a mother to use her muscles to assist in her delivery; other regional anesthetics prevent this.[3] *Local anesthetics* are for smaller areas and help block sensations as the baby moves through the birth canal. Procaine (Novocain) is often injected near the vaginal opening if an *episiotomy* has taken place. An episiotomy is an optional surgical procedure that enlarges the vaginal opening. Novocain permits the painless suturing of the episiotomy incision.

Cesarean Deliveries

Cesearean deliveries (cesarean sections, C-sections) now account for nearly 30% of all deliveries in the United States.[8] A cesarean delivery is a procedure in which the baby is surgically removed from the mother's uterus through the abdominal wall. Lasting up to 1 hour for the complete procedure, this type of delivery can be performed with the mother having a regional anesthetic or a general anesthetic. The dramatic increase in the use of cesarean deliveries is

cesarean delivery
surgical removal of a fetus through the abdominal wall.

A cesarean delivery.

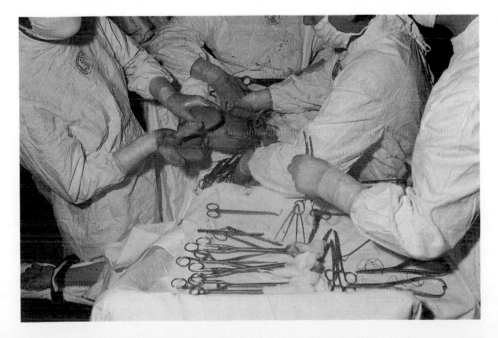

questioned by some medical experts, although others point to the need for this kind of delivery when one or more of the following factors are present[3]:

- The fetus is improperly aligned.
- The pelvis of the mother is too small.
- The fetus is especially large.
- The fetus shows signs of respiratory or cardiac distress.
- The umbilical cord is compressed.
- The placenta is being delivered before the fetus.

Although a cesarean delivery is considered major surgery, most mothers cope well with the delivery and postsurgical and postpartum discomfort. The hospital stay is usually a few days longer than for a vaginal delivery. The mother can still nurse her child and may still be able to have vaginal deliveries with later children. More and more hospitals these days are allowing the father to be in the operating room during cesarean deliveries. Fortunately, research indicates that early **bonding** between child, mother, and father can still occur in cesarean deliveries.

bonding
important, initial sense of recognition established between the newborn and those adults on whom the newborn will be dependent.

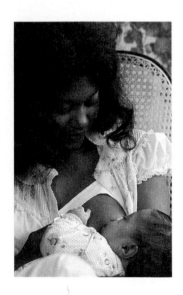

Breastfeeding

For a variety of reasons, mothers of newborns are being encouraged to breastfeed (nurse) their babies. The baby's nursing stimulates the release of the hormone oxytocin from the mother's pituitary gland. Oxytocin encourages the uterus to contract shortly after birth, but it also stimulates cells in the *mammary glands* of the breasts to release milk. This process is called *lactation*. Initially the child's sucking actions produce a watery clear fluid called *colostrum*, which is followed by milk in a couple of days.

Nursing has the advantage of providing a convenient, inexpensive, nutritionally complete diet for the infant. Furthermore, nursing provides the infant with an abundance of maternal antibodies that help fight infant infections and minimize allergic reactions—especially those of the digestive tract. Another advantage of breastfeeding is that it can provide a very close bonding experience between mother and child. Research indicates that women who nurse return more quickly to sexual activity than those who bottle-feed.[5]

Possible disadvantages of breastfeeding include the passage of toxic substances to the infant (drugs, nicotine, alcohol) that are ingested by the mother, lack of freedom for the mother, discomfort caused by engorged breasts and sensitive nipples, and reduced time spent with the baby by the father. Contrary to popular belief, breastfeeding is not an effective form of contraception. Clearly, whether to nurse or to bottle feed a baby depends on a host of factors that should be considered. Fortunately, most typical babies turn out to be healthy and happy regardless of how they were fed as infants. The choice is up to the parents.

Preparation for Birth

In the past expectant mothers (and fathers) were somewhat restricted in their attempts to play a major role throughout the pregnancy and delivery of their child. As long as the physician's prenatal examinations were normal, little information was given to the parents. Fathers were rarely seen in an obstetrician's office. Women were frequently told, "Everything is fine," and were instructed to come to the hospital as soon as they thought they were going into labor. At the hospital men sat anxiously in smoke-filled waiting rooms while their wives agonized through labor and then, often heavily sedated, delivered babies in sterile, impersonal surgical rooms. Indeed, the birthing process was perceived to be a painful, dreaded experience by many of its participants, except perhaps for the newborns, whose feelings could only be estimated.

Much of this picture has now changed, thanks largely to the pioneer efforts of three people. In the early 1930s, Dr. Grantly Dick-Read developed the concept that the fear of pain, and not the pain itself, was largely responsible for the discomfort and unpleasantness of childbirth. He believed that if expectant mothers were psychologically and physically prepared for childbirth and had a firm understanding of the biological events that would take place, they could actually enjoy the birthing experience, often without the use of drugs. Furthermore, Dick-Read developed a series of muscle-tension relaxation exercises that could help women during labor. Dick-Read was the first advocate for the value of fathers being present in the delivery room.[9]

The second widely known advocate of *prepared childbirth* (or natural, cooperative childbirth) was Dr. Fernand Lamaze. This French physician extended Dick-Read's muscle relaxation training to include techniques of breathing control, mental concentration, and proper birthing posture. Lamaze was a firm proponent of the role of the father in assisting the birth process.

Today expectant parents can elect to attend prepared childbirth classes during the last few months of their pregnancies. At these classes, parents can learn not only about the biological events relating to childbirth, but also about appropriate techniques, exercises, and positions that will help to reduce the fear and therefore the pain surrounding childbirth. These classes often include lectures, discussions, films, demonstrations, and visits to hospital obstetrical units. Typically, a small fee is charged for prepared childbirth classes.

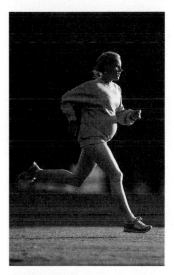

Keeping fit during pregnancy.

Most parents who deliver their children with this kind of training are overwhelmingly satisfied, even if their particular labor necessitated the use of medications or even an eventual cesarean section. The father's role appears to help establish an early bond between the *neonate* (newborn baby) and its father. Frequently the parents report their own relationship is strengthened as a result of a cooperative type of delivery.

The third contributor to changing attitudes toward childbirth is Dr. Frederick Leboyer. In his book *Birth Without Violence*, Leboyer advocated an alternate method of handling the newborn immediately after delivery.[10] Leboyer felt that most hospital delivery rooms were too noisy, too brightly lit, and excessively cold. He believed that these conditions were not very conducive to a smooth transition of the baby from its warm, wet, quiet, dark fetal home to the outside world. Leboyer advocated a much quieter, warmer delivery room—a place that was more dimly lit. He discouraged slapping the baby's bottom and immediately wrapping the baby and transferring it to the nursery or evaluation room. Leboyer preferred the practice of placing the baby (often by the father) in a warm water bath for at least a few minutes and then placing the baby in direct physical contact with the mother. Some hospitals and obstetricians permit (and encourage) the use of Leboyer techniques. Many parents report that newborn babies exposed to Leboyer techniques seldom cry after birth and appear to be calm and alert to both the father and mother.

birthing rooms
hospital facilities that serve as both a labor and a delivery room.

Another trend with regard to childbirth is the use of **birthing rooms** in many hospitals. For many years, pregnant women progressed through the lengthy first stage of labor in *labor rooms* and were then transferred to surgically equipped *delivery rooms* for the second and third stages of labor. These transfers generally were seen as an uncomfortable break in the continuity of the birth experience. Birthing rooms allow women in labor to go through the entire labor and delivery in one room. Typically birthing rooms are decorated in a homelike way, with pictures, televisions, wall hangings, carpets, and lounge chairs present in the room. Depending on hospital policy, fathers, and sometimes whole families, can be present in birthing rooms.

In many birthing rooms, women can complete the entire delivery in either a comfortable bed or in a modified surgical table called a *birthing chair*. This chair resembles a bed and can be modified to accommodate a variety of comfortable birthing positions.

Some hospitals permit mothers (and even families) to "room in" with newborn babies after they are delivered. Usually neonates are allowed to visit with their mothers and fathers only during limited hours. *Rooming in* allows unlimited (or near unlimited) visitation with newborns.

Although the practice is not generally accepted by the medical community, some parents choose to deliver their children in their own homes. This practice may be leveling off in popularity, primarily because of the recognized medical risks to the fetus and mother. In addition, most hospitals now permit many of the new birthing practices that are desired by many couples.

Birthing centers reflect yet another new trend in the management of pregnancy and birth. A birthing center is a nonhospital, homelike setting where pregnant women can opt for prenatal care, delivery, and postdelivery recovery. In 1987 about 200 of these centers were scattered around the United States. Many more were in the planning stage.[11]

registered nurse midwives
registered nurses (RNs) who have completed postgraduate education in the area of prenatal care and childbirthing and are licensed or certified to practice midwifery.

Birthing centers are staffed by a team of **registered nurse midwives** and birthing assistants **(lay midwives).** Generally located near fully equipped hospitals in case a medical emergency should arise, birthing centers accept only healthy, low-risk mothers as patients. Deliveries are made without the use of drugs, fetal monitors, forceps, or surgical procedures. Families are encouraged to be present during childbirth, and the short postpartum stay for mother and child is often a day or less.

lay midwives
persons who have received specialized training in midwifery but who do not possess the academic credentials of registered nurse midwives.

However, there is controversy in the medical community about birthing centers. Physicians and hospital professional associations are on record as opposing the concept of birthing centers because of maternal and fetal risk. They cite the high percentage of women who need to be transferred from birthing centers to regular hospitals because of medical complications during labor and delivery. Supporters of birthing centers counter by pointing to a high safety record and the significantly lower cost of the nonphysician, nonhospital prenatal care, and delivery.[11] Many states require birthing centers to be licensed.

BIRTH TECHNOLOGY

Technological advances continue to occur in the field of *obstetrics*. Not only have new procedures been developed, but also some common procedures have been modified. Included among these are:

- *Ultrasound.* Although ultrasound procedures have been around for years, a more restrictive set of guidelines now exists. No longer are ultrasound examinations being used simply to determine the sex of a child or to take a picture of the developing fetus. Now ultrasound is used primarily to determine the position and age of the fetus. This procedure is called for in about 30% of all pregnancies.

- *Pregnancy tests.* Pregnancy tests with greater sensitivity continue to be developed. The most recent type of serum pregnancy test (trade name Nimbus) allows a determination of pregnancy to be made within a week following conception. A near 100% accuracy has been reported.

- *Amniocentesis.* The human fetus develops within a fluid filled amniotic sac. Over the course of the pregnancy, cells and urine from the developing fetus accumulate within this fluid. Amniocentesis is a procedure in which a small quantity of amniotic fluid is drawn from the amniotic sac through a needle. The fluid is then analyzed for genetic abnormalities. The procedure is generally done around the sixteenth week of the pregnancy. The results obtained by amniocentesis can help those involved make decisions about pregnancy termination or medical care of the fetus.

- *Chorionic villi sampling (CVS).* One of the most important new technologies in the practice of obstetrics is an amniocentesis-like procedure known as chorionic villi sampling. CVS permits the microscopic examination of cells of the *chorionic villi* derived from the fetus. Chromosomes can be removed from these cells to be examined for genetic defects. Unlike amniocentesis (which cannot be done until the sixteenth week of pregnancy), CVS can be undertaken as early as the fifth week. If serious defects are found, a more simple pregnancy termination is possible.

- *Amniotic fluid level assessment.* It is now known that many fetuses who are developing abnormally produce less amniotic fluid than do normally developing fetuses. Ultrasound assessment of amniotic fluid levels allows for earlier intervention by the physician.

- *Fetal monitors.* Monitoring of fetal heart rate during labor is now considered less necessary than in the past, particularly when a low-risk delivery is anticipated; however, fetal monitoring is standard practice in some hospitals for all labors. It is now recognized that virtually all fetuses demonstrate frequent changes in heart rate during labor. In pregnancies that are progressing normally, these alterations do not always indicate the need for cesarean deliveries.[12]

- *Gender selection kits.* Although considered unreliable by many physicians, kits containing instructions and supplies for enhancing the likelihood of conceiving a male or female are again on the market. Based on a theory first appearing in the early 1970s, a new generation of parents can now study how the timing of intercourse, depth of penetration, and the presence or absence of female orgasm may help provide babies of a preferred sex.

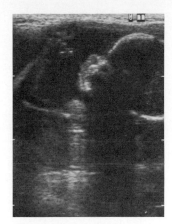

Ultrasound picture.

Infertility

Most traditional-age college students are interested in pregnancy prevention. However, increasing numbers of other persons are trying to do just the opposite: they are trying to become pregnant. It is estimated that about one in six couples has a problem with *infertility*. These couples wish to become pregnant but are unsuccessful. Medical experts indicate that between 1965 and 1982 infertility has doubled among couples of childbearing age.[13]

Why are couples infertile? The reasons are about evenly balanced between males and females. About 10% of infertility cases have no detectable cause. The major male complication is insufficient sperm production and delivery.[14] A number of approaches can be used to increase sperm counts. Among the simple approaches are the application of periodic cold packs on the scrotum and the replacement of tight underwear with boxer shorts. When a structural problem reduces sperm production, surgery can be helpful. Opinion is divided concerning whether increased frequency of intercourse improves fertility. Most experts (fertility endocrinologists) do suggest that couples have intercourse at least a couple of times in the week preceding ovulation.[14]

Males can also collect (through masturbation) and save samples of their own sperm to use in a procedure called *artificial insemination by partner*. Near the time of ovulation, the collected samples of sperm are then deposited near the woman's cervical opening. In a related procedure called *artificial insemination by donor*, the sperm of a donor is used. Donor semen is screened for the presence of pathogens, including the AIDS virus.

Causes of infertility in females center mostly on obstructions in the female reproductive tract and the inability to ovulate. The obstructions frequently result from tissue damage (scarring) caused by infections. Unchecked chlamydial and gonorrhea infections often produce fertility problems. In certain women, the use of IUDs has produced infections and PID; both of these increase the chances of infertility. Other possible causes of structural abnormalities include scar tissue from previous surgery, fibroid tumors, polyps, and endometriosis.[15] A variety of microsurgical techniques may correct some of these complications.

When a woman has ovulation difficulties, pinpointing the specific cause can be very difficult. Increasing age produces hormone fluctuations associated with lack of ovulation. Being significantly overweight or underweight also has a major impact on fertility. However, in women of normal weight who are not approaching menopause, it appears that ovulation difficulties are caused by failure of syncronization between the hormones governing the menstrual cycle. Fertility drugs can help alter the menstrual cycle to produce ovulation. Clomiphene citrate (Clomid), in oral pill form, and injections of a mixture of LH and FSH taken from the urine of menopausal women (Pergonal) are the most common fertility drugs available. Both are capable of producing multiple ova at ovulation.

For couples who are unable to conceive following drug therapy, surgery, and artificial insemination, the use of *in vivo fertilization and embryo transfer (IVF-ET)* is another option. This method is sometimes referred to as the "test tube" procedure. Costing around $5,000 per attempt, IVF-ET consists of surgically retrieving fertilizable ova from the woman and combining them in a glass dish with sperm. After several days, the fertilized ova are transferred into the uterus. At best, IVF-ET is successful for about 30% of couples wishing to establish a pregnancy.[15]

The newest test tube procedure is called *gamete intrafallopian transfer (GIFT)*. Similar to IVF-ET, this newer procedure deposits the retrieved eggs and sperm directly into the fallopian tubes. As this procedure becomes more refined, it is hoped that success rates higher than 30% will be possible.

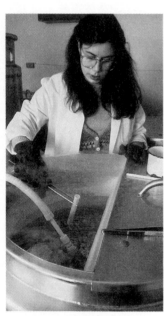

Freezing sperm for future use in artificial insemination.

Surrogate Parenting: The Case of "Baby M"

One of the most highly publicized surrogate parenting court cases involves the custody of an infant girl—"Baby M."

The case centered on the following situation: Mary Beth Whitehead, a mother of two, signed a contract agreeing to be artificially impregnated by William Stern. She promised to give the baby to William and Elizabeth Stern after delivery. For her efforts, May Beth Whitehead agreed to a $10,000 payment. However, after the baby was born, Ms. Whitehead decided to keep the child. When police arrived at the Whitehead home to take the baby, Ms. Whitehead handed her out a window to her husband and they all fled to Florida.

After a lengthy court battle, the Sterns recovered the baby—whom they call Melissa, the Whiteheads call Sara, and the court calls "Baby M."[16]

The initial court decision concluded that Baby M belonged to the Sterns since Ms. Whitehead had agreed to give up her parental rights. A February 1988 ruling by the New Jersey Supreme Court resolved some issues in the Baby M case.[17] The New Jersey court voided the contract between Ms. Whitehead and the Sterns, declaring it unenforceable. Visiting rights were, however, given to Ms. Whitehead.

More general questions pertaining to surrogate parenting will be answered in conjunction with forthcoming state and federal legislation.

Many important questions regarding surrogate parenting were raised by the "Baby M" case, including:

- Does the surrogate mother sell a service or a product?
- If a surrogate mother charges and is paid a fee, is this different from giving her "service" free of charge? Do her rights to the baby change?
- Do the persons who receive the services of a surrogate mother have the right to reject the baby if it is handicapped or otherwise unacceptable?
- Does the surrogate mother have a right to keep the child?

Surrogate parenting is another option that has recently been explored, although the legal and ethical issues surrounding this method of conception are not fully resolved. Surrogate parenting exists in a number of forms. Typically, an infertile couple will make a contract with a woman (the surrogate parent) who will then be artificially inseminated with semen from the expectant father. In some instances the surrogate will receive an embryo from the donor parents. The surrogate will carry the fetus to term and return the newborn to the parents. Because of the concerns about true "ownership" of the baby, surrogate parenting may not be a particularly viable option for many couples. The box above details the highly publicized surrogate parent case of "Baby M."

The process of coping with infertility problems can be an emotionally stressful experience for a couple. Hours of waiting in physician's offices, having numerous examinations, scheduling intercourse, producing sperm samples, and undergoing surgical or drug treatments place multiple burdens on a couple. Knowing that other couples are able to conceive so effortlessly adds to the mental strain. Fortunately, support groups exist to assist couples with infertility problems. Some of these groups are listed in the box on p. 478.

Where to Find Help

These agencies can provide you with information on infertility and give referrals to specialists in your area:

Resolve Inc.
P.O. Box 474
Belmont, MA 02178
(617) 484-2424

American Fertility Foundation
2131 Magnolia Avenue
Suite 201
Birmingham, AL 35256
(205) 251-9764

Center for Communications in Infertility
P.O. Box 516
Yorktown Heights, NY 10598
(914) 962-7140

Planned Parenthood Federation of America
810 Seventh Avenue
New York, NY 10019
(212) 541-7800

These agencies can provide help to prospective adoptive parents:

The National Adoption Center
1218 Chestnut Street
Philadelphia, PA 19107
(215) 925-0200

The National Committee for Adoption
P.O. Box 33366
Washington, DC 20033
(202) 638-0466

The North American Council on Adoptable Children
P.O. Box 14808
St. Paul, MN 55414
(612) 644-3036

Organization for United Response (OURS)
3307 Highway 100 North
Suite 203
Minneapolis, MN 55422
(612) 535-4829

What can one do to reduce the chances of developing infertility problems? Certainly the avoidance of infections in the reproductive organs is one crucial factor. Barrier methods of contraception (condom, diaphragm) with a spermicide reportedly cuts the risk of developing infertility in half. The use of an IUD should be avoided and the risk from multiple partners should be considered carefully. Men and women should be aware of the dangers from working around hazardous chemicals or consuming psychoactive drugs. Maintaining overall good health and having regular medical (and gynecological) checkups are also good ideas. Finally, since infertility is linked with advancing age, couples may not want to indefinitely delay having children.

SUMMARY

Becoming pregnant and bearing and rearing children can have a significant influence on the lives of young adults. Furthermore, raising a child from birth through 4 years of college can be a very expensive proposition. Thus it is important for potential parents to examine some of the reasons that people want to have children. Careful preparation may help young parents cope better with a variety of stressors associated with having and rearing children.

Even though there are many physiological obstacles that can reduce the chance of pregnancy, there are also many factors that encourage fertilization. Once a pregnancy occurs, accurate determination is made by testing for the hormone HCG (human chorionic gonadatropin) and observing the signs and symptoms of pregnancy. A pregnant woman must be concerned with many

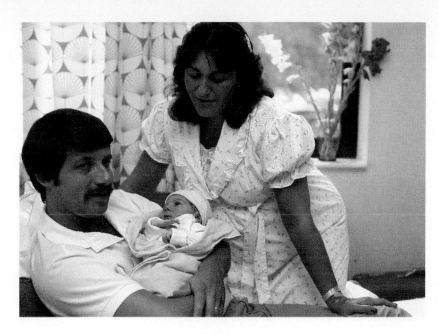

The new family.

agents that can affect fetal development, including drugs she ingests and environmental hazards to which she might be exposed.

The process of childbirth is typically an exciting experience for those involved. Labor is first recognized by several physical signs of the body. This chapter describes labor in its three recognizable stages: effacement and dilation of the cervix, expulsion of the fetus, and expulsion of the placenta. For a woman having her first baby, the entire birth process lasts an average of 12 to 16 hours.

Preparation for birth has changed greatly over the years. As a result of the efforts of pioneer childbirth educators, such practices as father-assisted deliveries, natural childbirth, and childbirth preparation classes are now common. New birth technologies, including those that deal with problems of infertility, are continually being developed.

REVIEW QUESTIONS

1 Identify the basic considerations presented in the chapter that should be considered by an individual or couple planning parenthood.
2 What are some of the obstacles and aids in fertilization presented in the chapter? Can you think of others that were not presented?
3 What kinds of tests are used to determine pregnancy?
4 Explain the formula for determining the due date.
5 Identify and describe the events that occur during each of the three stages of labor. Approximately how long is each stage?
6 What should a pregnant woman know about the following factors: anesthesia, medications, cesarean delivery, and breastfeeding? List some of the situations that might require a cesarean delivery.
7 Describe the advances that have been made over the years in preparation for childbirth.
8 Describe some of the recent advances in birth technology.
9 What can one do to reduce the chances of infertility?
10 Distinguish between IVF-ET and GIFT.

QUESTIONS FOR PERSONAL CONTEMPLATION

1 Do you think the trend to delay parenthood will change? What effects do you think starting parenthood at a later age has? How old do you want to be when you have your first child? Why?

2 Many couples are choosing not to have any children at all. How do you feel about such a choice?

3 Does having children automatically make you a responsible parent? If you think there are situations when couples should not have children, give some examples of these situations.

4 What are the responsibilities that a woman has to her fetus? If you knew you were pregnant, which of your health-related behaviors would you change? If a woman should not smoke, drink, or use other drugs during pregnancy, should these limitations also be placed on the fathers? Why or why not?

5 To what extent do you believe fathers should participate in the birthing experience? Why?

REFERENCES

1 Espenshade, TJ: The value of children, Interchange 6:4, 1977.

2 Hatcher, RA, et al: Contraceptive technology: 1986-87, ed 13, New York 1986, Irvington Publishers, Inc.

3 Jones, RE: Human reproduction and sexual behavior, Englewood Cliffs, NJ, 1984, Prentice-Hall, Inc.

4 Tortora, GJ, and Evans, RL: Principles of human physiology, ed 2, New York, 1986, Harper & Row Publishers, Inc.

5 Kaluger, G, and Kaluger, M: Human development, ed 3, Columbus, Ohio, 1984, Charles E Merrill.

6 Accutane alert: birth defects, The Harvard Medical School Health Letter 11:3, 1986.

7 Haas, K, and Haas, A: Understanding sexuality, St. Louis, 1987, Times Mirror/Mosby College Publishing.

8 Shiono, P, et al: Recent trends in cesarean birth and trial labor in the United States, The Journal of the American Medical Association 257:494-497, 1987.

9 Wilson, S, et al: Human sexuality: a text with readings, ed 2, St. Paul, MN, 1980, West Publishing Co.

10 Leboyer, F: Birth without violence, New York, 1980, Alfred A Knopf, Inc.

11 Birth centers are as safe as hospitals, USA Today, January 22, 1987, p 5.

12 Leveno, K, et al: A prospective comparison of selected and universal electronic fetal monitoring in 34,995 pregnancies, The New England Journal of Medicine 315:615-619, 1986.

13 Peterson, KS: The high costs of pursuing pregnancy, USA Today, February 26, 1985, p 1.

14 Infertility, The Harvard Medical School Health Letter 12:6-8, 1987.

15 Infertility in the woman, The Harvard Medical School Health Letter 12:5-8, 1987.

16 Pass laws to control all surrogate births, USA Today September 4, 1986, p 8a.

17 McQueen, M: Baby case is model for other states, USA Today February 4, 1988, p 1a.

ANNOTATED READINGS

Grollman, EA, and Sweder, GL: The working parent dilemma, Boston, 1986, Beacon Press.
Working parents, particularly single parents, and their children can experience a wide variety of feelings about parental absence from the home. The authors provide suggestions for minimizing the negative impact that limited parental contact can have on children.

Mattis, M: Single parent, how to have happy and healthy kids and an active social life, New York, 1986, Henry Holt and Co.
When a single parent begins to date, adjustments can be difficult for the child. Suggestions are provided on recognizing these signs of difficulty and how to respond to them.

Pruett, KD: The nurturing father, New York, 1987, Warner Books, Inc.
The author, a child psychologist at the Yale University Child Study Center, interviewed many stay-at-home fathers and discovered how important fathers are in affecting the lives of their children. The measurable benefits that fathers provide are discussed.

Mastering Tasks

s you read through this unit, you probably saw connections between the nature of your own sexuality and the four developmental tasks: identity, independence, responsibility, and social interaction. If you are a traditional-age student, these connections were probably based on your own personal experiences or those you anticipate in the future. Nontraditional students may have reflected on their past or current experiences, as well as those of their children.

▪ **Forming an Initial Adult Self-Identity** In your search to accomplish this particular developmental task, the same question keeps repeating itself: "Who am I?" As a young adult, or as an older person looking back on this period, you see yourself engaged in "writing a script" about who you are and who you will become in the near future. Certainly, this script will include information about your sexuality.

We would contend that to really know yourself, you must start to analyze the way you feel about aspects of your reproductive, genital, and expressionistic sexuality. Start asking yourself some important questions, such as: "What do I really want in a relationship?" "How much do I care about the feelings of my partner?" "Have I developed my personal code of ethics?" "Am I ready to become a parent?" "How might I improve my skills as a lover?" "To what extent am I familiar with contraceptive techniques?" "Am I happy with the way I express myself as a man or woman?" Answers to these kinds of questions will help you come to grips with your emerging adult self-identity.

▪ **Establishing a Sense of Relative Independence** For the majority of young adults, independence from the family encourages mobility. Mobility provides the opportunity for the experiences that allow you to achieve a fully developed adult gender identification. Living and working in new places and interacting with a variety of different individuals can function as stimuli to help broaden your gender schemas.

Thus being mobile allows you to see a wide range of masculine and feminine models. Some of these models you will appreciate more than others, yet we contend that you will learn something from them all. In much the same manner that college increases your pool of friends and presents alternative lifestyle experiences, your independence after college can further enhance this process.

▪ **Assuming Increasing Levels of Responsibility** Hand-in-hand with gaining independence goes the important task of increasing personal responsibility. In terms of a paired sexual relationship, how does one direct this responsibility? In our minds, the responsibility starts before the relationship begins. It is only beforehand that you have the opportunity to look carefully at your intent regarding the sexual standards you will follow.

You must ask yourself questions concerning your personal standards and your ability to adhere to these standards. You must address questions concerning contraceptive effectiveness, the likelihood of STDs, and possible pregnancy. Ignoring these issues can lead to disappointment for yourself and frustration for others. Fortunately, many individuals want to share their responsibility with their partners.

▪ **Developing the Skills for Social Interaction** A discussion concerning paired sexual relationships and the development of skills required for social interaction is very much like a description of the evolution of a friendship. In a growing friendship, new social skills are layered, level upon level. The evolving nature of the paired sexual relationship follows a similar pattern of growth and development in social skills.

A person engaged in dating relationships must develop insights, sensitivities, and responses that will be of value not only through courtship, but more importantly, in marriage. Social skills particularly relevant to mate selection include the ability to form and assess perceptions, to recognize the reward system around which you and your partner operate, to articulate your values, and to act on those values with integrity and consistency.

UNIT VI

At first, a unit that combines chapters on consumer health and the environment might seem unusual. Yet everything we do in life is in some way related to our environment. Each day we come into contact with our land, air, and water. Within our environment, we make health-related consumer decisions. Unit VI will focus on these kinds of decisions because they will affect the multiple dimensions of health.

▪ **Physical Dimension of Health** In a variety of ways, the physical dimension of health can be immediately influenced by consumer decisions. Your choice of a particular physician, for example, is prudent when you know that that physician specializes in the services you require and is able to restore physical function within a few days. Similarly, the choices you make concerning where you wish to live (perhaps in a location with clean air, clean water, and clean land) will have an impact on your physical health.

▪ **Emotional Dimension of Health** The impact of an overcrowded, highly industrialized society on our emotional health is not as evident as the impact on our physical health. However, when we are able to spend a few days in a pristine environment, we begin to understand how our surroundings affect our mental health. We appreciate natural sounds and natural odors. We delight in the unspoiled beauty of an uncluttered forest or a sparkling clear stream. The psychological benefits are refreshing and may remain with us for months or years.

On the other hand, our emotional health can be damaged when we see an environment gradually overcome by our society's greed and technological advancements. We easily feel stressed by overcrowding, congested traffic, polluted air, and constant noise. When we realize that beyond our own day-to-day battles, an environmental war continues to be waged, we may begin to feel guilty that we are remaining on the sidelines. Fortunately, as consumers, we will have opportunities to become involved in decisions that may preserve our environment and keep our emotional health intact.

▪ **Social Dimension of Health** Consumers are not born—they are made. They are shaped in part by their contact with others. The direction other people provide about the information, services, and products you use is a powerful factor in your development as a health-oriented consumer. Discussing your health needs with parents, friends, or health care professionals can help you to quickly and efficiently meet those needs.

▪ **Intellectual Dimension of Health** Understanding environmental concerns and consumer options is not a task for the unskilled mind. Trying to isolate causes of environmental pollution and preparing workable solutions are two extremely complicated tasks. Understanding the relationships among pollutants, humans, and our environment may require study in a variety of physical and biological sciences.

▪ **Spiritual Dimension of Health** The study of consumer information and environmental issues that relate to our health can be viewed from a spiritual dimension. We frequently hold much faith in the health products and medical services that we select. When we are ill, we may hope that a higher power is capable of working through our physician to make a correct diagnosis. As our health improves, the beauty that we begin to notice in the world is a tribute to our unending search for a deeper meaning to life.

As we search for solutions to complex environmental problems, we may be forced to make some difficult decisions. For example, will we someday force third world countries to use contraceptive measures or sterilization? Will we attempt to feed the world's hungry people? Will we continue to protect endangered species of plants and animals? Will we strive more forcefully for nuclear disarmament? To build a better world for future generations may be the biggest challenge in our spiritual commitment to serve others.

Consumerism
and Environment
Outside Forces Shaping
Your Health

CHAPTER 17

Consumerism
and Health Care
Making Sound Decisions

Key Concepts

Decisions you make about health-related information, services, and products have a direct influence on your health.

Consumers should analyze health-related information in terms of its validity and reliability.

Consumers receive health services from a variety of health care providers in many types of facilities.

The growing popularity of self-care places more responsibility for health care in the hands of the consumer.

Rising health care costs make it imperative that consumers carefully examine their health insurance coverage.

Health care products should be used in an informed and responsible manner.

Consumer fraud is common in the areas of drugs, foods, and devices.

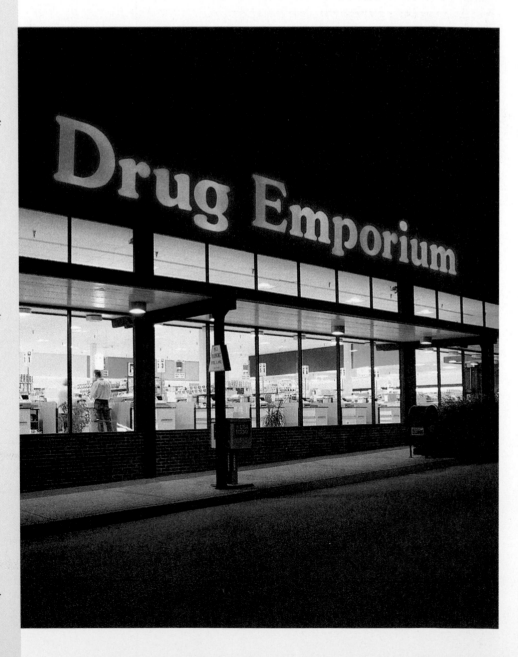

*H*ealth care providers often evaluate you by criteria pertaining to their area of expertise. The nutritionist knows you by the food you eat. The physical fitness professional knows you by your body type and activity level. And in the eyes of the expert in health-related consumerism, you are the product of the health information you believe, the health-influencing services you use, and the products you consume. When your decisions about health information, services, and products are made after careful study and consideration, your health will probably be improved. However, when your decisions lack insight, your health as well as your pocketbook may suffer.

HEALTH-RELATED INFORMATION

The Informed Consumer

To become an informed consumer, you must learn about services and products that improve health. Practitioners, manufacturers, and sales personnel use a variety of approaches to transmit their messages to you. Each approach is really an attempt to get you to buy a product or use a service. As watchdogs for potentially fraudulent claims and advertising campaigns, certain regulatory agencies and consumer groups monitor the source and nature of consumer information to protect you from ineffective or even dangerous services or products (see the box on p. 488. As a consumer, you should be aware that these agencies and groups are valuable sources of information.

Validity and Reliability

How closely does a product's claim agree with the best scientific evidence available? This question concerns the concept of **validity.** For the consumer dealing with health-related information, this is a particularly important criterion on which to base a decision.

To serve as a basis for health care decisions, information must be not only valid but also reliable—capable of predictable results time after time. Just as you always expect vaccinations to provide immunity, so too should valid information be applicable in each situation to which you relate it. Such is the dimension of **reliability** as it is associated with health-related information.

Sources of Information

As you have undoubtedly concluded from courses you have taken in various academic areas, information on a specific topic is not the sole property of one particular discipline. Such is certainly the case with health-related information. The sources for information on a particular health topic are as diverse as the number of people you know, the number of publications you read, and the number of experts you see or hear. At present no single agency or profession regulates the quantity or quality of the health-related information you receive. Therefore you and the health community share the responsibility for using information in the most constructive way. If you fail to become a skilled and discriminating user of information, your health will always be at risk from those who purposefully or innocently disseminate information lacking validity or reliability.

Thirteen diverse sources of health-related information are presented in the

validity
the accuracy and soundness of one's perceptions; scientific accuracy.

reliability
consistent performance.

485

Figure 17-1
When it comes to treating common health problems, where do we first turn for relief? The percentages shown total 106%, because some individuals choose more than one action.

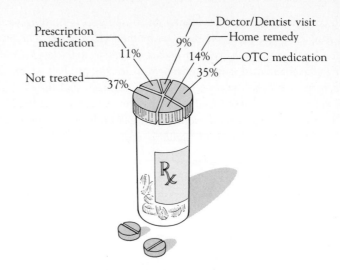

Prescription medication — 11%
Doctor/Dentist visit — 9%
Home remedy — 14%
OTC medication — 35%
Not treated — 37%

following discussion. You should quickly recognize that all are familiar sources, that some provide more valid information than others, and that some require more efforts to use effectively than others. Figure 17-1 shows the varied methods people choose to use when faced with health problems.

Family and friends

As most social workers would tell you, the first place most people go for assistance with a personal problem is to their family or friends. They also tend to seek health information from these familiar, readily available, and affordable sources.

From a consumerism point of view, the validity of information provided by a friend or family member may be questionable. Many persons are limited in their ability to understand or explain the application of technical information. Too often the information provided by family and friends is based on folk remedies that lack technical validity. Additionally, family members or friends may provide information they believe is in your best interests rather than providing factual information that may have a more negative impact on you.

Advertisements and commercials

Many adults spend a good portion of every day watching television, listening to the radio, and reading newspapers or magazines. Since many advertisements are health oriented, we should not be surprised to learn that these are major sources of information.

Although as consumers we may benefit from commercial messages, we should remember that the primary purpose of advertising is to sell products or services. In contrast to advertisements and commercials, the mass media routinely supplies public service messages that give valuable health-related information.

Labels and directions

Federal law requires that many consumer product labels contain specific information. The list in the margin gives an example of the kind of nutrition information you will find on food products.

Nutrition Information (Per Serving)

Serving size = 1 oz (1½ cup) corn flakes alone and in combination with ½ cup vitamin D fortified whole milk
Servings per container = 12

CORN FLAKES

	1 oz	with ½ cup whole milk
Calories	110	190
Protein	2 g	6 g
Carbohydrates	24 g	30 g
Fat	0 g	4 g

Percentage of U.S. Recommended Daily Dietary Allowance (U.S. RDA)

Protein	2	10
Vitamin A	25	25
Vitamin C	25	25
Thiamin	25	25
Riboflavin	25	35
Niacin	25	25
Calcium	*	15
Iron	10	10

*Contains less than 2% of the U.S. RDA of these nutrients.

When a drug is prescribed by your physician and provided by your pharmacist, a detailed information sheet describing the drug should be available. Information pertaining to the drug's chemical formulation, its mode of action, and its contraindications can be obtained from this sheet (see Figure 17-2). Generally your pharmacist will provide you with this information only when you request it.

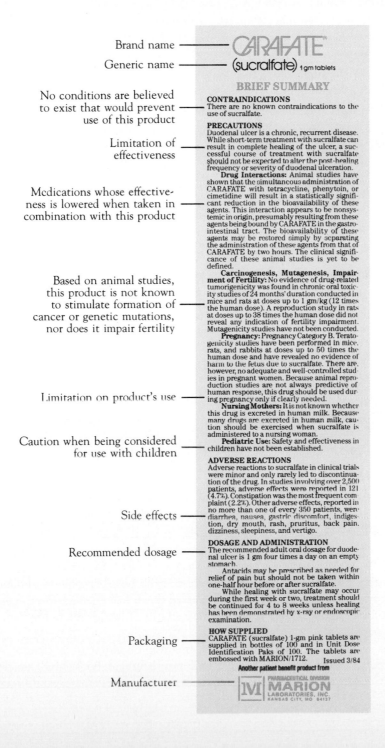

Brand name

Generic name

No conditions are believed to exist that would prevent use of this product

Limitation of effectiveness

Medications whose effectiveness is lowered when taken in combination with this product

Based on animal studies, this product is not known to stimulate formation of cancer or genetic mutations, nor does it impair fertility

Limitation on product's use

Caution when being considered for use with children

Side effects

Recommended dosage

Packaging

Manufacturer

CARAFATE®

(sucralfate) 1 gm tablets

BRIEF SUMMARY

CONTRAINDICATIONS
There are no known contraindications to the use of sucralfate.

PRECAUTIONS
Duodenal ulcer is a chronic, recurrent disease. While short-term treatment with sucralfate can result in complete healing of the ulcer, a successful course of treatment with sucralfate should not be expected to alter the post-healing frequency or severity of duodenal ulceration.
Drug Interactions: Animal studies have shown that the simultaneous administration of CARAFATE with tetracycline, phenytoin, or cimetidine will result in a statistically significant reduction in the bioavailability of these agents. This interaction appears to be nonsystemic in origin, presumably resulting from these agents being bound by CARAFATE in the gastrointestinal tract. The bioavailability of these agents may be restored simply by separating the administration of these agents from that of CARAFATE by two hours. The clinical significance of these animal studies is yet to be defined.
Carcinogenesis, Mutagenesis, Impairment of Fertility: No evidence of drug-related tumorigenicity was found in chronic oral toxicity studies of 24 months' duration conducted in mice and rats at doses up to 1 gm/kg (12 times the human dose). A reproduction study in rats at doses up to 38 times the human dose did not reveal any indication of fertility impairment. Mutagenicity studies have not been conducted.
Pregnancy: Pregnancy Category B. Teratogenicity studies have been performed in mice, rats, and rabbits at doses up to 50 times the human dose and have revealed no evidence of harm to the fetus due to sucralfate. There are, however, no adequate and well-controlled studies in pregnant women. Because animal reproduction studies are not always predictive of human response, this drug should be used during pregnancy only if clearly needed.
Nursing Mothers: It is not known whether this drug is excreted in human milk. Because many drugs are excreted in human milk, caution should be exercised when sucralfate is administered to a nursing woman.
Pediatric Use: Safety and effectiveness in children have not been established.

ADVERSE REACTIONS
Adverse reactions to sucralfate in clinical trials were minor and only rarely led to discontinuation of the drug. In studies involving over 2,500 patients, adverse effects were reported in 121 (4.7%). Constipation was the most frequent complaint (2.2%). Other adverse effects, reported in no more than one of every 350 patients, were diarrhea, nausea, gastric discomfort, indigestion, dry mouth, rash, pruritus, back pain, dizziness, sleepiness, and vertigo.

DOSAGE AND ADMINISTRATION
The recommended adult oral dosage for duodenal ulcer is 1 gm four times a day on an empty stomach.
Antacids may be prescribed as needed for relief of pain but should not be taken within one-half hour before or after sucralfate.
While healing with sucralfate may occur during the first week or two, treatment should be continued for 4 to 8 weeks unless healing has been demonstrated by x-ray or endoscopic examination.

HOW SUPPLIED
CARAFATE (sucralfate) 1-gm pink tablets are supplied in bottles of 100 and in Unit Dose Identification Paks of 100. The tablets are embossed with MARION/1712.   Issued 3/84

Another patient benefit product from

PHARMACEUTICAL DIVISION
M MARION LABORATORIES, INC.
KANSAS CITY, MO 64137

Figure 17-2
Pharmaceutical information inserts provide valuable consumer information.

Consumer Protection Agencies and Organizations

FEDERAL AGENCIES

1 Office of Consumer Affairs, Food and Drug Administration, U.S. Department of Health and Human Services, 5600 Fishers Lane, Rockville, MD 20857; phone: 301-443-5006

2 Bureau of Consumer Protection, Federal Trade Commission, Division of Advertising Practices or Division of Food and Drug Advertising, 6th St. and Pennsylvania Ave. N.W., Washington, DC 20580; phone: 292-523-3727

3 Fraud Division, Chief Postal Inspector, U.S. Postal Service, 475 L'Enfant Plaza, Washington, DC 20260

4 Consumer Information Center, Department SC, Pueblo, CO 81009

5 Consumer Product Safety Commission, Washington, DC 20207; hotline: 800-638-8326

CONSUMER ORGANIZATIONS

1 Consumers Union of the U.S., Inc., 256 Washington St., Mount Vernon, NY 10550; phone: 914-664-6400

2 The National Consumers' League, 1522 K St. N.W., Suite 406, Washington, DC 20005

BUSINESS ORGANIZATIONS

1 Health Insurance Institute, 1850 K St. N.W., Washington, DC 20006

2 Public Affairs Pamphlets, 381 Park Ave. S., Room 1101, New York, NY 10016

PROFESSIONAL ORGANIZATIONS

1 American Medical Association, 535 N. Dearborn, Chicago, IL 60610

2 American Hospital Association, 840 N. Lake Shore Dr., Chicago, IL 60611

3 American Pharmaceutical Association, Health Education Center Service, 2215 Constitution Ave. N.W., Washington, DC 20037

Many clinicians and health care institutions provide consumers with detailed directions applicable to their health problem. As a patient, you should study these directions and follow them closely.

Folklore

Ideas about health and information concerning health problems abound within the nonscientific community. Often passed down from generation to generation, this folklore about health is the primary source of health-related information for some people.

The validity of health-related information obtained from family members, neighbors, clerks in retail stores, and nontechnical books and articles about health is difficult to evaluate. As a general rule, however, we would recommend caution concerning the scientific soundness and, thus, the value of information from these sources. A blanket condemnation is not warranted, however, since folk wisdom is on occasion grounded in scientific soundness. Also, the intangible support provided by the suppliers of this information could be the best medicine some people need.

Testimonials

Since people feel strongly about sharing information that has proven beneficial to them, we include testimonials as a source of health information. The recommendations made by other people concerning a particular practitioner or health-related product may at first appear to be frivolous testimonials. Since they are frequently the basis for decision-making by others, we assign a small measure of validity to them as sources of health-related information. However, the grandiose testimonials that accompany the sales pitches of the medical quack or the "satisfied" customers appearing on television commercials should never be interpreted as valid endorsements.

Mass media exposure

Health programming on cable television stations, life-style sections in newspapers, health care correspondents appearing on national network news shows, and a growing number of health-oriented magazines are four examples of health-related information in the mass media. People have discovered that health is a vital component of well-being and they are seeking ever-increasing amounts of information. The media are, of course, responding to this need.

Although in general health-related information is presented well, it is presented with a brevity that is distracting. By and large, however, the consumer who desires more complete coverge of a health-related topic can obtain it by combining media sources. For instance, a topic introduced with only a few seconds of coverage on a cable news program may be covered with somewhat greater depth on the national network news and later be the focus of a television documentary. An example of this multifocused approach to health-related information is the coverage given to each new piece of evidence concerning the AIDS epidemic.

Practitioners

The health care consumer also receives much information from individual health practitioners and their professional associations. In fact, the *patient education* role is so clearly seen by today's health care practitioner that to find one who does not exchange some information with a patient would be unusual. Also, pamphlets, audio and video tapes, and other teaching aids are routinely found in practitioners' offices. Education enhances patient compliance with health care directives, which is important to the practitioner and the consumer.

A major development in the area of practitioner-provided information and patient education has been the evolution of the hospital as an educational institution. Wellness centers, chemical dependency programs, and sports medicine centers are becoming more common. In addition to generating information regarding particular biomedical needs, these centers promote wellness through a variety of methods and materials.

Patient education.

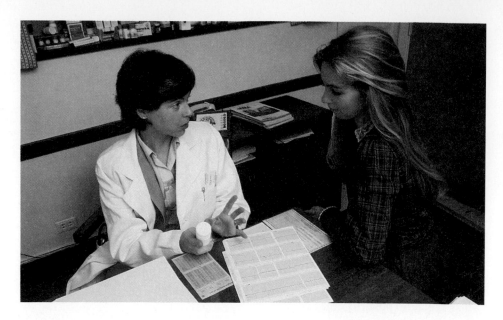

Medical reference books

It has been estimated that 60% of all households own at least one health (medical) reference book, such as *Woman's Health and Medical Guide,*[1] the *Physicians' Desk Reference,*[2] *Baby and Child Care,*[3] and other self-help books.

Personal computer programs and video cassettes featuring health-related information are rapidly becoming important sources of information for the consumer. As long as consumer demand for health care reference material remains, material will be developed to meet these needs.

Reference libraries

Even though a large percentage of households possess health-related reference material and health care professionals are dispensing more and more information to the consumer, public and university libraries continue to be much-used sources of health-related information. Reference librarians are consulted and audiovisual collections and printed materials are regularly used to answer health-related questions and broaden comprehension of the nature and role of health.

Consumer advocacy groups

A variety of nonprofit consumer advocacy groups patrol the health care marketplace, particularly in relationship to services and products. In conjunction with the overall advocacy missions, these groups produce and disseminate information designed to aid the consumer in recognizing questionable services and products. Large, well-organized groups such as The National Consumers' League and Consumers' Union and smaller groups at the state and local level champion the right of the consumer to receive valid and reliable information about health care products and services.

Voluntary health agencies

Volunteerism and the traditional approach to health care and health promotion are virtually inseparable. Few other countries boast so many national voluntary organizations, with state and local affiliates, dedicated to the enhancement of health through research, service, and public education. The American Cancer Society, the American Red Cross, and the American Heart Association are all voluntary health agencies. Consumers can, in fact, anticipate finding a voluntary health agency for virtually every health problem.

Many voluntary organizations focus on the dissemination of information through many avenues, including the support of curriculum development in public schools, provision of speakers for conventions and meetings, and distribution of printed and visual materials. These organizations are among the most active and effective sources of consumer information.

Although figures vary among voluntary agencies, the typical agency uses approximately 15% of its annual budget for public education.*[4] When direct services and monies for the support of research are added to the monies spent for education, the voluntary health agency is a cost-effective component of our health care system.

Government agencies

Although they will be mentioned again in conjunction with the regulation of products and services, governmental agencies are effective dispersers of information to the public. Through meetings and release of information to the media, agencies such as the Food and Drug Administration, Federal Trade Commission, United States Postal Service, and Environmental Protection Agency contribute to public awareness of health issues. Particularly in terms of labeling, advertising, and the distribution of information through the mails, government agencies also control the quality of information disseminated to the buying public. The various divisions of the National Institutes of Health regularly release research findings and recommendations pertaining to the clinical practices, which in turn reach the consumer through clinical practitioners.

In spite of their best intentions federal health agencies are often less effective than what the public deserves. A variety of factors including inadequate staff, poor administration, and lobbying by special interest groups prevent these federal agencies from enforcing the consumer protection legislation that exists. As a result, the public is left with a sense of false confidence regarding the consumer protection provided by the federal government.

State government also provides the public with health-related information. State agencies are primary sources of information, particularly in the area of public health and environmental protection. In addition to these agencies, state funding of universities is an important contribution to the basic research that generates health-related information for the consumer. State universities also train educators and health professionals, who in turn help consumers.

Qualified health educators

Health educators can be found working in a variety of settings and providing their services to diverse groups of individuals. *Community health educators* are found working with virtually all of the agencies mentioned in this section; *patient health educators* function in primary care settings; and *school health educators* are found at all educational levels. Increasingly, health educators are being em-

*Public and professional education expenses accounted for approximately 18% of the American Cancer Society's 1985 to 1986 budget!

The Value of Health Information Sources*

Rating scale: 1 Poor
             2 Below average
             3 Average
             4 Above average
             5 High

Source	Access	Validity	Reliability
Family and friends	5	1-5	1-5
Advertisements	5	2-5	2-5
Labels and directions	5	4-5	4-5
Folklore	2	2	2
Testimonials	5	3	3
Mass media	5	4	4
Practitioners	1-3	4-5	4-5
Medical reference books	3	4-5	4-5
References libraries	3	4-5	4-5
Consumer advocacy groups	4	4-5	4-5
Voluntary health agencies	4	5	5
Government agencies	4	5	5
Qualified health educators	4	4-5	4-5

Do you agree or disagree with the estimated ratings of these sources of information? Cite some reasons why you might rate these sources differently.

*These are only estimates of the value of these sources.

ployed in a wide range of wellness-based programs in community, hospital, corporate, and school settings. The box above lists the value of health information sources discussed.

HEALTH CARE PROVIDERS

The types and sources of health information just discussed can contribute greatly to the decisions we make as informed consumers. An understanding of the many health-related services available can add to our growth as wise consumers. The choices we make about physicians, health services, and medical payment plans will reflect our commitment to remain healthy and our trust in specific persons who are trained to keep us healthy.

Why We Consult Health Care Providers

Most of us seek care and advice from medical and health practitioners when we have a specific problem. A bad cold, a broken arm, or a newly discovered "lump" can make us realize that we need to consult health care professionals. Yet *diagnosis* and *treatment* are only two reasons why we might require the services of health care providers.

We might also use health practitioners for the purpose of *screening*. Screening is the examination of large numbers of people to discover particular diseases or health characteristics. Your earliest experience with screening may have been in elementary school, where physicians, nurses, audiologists, and dentists sometimes examine all children for normal growth and development patterns. As an adult, you might use the services of health care practitioners at a shopping center when you volunteer to be screened for hypertension or diabetes. Although screening should be considered much less precise than actual diagnosis, screening serves to identify people who should seek further medical examination.

Consultation is a fourth reason why knowledgeable consumers seek health care providers. A consultation is the use of two or more professionals to deliberate a person's specific health problem or condition. Consultations are especially helpful when a physician requires the opinion of a specialist. The use of an additional practitioner as a consultant can also help reassure patients who may have doubts about their own condition or about the abilities of their physician.

Prevention is a fifth reason why we might seek a health care provider. With the current emphasis on trying to stop problems before they begin, the use of health care providers for prevention is becoming more common. People want information about how to prevent needless risks and promote their health and are seeking such advice from physicians, nurses, dentists, exercise physiologists, health educators, and patient educators. The box below gives guidelines to follow when choosing a physician.

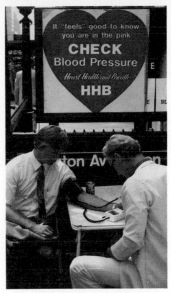

Screening for hypertension.

When Choosing a Physician. . .

When choosing a physician, ask yourself the following questions after your initial visit:
- Was I comfortable with the physician's age, gender, race, and national origin?
- Was I comfortable with the physician's demeanor? Did I find communicating with the physician to be understandable and reassuring? Were all my questions answered?
- Did the physician seem interested in having me as a patient?
- Is the physician's training and practice speciality in an area most closely associated with my present needs and concerns?
- Does the physician have staff privileges at a hospital of my preference?
- Does the physician's fee-for-service policy in any way exclude or limit my ability to receive necessary services?
- Did the physician take a complete medical history as a part of my initial visit? Was prevention, health promotion, or wellness addressed by the physician at any point during my visit?
- Did I at any point during my visit sense that the physician was unusually reluctant or anxious to try new medical procedures or medications?
- When the physician is unavailable, are any colleagues on call for 24 hours? Did I feel that telephone calls from me would be welcomed and responded to in a reasonable period of time?

If you have answered yes to the majority of these questions, you have found a physician with whom you should feel comfortable with.

Intern examining patient.

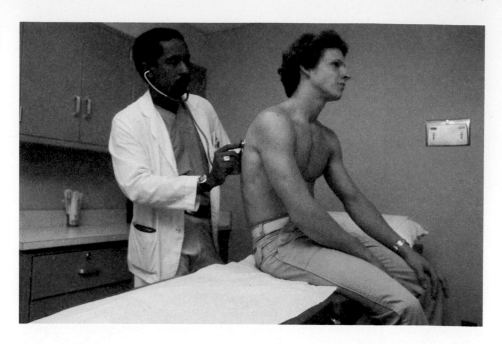

Another general reason why we consult health practitioners is in the broad area of *research*. We might seek the service of a medical research scientist when we have a critical question in a relatively unexplored area of knowledge. We also might require the help of a health care provider in interpreting the results from conflicting research reports. We might also come into contact with health care practitioners for research reasons if we were to volunteer to be a subject in experiments related to medical care, drug therapy, exercise physiology, or health education.

Allopathic and Osteopathic Physicians

Allopathy

Allopathy refers to a system of medical practice in which specific remedies (often in the form of drugs or medicines) are used to produce effects different from those produced by a disease. For example, physicians prescribe antibiotics to produce effects in a patient that are different from those produced by a bacterial infection.

The practitioners who subscribe to allopathy are already familiar to you. Medical physicians are health professionals who have earned the degree of M.D. (Doctor of Medicine) from accredited medical schools. The training required to become a medical physician is long and arduous. Usually, 4 years of undergraduate college preparation is required. There is a heavy emphasis on the sciences—biology, chemistry, mathematics, anatomy, and physiology. Most undergraduate schools have a prescribed pre-med course of study for students to follow.

Once accepted into medical school, students generally spend 4 more years in intensive training, which includes advanced study in the medical sciences and clinical practices. Medical students put in long hours in science laboratories and clinical settings, often working closely with physician-instructors in teaching hospitals.

Upon graduation from medical school, the students are awarded the M.D. degree and then take the state medical license examination. If the physicians pass this test, they will be permitted to practice medicine. For the next year or two, most newly licensed physicians will complete an *internship* at a hospital. During this period, the intern will gain experience in various clinical areas, including surgery, pediatrics, emergency medicine, internal medicine, and obstetrics.

If physicians decide to specialize in one particular area, they can elect to take additional training as *resident* physicians. Residency periods vary in duration, but all are geared toward helping the physicians to pass further examinations in the specialty area, after which they are allowed to practice medicine as board-certified specialists. The American Board of Medical Specialists recognizes the specialties listed in the box below.

Medical Specialties

The American Board of Medical Specialties is a nonprofit organization that represents 23 medical specialty boards.* Each board is composed of expert physicians already qualified in a particular field. These specialty boards evaluate physicians who wish to practice in a specific area of medicine. Some of the more common specialty areas consumers might encounter are listed below.

Specialty	Scope of Practice
Allergy	Treatment of sensitivity disorders
Anesthesiology	Use of drugs to sedate or anesthetize
Cardiovascular surgery	Various forms of heart surgery
Dermatology	Skin diseases and disorders
Emergency medicine	Care of accident victims
Family practice	Broad-based family medical care
Geriatrics	Diseases and disorders of the elderly
Gynecology	Female reproductive health care
Internal medicine	Nonsurgical treatment of internal organ systems
Neurology	Diseases and disorders of the nervous system
Nephrology	Kidney diseases and disorders
Obstetrics	Prenatal care and child delivery
Oncology	Treatment of unusual growths and tumors
Orthopedic surgery	Surgery for structural disorders of the bones and joints
Otorhinolaryngology	Ear, nose, and throat problems
Psychiatry	Mental and emotional diseases or disorders
Pediatrics	Childhood health concerns
Radiology	Use of radiation to diagnose and treat diseases and injuries
Urological surgery	Surgery for urinary tract diseases and male reproductive dysfunctions

*Governed by these 23 medical boards are 85 practice specialties.

Osteopathy

The medical practice of *osteopathy* has undergone a remarkable change since its inception in the late 1800s. Originally, osteopaths attempted to cure diseases and promote health by the manipulation of the body's musculoskeletal system. They were understandably known as "bone doctors" and were frequently called upon to set fractured bones. The educational preparations for osteopaths was much less rigorous than that for traditional medical physicians. For years osteopaths could only work in private practice and at special osteopathic hospitals.

Today the gap between osteopaths and traditional medical physicians is virtually nonexistent. Osteopaths must now complete similar courses of undergraduate and medical school study, although this study is done at 1 of the 15 schools of osteopathy in the United States.[5] Osteopaths also now can use all the therapy methods that have been traditionally reserved for medical physicians. Also, osteopaths can be licensed in the same specialties as medical physicians.

Nonallopathic Health Care Providers

Nonallopathic health care providers use a variety of quasi-medical practices that are not supported by the bulk of traditional medical thinking. Some of the more common nonallopathic practitioners include chiropractors, naturopaths, and those who practice acupuncture.

As osteopaths thought nearly 100 years ago, *chiropractors* still believe that most health disorders stem from the unusual alignments of the bones, primarily those in the spinal column. Chiropractors use x-ray films to locate what they believe are improperly aligned vertebrae (subluxations), which place a strain on the spinal cord. Chiropractors believe that by manipulating the vertebral column they can cure people of a variety of aliments. Traditional medical practitioners contend that much of the recent popularity of chiropractors comes from their reduced fees, their "hands-on" approach to therapy, and the **placebo effect.**

placebo effect
improved status of one's health attributable only to the belief that one is being helped.

Within the past 20 years, academic standards at some of the 4-year chiropractic colleges have improved considerably. Today, chiropractic school graduates have taken many of the same basic science courses taken by medical school students. Any blanket condemnation of chiropractors would be inappropriate, especially since significant numbers of people claim to have been helped by chiropractic care and would recommend chiropractic care to others. Medicare and many insurance companies provide reimbursement for chiropractic care.

Clearly there are limits to the types of health care chiropractors can provide. For example, chiropractors do not give immunizations, perform operations, prescribe prescription drugs, or conduct sophisticated laboratory analyses of human tissue. These limitations must be recognized by both chiropractors and their clients.

Naturopaths believe in the use of natural therapies for victims of disease or illness. Most naturopaths have had some training at naturopathic institutes, but many people operate as self-proclaimed naturopaths. Naturopaths advocate the use of natural foods, food supplements, sunshine, exercise, and water to help sick people return to normal functioning. Some health food stores employ salespeople who try to combine a limited understanding of philosophy, anatomy, and physiology with an interest in "natural health" to convince buyers of the value of their store's extracts and supplements. Although not trained as naturopaths, these people are advocates for a naturopathic approach to self-care.

Persons who practice *acupuncture* must also be referred to as nonallopathic health care providers. Acupuncture is an ancient Chinese medical practice of inserting fine-gauge needles at specific points throughout the body. Insertion of these needles is thought to stimulate improved energy flow throughout the body to cure disease, reduce chronic pain, or anesthetize a body part. Many medical scientists question the validity, reliability, and safety of acupuncture. To a limited degree, some physicians are working with acupuncturists in a combined therapeutic approach to medical problems. Acupuncture appears to be most effective in persons who believe that it will be effective.

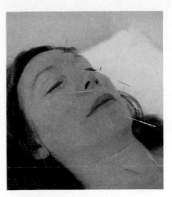

Acupuncture.

Limited Health Care Providers

We receive much of our health care from medical physicians. However, most of us also use the services of various health care specialists who also have advanced graduate level training. These specialists are labeled "doctors" by colleges, their professional associations, and their state licensing agencies. Although not certified as medical physicians, they nevertheless have had extensive training and command attractive salaries. Among these professionals are dentists, psychologists, podiatrists, and optometrists.

A *dentist* (Doctor of Dental Surgery, D.D.S.) is trained to deal with a wide range of diseases and impairments of the teeth and oral cavity. Most dentists undergo rigorous undergraduate predental programs that emphasize the natural sciences, followed by 3 or 4 additional years of graduate study in dental school. State licensure examinations are then required. As with medical physicians, dentists can also specialize in fields ranging from *oral surgery* to **orthodontics** to **prosthodontics.** Dentists are also permitted to prescribe therapy programs and drugs that pertain to their practices (primarily analgesics and antibiotics).

When we are in need of services related to improving or understanding our behavior patterns or perceptions, we might consult a *psychologist*. Over 40 states have certification or licensing laws that prohibit unqualified persons from using the term "psychologist." Many states also have special requirements before people can list themselves as health service providers.

It is important for a consumer to examine the credentials of a psychologist. Legitimate psychologists have received advanced graduate training (often leading to the Ph.D. or Ed.D. degree) in clinical, counseling, industrial, or school psychology. Furthermore, these practitioners will have passed state certification examinations and, in many states, will have met further requirements that allow them to offer health services to the public. Psychologists may have special interests and credentials from professional societies in individual, group, family, or marriage counseling. Some are certified as sex therapists.

Increasing numbers of psychologists also have special credentials from institutes or associations that train psychologists in the use of special counseling approaches, including hypnosis and biofeedback. Unlike *psychiatrists*, who are medical physicians, psychologists cannot prescribe or dispense drugs. They may refer to or consult with medical physicians about clients who might benefit from drug therapy. However, only physicians may prescribe medications.[6]

orthodontics
dental specialty that focuses on the proper alignment of the teeth.

prosthodontics
dental specialty that focuses on the construction and fitting of artificial appliances to replace missing teeth.

Eye examination.

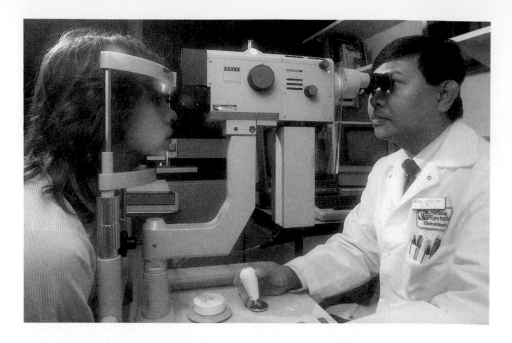

Podiatrists are specialists who treat relatively minor foot ailments. They are not board-certified medical physicians, and their training period is usually shorter than that of medical physicians. Foot disorders that podiatrists treat include corns, bunions, enlarged calluses, and structural abnormalities. Podiatrists perform foot surgery, prescribe appropriate medicines, and prescribe corrective shoes or special exercises for structural defects.

As a byproduct of the running craze in this country, the stature of podiatrists has received a large boost in recent years. Runners, shoe designers, and sports medicine personnel, including physicians, frequently consult podiatrists for their expert advice on the structure of running shoes and shoe inserts. These shoe products are designed to improve the wearability of running shoes; to prevent alignment injuries of the ankle, knee, and hip; and to prevent foot injuries.

Eye specialists fall into three specific categories. Ophthalmologists, formerly called oculists, are medical physicians who have chosen the care of eye disorders as a specialty. They can prescribe drugs and perform eye surgery if necessary to correct eye diseases or defects, including major **refractory errors** and eye muscle imbalances.

Optometrists are eye specialists who deal primarily with vision problems associated with refractory errors. They examine the eyes and prescribe glasses or contact lenses to correct visual disorders. Sometimes optometrists also attempt to correct certain ocular muscle imbalances with specific exercise regimens. Optometrists must complete rigorous undergraduate training and additional years of coursework at one of 16 accredited colleges of optometry in the United States or two Canadian colleges before taking a state licensing examination.[7]

Opticians are technicians who manufacture and fit eyeglasses or contact lenses. Although they are rarely licensed by a state agency, they perform the important function of grinding lenses to the precise prescription designated by an optometrist or ophthalmologist. To save money and time, many consumers take an optometrist's prescription for glasses or contact lenses to a large-volume retail store that deals exclusively with eyewear products.

refractory errors
incorrect patterns of light wave transmissions through the structures of the eye.

Nurse Professionals

Nurses constitute a large group of health professionals who practice in a variety of settings. Frequently, the responsibilities of nurses vary according to their academic preparation. Registered nurses (RNs) are academically prepared at two levels: (1) the technical nurse, and (2) the professional nurse.[8] The technical nurse is educated in a 2-year associated degree program. The professional nurse receives 4 years of education and earns a bachelor's degree. Both technical and professional nurses must successfully complete state licensing examinations before they can practice as RNs. At the present time, there is a critical shortage of professional nurses in the United States.[9]

Many professional nurses continue their education and earn master's and doctoral degrees in nursing or other health-related fields. Some professional nurses specialize in a clinical area (such as pediatrics, gerontology, or school health) and become certified as *nurse practitioners*.

Licensed practical nurses (LPNs) are trained in hospital-based programs ranging from 12 to 18 months. Because of their brief training, LPNs scope of practice is limited. Most LPN training programs are gradually being phased out.

Allied Health Care Professionals

Our primary health care providers are supported by a large group of *allied health care professionals*, who often take the responsibility for highly technical services and procedures. Such professionals include respiratory and inhalation therapists, radiological technologists, nuclear medicine technologists, pathology technicians, general medical technologists, operating room technicians, emergency medical technicians, registered nurse midwives, physical therapists, occupational therapists, dental technicians, physician assistants, and dental hygienists. Depending on the particular field, the training for these specialty support areas can take from 1 to 5 years of post–high school study. Most allied health care professionals must also pass state or national licensing examinations.

SELF-CARE

The emergence of the **self-care movement** indicates that many of us are becoming more responsible for the maintenance of our health. Acting individually or in groups, we are developing the expertise to prevent or manage numerous types of illness, injuries, and conditions. We are learning to assess our health status and treat, monitor, and rehabilitate ourselves in a manner that was once thought possible only with the direct help of a physician or some other health care specialist. Table 17-1 gives examples of home health test kits.

self-care movement trend toward individuals taking increased responsibility for prevention or management of certain health conditions.

The benefits of this movement are that self-care can (1) lower our health care costs, (2) be effective care for particular conditions, (3) free physicians and other health care specialists to spend time with other clients, and (4) enhance our interest in health-related activities.

In what situation is self-care an appropriate alternative to professional care? We can identify three areas. First, self-care may be appropriate for certain acute conditions that have familiar symptoms and are **self-limiting.** Common colds and flu, many home injuries, sore throats, and nonallergic insect bites are often easily managed with self-care.

self-limiting self-correcting.

Table 17-1   **Home Health Test Kits**

Brand Name	Manufacturer	How It Works	Time for Results	Price	Stated Accuracy
Pregnancy					
e.p.t. Plus	Warner-Lambert Company	Urine is dropped into test tube containing chemicals and monoclonal antibodies—pink color indicates presence of urinary HCG	10 minutes	$11	98%
Advance	ORTHO Pharmaceutical Corporation	A dipstick test using monoclonal antibodies—blue color indicates presence of urinary HCG	30 minutes	$10 to $12	98%
Acu-test	Beecham Products	Ring forms on bottom of test tube containing a few drops of urine to indicate presence of HCG	2 hours	$11 for single test, $16 for double test	98%
Diabetes: Urinary Glucose Self-Monitoring					
Tes-Tape	Eli Lilly and Company	A strip of tape is dipped into urine; the color is then compared to chart to indicate blood sugar level	A few seconds	$6.50 for 100 strips	96%
Clinitest	Ames Division of Miles Laboratories	A pill is dropped into urine; the color is then compared to chart to indicate blood sugar level	15 seconds	$6 for 100	99%
Diabetes: Blood Glucose Self-Monitoring					
Reagent strips	Various	A drop of blood is placed on reagent strip, the color change is then compared to chart to indicate blood sugar level	2 minutes	$30 to $50 for bottle of 100	96%
Glucometer II	Ames Division of Miles Laboratories	A drop of blood on reagent strip is inserted into electronic digital meter to measure blood sugar level.	1 to 2 minutes	$150	99%

Brand Name	Manufacturer	How It Works	Time for Results	Price	Stated Accuracy
Blood Pressure Monitors					
Various	Various	Blood pressure cuff and dial	5 minutes	$25 to $50	Same as in doctor's office
Various	Various	Electronic monitor recognizes heart sounds from inflated cuff and gives digital readout of blood pressure	2 minutes	$50 to $240	Same as in doctor's office
Early Colon Cancer					
ColoScreen Self-Test	Helena Laboratories, Inc.	Pad dropped in toilet turns reddish if blood in stool	30 seconds	$7	As effective as lab test
Early Detector	Warner-Lambert Company	Chemically treated tissue paper turns blue if blood in stool	1 minute	$4.99 to $6.99	As effective as lab test
Hemoccult Home Test	Menley & James Laboratories	A paper side turns blue if blood in stool sample	15 minutes	$7.49	As effective as lab test
Ovulation					
Ovutime	ORTHO Pharmaceutical Corporation	A dipstick test turns blue when mixed with urine and chemicals containing monoclonal antibodies for urinary LH	60 minutes	$35 for 6	96%
First Response	Tambrands, Inc.	Urine dropped into solution in test tube turns blue to indicate LH	20 minutes	$25 for 6	85% to 99%
Urinary Tract Infections					
Microstix-Nitrite	Ames Division of Miles Laboratories	Test strip dipped into urine changes color to indicate nitrite	30 to 40 seconds	$39 for 25	94% (with 3 consecutive morning specimens)
Venereal Disease: Gonorrhea					
V.D. Alert	Medical Frontiers, Inc.	Urethral sample collected on slide and mailed to lab	Within 2 days	$14 to $19	96%

When Using Home Tests. . .

- Check expiration date (chemicals lose potency and results could be affected)
- Store products as directed (they can be affected by heat and cold)
- Read labels and package inserts carefully; follow directions exactly
- Keep accurate test results
- Follow directions for positive, negative, and unclear results
- Use a stopwatch if precise timing is necessary
- Ask your pharmacist or physician for information when questions arise

A second area in which we might use self-care is therapy. For example, many people are now administering allergy shots and continuing physical therapy programs in their homes. Asthma, diabetes, and hypertension are also conditions that can be managed or monitored with self-care. The assistance of such groups as Alcoholics Anonymous, United Ostomy Association, and Mended Hearts also helps many persons to care for certain chronic conditions.

A third area in which self-care has appropriate application is health promotion. Weight loss programs, physical conditioning activities, and stress reduction programs are particularly well suited to self-care. In most communities a variety of organizations specialize in these areas of health promotion, including Weight Watchers, Parents Without Partners, and YMCA/YWCA fitness clubs.

People interested in practicing more self-care must be skilled consumers. The self-care marketplace is growing very rapidly and is expected to be a multibillion dollar industry by the end of the decade. A variety of books, groups, and self-care equipment is becoming available for the consumer. The box on p. 503 gives common medical tests and screening procedures that may lend themselves to self-care. Such equipment as blood pressure–measuring instruments, stethoscopes, and diagnostic kits as well as over-the-counter drugs can represent significant investments. Clearly, your money, time, and willingness to develop expertise are important components in this growing area of health care consumerism.

HEALTH CARE FACILITIES

Most of us have a general idea of what a hospital is. However, all hospitals are not alike. They usually fall into one of three categories—private, public, or voluntary hospitals. *Private hospitals* (or proprietary hospitals) function as profit-making hospitals. They are not supported by tax monies and usually only accept clients who can pay all of their expenses. Although there are some exceptions, these hospitals are generally smaller than tax-supported voluntary hospitals. Commonly owned by a group of business investors, a large hospital corporation, or a group of physicians, these hospitals sometimes limit their services to a few specific types of illnesses.

Public hospitals (also called governmental or tax-supported hospitals) are supported primarily by tax dollars. They can be operated by government agencies at the state level (such as state mental hospitals) or at the federal level (such as the Veterans Administration Hospitals and various military service hospitals such as Walter Reed Army Hospital). Large county or city hospitals are frequently public hospitals. Routinely, these hospitals serve indigent segments of the population. They also function as *teaching hospitals*.

The most commonly recognized type of hospital is the *voluntary hospital*. Voluntary hospitals are maintained as nonprofit, public institutions. Often supported by religious orders, fraternal groups, or charitable organizaitons, these hospitals usually offer a wider range of comprehensive services than do private hospitals or clinics. Many voluntary hospitals have established **wellness centers,** which provide both rehabilitation and preventive medicine. Voluntary hospitals are supported by patient fees and contributions from the community.

Regardless of the type of hospital that you are a patient in, you have a variety of rights. These are, of course, intended to protect you from unnecessary harm and financial loss. The hospital too can expect your cooperation as a patient. In the box on p. 504, you will find these relationships more fully explained.

wellness centers
units within hospitals or clinics that provide a wide range of rehabilitation, disease prevention, and health enhancement programs

Common Medical Tests and Screening Procedures

Following are some of the common medical tests and screening procedures that often compose the medical and self-care assessment first received by young adults.

PROCEDURE	PURPOSE	SETTING FOR TEST	
Breast examination	To detect lumps, thickenings, or fluid-filled cysts within tissue of the breast	Medical	Self-care
Blood pressure measurement	To detect the presence of hypertension	Medical	Self-care
Body fat measurement	To determine the percentage of body fat	Medical	Self-care
Dental evaluation	To detect dental caries, periodontal disease, or other abnormalities of the oral cavity	Dental	
Pap smear	To microscopically examine cervical cells	Medical	Limited self-care*
Pelvic examination	To visually and manually examine the vagina, cervix, and uterus	Medical	Self-care
Pregnancy test	To detect the presence of the hormone HCG, suggestive of pregnancy	Medical	Self-care
Testicular examination	To detect the presence of tumors in the tissues of the testicles	Medical	Self-care

Following are some common medical tests and screening procedures that often compose the medical and self-care assessment first received by older adults or by persons who have specific conditions requiring ongoing assessment.

PROCEDURE	PURPOSE	SETTING FOR TEST	
Blood glucose test	To determine the level of glucose in the blood	Medical	Self-care
Blood lipid study	To determine the amount and type of cholesterol and triglycerides in the blood	Medical	Limited self-care*
Complete blood count	To determine the number and type of cells and other formed elements within the blood	Medical	
Electrocardiogram	To study the electrical activity of the heart	Medical	Limited self-care*
Exercise stress test	To measure the heart's work capacity	Medical	Limited self-care*
Fecal blood	To detect the presence of blood within the feces (stool)	Medical	Limited self-care*
Mammography	To detect breast tissue masses and other abnormalities through the use of an x-ray examination	Medical	
Sigmoidoscopy	To visually examine the rectum and lower portion of the colon	Medical	
Urinalysis	To detect the presence of sugar, protein, and other substances within the urine	Medical	Limited self-care*

*Limited self-care: For those procedures identified as limited self-care, some aspect of the procedure may be undertaken without direct medical supervision, either individually or with a support group. However, evaluation and interpretation usually involve the expertise of a laboratory or other facility that by itself must be directed by a medical practitioner.

NOTE: The frequency at which these assessment procedures are undertaken depends on a number of factors. You should consult your medical practitioner to determine when these screenings are appropriate for you.

Rights: The Patient's and the Hospital's

As a patient, you can expect from the hospital:
To be treated with respect and dignity
To be afforded privacy and confidentiality consistent with federal and state law, institutional policies, and the requirements of insurance carrier
To be provided services upon request, so long as they are reasonable and consistent with appropriate care
To be fully informed of the identity of the physicians and staff providing care
To be kept fully updated as to your condition, including its management and your prognosis for recovery
To be listened to regarding your concerns over the type and extent of care received

As a patient, the hospital can expect you:
To keep all appointments
To provide all background information pertinent to your condition
To treat hospital personnel with respect
To ask questions and seek clarification about matters pertaining to your condition
To maintain the treatment indicated by your physician
To provide information needed in providing the fullest insurance coverage and to raise questions concerning hospital charges

As a patient, you may at anytime:
Refuse treatment
Seek a second opinion
Discharge yourself from the hospital

Other health care facilities include *clinics* (both private and tax supported), *nursing homes* (most of which are private enterprises), and *rehabilitation centers*. Rehabilitation centers are often supported by charitable organizations devoted to the care of chronically ill or handicapped persons, orthopedically injured persons, or burn victims.

Within recent years a number of private, 24-hour drop-in medical emergency and surgical centers have emerged. These clinics hire their own professional staffs of physicians, nurses, and allied health professionals. They provide direct competition with the larger hospital-based facilities. Some clinics specialize in women's health needs, including gynecological care, prenatal care, and childbirth services. If these organizations can provide low-cost, high-quality care, we can expect to see more of them in the future.

HEALTH SERVICE REIMBURSEMENT

Despite a decline in the inflation rate during the 1980s, the cost of health care in the United States has risen at a double-digit pace. In 1985, we spent $425 billion for health care. It has been estimated that in 1990 this figure will balloon to $625 billion.

Who pays for health care? We all do, in many different ways. We can pay directly out of our pockets for health-related products, services of health care professionals, and use of health care facilities. Other ways we finance health care are more indirect. For example, portions of our local, state, and federal taxes also help shoulder the health care bill.

Most businesses pay some or all of the cost of health insurance for their employees. Many employees consider this "free" health care, but usually their health insurance is just one part of an overall compensation package. Their company-paid health insurance is probably supported by lower employee salaries and increased costs of business products and services for the consumer. The old saying that "there's no such thing as a free lunch" is especially true when it comes to financing health care.

Health Insurance

Health insurance is a financial agreement between an insurance company and an individual or group for the payment of health costs. After paying a premium to an insurance company, the policy holder is covered for specific benefits. Each policy is different in terms of coverage for illness and injuries. Consumers must make real efforts to understand the provisions of their insurance contracts.

Merely having an insurance policy does not mean that all of your health care expenses will be covered. Most health insurance policies require various forms of payments on the part of the policy holder, which include provisions for deductible amounts, fixed indemnity benefits, coinsurance, and exclusions.

A *deductible* amount is an established amount that the insuree must pay before the insurer reimburses for services. For example, if you have been billed for $500 worth of services, your policy might require you to pay $200 before the insurance company will pay the other $300. Usually, the lower the deductible amount is, the higher your premiums will be.

A policy with *fixed indemnity benefits* will pay only a specified amount for a particular procedure or service. If your policy pays only $1,000 for an appendectomy and the actual cost of your appendectomy was $1,500, then you owe the health care providers $500. A policy with full service benefits, which pays the entire cost of a particular procedure or service, may well be worth the extra cost.

Policies that have *coinsurance* features require that you and the insurance company share the costs of certain covered services, usually on a percentage basis. One standard coinsurance plan requires that you pay 20% of the costs above a deductible amount, while the company pays the remaining 80%.

An *exclusion* refers to a service or expense that is not covered by your policy. Elective or cosmetic surgical procedures, unusual treatment protocols, prescription drugs, and certain kinds of consultations are common exclusions in many policies. Coverage for illness and injuries you already have at the time you purchase your policy (preexisting conditions) often is excluded. Also, injuries incurred during high-risk activities (ice hockey, hang gliding, mountain climbing, intramural sports) might not be covered by a policy. The best advice is to read your policy carefully to find out how broad your coverage is.

Health insurance can be obtained through *individual policies* or *group plans*. Group health insurance plans usually offer the widest range of coverage at the least expensive price and often are purchased by companies for their employees.

Fortunately, no employee is refused entry into a group insurance program. However, when employees leave the company, they often lose their group health insurance coverage. Two large, nonprofit companies that deal primarily with group plans are the Blue Cross and Blue Shield companies.

Individual policies are purchased by one person (or a family) from an insurance company. These policies are often much more expensive than group plans and may provide much less coverage. Persons who do not have access to a group plan should still attempt to secure individual policies, since the financial burdens resulting from a major accident or illness that is not covered by some form of health insurance can be devastating.

We have noticed that many students in our classes have no understanding of their health insurance. Many students think they are covered by their parents' policies, although some policies exclude coverage for children when they move away from their parents' home or when they reach age 18 or 21 years. Some students think they are covered automatically when they enroll at a college or university. However, health insurance often must be purchased individually, although it may be available for students through their schools at reduced rates. One critical time is immediately after graduation. There may be a lag of a few months before graduate school or full employment when students are not covered by any health insurance policy. It is important that these persons seek an extension of an existing policy or purchase a short-term, low-cost policy from a private insurance company. The box on p. 507 gives some health insurance consumer questions to consider before purchasing a policy.

From whom should you purchase a health insurance policy? That depends on your personal situation. As we already stated, you should first find out if you are covered by an existing policy. If you are not, shop around to find a policy that suits your needs. The box on p. 508 details various types of health insurance. There are hundreds of private commercial insurance companies that can offer you a policy. After examining some policies, you could next locate a book called *Best's Insurance Reports* to check for (among other things) the various companies' *return rates*. A return rate reflects the percentage of premiums that the company returns in benefits to insured policy holders. As a rule of thumb, you should look for a company with a high return rate—certainly at least 50%.

Health Maintenance Organizations

The emergence of *health maintenance organizations (HMOs)* during the past 10 years lends testimony to the fact that health care and preventive medicine can go hand in hand. HMOs are health care delivery plans under which health care providers agree to meet the covered medical needs of subscribers for a prepaid amount of money. For a fixed monthly fee, enrollees are given comprehensive health care with an emphasis on preventive health care. Enrollees receive their care from physicians, specialists, allied health professionals, and educators who are hired or contractually retained by the HMO. More than 100 HMOs currently exist in the United States.

One of the greatest advantages offered by HMOs involve *cost containment.*[10] Since all of the medical services within an HMO are centralized, there is little duplication of facilities, equipment, or support staff. Central filing of records allows several HMO physicians to have access to a single client's record file.

Health Insurance: Consumer Questions

Before you purchase a health insurance policy, ask yourself the following questions. The more questions you can answer with a "yes," the better you should feel that the policy you select is right for you.

GENERAL QUESTIONS

Do I really need an individual insurance policy?

Am I already covered by a group insurance policy?

Is the insurance company I'm considering rated favorably by *Best's Insurance Reports* or my state insurance department?

Have I compared health insurance policies from at least two other companies?

Does this company have a "return rate" of 50% or more?

Can I afford this insurance policy?

Do I understand the factors that might raise the cost of this policy?

SPECIFIC QUESTIONS

Do I clearly understand which health conditions are covered and which are not?

Do I clearly understand whether I have fixed indemnity benefits or full service benefits?

Do I clearly understand the deductible amounts of this policy?

Do I clearly understand when the major medical portion of this policy starts?

Do I clearly understand all information in this policy which refers to exclusions and preexisting conditions?

Do I clearly understand any disability provisions of this policy?

Do I clearly understand all information concerning both cancellation and renewal of this policy?

This saves time, administrative costs, and the overlapping of care. Furthermore, the central filing of client records lessens the chance that a patient might experience an accidental drug interaction. HMOs also routinely use health promotion activities to encourage clients to practice illness prevention.[11] All of these approaches can help lower health care costs.

One major criticism directed at HMOs is the potential lack of close physician/patient relationships. In many HMOs a client may have more than one physician. However, in most HMOs clients may select their primary practitioner if they are willing to schedule appointments well ahead of time.

Additional new approaches to reducing health costs involve the formation of *independent practice associations (IPAs)* and *preferred provider organizations (PPOs).*[12] An IPA is a modified form of an HMO that uses a group of doctors who offer prepaid services out of their own offices and not in a central HMO facility. IPAs have been viewed as "HMOs without walls." A PPO is a group of private practitioners who sell their services at reduced rates to insurance com-

Health Insurance: Types of Coverage

When considering a policy you should evaluate the following types of coverage.

Hospital. Hospital coverage refers to insurance that covers inpatient hospital expenses. With hospital expenses exceeding $600 per day, you want to be certain that your policy provides for this expense.

Surgical. Surgical coverage provides for the fees surgeons charge for specific surgical care.

Regular medical. Regular medical insurance covers physicians' fees for nonsurgical care. Often maximum benefits are specified for certain types of nonsurgical procedures.

Major medical. Major medical coverage is for unusually large, often unpredictable, medical expenses. Major medical coverage is designed to extend beyond a health insurance policy's regular medical coverage. Although major medical benefits have very high maximum benefit limits (often hundreds of thousands of dollars), these benefits are often paid on a coinsurance basis. Thus you may pay a portion of the medical expense.

Dental. Initial coverage provides for various types of dental care.

Disability. Disability insurance (also called income protection insurance) provides for income lost because of your inability to work after an illness or injury.

panies. When policy holders choose a physician who is in that company's PPO, the insurance company will pay the entire physician's fee. When a policy holder selects a non-PPO physician, the insurance company will pay only a portion of that physician's fee.

Government Insurance Plans

Medicare
contributory governmental health insurance, primarily for persons 65 years of age or older.

Created in 1965 by amendments to the Social Security Act, **Medicare** and Medicaid represent governmental types of health insurance. Medicare provides health care reimbursements primarily for persons aged 65 years or older.[13] Medicare is a *contributory program*—that is, through their working years, all employed citizens contribute a portion of their salaries (through Social Security taxes) to the Medicare fund. When they reach age 65 years, some of their health care expenses are covered by Medicare. Your parents or grandparents may be covered by Medicare. Regardless of their age, persons that require kidney dialysis are covered by Medicare.

Medicare is actually composed of two parts. Medicare A is basically a hospital insurance program. Medicare B is a voluntary program (for which the subscriber must pay a monthly fee) that supplements Medicare A. Medicare B provides regular medical insurance that covers a broad range of physicians' fees and other health care services. Both Medicare plans are subject to yearly changes in coverages and administrative procedures. With health care costs rising and Medicare coverages being increasingly restricted, many senior citizens find it necessary to purchase additional health insurance through private health insurance policies or group plans. Senior citizens should carefully evaluate these policies to be certain that they need the coverage that extends beyond medicare coverage.

Medicaid is a *noncontributory program* for citizens who are receiving other types of public welfare assistance. It is designed to provide both medical and hospital coverage. Unlike Medicare, Medicaid has no age requirements and is administered cooperatively through federal and state agencies.

Because of the bureaucracy currently surrounding these two governmental insurance programs, a number of private physicians and voluntary hospitals are reluctant to accept Medicaid and Medicare clients. A major concern now seems to be how the United States can provide proper health care for all of its citizens, including the aged, economically disadvantaged, and those whose life savings can be quickly depleted by a catastrophic illness. Currently, the federal government is considering ways to prevent its citizens from incurring huge medical expenses through the use of *catastrophic health insurance*.

Some believe that *national health coverage* can be the solution. Forms of national health coverage exist in Canada, England, and Sweden. In these countries, citizens receive "cradle to grave" health care. This coverage is supported through high rates of taxation.

One of the more recent attempts at cost containment in the area of health care is the *prospective pricing system* established in 1984 by the federal government. Under this system, Medicare reimbursements to hospitals are based upon 467 *diagnosis-related groups (DRGs)* rather than on the costs accrued by the hospitals. Each hospital stay is now assigned a DRG classification, and reimbursement to the hospital is based on that classification. This system encourages hospitals to deliver services at or below the DRG payment schedule.

Medicaid
noncontributory governmental health insurance for persons receiving other types of public assistance.

HEALTH-RELATED PRODUCTS

As you might imagine, prescription and over-the-counter drugs constitute an important part of our discussion of health-related products. The area of health care quackery, the most insidious source of health-influencing products and services, will also be considered.

Prescription Drugs

Caution: Federal law prohibits dispensing without prescription.

This FDA warning appears on the labels of approximately three-fourths of all medications. Prescription drugs must be ordered for us by a licensed practitioner. Because these compounds are legally controlled and may require special skills in their administration, our access to these drugs is limited.

Although over 2,500 compounds listed in the current edition of the *Physicians' Desk Reference* represent the drugs that can be prescribed by a physician, only 200 drugs make up the bulk of the 750 million new prescriptions and 780 million refills ordered each year.[14] The most frequently prescribed drugs are oral contraceptives and drugs used to treat infections, hypertension, gastric ulcers, pain, arthritis, and anxiety.[15] Working through physicians and pharmacists, pharmaceutical companies contribute to the improvement of health while gen-

In a few states, pharmacists are permitted to prescribe certain prescription drugs for minor illnesses. What is your opinion of this?

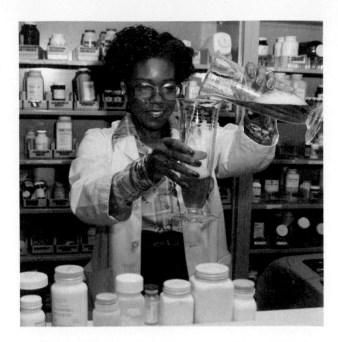

erating sales in excess of $30 billion per year. Health care dollars spent for prescription drugs account for 13% of the total health care costs accrued by Americans.[16]

Research and development of new drugs

As a consumer of prescription drugs, you may be curious about the process by which drugs gain FDA approval for marketing. The rigor of this process may be why fewer than 25 new drugs are added to our national pharmacopoeia each year and why the price of an average prescription is about $12.[14]

On a continuous basis, the nation's pharmaceutical companies are exploring the molecular structure of various chemical compounds and the chemical composition of *biologicals* in an attempt to discover important new compounds with desired types and levels of biological activity. (See the margin at left for an example of the molecular structure of a chemical compound.) Once these new compounds are identified, extensive in-house research with computer simulations and animals is required to determine whether clinical trials with humans are warranted. Of the 125,000 or more compounds under study each year, only a few thousand will receive such extensive preclinical evaluation. Even fewer of these are then taken to the FDA to begin the evaluation process necessary to gain approval for further research with humans. Once a drug is approved for clinical trials, the chemical companies can secure a patent, which prevents the drug from being manufactured by other companies for the next 17 years.

Over the course of approximately 7 years, a pharmaceutical company must supply the FDA with extensive information[14] pertaining to (1) the biological source of the new compound, (2) the steps required to manufacture the compound, (3) animal studies conducted by the company, (4) proposed clinical studies, (5) credentials of the physicians who will be involved in the clinical studies, (6) prior research on the drug, and (7) patient consent. The company must also agree to inform the FDA of all pertinent information as it is generated.

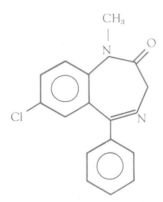

Valium (diazepam)

7-chloro-1,3-dihydro-1-methyl-5-phenyl-2H-1,4-benzodiazephin-2-one

Clinical studies with humans will be performed during the last 3 to 4 years of the 7-year period. The $70 million price tag for bringing a new drug into the marketplace reflects this slow, careful process.[14] If this 7-year process goes well, a pharmaceutical company will enjoy 10 years of protected retail sales.

Although there are claims that there is too much "lag time" involved in the FDA's drug approval process, the majority of Americans believe that the safety and effectiveness of new prescription drugs is of more importance than the time it takes to produce them. Within the last couple of years, however, a speeded-up process has been approved by the FDA for drugs that might be helpful against certain catastrophic diseases, such as AIDS, Alzheimer's disease, and some forms of cancer. However, there are many restrictions on the use of these special drugs (such as which patients may use them and which physicians may administer them). Furthermore, pharmaceutical companies are not permitted to make a profit on these drugs until additional evaluations are completed.

Generic versus brand name drugs

When a new drug comes into the marketplace, it carries with it three names: its **chemical name,** its **generic name,** and its **brand name.** While the 17-year patent is in effect, no drug with the same chemical formulation can be sold. When the patent expires, other companies can manufacture an equivalent chemical and market it under its original generic name. Because extensive research and development are not necessary at this point, the production of generic drugs is far less costly than the initial development of the brand name drug. However, some concern exists over whether certain generic drugs have the same levels of **bioavailability** as brand name drugs.

Nearly all states allow pharmacists to substitute generic drugs for brand name drugs, as long as the prescribing physician approves. Clearly, it is to the consumer's advantage to request the less expensive generic drug. In addition to substituting generic drugs for brand name drugs, pharmacists in a few states are permitted to prescribe certain drugs. What is your opinion about allowing pharmacists to engage in even limited diagnosis?

Over-the-Counter Drugs

When did you last take some form of medication? For many of you the answer might be, "I took aspirin this morning." In making this decision, you engage in self-diagnosis, determine a course for your own treatment, self-administer your treatment, and free a physician to serve a person whose illness is more serious than yours. None of this would have been possible without readily available, inexpensive, and effective over-the-counter (OTC) drugs.

In comparison to the 2,500 prescription drugs available, there are perhaps as many as 300,000 different OTC products, routinely classified into 26 different families (such as cold products and laxatives) (see the list in the margin on p. 512). Like prescription drugs, nonprescription drugs are regulated by the FDA. However, for OTC drugs the marketplace is a more powerful determinant of success.

Today OTC drugs are classified into three categories on the basis of the *safety* and *effectiveness* of their *active ingredients:* category I, drugs that have been determined to be safe and effective; category II, drugs that have not been determined to be safe and effective; and category III, drugs whose supporting data do not

chemical name
name used to describe the molecular structure of a drug.

generic name
common or nonproprietary name of a drug.

brand name
specific patented name assigned to a drug by its manufacturer.

bioavailability
speed and extent to which a drug becomes biologically active within the body; bioavailability for a drug varies between individuals and within a given individual over the course of time.

Categories of Over-the-Counter (OTC) Drugs

Antacids
Antimicrobials
Sedatives and sleep aids
Analgesics
Cold remedies and antitussives
Antihistamines and allergy
    products
Mouthwashes
Topical analgesics
Antirheumatics
Hemantinics
Vitamins and minerals
Antiperspirants
Laxatives
Dentifrices and dental products
Sunburn treatments and
    preventives
Contraceptive and vaginal
    products
Stimulants
Hemorrhoidals
Antidiarrheals
Dandruff and athlete's foot
    preparations
Bronchodilators and
    antiasthmatics
Antiemetics
Ophthalmics
Emetics
Miscellaneous internal products
Miscellaneous external products

consumer fraud
marketing of unreliable and
ineffective services, products, or information under
the guise of curing disease or
improving health; quackery.

clearly establish safety and effectiveness. Category III drugs have a limited period in which to establish safety and effectiveness.[14] The FDA's drug classification process also allows some OTC drugs to be made stronger and some prescription drugs to become nonprescription drugs (a recent example is ibuprofen).

The current labeling of OTC drugs also reflects the regulatory process described above. The labels must clearly state the type and quantity of active ingredients, alcohol content, side effects, instructions for appropriate use, and warnings against inappropriate use. Unsubstantiated claims must be carefully avoided in advertisements for these products.

As a typical consumer, you will probably purchase a variety of these OTC medications. We could not possibly describe products in all 26 general families of OTC drugs. Instead, we have chosen to include information concerning products frequently of interest to our students. Appendix 1 lists acne products, products for colds and coughs, deodorants and antiperspirants, dental hygiene products, pain relievers, and sun tanning products.

Cosmetics

Concern over the safety of cosmetics has existed for over 50 years. Hyperallergic reactions, bacterial infections, and the presence of carcinogens and teratogens (agents that cause birth defects) remain at the center of this concern. Because cosmetics are not generally classified as drugs, their regulation is limited in terms of FDA involvement. Legislation is regularly proposed that would increase the ability of the FDA to better control this important segment of the personal care retail trade.

In a recent action by the FDA, manufacturers that claimed their products delayed or reversed the aging process were ordered to remove the unproven claims from their advertisements and commercials. Retin-A, the prescription drug that has been shown to reverse some age-related changes to the skin, was not, of course, included in this action.

HEALTH CARE QUACKERY AND CONSUMER FRAUD

A person who earns money by marketing inaccurate health information, unreliable health care, or ineffective health products is called a fraud, quack, or charlatan. **Consumer fraud** flourished with the old-fashioned medicine shows of the late 1800s. During medicine shows, self-proclaimed "doctors" would sell their tonics and potions (primarily alcohol based) from covered wagons, often to gullible people who wanted cures for everything from gout to rheumatism.

Unfortunately, consumer fraud still flourishes. One need look no further than large city newspapers to see questionable advertisements for disease cures and weight loss products. Quacks have found in health and illness the perfect avenues to realize maximum gain with minimum effort.

When people are in poor health they may be afraid of dying. So powerful are their desires to live and be free of suffering that they are vulnerable to promises of health improvement and life extension. Even though many persons have great faith in their physicians, they also would like to have access to "experimental" treatments or products touted as being superior to currently available therapies. When fortified with the promise of "real help," people are willing to set aside traditional medical care.

Stocking Your Medicine Cabinet

A well-supplied medicine cabinet can be a valuable aid in maintaining a high level of health. How well supplied is yours?

SUPPLIES

Absorbent cotton

Adhesive bandages of assorted sizes

Adhesive tape

Dosage spoon (common household teaspoons are rarely the correct dosage size)

Elastic bandage

Eye cup for flushing objects out of the eye

Fever thermometer, including rectal type for a young child

First aid manual

Heating pad

Hot water bottle

Ice bag

Small blunt-end scissors

Sterile gauze in pads and a roll

Tweezers

Vaporizer or humidifier

NONPRESCRIPTION DRUG ITEMS

Analgesic—aspirin and/or acetaminophen. Both reduce fever and relieve pain; only aspirin can reduce inflammation.

Antacid

Antibacterial topical ointment

Antidiarrhetic

Antiseptic solution

Burn ointment

Calamine for poison ivy and other skin irritations

Cough syrup—nonsuppressant type

Decongestant

Emetic (to induce vomiting)—syrup of ipecac and activated charcoal to induce vomiting. Read the instructions on how to use these products.

Hydrocortisone creams for skin problems

Petroleum jelly as a lubricant

The medicine cabinet might also include antinausea medication if any family member is prone to motion sickness, a laxative, and some liniment. Seasonal items, such as insect repellents and sunscreens, round out the list.

In another sense, many victims of consumer fraud participate in their own demise. Since the days of the medicine shows, the quack has recognized that many persons have a measure of gullibility, blind faith, impatience, superstition, ignorance, or hostility toward professional expertise. The fraud provides an answer for those who believe in miracle cures.

Regardless of the specific motivation that leads people into consumer fraud, the outcome is frequently the same. First, the consumer suffers financial loss. The services on products provided are grossly overpriced and the consumers have little recourse to help them recover their money. Second, the consumers often feel disappointed, guilty, and angered by their own carelessness as consumers. Finally, consumer fraud may lead to unnecessary suffering. Far too frequently, premature deaths result from the faith that consumers place in the fraud products or services.[17]

Three areas seem particularly attractive for those who engage in health fraud. *Drugs* are often favorite **nostrums.** Because of the AIDS crisis in the late 1980s, nostrums that are touted as cures for AIDS or as boosters to the immune system are being vigorously promoted. Among these are rattlesnake venom capsules,

nostrums

ineffective medications or products sold by quacks.

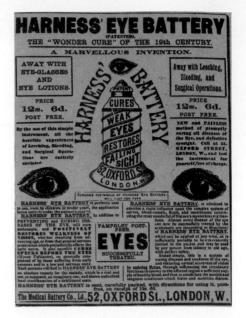

Early quackery as it appeared in the late 1800s.

extracts from geraniums, bleach-based bathing preparations, and a variety of products made from herbs. Other popular nostrums claim to inhibit tumor growth or to lower serum cholesterol.

Because many persons are overweight and a growing number of us are concerned about the quality of our diets, *food* is a second major area for health fraud. Weight reduction diets, promotion of health through certain natural and organic foods, and medical cures through dietary changes (particularly for cancer and arthritis) are a part of this area of health fraud. For example, some current food supplements claim to reduce arthritis by the ingestion of celery oil. Fraudulent diets are not only nutritionally unsound and expensive, but they also present the potential for serious damage to the body. Particularly for persons whose health is already compromised by illness, these diets may be capable of worsening health or causing death.

The third major area of health fraud involves health *devices* designed to diagnose or treat physical problems. For example, a number of current weight loss plans involve the use of placebo devices (such as ear molds, adhesive strips, ear staples, or tiny metal disks) combined with a diet plan that allows the daily consumption of only 500 to 1,000 kilocalories per day. These plans do nothing in and of themselves—they just stick to you. People who adhere to these plans will lose weight, but not because of the technology of the device. Sadly, it is relatively easy to get certain people to believe that a useless piece of equipment is at the forefront of medical science. Abraham Lincoln must have known a lot about consumer behavior when he said that "you can fool some of the people all the time."

HOW TO BECOME A SKILLED CONSUMER

After this discussion of health-influencing information, services, and products, you should be a wiser, more prepared consumer. However, information alone is not enough. We would like to offer six suggestions that may help you become a more skilled assertive consumer.

- *Prepare yourself for consumerism.* In addition to this personal health course, your university may offer a course on consumerism. Trade books on a variety of consumer topics are available in the library as well as in bookstores. Consumer protection agencies can provide direction in selected areas. Governmental agencies may also provide assistance for your consumer choices.
- *Engage in comparative shopping.* In our free enterprise system, virtually every service or product can be duplicated on the open market. Very few "one-of-a-kind" items exist. Take the time to study your choices before purchasing a product or sevice.
- *Insist on formal contracts and dated receipts.* Under the consumer laws in most states, you have a limited period in which to void a contract. Formal documentation of your actions as a consumer will provide you with the maximum protection available.
- *Obtain written instructions and warranties.* Be certain of the appropriate use of any product you purchase. If you inappropriately use a product, you might void its warranty. Be familiar with what you can reasonably anticipate from the purchases you make. Also, be aware that a written warranty supersedes any verbal assurances a salesperson might make.
- *Put your complaints in writing.* There is no substitute for a carefully constructed record of your complaints. By having accurate records of the names and addresses of all persons and companies with whom you have done business, you will be able to document your actions as a consumer.
- *Press for resolution of your complaints.* As a consumer, you are entitled to valid and reliable products and services. If your consumer complaints are not resolved, legal recourse through the courts is available. You should not hesitate to assert your rights, not only for your own sake, but for consumers who might subsequently become victims.

Consumerism is an active relationship between you and a provider. If the provider is competent and honest and you are an informed and active consumer, both of you will profit from the relationship. However, if the provider is not competent or honest, you can protect yourself by following these six suggestions.

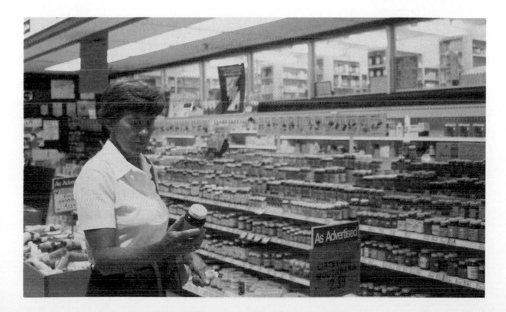

An informed consumer.

Health Consumer Skills

Circle the selection that best describes your practice. Then total your points for interpretation of your health consumer skills.

1 Never
2 Occasionally
3 Most of the time
4 All of the time

1 I read all warranties and then file for safekeeping.	1	2	3	4
2 I read labels for information pertaining to the nutritional quality of food.	1	2	3	4
3 I practice comparative shopping and use unit pricing, when available.	1	2	3	4
4 I read health-related advertisements in a critical and careful manner.	1	2	3	4
5 I challenge all claims pertaining to secret cures or revolutionary new health devices.	1	2	3	4
6 I engage in appropriate medical self-care screening procedures.	1	2	3	4
7 I maintain a patient-provider relationship with a variety of health care providers.	1	2	3	4
8 I inquire about the fees charged before using a health care provider's services.	1	2	3	4
9 I maintain adequate health insurance coverage.	1	2	3	4
10 I consult reputable medical self-care books before seeing a physician.	1	2	3	4
11 I ask pertinent questions of health care providers when I am uncertain about the information I have received.	1	2	3	4
12 I seek second opinions when the diagnosis of a condition or the recommended treatment seems questionable.	1	2	3	4
13 I follow directions pertaining to the use of prescription drugs, including continuing their use for the entire period of the prescription.	1	2	3	4
14 I buy generic drugs when they are available.	1	2	3	4
15 I follow directions pertaining to the use of OTC drugs.	1	2	3	4
16 I maintain a well-supplied medicine cabinet.	1	2	3	4

Your total points _____

Interpretation

16-24 points   A very poorly skilled health consumer

25-40 points   An inadequately skilled health consumer

41-56 points   An adequately skilled health consumer

57-64 points   A highly skilled health consumer

SUMMARY

The choices you make concerning health care information, services, and products direclty influence your health. If your consumer decisions are made after careful consideration, your health will probably be improved. Fortunately, health-related information is available from many diverse sources. It is important for you to consider the validity and reliability of health information and to evaluate how the information applies to your unique situation.

We often seek health care when we have a specific problem and need diagnostic and treatment services. The wise consumer is aware that there are other sound reasons to seek health care and a wide range of professionals who can offer health-related services. These services are available in a number of different health care facilities.

The growing self-care movement encourages consumers to be responsible for the maintenance and promotion of their health. The advantages of self-care include reduced health care costs and an increased focus on preventive health practices. Self-care can be undertaken through individual or group efforts.

Rising health care costs encourage consumers to look carefully at their health care insurance plans, particularly in regard to coverage for hospital, surgical, regular medical, major medical, and disability services. HMOs, IPAs, and PPOs represent new organizational approaches that attempt to lower health care costs.

The wise health care consumer purchases and uses prescription and over-the-counter drugs intelligently. Intelligent use involves understanding the difference between generic and brand name forms of prescription drugs and carefully reading the labels on over-the-counter drugs.

Because people desire to be healthy and free of pain, they can become targets for consumer fraud. Unfortunately, quackery can easily cause financial loss, disappointment, guilt, anger, and unnecessary suffering. Consumers should be aware that there are three areas that are particularly attractive to the health quack: drugs, foods, and health care devices.

Consumerism is a shared responsibility between the health care community and the consumer. In this chapter we have suggested six key steps that may help you become a more skilled consumer.

REVIEW QUESTIONS

1 Explain the concepts of validity and reliability as they are associated with health-related information.

2 Identify and describe some sources of health related information presented in this chapter. What factors should one consider when using these sources?

3 Point out the similarities between allopathic and osteopathic physicians. What is a nonallopathic health care practitioner? Give examples of each type of nonallopathic practitioner.

4 Describe the services that are provided by the following limited health care providers: dentists, psychologists, podiatrists, optometrists, and opticians. Identify several allied health care professionals.

5 In what ways is the trend toward self-care evident? What are some reasons for the popularity of this movement?

6 Identify and describe three general categories of hospitals. What new types of health care facilities are emerging in our society?

7 What is health insurance? Explain the following terms relating to health insurance: deductible amount, fixed indemnity benefits, full service benefits, coinsurance, exclusion, and preexisting illnesses.

8 What is a health maintenance organization? How do HMO plans reduce the costs of health care? What are IPAs and PPOs?

9 What do the chemical name, brand name, and generic name of a prescription drug represent? OTC drugs are categorized according to what two factors?

10 What is health care quackery? What can a consumer do to avoid consumer fraud?

QUESTIONS FOR PERSONAL CONTEMPLATION

1 How do you rate yourself as an informed consumer of health information, services, and products? What sources of health information have you used in making decisions? Do you believe you made wise choices based on the sources you used? What sources do you think you will use in the future? Explain your answer.

2 What health care providers have you relied on for health care in the past? Do you think your providers will change in the future? Are there any types of providers mentioned in this chapter whom you would not choose to consult? Explain your answer.

3 Illness prevention is one of the services for which you might seek a health care provider. Have you ever paid for information that would help you to prevent health problems? If you have not, would you in the future? Why do you think it is difficult to get people to seek help for preventive care when it is usually less expensive than treatment services?

4 College students are often encouraged to buy life insurance. Is life insurance more important than health insurance for young adults? Explain your answer.

5 When you read a newspaper or magazine, do some advertisements seem questionable to you? What makes these advertisements seem less than legitimate? What makes them so appealing to many people?

REFERENCES

1 Cooper, P: Better Homes and Gardens woman's health and medical guide, New York, 1981, Better Homes & Gardens.

2 Physicians' Desk Reference, ed 42, Oradell, NJ, 1988, Medical Economics Company.

3 Spock, B, & Rothenberg, M: Dr. Spock's baby and child care, Fortieth anniversary ed, New York, 1985, EP Dutton.

4 American Cancer Society: Cancer facts 1987, New York, 1987, The Society.

5 American Association of Colleges of Osteopathic Medicine: Colleges of osteopathic medicine accredited by the American Osteopathic Association, Chicago, 1987, The Association.

6 Zimmerman, JS, Ph D: Former President, Indiana Psychological Association, Personal interview, January 6, 1988.

7 Association of Schools and Colleges of Optometry, office of the executive director, Personal interview, December 15, 1987.

8 American Nurses' Association: The scope of nursing practice, NP-72 15M 6, 1987.

9 Nurses: Few and fatigued, Newsweek, 60:59-61, June 29, 1987.

10 Manning, WG, et al: A controlled trial of the effect of a prepaid group practice on use of services, New England Journal of Medicine 310:1505-1510, 1984.

11 Green, LW, and Anderson, CL: Community health, ed 5, St. Louis, 1986, Times Mirror/Mosby College Publishing.

12 Mangan, KS: New health insurance options in academe vie with traditional plans, The Chronicle of Higher Education 33:48, 8-12, 1987.

13 US Department of Health and Human Services, Social Security Administration: What you should know about Medicare, SSA pub no 05-10043, Washington, DC, 1987, US Government Printing Office.

14 Ray, O, and Kisr, C: Drugs, society, and human behavior, ed 4, St. Louis, 1987, Times Mirror/Mosby College Publishing.

15 Lawton, D, MD: Personal interview, December 15, 1987.

16 Top 200 pharmaceutical drugs, Drug Store News 9:8-12, 1987.

17 Cornacchia, HJ, and Barrett, S: Consumer health: a guide to intelligent decisions, ed 4, St. Louis, 1989, Times Mirror/Mosby College Publishing.

ANNOTATED READINGS

The Columbia University College of Physicians and Surgeons Complete Home Medical Guide, New York, 1985, Crown Publishers, Inc.

A family medical guide considered by many to be the best health reference book currently available. Content focuses on many common illnesses, pregnancy, first aid, diagnostic tests, and medical examinations.

The good housekeeping family health and medical guide, New York, 1986, Hearst Books.

A highly usable and not too technical reference book. Questions regarding many health concerns are addressed. Chapters on various medical specialities and nutrition that are commonly missing from other home medical reference books are features.

Lewith, GT, and Lewith, NR: Modern Chinese acupuncture, New York 1983, Thorsons Publishers, Inc.

Basic principles of Chinese traditional medicine, principles of therapy, and therapy of some common diseases using modern acupuncture methods are discussed. Other topics include tongue and pulse diagnosis; ear, scalp, and hand acupuncture; and how acupuncture is used as an anesthetic.

Vickery, DM, and Fries, JF: Take care of yourself: the consumer's guide to medical care, New York, 1986, Addison-Wesley Publishing Co, Inc.

A basic home medical guide that is written in a less technical manner than many other popular health reference books. Chapters cover several common health problems, home medical care, and risk reduction behavioral change.

Winter, R: A consumer's dictionary of cosmetic ingredients, New York, 1984, Crown Publishers, Inc.

Provides information about the new ingredients used in cosmetics to help you determine the "desirability or toxicity" of your cosmetics. Information covers preservatives, coloring agents, flavorings, fragrances, and processing agents. A good book for persons concerned about the safety of their cosmetics.

CHAPTER 18

Environment
Influences From the World Around Us

Key Concepts

The environment influences our health in significant, though often unnoticed, ways.

Our personal health decisions can have a major impact on our increasingly polluted environment.

Air pollution is caused by gaseous and particulate pollutants.

Water pollution makes it difficult to maintain a safe and plentiful water supply.

Land pollution is caused by solid and chemical waste products.

Radiation and noise can produce a variety of detrimental health effects.

Overpopulation produces crisis situations for many people and presents a major threat to world health.

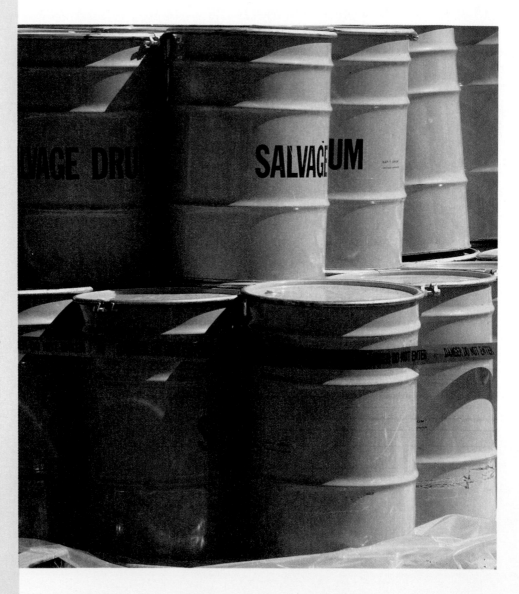

Throughout this book you have read about areas of health over which you have significant control. For example, you select the foods you eat, how much alcohol you consume, and how you want to manage the stressors in your life. You make many of these kinds of decisions on a daily basis, often subconsciously.

The study of the environment and its impact on your health provides an interesting contrast to the daily controls you have on your own health. Perhaps because of the natural processes of life and death and the vital role the environment plays, we are inclined to think that we cannot make personal health decisions concerning it. We are such a part of our environment that we may unconsciously ignore it, especially when we are more directly faced with college courses, personal relationships, growing families, and financial worries. In light of our primary concerns, it is not surprising that we tend to forget our environment's impact on us as well as our ability to have our say in its conservation or destruction.

TRANSITION TO A POSTINDUSTRIAL SOCIETY

Before the industrial revolution our environmental resources supported the physical well-being of most people. The air was crisp, the water was clean, and the land was fertile. When forms of pollution occurred, they were the results of natural events, such as floods, dust storms, forest fires, and volcanos. Agrarian living was the rule in this decentralized society. When the industrial revolution occurred at the turn of the century, many people moved to the large cities where factory labor was needed. Population growth in urban areas increased significantly faster than did growth in rural communities.

These major shifts produced problems for the health of the country. Segments of our population were subjected to overcrowding, poor sanitation and waste disposal, industrial waste, and environmental pollutants of various kinds. Over time it became clear that life in the urban centers was more precarious than that in rural areas. A few people returned to rural areas, but the majority were economically unable to move. They remained in large cities, close to the industrial centers that promised a "better tomorrow."

From an environmental point of view, this better day has not arrived. Our environment has deteriorated: our air is polluted, our fresh water is scarce, and our land is filled with toxic chemicals. Although our society is rapidly moving toward the high technology of a postindustrial society, our natural resources are dwindling to the point where even our own technologies may not be able to reduce the negative impact on our health. Let us examine our environmental issues, starting with air pollution.

AIR POLLUTION

If you think that air pollution is a modern concern reflecting technology that has gone astray, we would remind you that our air is routinely polluted by nature. Sea salt, soil particles, ash, dust, soot, microbes, assorted trace elements, and plant pollens are consistently found in the air we breathe.

Pollution caused in part by humans also has a long history. From the fires that filled our ancestors' caves with choking smoke, through the "killer fogs" of nineteenth century London, to the dust storms of the Great Depression, humans

521

A familiar source of air pollution.

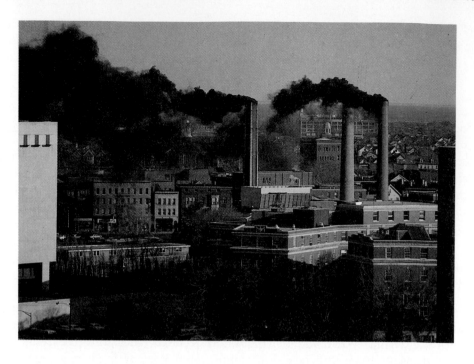

have contributed to air pollution. Only since World War II, however, has air pollution become a widely recognized concern in North America.

Sources of Air Pollution

The sources of our modern air pollutants are familiar to you. A leading source is the internal combustion engine.[1] Automobiles, trucks, and buses contribute a variety of materials to the air, including carbon monoxide and hydrocarbons. Industrial processes, domestic heating, refuse burning, and use of pesticides and herbicides contribute to our air pollution problem.

Gaseous pollutants

The pollutants dispersed into the air by the sources just identified are generally in the form of gases, including carbon dioxide and carbon monoxide. Carbon dioxide is the natural byproduct of combustion and is produced whenever fuels are burned. According to many scientists, increasing levels of carbon dioxide may result in a **greenhouse effect**. A greenhouse effect would cause the Earth's surface temperature to increase. An increase of only a few degrees Farenheit could produce significant increases in violent storms, unbearably hot summer days, and prolonged droughts.[1]

Carbon monoxide, the colorless and odorless gas produced when fuels are burned incompletely, has already been discussed in conjunction with cardiovascular disease (see Chapter 10). Also occurring in gaseous form are methane, from decaying vegetation; the terpenes, produced by trees; and benzene and benzopyrene, produced by incomplete combustion of many types of hydrocarbons, which may cause cancer when taken into the respiratory system.[2]

The nitrogen compounds nitric oxide and nitrogen dioxide and the sulfur compounds sulfur dioxide and sulfur trioxide are pollutants produced by a variety

greenhouse effect
warming of the Earth's surface that is produced when solar heat becomes trapped by layers of carbon dioxide and other gases.

of industrial processes, including the burning of high sulfur–content fuels (especially coal). When they combine with rain, nitrogen dioxide, sulfur dioxide, and sulfur trioxide convert to nitric acid and sulfuric acid. The destruction of aquatic life and vegetation in the eastern United States and Canada can be traced to **acid rain** and **acid fog.**[1] In addition, nitrous oxides, in combination with sunlight, generate the photochemical **smog,** common to major urban areas, particularly Los Angeles.

An environmental concern currently being studied is the destruction of the ultraviolet light–absorbing **ozone layer.**[3] Nitrous oxides and materials containing **chlorofluorocarbons (CFCs)** are believed to be capable of destroying this protective ozone layer within the stratosphere. Nitrous oxides come from the burning of fossil fuels like coal and gasoline. CFCs are used in air conditioners, many fast food containers, insulation materials, and solvents. As food containers and other packaging products deteriorate because of weathering, CFCs are released into the atmosphere. Upon reaching the stratosphere, the CFCs undergo the conversion shown in Figure 18-1. In 1978, freon gas (a CFC) was banned from use as a propellant in the United States, but not in most other countries.

With holes in the ozone layer already evident periodically in the Antarctic and the Arctic, the threat of increased ultraviolet radiation reaching inhabited areas is growing. The primary health dangers that are anticipated are increased skin cancers and cataracts.

Concern over indoor air pollution, particularly the presence of *formaldehyde,* is increasing within the scientific community.[4] Released from many common building materials and home furnishings, formaldehyde may be responsible for many subclinical complaints of illness and fatigue. Air sample studies are currently being undertaken to determine the extent of this pollutant. Environmentalists and health officials remain concerned over the presence of *asbestos* in insulation and other building materials. Asbestos is known to cause lung cancer.

acid rain
rain that is more acidic (lower pH) than that normally associated with rain.

acid fog
fog composed of water droplets that are more acidic (lower pH) than that normally associated with fog.

smog
air pollution comprised of a combination of smoke, photochemical compounds, and fog.

ozone layer
layer of triatomic oxygen that surrounds the Earth and filters much of the sun's radiation before it can reach the Earth's surface.

chlorofluorocarbons (CFCs)
gaseous chemical compounds that contain chlorine and fluorine.

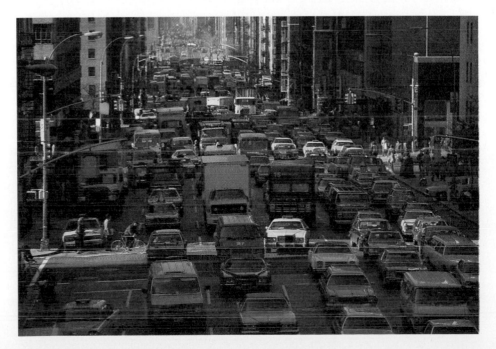

Automobiles are a principal source of air pollution.

Figure 18-1
Process in which ozone is destroyed.

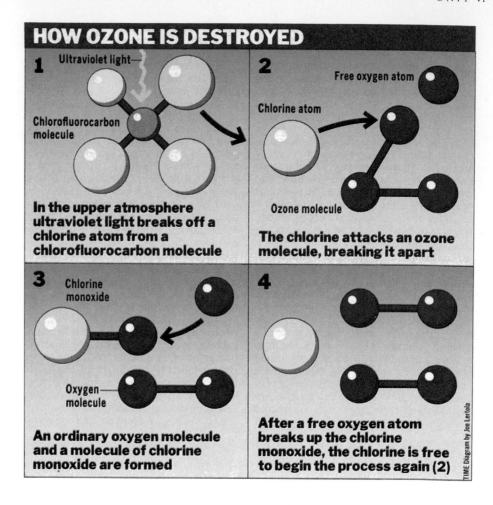

Another indoor air pollutant is cigarette and cigar smoke. The presence of tobacco smoke in the home or office not only is a health concern (see Chapter 9) but also requires that large office buildings and other public facilities be ventilated more thoroughly than would otherwise be necessary. Of course, this raises utility and maintenance costs.

Particulate pollutants

There are many *particulate pollutants*, including both naturally occurring materials and particles derived from industrial processes, mining, and agriculture. Inhalation of particulate matter can cause potentially fatal respiratory diseases, including *silicosis* from quartz dust, *asbestosis* from asbestos fibers, and *byssinosis* from cotton fibers. These conditions are frequently seen among workers in related industries. For the population in general, and especially for cigarette smokers, particulate matter in the air contributes to respiratory distress, including bronchitis and emphysema (see Chapter 9).

Trace mineral elements, including lead, nickel, iron, zinc, copper, and magnesium, are also among the particles polluting the air. Chronic lead toxicity is among the most serious health problems associated with this form of air pollution. Legislation requiring the use of nonleaded gasoline was an important step toward reducing the levels of lead in the air. Those persons who must live or work in areas that have higher than acceptable levels of lead in the air may sustain damage to hemoglobin, their gastrointestinal tracts, or their central nervous systems. Lead toxicity is disproportionately seen in young, low-income, minority children.

Influence of Climatic Factors

In addition to the gases and particulate matter in our polluted air, two climatic conditions worsen air pollution: *insufficient wind,* which restricts dispersal of the pollutants, and *highly stable air,* into which the pollutants cannot escape. Insufficient wind flow is frequently associated with high barometric pressure and land masses that block the movement of air into an area. High air stability occurs when the air surrounding a source of polluted air is warmer than the polluted air that is attempting to move upward to disperse.

Highly stable air can produce **thermal inversion.**[1] Thermal inversion occurs when a large layer of warm stable air develops above a layer of polluted cooler air, trapping the pollutants beneath it. Should an inversion develop in an area

thermal inversion
whether conditions in which a layer of warm stable air forms above a cooler, polluted layer, inhibiting dispersal of pollutants.

Main Targets of Major Pollutants in the Human Body

Body Part	Pollutants
Brain and nerve tissue	Carbon monoxide, hydrogen sulfide, lead, manganese, mercury
Nasal cavity and sinuses	Arsenic, cadmium, chromium, nickel
Respiratory passages and lining of chest cavity	Asbestos, ammonia, carbon, chlorine, cobalt, house dust, formaldehyde, fungi, hydrogen sulfide, nickel carbonyl, nitrogen oxides, ozone, pollen, quartz, silica, sulfur oxides, thiocyanate
Alveoli (of lungs)	Asbestos, beryllium, cotton fibers, hair sprays, magnesium, manganese, zinc
Heart and blood	Carbon monoxide
Blood vessels	Cadmium, fluoride
Teeth	Fluoride
Bone	Fluoride, lead, strontium-90
Skin	Arsenic, beryllium, chromium, formaldehyde, nickel, resins
Thyroid gland	Cobalt, iodine-131
Liver	Chlorinated hydrocarbons, selenium
Kidney	Cadmium, mercury
Gastrointestinal tract	Arsenic, fluoride, lead, mercury, vanadium, zinc
Adipose tissue	Chlorinated hydrocarbons

that is inclined to have poor air circulation, the cooler lower layer of air can become extremely polluted. During periods of thermal inversion, respiratory function declines rapidly in elderly persons and persons with respiratory disease.

The greater Los Angeles basin is the archetype of an inversion "haven"; abundant sunshine heats the air over the city, and the nearby mountains reduce wind flow. These forces join to bury the city in heavy smog several times each year.

Health Implications

Because of the multifaceted nature of many health problems, it is difficult to assess clearly the impact of air pollution on health. Age, gender, genetic predispositions, occupation, residency, and personal health practices complicate this assessment. Nevertheless, air pollution may severely affect health problems for elderly persons, persons who smoke or have respiratory conditions such as asthma, and persons who must work in polluted air. Fortunately, since 1975 enforcement of air quality standards has reduced levels of five major air pollutants—lead, carbon monoxide, smog, sulfur dioxide, and particulate matter.[5]

WATER POLLUTION

Although water is the most abundant chemical compound on the Earth's surface, we are finding it increasingly difficult to maintain a plentiful and usable supply. Water pollution is depriving us of the water we need to meet our personal demands (drinking, cooking, bathing, and recreation) as well as agricultural and industrial requirements.

Yesterday's Pollution Problem

Like air pollution, water pollution is not solely a phenomenon of twentieth century overpopulation or unchecked technology. Nature has, in fact, routinely polluted our surface and ground water with minerals leeched from the soil, acids produced by decaying vegetation, and the decay of animal products. Also, people have polluted their own water supplies. Waterborne contaminants that resulted in outbreaks of dysentery, typhoid fever, cholera, and infectious hepatitis can be traced to poor sanitation practices in centuries past. As recently as one generation ago, people living in rural areas occasionally found that their feed lots, chicken coops, and septic tank systems polluted their water supplies.

Today's Pollution Problem

In addition to the natural sources of water pollution already described, today's water sources are often damaged by pollutants derived from agricultural, urban, and industrial sources. Most of these pollutants are either biological or chemical products, and many can be either removed from the water or brought within acceptable safety limits. For some pollutants, however, management technology has been only partially successful or is still being developed. We can certainly expect an increase in the cost of producing the 200 gallons of water each of us needs on a daily basis.[6]

Sources of Water Pollution

Pathogens

Pathogenic agents, in the form of bacteria, viruses, and protozoa, enter the water supply through human and animal wastes. Communities with sewage treatment systems designed around a combined sanitary/storm system can, during heavy rain or snow melt, allow untreated sewage to rush through the processing plant. In addition, pathogenic organisms can enter the water supply when sewage is flushed from boats. Even swimmers can contribute pathogens to our water sources.

Pathogenic agents are also introduced into the water supply from animal wastes at feed lots and at meat processing facilities. Pet droppings have also been found contaminating water supplies.

Sewage treatment plants and public health laboratories routinely test for the presence of pathogenic agents. The presence of coliform bacteria indicates human or animal feces.

Biological imbalances

Aquatic plants tend to thrive in water rich in nitrates and phosphates. This overabundance leads to **eutrophication,** which can render a stream, pond, or lake unusable.

During hot, dry summers aquatic plants die in large amounts. Since the decay of vegetation requires aerobic bacterial action, the *biochemical oxygen demand* will be high.[2] To satisfy the biochemical oxygen demand, much of the water's oxygen is used. When such a condition exists, fish may be killed in great numbers. **Putrefaction** of the dead fish not only further pollutes the water, but also fouls the air.

Contamination of water by nitrates and phosphates can occur in a number of unintentional ways. In rural areas run-off from fields carries fertilizers into the water supply. Animal wastes contribute nitrogen and phosphorus to the water supply. Manure spread on fields can be leeched by rain and snow melt and thus reach streams and ground water supplies.

In addition, many nitrates and phosphates pass through sewage treatment facilities without being altered. Some detergents used in homes and industries contain phosphates that can pass undegraded through all but the most extensive sewage treatment process. Recognizing this problem, some states have banned the use of detergents containing phosphorus.[7]

Toxic substances

Of the pollutants found in today's water supply, perhaps none are of greater concern than toxic chemical substances. These chemical toxins, including metals as well as hydrocarbons, are dangerous because they have the ability to enter the food chain. When they do so, their concentration per unit of weight increases with each life form in the chain. This increase is called *biological magnification.*[2] By the time humans consume the fish that have fed on the contaminated lower forms of aquatic life, the toxic chemcials have been concentrated to dangerous levels.

Among the important toxic substances is *mercury,* in the form of methyl mercury. Derived from industrial wastes, methyl mercury is ingested and concen-

eutrophication
enrichment of a body of water with nutrients, which causes overabundant growth of plants.

putrefaction
decomposition of organic matter.

trated by shellfish and other fish. When humans eat these fish regularly, mercury levels increase to the point that hemoglobin and central nervous system function can be seriously altered. Death from mercury poisoning is well documented.[1]

A variety of other metals have also been found in North American rivers and lakes. Arsenic, cadmium, copper, lead, and silver are all capable of entering the food chain. In many cases, only very low levels of these metals need to be ingested before changes in health become evident.

Of the wide variety of agricultural products currently used on American and Canadian farms, **pesticides** are among the most toxic. Containing more than 1,800 different chemical compounds, pesiticides deliver a diverse array of chemicals to our water supplies.

Most serious of the toxic chemicals found in our water are the *chlorinated hydrocarbons,* including dichlorodiphenyltrichloroethane (DDT), chlordane, and chlordecone (Kepone). An incident involving Kepone (in Hopewell, Virginia) resulted in serious illnesses, including sterility, to workers in a chemical plant producing this powerful roach killer.[2] Kepone contamination of the nearby James River also destroyed aquatic life and commercial fishing. The **mutagenic, carcinogenic,** and **teratogenic** effects of these hydrocarbon products need further scientific exploration.

Polychlorinated biphenyls (PCBs) are a second group of hydrocarbons causing a great deal of concern because of their presence in the water supply.[1] PCBs are, on the basis of their chemical structure, very stable, heat-resistant compounds that have been used extensively in transformers and electrical capacitors. In many areas of the country, discarded electrical equipment has broken open and released PCBs into the surrounding water supply. Tests are now being conducted at these dump sites to determine the extent of contamination. Studies on persons who have been exposed to high levels of PCBs in drinking water are being undertaken. Relatively little is known concerning long-term exposure to these hydrocarbons. In laboratory animals, PCBs produce liver and kidney damage, gastric and reproductive disorders, skin lesions, and tumors.[1] The U.S. **Environmental Protection Agency (EPA)** has ordered all PCBs in electrical transformers be removed by 1990.

Miscellaneous sources

Three additional types of pollution that affect our water are important, although their impact on human health is not fully understood. The pollution from these sources is detrimental to aquatic life, alters the aesthetic value of our waterways, and reduces recreational use of our rivers, lakes, and shores.

Oil spills include not only the major spills resulting from tanker accidents, but also spills that occur on inland waters and those that result from the seeping of crude oil from the ground. Any kind of oil spill can foul our water. Fish, aquatic plants, sea birds, and beaches can be damaged by both surface oil film and tar masses that float below the surface or roll along the ocean bottom.

The costly vacuuming of oil, the use of detergents to break up oil slicks, and, eventually, the consumption of oil by bacteria can perhaps return polluted water to a more normal state.

Power plants that use water from lakes and rivers to cool their stream turbines cause *thermal pollution.* When this heated water is returned to its source, temperatures in the water may rise significantly. As temperatures increase, the oxy-

pesticide
agents used to destroy pests.

mutagenic
capable of promoting genetic alterations in cells.

carcinogenic
related to the production of cancerous changes; property of environmental agents, including drugs, that may stimulate the development of cancerous changes within cells.

teratogenic
capable of promoting birth defects.

Environmental Protection Agency (EPA)
federal agency charged with the protection of natural resources and the quality of the environment.

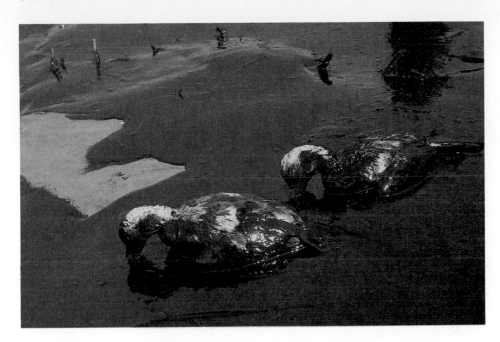

Oil spills damage water supplies and destroy wildlife.

gen-carrying capacity of the water decreases and the balance of aquatic life forms is altered. In water that is raised only 10° C (18° F) entire species of fish can disappear and aquatic plants can proliferate out of control.[8]

Sediments in the form of sand, clay, and other soil constituents regularly reach waterway channels. Rivers, lakes, reservoirs, and oceans serve as settling basins for these sediments. As land is cleared for agriculture and commercial development, the effects of sedimentation grow. Water that is polluted by these sediments is deprived of sunlight. Thus plant life is reduced and the water channels eventually become filled as the materials settle. If cleared land areas cannot be returned to vegetative cover, then dredging may be required to keep the waterway usable, although this is an expensive and relatively ineffective response.

Effects on Health

When our water becomes polluted, its quality falls below acceptable standards for its intended use, and some aspects of our health will be negatively influenced. Polluted water is associated with disease and illness, but it also distresses us emotionally, limits our social activities, and challenges us intellectually and spiritually to be more active stewards of our environment.

LAND POLLUTION

Since we live, work, and play on land, it may be difficult to believe that land constitutes only about 30% of the Earth's surface. The rest is, of course, water. When we consider the rivers, streams, marshes, and lakes found on our land surfaces, our land surface seems even smaller. Uninhabitable land areas, such as swamps, deserts, and mountain ranges, further reduce the available land on which we humans can live. Our land is a precious commodity—one that we have taken for granted.

The effects of our growing population on our limited land resources are becoming more evident. However, the greatest impact on our land comes from the products our society discards: solid waste products and chemical waste products.

Solid Waste

The trash that is collected on a weekly basis from our homes is composed primarily of disposed products used in the packaging of food and commercial items. Turk and Turk[7] estimate that if we were to accumulate all the municipal waste collected in the United States in 1 year, it would fill an area 55 square miles to a depth of nearly 5 yards.

Although numerous, our municipal waste sources make up only a fraction of the types and amounts of solid wastes we discard in this country. Agricultural wastes (three-quarters of which is manure), mining wastes (including mine tailings), and industrial wastes (including manufacturing debris) contribute much more to our solid waste problem than does municipal trash.

All four types of waste require some form of disposal. Municipal waste is collected and disposed in one of four ways.[7]

- *Open dumping.* Trash is compacted and dumped on a dump site. Unattractive and potentially harmful, open dumps are discouraged near urban areas but are still relatively common in rural areas.
- *Sanitary landfill.* Trash is compacted and buried in a man-made pit. Each day, a layer of soil is pushed over the trash to encourage decomposition, reduce unpleasant odors, and keep animals away.
- *Incineration.* Trash can be burned. This process can provide a fuel source for a community and offset the costs of expensive landfill. The effects on our air might be significant, however.
- *Ocean dumping.* Ocean dumping is a method of trash disposal that many seacoast cities use. Trash is transported by barges to offshore dump sites along the ocean bottom. Marine biologists express concern that this practice changes the natural habitat for numerous marine plants and fish.

Sanitary landfill.

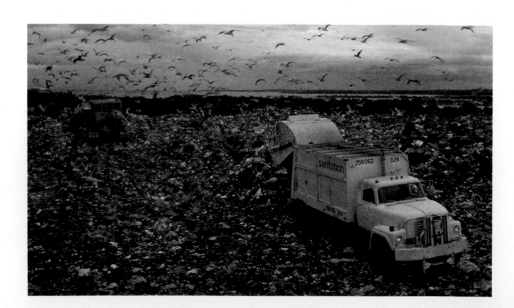

National attention was directed to the problem of municipal waste when a barge loaded with 3,200 tons of garbage left New York City to search for a site for disposal. In a period of seven weeks, the garbage barge was turned away by six states and three countries before finally returning to its port of origin for disposal. This dramatic example of the difficulty of waste disposal speaks to the need for heightened recycling efforts.

Our ability to solve our solid waste disposal problems may depend on converting many of our throwaway items into recyclable ones. It has been difficult to convince both manufacturers and the public that many of our solid waste products should be recycled. Efforts to recycle glass, aluminum, paper, and plastics have not been wholly embraced by our society, although a few communities have initiated very successful recycling programs. Are you aware of recycling programs on or near your campus?

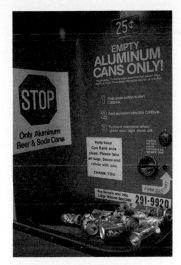

Financial incentives can encourage recycling.

Chemical Waste

According to many environmental consumer group leaders, the quality of our lives is deteriorating, in part, because of the unsafe disposal of hazardous chemicals from industrial and agricultural sources.

Perhaps the damage done to the Love Canal region of Niagara Falls, New York, has brought the fear of chemical dump sites to the forefront of the American public. The toxic waste dump site discovered in the Love Canal area was linked directly to a variety of health problems suffered by the area residents. It is estimated that there could be as many as 18,000 toxic waste dump sites sprinkled across the country.[9] Because it costs much more money to detoxify, recycle, and reuse toxic chemical products than to dump them, too many chemical companies have been more than willing to furtively and unlawfully bury their chemical wastes.

Future Love Canal–type incidents can be prevented if major governmental efforts identify hazardous dump sites, decontaminate them, and prosecute negligent companies. The EPA, through the use of monies from its $10 billion *Superfund,* is supporting the cleanup of approximately 1,000 toxic waste disposal sites in various parts of the country.[1] Additionally, state government agencies are active in the licensing and inspection of toxic waste disposal facilities. Court decisions have also forced certain negligent operators to clean dump sites and pay fines. Hopefully, inappropriate disposal of toxic wastes will decline, but who can estimate the extent of damage already done?

Debate continues over the damages attributed to the chemical **dioxin.** Found in the Agent Orange **herbicide** used in the Vietnam War, dioxin is believed by many veterans' groups to be responsible for numerous health problems seen among Vietnam veterans, including birth defects in their children. A federal court decision in 1984 tentatively approved a compensatory settlement of $180 million to Agent Orange victims.[10] Research studies published at the same time of this court decision, however, failed to identify relationships between exposure to dioxin and serious health problems.[11,12] More recent studies suggest a correlation between Agent Orange exposure, lymph node tumors, and birth defects.[8]

The disposal of dioxin-based herbicides in landfills in various areas of the country remains a source of concern. The presence of dioxin in the soil and in ground water supplies may prove to be a more serious threat than that associated with its use in Agent Orange.

dioxin
powerful and potentially harmful chemical compound found in some herbicides.

herbicide
chemical compound used to kill vegetation.

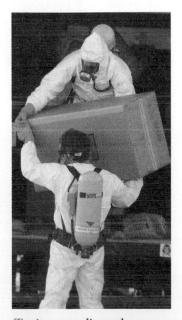

Toxic waste disposal.

Pesticides

Since Rachel Carson[13] wrote her now-classic book *Silent Spring* in 1962, the public has been aware of the potential dangers associated with the use of some pesticides. Although Carson's primary concern was with the pesticide DDT, a number of other hazardous pesticides have since been removed from the marketplace. Tighter controls established by the EPA have restricted the availability of other less hazardous pesticides. Clearly, farmers need to use effective poisons to save their crops from insect destruction. However, equal concern seems to be focused now on the effects of pesticides on water supplies, soil quality, animals, other insects, and humans. Figure 18-2 shows the delicate balance between the factors within an **ecosystem**. Harmful agents, such as pesticides, can enter an ecosystem and effect the entire food chain.

One pesticide that recently received careful scrutiny was *ethylene dibromide* (EDB). EDB has been sprayed on fruit and grain crops and grain-processing equipment. In 1984 when scientists discovered that EDB could be a powerful cancer-causing agent in humans, the EPA banned its use.[14]

The world's worst industrial accident took place at a pesticide plant in Bho-

ecosystem
an ecological unit made up of both animal and plant life that interact to produce a stable system.

Figure 18-2
An example of an ecosystem. Some pesticides do not harm the food chain.

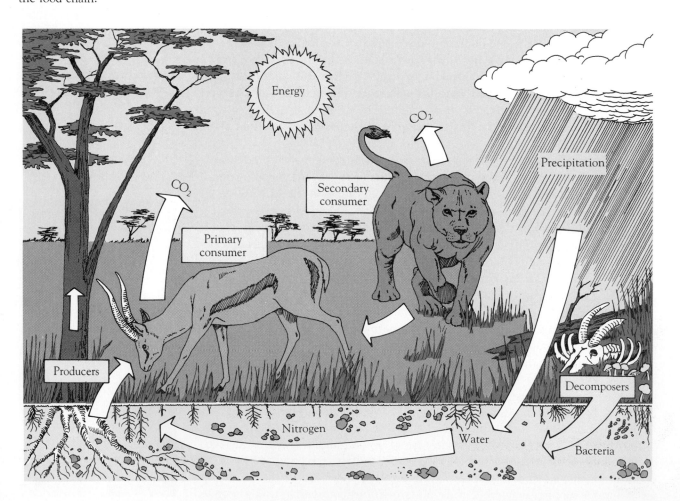

pal, India. In December 1984, the Union Carbide India Limited pesticide plant accidentally emitted over 16 tons of the chemical methyl isocyanate vapor into the air of neighborhoods adjacent to the plant. Within a few days, approximately 2,500 people died and between 80,000 and 90,000 others were injured—many with lung damage, eye injuries, and liver and kidney disorders. This tragedy reminds us of the precarious relationship between our expanding technology and our immediate environment.

RADIATION

We live in the nuclear age. Actually, our society has been in the nuclear age since the atomic bomb was first developed at the end of World War II and subsequently dropped on the Japanese cities of Hiroshima and Nagasaki. Scientists then discovered that by bombarding the nucleus of a heavy element (such as uranium) with neutrons, they could actually split the atom's nucleus and cause the release of vast amounts of energy. This process, called *atomic fission*, has brought with it both great hopes and concerns for the future.

The hopes for nuclear energy primarily lie in its enormous potential for us to reduce our dependency on fossil fuels as energy sources. Also, nuclear energy can (and already does) improve our industrial and medical technology, as evidenced by an expanding use of radioactive materials in the diagnosis and treatment of various health disorders. Some physicians now specialize in "nuclear medicine." A new allied health professional certification also exists in nuclear medicine technology.

The two greatest concerns over nuclear energy are (1) the negative health effects that come from day-to-day exposure to radiation and (2) the potential for nuclear war and subsequent global catastrophe. Fission produces not only great energy, but also **ionizing radiation** in the form of radioactive particles. These particles affect our health when they enter our bodies. *Alpha particles,* although not capable of penetrating the skin through particle streams called alpha rays, can pose a health threat if they are either inhaled or ingested. *Beta particles,* which have better penetrating power than do alpha rays, can disrupt the organization of human body cells by damaging the molecules that make up living protoplasm. *Gamma rays* are streams of radioactive particles that have the greatest ability to penetrate deeply into body tissue and produce significant damage.

ionizing radiation
form of radiation capable of releasing electrons from atoms.

We are already exposed to various forms of ionizing radiation on a daily basis, through natural radiation, including ultraviolet radiation from the sun and natural radioactive mineral deposits, and man-made radiation, including waste from nuclear reactors, industrial products, x-ray examinations, and **nuclear fallout.** Most of these exposures we get on a daily basis produce negligible health risks. Although it is clear that no kind of radiation exposure is good for you, safe levels of exposure are difficult to determine.

nuclear fallout
radioactive debris that reaches the Earth's surface after a nuclear explosion.

Health Effects of Radiation Exposure

The health effects of radiation depend on many factors, including the duration, type, dose of exposure, and individual sensitivity. Clearly, heavy exposure (as in a nuclear explosion or major nuclear accident) can produce **radiation sickness**

radiation sickness
illness characterized by fatigue, nausea, weight loss, fever, bleeding from mouth and gums, hair loss, and immune deficiencies, resulting from overexposure to ionizing radiation.

or immediate death. Lesser exposures can be quite harmful as well, as Dasmann states[15]:

In lesser, but still heavy doses, from heavy atmospheric fallout, from nuclear plant accidents, and the like, it can cause radiation sickness, from which most people will die more slowly. In still small amounts, it can cause cancer, which takes longer to kill. If it strikes egg or sperm cells, fertilized eggs, embryos, or fetuses, it can cause genetic abnormalities. No ionizing radiation is good for you.

From a health perspective the message is clear. Avoid any unnecessary exposure to radioactive materials. Make it a point to question the value of diagnostic x-ray examinations, especially routine dental and chest x-ray studies and mammograms. Routine x-ray studies have been discouraged by numerous professional societies and consumer groups. Furthermore, if your skin is fair, you should limit your exposure to solar radiation.

Threat of Nuclear War

Aside from the physical threats that may result from exposure to nuclear radiation, the fear of a nuclear war seems to be increasing with each decade. At a time when the world political and economic situation has become more turbulent and unpredictable, more countries are acquiring the technology not only to produce nuclear energy for peaceful purposes, but also to manufacture nuclear weapons.

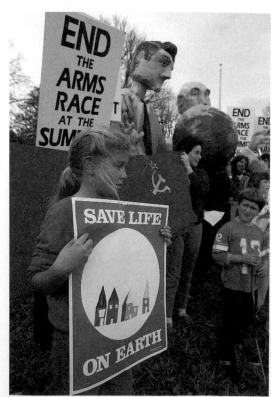

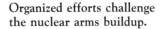
Organized efforts challenge the nuclear arms buildup.

A Nuclear Autumn

Many questions about the validity of the nuclear winter hypothesis have emerged since its introduction in 1984. Using complex computer models, other scientists have concluded that the effects of a limited nuclear war might not produce the profound changes leading to a nuclear winter. Rather, they predict a less devastating scenario that is called "nuclear autumn." In a nuclear autumn, global temperature decreases would be less than in a nuclear winter. Worldwide, fewer people would die from starvation, and agricultural production could resume more quickly. Regardless of which situation results from a nuclear engagement, the effects would be catastrophic. The question of total annihilation versus "survival of a few" should not deter us from pursuing nuclear disarmament.

The nuclear weapons buildup has escalated to the point that world superpowers have the capability to destroy the Earth (as we know it) many times over. The possibility of our survival after nuclear war appears to be remote, since the damage to the balance of nature would be overwhelming.

This damage is reflected in the concept of **nuclear winter.** Popularized by astronomer Carl Sagan and environmentalist Paul Ehrlich, this concept hypothesizes a lowering of atmospheric temperature by 30° C (54° F) or more for a period of several months following a major nuclear exchange.[16] This decrease in temperature would result from a loss of solar energy due to a thick layer of smoke, dust, and debris. This temperature change would destroy most forms of life, including the human race. Some scientists suggest that the nuclear winter theory is too drastic, and that a less severe "nuclear autumn" may occur (see the box above).

As yet, political attempts at nuclear disarmament and eventual arms reduction have not been especially fruitful, although they are ongoing. In 1988 the SALT (Strategic Arms Limitation) Treaty was signed by the United States and the Soviet Union. Arms limitations negotiations are continuing. One major thrust that seems to be exerting pressure on the superpowers is the peace (or antinuclear) movement. Especially active in Western European countries through such groups as the Green Party (West Germany) and the Committee for Nuclear Disarmament (England), the peace movement serves as a voice of conscience. By actively resisting nuclear buildup and by educating the world's publics about the consequences of nuclear accidents or nuclear war, this movement has grown to an extent that it cannot be ignored. In the United States and Canada, the peace movement is represented by such groups as Ground Zero, Nuclear Weapons Freeze Committee, Physicians for Social Responsibility, and Union of Concerned Scientists.

On a less visible level, certain elected government officials are strong supporters of reducing the global nuclear buildup. You may decide to become involved in the activities of these people as part of a personal stand against nuclear war.

nuclear winter
the lowering of atmospheric temperature caused by the loss of solar heat resulting from dust covering produced during nuclear war.

Nuclear power plant.

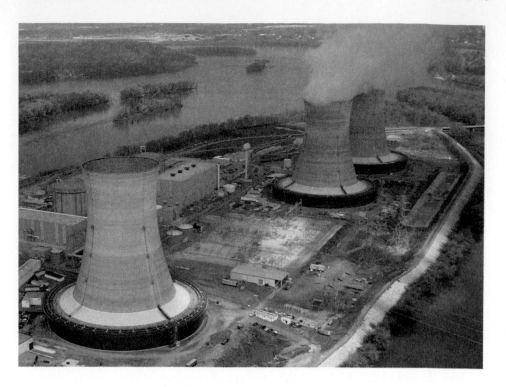

Nuclear Reactor Accidents and Waste Disposal

To generate the nuclear energy to produce electrical energy, more than 100 nuclear power plants have been constructed in North America. Built mostly by utility companies, these nuclear power plants were designed to produce electrical energy in an efficient, economical, and safe manner. Much public criticism has been directed at these power plants, claiming that their safety and efficiency have not been documented.

The safe disposal of nuclear waste is a major problem that also has not been fully solved. The byproducts of nuclear fission remain radioactive for many years. Although the current method for disposing of these wastes is to bury them, the question of eventual leakage into our environment is a valid one.

Some have suggested transporting nuclear waste into outer space or dumping it in uninhabited areas of the Artic or Antarctic. Neither approach seems feasible for now. Two more plausible methods are (1) above-ground storage in concete-enclosed steel tanks and (2) the conversion (transmutation) of dangerous waste into less dangerous byproducts.[9]

Furthermore, construction costs and safety features of nuclear reactor sites are being questioned by prominent laypersons and scientists. Who will pay for the construction cost overruns? Who will pay for the cleanup of an accident at a reactor site? How real is the possibility of a major accident at a nuclear reactor site in the U.S.? Could a terrorist attack result in a nuclear catastrophe? These questions do not have simple answers.

Proponents of nuclear power maintain their stance that not one person in the U.S. has died as the result of a power plant accident. They point to a spotless safety record and reiterate that our fossil fuel supply is limited. Supporters of the nuclear industry feel that a public commitment to establishing more nuclear reactors is important for the future of our country. Currently, nearly 20% of our electrical energy is generated by nuclear power. Would an increased reliance on nuclear power place us at greater risk for a major accident? The debate continues.

Perhaps some of the answers to the above questions were obtained on April 26, 1986, when a **meltdown** occurred at the Chernobyl nuclear power plant in the Soviet Union. Human error was responsible for creating a situation in which excessive heat was allowed to build up in the core of the nuclear reactor. The resultant explosion instantly killed two people and hospitalized 500. Eventually 29 people died. Radioactive fallout descended mostly on Europe, but was reported throughout the world (see Figure 18-3). Although Chernobyl's remaining victims are expected to live, it is projected that they will have slightly higher instances of cancer and that their offspring could experience slightly increased chances of genetic defects.[17]

meltdown
the overheating and eventual melting of the uranium fuel rods in the core of a nuclear reactor.

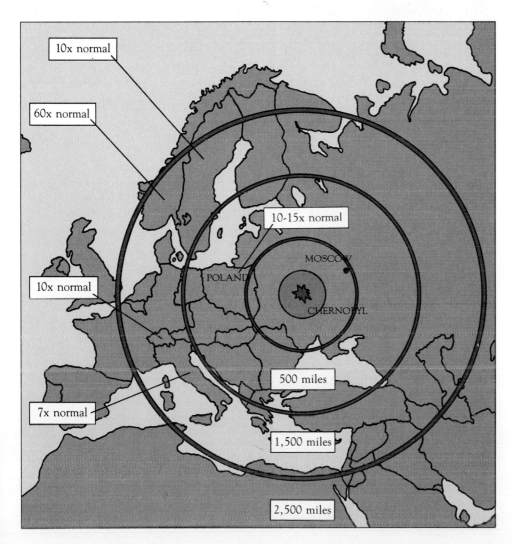

Figure 18-3
Radiation levels emitted after the Chernobyl nuclear accident.

Personal Assessment

Estimate Your Exposure to Radiation

Calculate your average annual exposure to radiation by filling in the blank spaces in the column on the right.

Radiation Source	Estimated Annual Dose (in millirems)
NATURAL RADIATION	
Cosmic rays from space	
At sea level	__40__ (U.S. average)
Add 1 mrem for each 100 feet you live above sea level	_____ (Your Risk)
Radiation in rocks and soil (ranges from 30-200)	__55__ (U.S. average)
Radiation from air, water, and food (ranges from 200-400)	__25__ (U.S. average)
RADIATION FROM HUMAN ACTIVITIES	
Medical and dental x-rays and treatments	__80__ (U.S. average)
Working or living in a stone or brick building (add 40 for each, if applicable)	_____ (Your risk)
Smoking one pack of cigarettes per day (add 40 mrem)	_____ (Your risk)
Nuclear weapons fallout	__4__ (U.S. Average)
Air travel: add 2 mrem a year for each 1500 miles flown	_____ (Your risk)
TV or computer screens—add 4 mrem/year for each 2 hours of exposure per day	_____ (Your risk)
Occupational exposure (depends on occupation)	__0.8__ (U.S. Average)
Living next to a nuclear power plant (boiling water reactor, add 76 mrem; pressurized water reactor, add 4 mrem)	_____ (Your risk)
Living within 5 miles of a nuclear power plant (add 0.6 mrem)	_____ (Your risk)
Normal operation of nuclear power plants, fuel processing, and research facilities	__0.1__ (U.S. average)
Miscellaneous—industrial wastes, smoke detectors, certain watch dials	__2__ (U.S. average)
Your total points	_____

Interpretation

The average annual exposure per person in the United States is 230 mrem. Of this, 130 mrem comes from natural radiation and 100 mrem comes from human activities. Your exposure may be considerably higher than this depending on your place of residence, water supply, medical tests and treatments, occupation, and specific health behaviors, including smoking and exposure to sun.

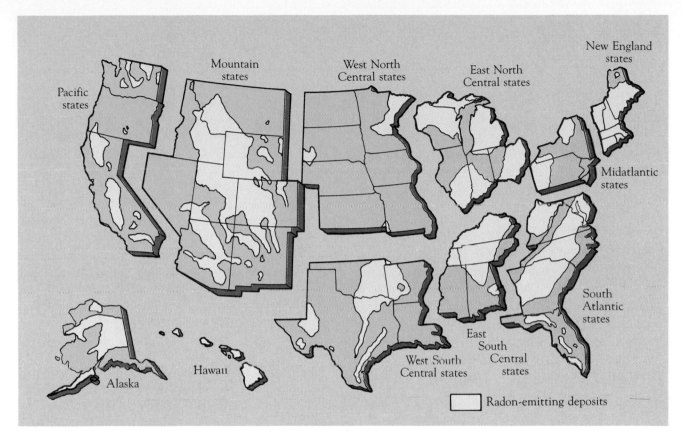

Radon Gas

Perhaps the form of radiation exposure that strikes closest to home is **radon gas**. Released from underlying rock formations and stone building materials, this radioactive gas is being found in unacceptably high levels in well-insulated structures. Radon gas concentrations within the stagnant air of energy-efficient "airtight" homes, schoolrooms, and buildings exceed those found in less well-insulated dwellings. The EPA estimates that 20,000 of the 130,000 deaths from lung cancer are caused by exposure to radon gas. Figure 18-4 shows radon gas deposition in the United States. Homeowners can purchase inexpensive kits that test their homes' level of radon gas. In homes that have unacceptably high levels of radon gas (estimated to be 12% of all homes in the United States), the cost of installing adequate ventilation systems may range from approximately $300 to $5,000.[18]

Figure 18-4
Mineral deposits in the U.S. that emit radon.

radon gas
a naturally occurring radioactive gas produced by the decay of uranium.

NOISE POLLUTION

In much the same fashion that a weed is an unwanted plant that can ruin our lawn, noise is an undesirable sound that can be detrimental to our overall health. Today's world is characterized by noise whose loudness and unrelenting presence are not only unpleasant but also dangerous to our health. Noise can reduce our hearing acuity, disrupt our emotional tranquility, infringe upon our social interactions, and interrupt our concentration.

Noise-Induced Hearing Loss

Sound, or a wave of compressed air molecules moving in response to a pressure gradient, is characterized by two qualities—*frequency* and *intensity*. Intensity is primarily responsible for the loss of **auditory acuity** experienced by many persons living in noise-polluted environments. Intensity of sound exceeding 80 to 85 *decibels* (1,200 to 4,800 cycles per second frequency range) can cause hearing damage.[2] The box on p. 541 shows sound intensity associated with several common environmental sound sources. How many of these daily sounds are familiar to you?

The interpretation of a sound (hearing) is a sophisticated and sensitive physiological process involving the progressive conversion of acoustical energy to mechanical energy, then to hydraulic energy, and, finally, to electrochemical energy. Electrochemical energy is subsequently transmitted by the acoustic nerve to the brain for interpretation. The destructive influence of exposure to sounds of high intensity lies in the destruction of special *hair cells* in the *cochlea* that are responsible for converting hydraulic energy into electrochemical energy. Rock music, jet engine noise, vehicular traffic, and a wide range of industrial noises can collapse these sensitive cells. Ironically, the cells that are damaged are those responsible for hearing the high-frequency sounds associated with normal conversation. Thus the environmental sources of noise rob you of your ability to hear sound of a far greater value—the sound of the unamplified human voice.

The damage just described is initially reversible. However, with continued exposure, the changes in the sensitive cells of the inner ear become permanent. Because the hearing loss inflicted by intense environmental sound is so serious, **audiologists** are now stating that most persons older than 15 years are no longer capable of having *maximum auditory acuity*.

auditory acuity
clarity or sharpness at which a particular sound can be heard.

audiologists
health care professionals trained to assess auditory function.

Urban noise pollution.

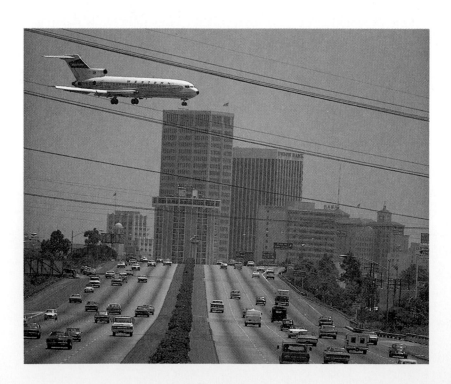

Noise Pollution and its Effects on Hearing

The loudness of sounds is measured in decibels (dB). Sound intensity is determined logarithmically, not arithmetically. Each increase of 10 dB produces a tenfold increase in sound intensity. Thus 30 dB has 10 times the intensity of 20 dB, 40 dB has 100 times the intensity of 20 dB, and 110 dB sounds 10 times as loud as 100 dB. Hearing damage depends on the dB level and the length of exposure. Presented below are dB ranges, common sources, and effects on hearing.

Decibel	Common Sources	Effect on Hearing
0	Lowest sound audible to human ear	
30	Quiet library, soft whisper	
40	Quiet office, study lounge, bedroom away from traffic	
50	Light traffic at a distance, refrigerator, quiet conversation, gentle breeze	
60	Air conditioner at 20 feet, normal conversation, sewing machine	
70	Busy traffic, noisy office or cafeteria	Annoying, and may start to affect hearing if constant
80	Heavy city traffic, alarm clock at 2 feet, typical factory	Start to affect hearing if exposed more than 8 hours
90	Truck traffic, noisy home appliances, shop tools, lawn mower	Temporary hearing loss can occur in less than 8 hours
100	Chain saw, pneumatic drill (jackhammer), loud motorcycle or farm equipment	Unprotected exposure for 2 hours can produce serious damage to hearing
120	Rock band concert in front of speakers, sandblasting, loud thunderclap	Immediate danger threat
140	Shotgun blast, jet plane from 50 feet	Immediate pain threat; any length of exposure is dangerous
180	Rocket pad area during launch (without ear protection)	Immediate, irreversible, and inevitable hearing loss

Noise as a Stressor

In addition to the damaging effects of noise on auditory acuity, the role of noise as a stressor has long been recognized. Indeed, the absence of noise (silence) and prolonged noise are both proven techniques to break the will of prisoners during war. Recently, however, attention has shifted to the role of noise in terms of the stress response, studied in Chapter 3. In people stressed by unrelenting noise, the enhanced epinephrine output contributes to hypertension and other stress-related health problems.

Noise Pollution Reduction

Beyond giving your political support to legislation and enforcement policies designed to reduce environmental noise pollution, what can you do to lessen the degree of noise pollution in your life? The box on p. 541 lists common noise sources and their effect on hearing. The suggestions appearing below are only a few of the recommended approaches:

- Limit your exposure to highly amplified music. The damage from occasional exposure to sound intensity between 110 and 120 decibels can be reversible. Daily exposure, however, will result in permanent hearing loss.
- Reduce the volume on your portable headsets. When others can hear the music coming through your headset while you are wearing it, you should probably turn down the volume.
- Wear ear plugs (wax or soft plastic) and sound-absorbing ear muffs when using firearms or operating loud machinery.
- Maintain your automobile, motorcycle, or lawn mower exhaust systems in good working order.
- Furnish your room, apartment, home, and office with sound-absorbing materials. Drapes, carpeting, and cork wall tiles are excellent for reducing both interior and exterior noises.
- Establish noise reduction as a criterion in selecting a site for your residence. An apartment complex near a freeway or airport or property near an interstate highway may prove to be less than desirable.

Since you are a person with a lifetime of hearing ahead, noise pollution reduction deserves your participation and your support.

WORLD POPULATION GROWTH

Population Growth

World Population Growth Between 1950 and 2000 (in billions):

Developed countries	Undeveloped countries	TOTAL
0.832	1.732	2.564
1.268	4.891	6.159

It is difficult for many of us to grasp the significance of the population projections for the turn of the century—now less than 12 years in the future. From a global perspective, for every two persons on Earth in 1975, there will be three by the year 2000. This is a 50% increase in population! Forecasts by *The Global 2000 Report to the President of the U.S.* place the world population at over 6 billion at the turn of the twenty-first century.[19]

Effects of Unchecked Growth

Perhaps these figures have little impact on most of us in Western society because we have never really felt the consequences of overcrowding to the extent that some underdeveloped countries have. Our growth increase is projected to be much slower than the rates in other countries. Our technology and economic systems have, by and large, been able to help us avert the major population-related crises that have occurred in the less developed countries. Certainly our own overcrowding has led to pollution, congested cities and freeways, and sprawling suburban areas. For underdeveloped countries, however, the population explosion has led directly to human misery—misery that nearly defies description.

Understandably, it is estimated that 90% of the world population growth by the year 2000 will take place in these less developed countries—third world countries that can least afford to accommodate such population increases. Population experts use such adjectives as "enormous," "catastrophic," and "overwhelming" when they write about the effects of this population explosion in less developed countries. The following are among the predicted effects[19]:

- There will be fewer resources, with enormous declines in fresh air, fresh water, forest land, agricultural land, and forage land. By the year 2000, some experts project a loss of between 15% and 20% of the Earth's total species of plants and animals.
- Food prices will double.
- Energy costs will soar.
- The economic gap between rich and poor countries will become magnified.

These effects will, of course, become most pronounced in the health of the people in underdeveloped countries. *The Global 2000 Report*[19] states in a succinct, dispassionate fashion that:

Hunger and disease may claim more lives—especially lives of babies and young children. More of those surviving infancy may be mentally and physically handicapped by childhood malnutrition.

R.F. Dasmann,[15] in his text *Environmental Conservation,* paints an even more desperate view of the future:

One thing is certain. Population growth of the magnitude we have seen in recent years will not continue. Either people will begin to die in greater numbers than any of us would care to contemplate, or they will learn to limit birth rates. There are no other ways. We are reaching the end of the line.

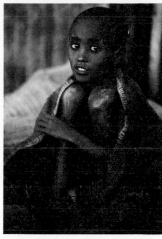

An innocent victim of world hunger.

Answers to the Problem

On paper, the answers to population growth seem relatively simple. *The Global 2000 Report* has recommended that the developed countries help underdeveloped countries to improve social and economic conditions, reduce birth rates, manage resources, and protect the environment. However, the principal problem is achieving sufficient cooperation in a world that currently has few effective mechanisms for solving complex problems. Compounding this problem are the facts that some religions prohibit the use of contraception, some countries promote

Live Aid for Africa involved worldwide support.

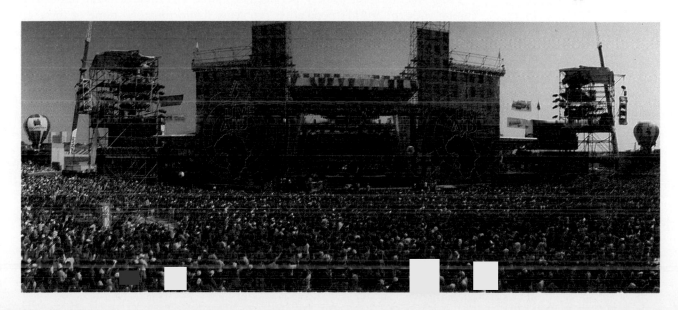

Personal
Assessment

Environmental Ethics

Indicate your level of agreement for each of the following statements. Total your points and check the interpretation following the quiz.

1   Disagree
2   Undecided
3   Agree

Humans are more valuable than any other aspect of nature.	1	2	3
Natural resources exist for human consumption.	1	2	3
Success is measured by production and consumption of material goods.	1	2	3
Human ingenuity will ensure that adequate resources will exist in the future.	1	2	3
Science and technology is capable of shaping an environment to meet all human needs.	1	2	3
Humans have a right to the highest standard of material living.	1	2	3
The major purpose of government is to ensure that its citizens have access to everything they desire.	1	2	3
The ideal person is a self-made person who does as he or she wants.	1	2	3

Your total points _____

Interpretation

8-12 points   Reflects an ethic of environmental stewardship
13-20 points   Reflects an undecided ethical standard
21-24 points   Reflects an exploitive environmental ethic

population growth for political reasons, and many of the world's poor people have little education and even less access to family planning services.

From our Western society perspective, there are three general options for coping with the world's population problems. Unfortunately, none of these options can guarantee success. The first option is to become considerably more involved in other countries' efforts to control population rates, as *The Global 2000 Report* suggested. This approach lacks support because of its expense.

A second option is to continue our "middle ground" efforts (such as the fragmented approaches to control world population and hunger by certain government, religious, and volunteer programs). These efforts clearly are not solving the problems. Although well-intentioned, these efforts reach only a small portion of the affected populations.

A third choice—to isolate ourselves—may be the only realistic choice that we will have by the turn of the twenty-first century. This alternative would make each country solely responsible for its own economic and human hardships. Certainly, this action could produce horrible, perhaps heinous consequences, but it might be the only way the Earth can be saved during your lifetime or the lifetimes of your children. We may find ourselves caught between a potentially immoral decision (to isolate ourselves), an implausible decision (to maximize our aid to other countries), and an ineffective decision (to continue our current efforts).

SIMPLIFYING OUR ENVIRONMENT

How often have you heard people yearn for a return to the "good old days"? They reminisce about times when people once moved more slowly, cared more for their neighbors, and appreciated their natural resources. After listening to these nostalgic impressions, you could believe that our society was once almost idyllic—with little or no pollution, population concerns, or threats of nuclear accidents.

Certainly it is nice to dream, but it is doubtful that our advancing technology and exploding worldwide population will permit us to find such an ideal world. Instead, we need to focus on finding the appropriate balance between technological growth and environmental deterioration. Perhaps, some of the organizations listed in the box below can help us in our efforts.

We must learn to think beyond the present. Each decision we make for the future should be considered in light of its influence on our environmental systems. If our future decisions are based solely on financial gain or personal convenience, we will be committing a monumental disservice to our children and future generations.

Organizations Related to Environmental Concerns

FEDERAL DEPARTMENTS, AGENCIES, AND OFFICES

1 Environmental Protection Agency, 401 M St. S.W., Washington, DC 20460; phone: 202-382-2090

2 Council on Environmental Quality, 722 Jackson Pl. N.W., Washington DC 20503; phone: 202-395-5750

3 Department of Energy, Forrestal Bldg., 1000 Independence Ave. S.W., Washington, DC 20585; phone: 202-586-6210

4 Department of Interior, Interior Bldg., C St. (between 18th and 19th) N.W., Washington, DC 20240; phone: 202-343-1100

5 National Oceanic and Atmospheric Administration, Rockville, MD 20852; phone: 301-433-8910

6 United States Fish and Wildlife Service, Washington, DC 20240; phone: 202-343-4717

NATIONAL ORGANIZATIONS

1 National Wildlife Federation, 1412 16th St. N.W., Washington, DC 20036-2266; phone: 202-797-6800

2 Sierra Club, 730 Polk St., San Francisco, CA 94109; phone 415-776-2211

3 Cousteau Society, Inc., World Headquarters, 930 W. 21st St., Norfolk, VA 23517; phone: 804-627-1144

CANADIAN ORGANIZATIONS

1 Environment Canada, Ottawa, Ontario K1A 1G2; phone 819-997-1441

2 Conservation and Protection Service, Place Vincent Massey, Hull, P.Q. Ottawa, Ontario K1A OE7; phone 819-997-1575

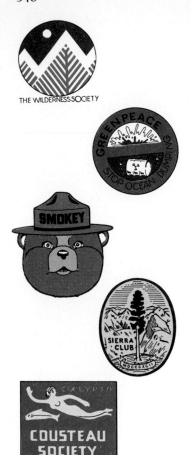

Your Role in Creating a Sustainable Environment

As we search for solutions to complex environmental problems we may have to make some difficult decisions. For example, will third world populations be forced to use contraception or sterilization? Will we attempt to feed the world's hungry people? Will we continue to protect endangered species of plants and animals? Will we strive more forcefully for nuclear disarmament? Can we commit ourselves to cleaning up all of our toxic waste sites? Answers to these complex questions regarding *stewardship* will probably be based not only on our knowledge but also on our moral predispositions.

Answers to these sorts of complex questions can come from recognizing the value of a *sustainable environment.* This environment will be developed only when individuals and groups are willing to:

- Evaluate their environment
- Become environmentally educated
- Choose a simpler, less consumption-oriented lifestyle
- Recognize the limitations of technology in solving problems
- Become involved in environmental protection activities
- Work with people on all sides of environmental issues[1]

These suggestions might sound abstract for a person confronted with a local environmental problem. However, each of these steps can be applied to a local situation with only limited modifications. The PCB soil contamination in Indiana, the nerve gas weapons storage in Kentucky, the toxic waste site cleanup in Missouri, and the transportation of nuclear waste materials in California and other states represent local issues to which these steps can be applied. Are you committed enough to a sustainable environment to practice these steps?

SUMMARY

It is important for us to recognize the impact our personal decisions have on the future of our environment. The manner in which we care for our environment will reflect how much we value our health.

Pollution affects all aspects of the environment; air, water, and land. Gasseous and particulate matter combine with climatic conditions to boost air pollution to unhealthy levels. Biological and chemical wastes reduce our usable water supply. Solid waste and chemical waste products damage our land. Indoor air pollution, including radon gas, is a growing concern. If not monitored carefully, all of these pollutants can pose risks to our health.

The nuclear age threatens our environment with radiation and nuclear energy. The two greatest concerns over nuclear energy are the negative health effects of radiation and the possibility of nuclear war.

Another environmental pollutant is noise. Since noise can impair our overall health, it is important that we learn to practice noise reduction.

Overpopulation presents a major threat to a healthy world environment. People in underdeveloped countries are especially affected by overpopulation. Approaches to solving this problem are often hampered by political and religious ideologies. A sustainable environment raises many difficult questions. This environment will be achieved only when the majority of people adopt the practices described above.

REVIEW QUESTIONS

1 How has the shift to a postindustrial society increased the pollution of our environment?

2 What are the leading sources of air pollution in our society? What two major categories of pollutants contribute to air pollution? Define the greenhouse effect. What two climatic conditions play an important role in bringing air pollution to serious levels? Explain how these conditions magnify the air pollution problem.

3 Explain the role of nature in water pollution. How have people polluted their own water supplies? Identify and explain a variety of water pollutants presented in this chapter.

4 What are the two types of waste products that have the greatest impact on land pollution? Identify and explain the four ways that municipal waste is collected and disposed. Why has toxic chemical pollution continued despite the recognized health hazards? What role have pesticides played in environmental pollution?

5 What are some of the principal concerns over nuclear energy? Identify the health effects of radiation exposure. How can you avoid unnecessary exposure to radioactive materials? What is radon gas?

6 Identify the detrimental effects that noise pollution has on our health. Identify some of the approaches you may take to reduce noise pollution.

7 What are the predicted effects of overpopulation? What segments of the world are most seriously affected by overpopulation? Why? What solutions are recommended to solve these problems?

QUESTIONS FOR PERSONAL CONTEMPLATION

1 Consider how you treat the environment on a day-to-day basis. In what ways can you become a better steward of the environment? What are your responsibilities when you see others harming the environment?

2 How do you feel about radiation and the possibility of nuclear war? What do you think life on Earth would be like after a nuclear war? What steps can you take to help prevent a nuclear war?

3 As a college student, you are probably exposed to considerable noise. In what ways do you contribute to noise pollution? Do you believe that other kinds of pollution are more significant than noise pollution? In the future, do you plan to reduce your exposure to noise?

4 Imagine that you are in a very crowded room. Someone locks the door and tells you that you must stay in there for 1 year. What kinds of problems do you foresee? Can you think of ways these problems might be avoided without people leaving the room? How does this hypothetical situation differ from the problem of overpopulation? In what ways do you feel this problem can be solved?

REFERENCES

1 Miller, G: Living in the environment ed 5, Belmont, Calif, 1988, Wadsworth, Inc.

2 ReVelle, P, and ReVelle, C: The environment: issues and choices for society, ed 3, Boston, 1988, Willard Grant Press.

3 Botkin, D, and Keller, E: Environmental studies: earth as a living planet, Columbus, Ohio, 1987, Merrill Publishing Co.

4 Godish, T: Indoor air pollution in offices and other nonresidential buildings, Journal of Environmental Health 48:190-195, 1986.

5 US Environmental Protection Agency: Trends in the quality of the nation's air, Washington, DC, 1984, US Government Printing Office.

6 Moon, R: Representative of the Indiana-American Water Co, Personal interview, December 29, 1987.

7 Turk, J, and Turk, A: Environmental science, ed 3, Philadelphia, 1984, WB Saunders Co.

8 Chiras, D: Environmental science: a framework for decision making, ed 2, Menlo Park, Calif, 1988, The Benjamin-Cummings Publishing Co.

9 EPA Fights Hazardous Waste: Interview with Lee Thomas, Assistant Administrator for the EPA Solid Waste and Emergency Response, EPA Journal, 10:4-7, 1984.

10 McGowan, J: Agent Orange: payment pleas begin today, USA Today September 26, 1984, p 4a.

11 Erickson, J, et al: Vietnam veterans' risk for fathering babies with birth defects, The Journal of the American Medical Association 252:903-912, 1984.

12 Suskind, R, and Hertzberg, V: Human health effects of 2, 4, 5-T and its toxic contaminants, The Journal of the American Medical Association 251:2372-2380, 1984.

13 Carson, R: Silent spring, Boston, 1962, Houghton Mifflin Co.

14 EDB risk is real: get it out of food, USA Today, January 16, 1984, p 8a.

15 Dasmann, RF: Environmental conservation, ed 5, New York, 1984, John Wiley & Sons, Inc.

16 Ehrlich, PR, et al: The cold and the dark: the world after nuclear war, New York, 1984, WW Norton & Co., Inc.

17 Gale, RP: Immediate medical consequences of nuclear accidents: lessons from Chernobyl, The Journal of the American Medical Association 258:625-628, 1987.

18 Radon: no threat to sneeze at, US News & World Report, August 25, 1986, p 10.

19 Barney, GO: The global 2000 report to the President of the US: entering the 21st century, vol 1, New York 1980, Pergamon Press, Inc.

ANNOTATED READINGS

Bergin, EJ, and Grandon, RE: The American survival guide: how to survive in your toxic environment, New York, 1984, Avon Books.

Information on PVC, PCB, dioxin, asbestos, formaldehyde, and pesticides is presented. The book also discusses common myths about toxic chemicals (what they are, who is using them, and how to avoid them) and explains how to evaluate your own workplace and the warning signs of toxic poisoning. It includes appendices of state agencies, consulting firms, and superfund sites.

Boyle, RH, and Boyle, AR: Acid rain, New York, 1983, Schocken Books, Inc.

Discusses the causes of acid rain, the scope of the problem, and the effects of the problem on humans, wildlife, water, and our culture. It presents a view of the political delays and industrial arguments that have prevented the problem from being solved and also proposes some solutions.

National Wildlife Federation: Conservation directory 1988, ed 33, Washington, DC, 1988, The Federation.

A comprehensive list of international, national, regional, and state organizations, agencies, and officials concerned with natural resource use and management. It includes addresses, phone numbers, services, and names of officers for each organization.

Ehrlich, PR, et al: The cold and the dark: the world after nuclear war; the long-term consequences of nuclear war, New York, 1984, WW Norton & Co, Inc.

Presents a scientific view of the world after a nuclear war. It describes what a nuclear winter is, and the destructive results on plants, animals, and humans. Presents the atmospheric, climatic, and biological consequences of even a small nuclear conflict. Includes a dialogue between U.S. and Soviet scientists.

Epstein, SS, et al: Hazardous waste in America: our number one environmental crisis, San Francisco 1982, Sierra Club Books.

Explains what hazardous wastes are, how they threaten our lives and our environment, and why our industries produce these wastes. They also provide information on how congress writes laws to protect the public and how they are enforced. Case studies are presented and 14 appendices of references are included. One of the appendixes is a directory of 8,000 hazardous waste dump sites.

Wattenberg, BJ: The birth dearth, New York 1987, New York, Pharos Books.

Is the United States reproducing too slowly? Will we some day face a shortage of workers, taxpayers, consumers, and soldiers? This book suggests that, in fact, we might be reproducing too slowly. Approaches to counter the current trend in low reproduction are presented.

Throughout Unit VI we have explored the health-related issues of consumerism and the environment. Now we will relate these topics to the important developmental tasks of identity, independence, responsibility, and social interaction. Although each of you will be in a particular setting with unique opportunities, we believe that this exploration will be beneficial to you.

■ **Forming an Initial Adult Self-Identity** Whether we are able to admit it or not, we all want to find out "who we are." To develop the confidence to face the world and to contribute to its improvement require that we come to grips with our personal strengths and limitations. Although it may be valuable to be able to understand and analyze others, it is much more significant that we discover, develop, and define our own identity. Examining our attitudes and behaviors about health consumerism and the environment can help us learn about ourselves.

In the area of self-care, you can examine how you value and manage your health; we learn about ourselves as we consider how we take care of ourselves when we are ill. Are you a person who must always visit a doctor when ill, or are you able to cope reasonably well with self-limiting conditions? Are you a skilled consumer in purchasing prescriptions or over-the-counter medications? How frequently do you promote your own health by eating properly, exercising, and getting adequate rest? Honest answers to these kinds of questions will help you understand your unique identity.

■ **Establishing a Sense of Relative Independence** Gaining a sense of independence can be a refreshing, exciting experience for most young adults. For traditional-age students, becoming independent from your family provides the chance for you to undertake new and diverse experiences. Relocation, employment, and new friendships will propel you into consumer involvement on a scale greater than that required while you were at home or in college.

Besides choosing new health care providers, you will independently obtain the insurance needed to pay for these services. Health insurance and disability insurance are critical investments you must make. Independence often brings with it new acquaintances who may attempt to push you into areas of consumerism for which you have no legitimate need. Start preparing yourself now to live and work among people who will try to influence your consumer perspectives.

■ **Assuming Increasing Levels of Responsibility** Along with the independence gained through adulthood comes a new kind of freedom—the freedom to decide for yourself which kinds of social issues you want to become involved with. Of course, a number of emerging, independent adults may feel that their responsibilities lie only with themselves. However, a new kind of activism seems to be emerging from young adults as we move into the 1990s. The self-indulgence of the early 1980s may have run its course. Volunteerism is on the rise in movements that feed the hungry, provide shelter for the homeless, improve literacy, and protect the environment. Will you be a participant?

■ **Developing the Skills for Social Interaction** Regardless of whether we are involved in decisions related to our environment or our consumer choices, we frequently make these decisions with other individuals, companies, or agencies. Our social skills help us convey our needs, interpret directions, and voice our concerns. Effectively speaking, listening, writing, reading, and working cooperatively with others are the tools we need to refine as we work to improve our health or the health of others.

Sometimes in the areas of consumerism and environment, the social interactions we have with others may not always be pleasant. For example, voicing a complaint about a health-related product may require a face-to-face confrontation with a store manager. Speaking up at a public debate on a local environmental issue might be intimidating. Poise, tact, and a degree of assertiveness may be beneficial in both of these situations. Fortunately, these social skills can be developed and sharpened with practice.

UNIT VII

The last unit examines two topics that many traditional-age students initially prefer not to study: aging and death. These topics seem to run counter to a culture that idolizes youth, vitality, and health. However, as you will discover, most midlife and elderly adults are relatively satisfied and pleased with their movement into new segments of the life cycle. Understandably, the content of Unit VII is closely related to each of the five dimensions of health.

- **Physical Dimension of Health** The inevitability of aging and death is beyond questioning. Unless we die suddenly at an early age, most of us will go through years of relatively good physical health before we reach a period of gradual decline. Eventually we will experience an extended period of failing health. Our deaths will probably result from a chronic health condition that our bodies cannot successfully overcome. The prospect of our decline and eventual death can seem unpleasant to contemplate.

The above scenario is somewhat depressing because it has packed 50 to 60 years of physical change into one short paragraph. Overall, the physical changes described are those of decline, but this one-sided view neglects the fact that many persons today enjoy their highest levels of physical health late in life. As a part of a larger societal movement toward exercise, weight management, smoking cessation, and moderation in alcohol use, today's older adults often indicate that they are physically healthier than they were just a few years ago. This is an optimistic sign for young and old alike.

- **Emotional Dimension of Health** The events associated with aging and death often influence the emotional dimension of health. The independence of grown children and the move to retirement can tax one's emotional health. Even the lack of change in life experience can influence how an aging person feels. For some persons, a life that continues unchanged will be seen as positive and stable, whereas for others it will produce stress or changes in mood, outlook, and self-perception.

Another powerful stressor to the emotional dimension of an older person's health is the death of a spouse or close friend; this event reminds aging people that their lives are limited, and a major challenge to their emotional stability often takes place.

- **Social Dimension of Health** Three significant challenges to the social dimension of health for older persons are the independence of their children, the death of a spouse or close friend, and the evolution of the neighborhood or town in which they live. When these events occur, many familiar, comfortable social relationships can be strongly influenced. Older persons may not have the interest and skill to replace these social contacts. Here is where a younger person can be quite helpful. You can do your best to fill the void created by these personal and social changes.

- **Intellectual Dimension of Health** Intellectual activity holds value to the overall health of older individuals. Contrary to popular assumption, older persons do not experience a major loss in their intellectual capacities. Fortunately, persons who continue intellectual activity also tend to continue physical activity and social involvement and thus maintain their health resources.

- **Spiritual Dimension of Health** The maturing of the spiritual dimension of health centers on an inward search that is evident in the form of overt behaviors. You can support an older person's need for introspection by recognizing his or her desire to, for example, participate in religious services, visit an art gallery, or attend a musical concert. You can be genuinely interested in an older adult's recollections of past experiences. Your willingness to discuss such topics as dying and death can also help an older person in the inward search for meaning.

Probably no other topic in this book is tied as closely to the spiritual dimension of health as dying and death. Perhaps this is true because dying and death are mystical phenomena which provide the perfect avenue for an examination of our spiritual existence.

Growing Older

Balancing Your Future
with Your Past

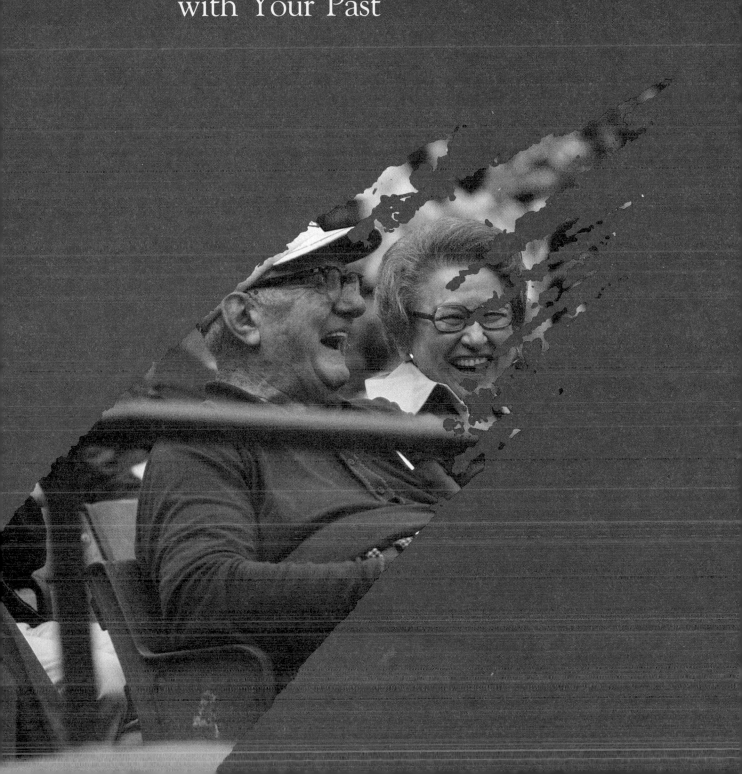

The Maturing Adult
Growing Older in America

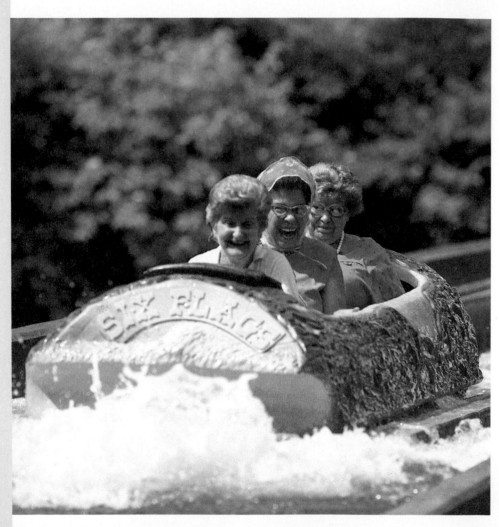

W hat does it mean to be growing, developing, and aging? It probably depends on your perspective. For traditional-age college students, growing and developing are usually positive experiences. They reflect a movement in the direction of future resources, recognition, and opportunity. Aging, in contrast, is perceived more negatively. Aging reflects a movement away from the very accomplishments and abilities toward which young people strive.

For college students who are in midlife (between 45 and 65 years of age) or are elderly (older than 65 years), all three terms might be equally positive. Growing and developing imply a potential for improvement, whereas aging reflects maturation, valuable insights, and sharpened skills.

In this chapter we will consider growing, developing, and aging in terms of the second half of the life cycle. Regardless of your perspective (as a traditional-age or nontraditional-age student), we hope that you will be able to visualize this time span as a potentially meaningful one.

AN OPTIMISTIC VIEW OF AGING

It is not uncommon for our students to find the study of the aging process some-what depressing. With each passing day, semester, or year, they realize that they are getting closer to "old age," and may consider it a frightening prospect. Certainly, such a perspective can become a self-fulfilling prophecy.

Perhaps we can dispel some of these fears by reporting that most of the stereotypes of old age have little factual foundation. Growing old does not have to be unenjoyable. In fact, most older people report that they are generally happy and satisfied. Intelligence, creativity, attractiveness, physical fitness, and sexual intimacy can all last a lifetime, as long as people continue to participate in the activities that enhance these qualities.

The phrase "use it or lose it" may be a good focus for you as you move through your life cycle. Rather than deny your aging, keep a positive attitude. By looking beyond the stereotypes of aging and by participating in growth-enhancing activities, your movement through life's stages will be enjoyable and meaningful.

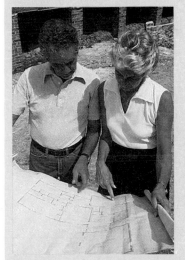

Planning for the future is important throughout life.

DEMOGRAPHIC ANALYSIS OF AGING

Data provided by the federal government allow us to observe our aging population in light of many variables, including representation within the total population, marital status, income, level of education, and living arrangements. This demographic information provides interesting generalizations about our older citizens.

Data for 1985 indicate that 75 million of our 241.5 million citizens were over the age of 45 years. 9.0 million are between 75 and 85 years, 2.8 million are over 85 years of age, and 25,400 are over 100 years of age.[1] Of these 75 million, more than one third (29 million) were over the age of 65 years. When viewed as a percentage of the total population, nearly 12% of our citizens are over 65, while nearly one third (31%) are middle aged (between 45 and 65 years) or older.[2] Figure 19-1 depicts the growth of older people between 1987 and 2025.

In our discussion of marriage in Chapter 14 we indicated that approximately 80% of adults marry, and that remarriage often follows divorce. This tendency

Figure 19-1
The population growth of older people.

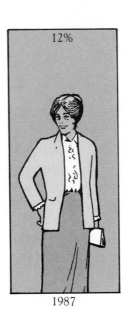
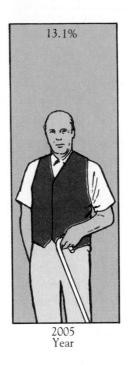
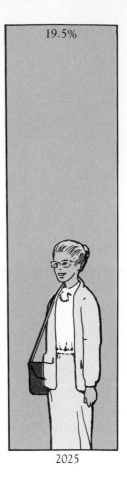

19.5%

13.1%

12%

1987   2005   2025
              Year

holds true for men 45 to 74 years of age. Just over 80% of men between 45 and 74 years of age are married. Approximately 70% of men above 76 years of age are married.[2]

In comparison to men, women are far less likely to be married during the second half of the life cycle. Although approximately 75% of women at age 45 years are married, by retirement age only 50% have a husband.[2] This rate primarily reflects not divorce or singlehood, but the fact that men die at a younger age than women.

Where do the older members of our population live, and under what arrangements? Census data reveal that California, New York, Florida, and Texas lead the other states in terms of the absolute number of older persons. When viewed in terms of a state's total population, the highest percentages of retirement-age persons are found in Florida, Rhode Island, Pennsylvania, Iowa, and Arkansas.[2] Can you speculate why these states are so attractive to the elderly?

Regardless of where older citizens choose to reside, they are strongly inclined to live in a household setting. Whether living alone, with a husband or wife, or with a grown son or daughter, almost all retirement-age persons live in a household as opposed to a nursing home, hospital, or **extended care facility**[2] (see Figure 19-2). Even when husbands die prematurely, most widows choose to spend their remaining years in familiar household surroundings.

extended care facility institution designed to provide long-term medical or custodial care for persons who do not require hospitalization.

Contrary to what some younger persons might believe, only a small percentage (5%) of the elderly are permanently institutionalized.[3] Nursing homes serve as primary alternatives to a household setting only when the needs of the elderly cannot be met by themselves, their families, or their friends.

Regardless of where you live or how old you are, living requires an income sufficient to meet the most basic demands. Food, clothing, shelter, and health care costs can quickly deplete the income of older persons after they retire from the work force.

There is a progressive decline in income experienced by persons as they move through the second half of the life cycle (see Figure 19-3). Income for a single person drops nearly 44% between ages 55 and 80 years, whereas income earned by a couple drops 64% between ages 55 and 80 years. Certainly some of this decline is a result of retirement. Unfortunately, social security payments alone are rarely sufficient to meet the financial needs of older persons. According to 1985 figures, the median income for families whose head of household is 65 years

Figure 19-2
Current living arrangements of the elderly.

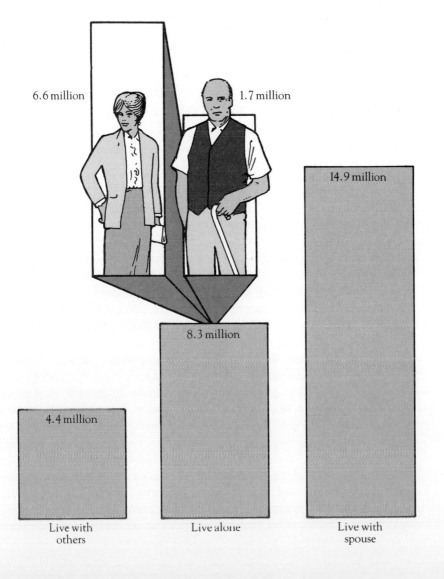

6.6 million

1.7 million

14.9 million

8.3 million

4.4 million

Live with
others

Live alone

Live with
spouse

Figure 19-3
Income decreases as
we age.

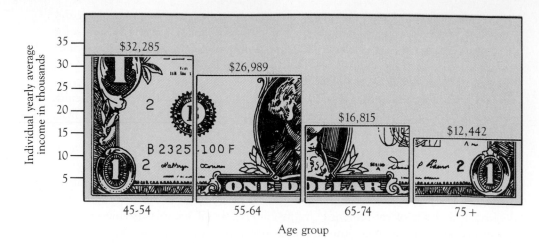

or older was $19,162.[2] Only older adults who save money regularly, invest wisely, or establish personal pension plans at a younger age can live comfortably in our current economic times. Have you started to plan for your own retirement?

A final demographic characteristic of the elderly is the increasing amount of formal education they have. Census Bureau data from 1985 reveal that nearly 48% of people over 65 years of age have completed high school and 9% have completed 4 or more years of college. Hopefully, this increased level of education is enhancing the quality of the elderly years.

AGING PHYSICALLY: A PROCESS OF DECLINE

Regardless of the emotional, social, intellectual, and spiritual gains that occur during the adult years, physical decline is inevitable. From the fourth decade onward, a gradual decline in vigor and resistance eventually gives way to various types of dysfunction. In the opinion of many authorities, people do not die of old age. Rather, old age worsens specific conditions responsible for death. This process of decline can be described on the basis of predictable occurrences[4]:

- *Change is gradual.* In aging, there are gradual changes in structure or function whose presence predates the diagnosis of the specific condition.
- *Individual differences occur.* When two people of the same age are compared for the type and extent of change that has occurred with age, marked differences can be noted. Even within the same person, different systems decline at differing rates and to varying extents.
- *Greatest change is noted in areas of complex function.* In physiological processes involving the interplay of two or more major body systems, the most profound effects of physiological aging can be noted.
- *Homeostatic decline occurs with age.* Regardles of whether a diagnosable disease process exists, becoming older is associated with a growing difficulty in maintaining homeostasis. In the face of stressors, the older adult's system takes longer to respond, does not respond with the same magnitude, and may take longer to return to baseline.

Like growth and development, aging is predictable yet unique for each person.

Tissue, Cellular, and Subcellular Theories

Scientists are currently seeking an explanation of why organs become dysfunctional. Many diverse theories that focus on tissue changes, cellular changes, and subcellular changes have been proposed.[5,6]

- **Collagen cross-linking.** Collagen, the molecular building material of connective tissue, appears to undergo progressive structural change with age. Because of the importance of this tissue to the structure of many important organs, collagen changes eventually alter the organ's function.

- *Loss of cellular homogeneity.* As tissue regenerates, there is a loss of order in the tissue caused by subtle changes in the size, shape, and function of the replacement cells. Eventually, the tissue becomes so altered that its own function may be lost. This results in a pathological process in the organ.

- *Accumulation of harmful waste products.* Over time, metabolic efficiency within the cells decreases. Faulty oxidation of *metabolites* results in the production of toxic products, including *lipofuscin,* a pigment found in the tissue of the elderly at autopsy. *Amyloid,* a protein-related waste, is also found and probably represents altered oxidation processes.

- *Accumulation of faulty protein.* Whether resulting from defective prescription for the composition of the protein or faulty synthesis in the *ribosomes,* the cells of the elderly may produce defective proteins. Enzymes, hormones, and cellular structures requiring protein are negatively affected. Thus organ systems begin to decline.

- *Error accumulation hypothesis.* The growth and maintenance of tissue require the continuous duplication of cells. The genetic message contained in the DNA of each cell must be replicated, and each division exposes the genetic material to insults of various types. At some point tissue function too is altered and organ systems begin to falter.

- *Programmed aging.* The most hypothetical construct to account for the aging process suggests that a primitive "script" is written into the genetic message contained in each cell. A biological clock controls the *doubling rate* of each tissue type. The maximum time available to any person is reflected in the concept of the "life span."

collagen cross-linking
An alteration in the normal alignment of collagen strands; causes a loss of normal elasticity.

Sexuality and Aging

Frequently, our students are concerned about how aging affects sexuality. This is understandable because we live in a society that idolizes youth and demands performance. Many college students become anxious about growing older because of what they think will happen to their ability to express their sexuality. Interestingly, students are willing to accept other physical changes of aging (such as the slowing down of basal metabolism, reduced lung capacity, and even wrinkles) but not those changes related to sexuality.

Most of the research in this area suggests that older people are quite capable of performing sexually. As with other aspects of aging, certain anatomical and physiological changes will be evident, but these changes do not necessarily reduce one's ability to enjoy sexual activity. Most experts in sexuality report that many older persons remain interested in sexual activity. Furthermore, persons

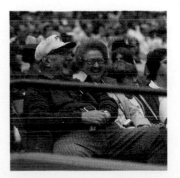

Enjoying the later years.

Sexual attraction continues throughout the adult years.

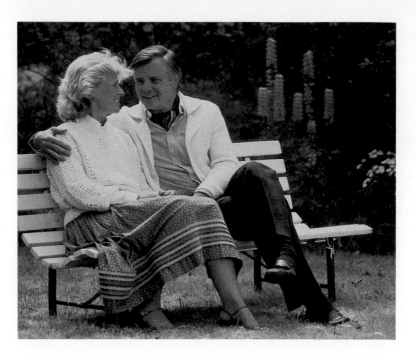

who are exposed to regular sexual activity throughout a lifetime report being most satisfied with their sex lives as older adults.

As people age, the likelihood of alterations in the male and female sexual response cycles increases. In the postmenopausal female, vaginal lubrication commonly begins more slowly and the amount of lubrication is usually diminished. However, clitoral sensitivity and nipple erection remain the same as in earlier years. The female capacity for multiple orgasms remains the same, although the number of contractions that occur at orgasm typically is reduced.[7]

In the older male, physical changes are also evident. This is thought to be caused by the decrease in the production of testosterone between the ages of 20 and 60 years. After age 60 or so, testosterone levels remain relatively steady. Thus many males, despite a decrease in sperm production, remain fertile into their eighties. Older males typically take longer to achieve an erection (however, they are able to maintain the erection longer before ejaculation), have fewer muscular contractions at orgasm, and ejaculate less forcefully. The volume of seminal fluid ejaculated is typically less than in earlier years and its consistency is somewhat thinner. The resolution phase is usually longer in older males.[7] In spite of these gradual changes, some elderly males engage in sexual intercourse with the same frequency as do much younger males.

HEALTH CONCERNS OF MIDLIFE ADULTS

The period between 45 and 65 years of age brings with it a variety of subtle changes in the body's structure and function. When life is busy and the mind is active, these changes are generally not evident. Even when they become evident, they are not usually the source of profound concern. Your parents, older students in your class, and persons with whom you will be working are, nevertheless, experiencing these changes[5]:

Loss of some musculoskeletal integrity
Decrease in bone mass and density
Increase in vertebral compression
Degenerative changes in joint cartilage
Increase in adipose tissue—loss of lean body mass
Decrease in capacity to engage in physical work
Decrease in visual acuity
Decrease in basal energy requirements
Decrease in fertility
Decrease in sexual function

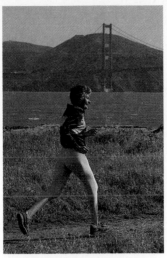

An active midlife adult.

For some midlife adults these health concerns can be quite threatening. Especially for those who view aging with apprehension and fear, these changes can spawn a variety of "youthful" acquisitions—a new wardrobe, a sports car, a new haircut, new makeup, or a new hair color. Some middle-age persons reject these physical changes and convince themselves they are sick. Indeed, *hypochondriasis* is much more common among midlife persons than among young people.

Conditions and Diseases

Although many of the illnesses and disease processes that affect midlife persons have been discussed in earlier chapters of this textbook, several pertain to this discussion because they are serious and may often be seen for the first time at this stage of life. Also, the fullest expression of these conditions may occur in midlife or the elderly period.

Obesity

In many regards, adult onset obesity (see Chapter 6) may be the most serious condition to affect the midlife person. Although a relatively small number of young adults are 10% or more above their desirable weight, 30% to 35% of all men and of all women between 51 and 64 years of age are obese.[8] Indeed, obesity makes its "grand appearance" during midlife. The seriousness of adult onset obesity stems from the conditions associated with it. Coronary artery disease, hypertension, diabetes, varicose veins, proneness to accidents, gallstones, osteoarthritis, and hernias are just a few of the conditions that often develop with obesity.

Even maintaining normal weight through the midlife years cannot ensure freedom from the conditions mentioned. However, the chances of developing these conditions are reduced if one can maintain reasonably normal weight.

Hypercholesterolemia and hypertriglyceridemia

For most adults, it is probable that abnormal elevations in serum cholesterol (hypercholesterolemia) and serum triglycerides (hypertriglyceridemia) are first identified during the midlife period. These conditions are assumed to be important links in the development of atherosclerosis. As you will recall from your study of Chapter 10, atherosclerosis results in the progressive closing of arterial lumens, particularly in the coronary arteries. Plaque, the atherosclerotic buildup, consists of lipids derived from fats circulating in the blood. Thus the control of these two conditions is critically important in the management of cardiovascular disease.

Physical activity is important in controlling essential hypertension.

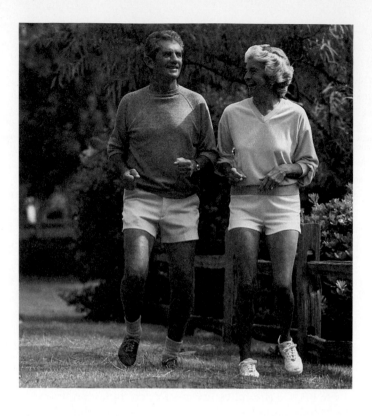

Essential hypertension

Hypertension, or consistently high blood pressure, affects approximately 15% of the American population. Of persons with hypertension, 90% have a form known as *essential hypertension,* and the remainder have **secondary hypertension.**[9] Although the exact cause of essential hypertension is not known, it seems to be caused by chronic constriction in the small peripheral arteries that control blood pressure. Age, family history, race, dietary practices, tension level, and activity level all relate to this condition.

secondary hypertension high blood pressure that results from a specific cause or pathological event; pathological hypertension.

Although essential hypertension does not occur only in persons between the ages of 45 and 65 years, the majority of cases are first identified within this age range. It is possible that you or a classmate may already have essential hypertension. When did you last have your blood pressure checked?

Essential hypertension can be a major risk to health and should be taken seriously. Control of hypertension by means of antihypertensive drugs, diuretic drugs, dietary changes, relaxation techniques, and exercise is usually successful. (See Chapter 10 for a further examination of this "silent killer.")

Menopause

Menopause is not a pathological problem, but it can become an important health concern for women of midlife age who are experiencing unpleasant side effects resulting from this natural cessation of ovarian hormone production.

As we described in Chapter 13 the cyclic production of follicle-stimulating hormone and luteinizing hormone by the anterior pituitary, leading to estrogen and progesterone production by the ovarian follicles, forms the basis of female reproductivity. However, for women of midlife age, the reproductive system undergoes a gradual cessation of oogenesis and menstruation, generally between 45 and 55 years of age.

As ovarian function and hormone production diminish, a difficult period of adjustment must be made by the hypothalamus, ovaries, uterus, and other estrogen-sensitive tissues. The degree to which **hot flashes,** vaginal wall dryness, depression and melancholy, breast changes, and even the uncertainty of fertility are problematic will determine the extent to which menopause is a "health problem" for a midlife woman. Fortunately, most physicians are aware of the value of various therapies, including low-dose estrogen replacement.

hot flashes
temporary feelings of warmth experienced by women during and following menopause, caused by blood vessel dilation.

Osteoporosis

Osteoporosis, a debilitating condition in which calcium is lost from the bone tissue and bone mass is depleted, affects 30% of the elderly population.[10] Occurring far more frequently in women than in men, this condition accounts for many of the hip fractures so common among elderly women. Unfortunately, recovery from a hip fracture (actually a fracture of the neck of the femur) can be lengthy and difficult. For some older persons the rigor of hip surgery and the prolonged period of recovery are too traumatic and death occurs. In fact, 15% of women who suffer hip fractures die within 3 months.[11] Osteoporosis is therefore a potentially life-threatening condition. (For additional information about osteoporosis, see Chapters 5 and 11.)

Osteoarthritis

Osteoarthritis, or degenerative arthritis, is most frequently seen for the first time in persons over the age of 40 years. In persons with this form of arthritis, the joint cartilage undergoes degenerative changes, loses its elasticity, and becomes frayed and eventually bonelike (ossified). The joints most often affected are those of the hips, knees, fingers, and vertebral column. Once osteoarthritic joint changes occur, deformity, swelling, and restricted movement are frequently observed. Inflammation and pain are relatively minor when compared with the pain of rheumatoid arthritis. Rheumatoid arthritis, also seen in midlife and elderly adults, is described in Chapter 11.

Although the exact cause of a person's osteoarthritis is often difficult to determine, trauma, excessive use of the joint, or metabolic and endocrine dysfunction are possible explanations. Treatment of osteoarthritis most often involves the use of aspirin or ibuprophen (not acetaminophen), rest, weight loss, and reduction of strenuous activity. In addition, the local application of heat and *hydrotherapy* may be employed.

When it is well managed, osteoarthritis is not usually a serious health problem. However, it still restricts the individuals and thus may reduce their involvement in some activities or reduce their participation in valuable midlife physical fitness programs.

Type 2 (non-insulin-dependent) diabetes mellitus

Of the several physial health problems that may appear for the first time during midlife, type 2 diabetes mellitus, formerly called adult onset diabetes, is among the most serious. It involves the body's inability to transport glucose through the cell wall and into the cell for conversion into energy. In a person with type 2 dibetes, insulin, the pancreatic hormone necessary for this transport to occur, is still produced. However, the insulin receptors in the cell wall are insensitive to its presence, which prevents it from performing in its normal manner.[12] Thus the insulin present cannot function and the body excretes the excess glucose. A more detailed description of diabetes mellitus, in both the type 1 (insulin-dependent or juvenile onset diabetes) and type 2 forms, can be found in Chapter 11.

Careful management of type 2 diabetes is important in the prevention of short- and long-term difficulties. Mismanagement involving an imbalance between dietary intake and energy expenditure could result in the sudden onset of **hypoglycemia.** Long-term difficulties including cardiovascular complications, impaired peripheral circulation, visual impairment, and decreased kidney function result when mismanagement becomes more frequent.

For the midlife person who has a family history of type 2 diabetes mellitus and who is developing a problem with excessive weight, diabetes mellitus could develop. Type 2 diabetes is most frequently controlled through careful dietary practices and the use of a drug that promotes insulin's effectiveness.

Endogenous depression

Of the two forms of depression discussed in Chapter 11, **endogenous (primary) depression** is frequently seen for the first time in midlife. As you will recall, endogenous depression creates a debilitating emotional state within the individual but is not caused by any clearly identifiable life experiences. To the observer the depressed person does not seem to have anything to be depressed about. Nevertheless, depression, labored speech, lack of vitality, and hypochondriasis are typically evident.

The current explanation of endogenous depression is that it is genetically based condition in which the brain is unable to properly use one of two **neurotransmitters.**[13] As a result the central nervous system is insufficiently stimulated, and a depressed mood follows. Medical management of endogenous depression centers around the use of electroconvulsive shock therapy and the use of tetracyclic antidepressant drugs. Although psychotherapy may be employed in a supportive measure, endogenous depression is not often successfully managed by the techniques that work successfully with **exogenous depression.**

Cancer

The diagnosis of cancer becomes increasingly more probable in the midlife years. Because cancer is a progressive disease that usually requires years of cellular doublings before clinical signs appear, it is understandable that the midlife period is closely associated with cancer diagnosis. Furthermore, by midlife, exposure to carcinogenic agents has been sufficiently prolonged for its effects to be seen.

Certain types of cancer are most prevalent during this period. Midlife men most frequently die of lung, colon-rectum, and prostate cancers. Midlife women most frequently die of lung, breast, and colon-rectum cancers.[14] During the past decade, the incidence of lung cancer in women has risen so dramatically that it now surpasses breast cancer as the leading cancer killer among middle-aged women.

hypoglycemia
condition in which too little glucose circulates in the bloodstream.

endogenous (primary) depression
form of depression caused by the chemical makeup of an individual; a depression resulting from a genetically based abnormal production of neurotransmitter chemicals.

neurotransmitter
chemical messengers released by neurons that permit impulses to be transferred from one nerve cell to another.

exogenous depression
form of depression that results from factors outside the individual; secondary depression.

DEVELOPMENTAL TASKS OF THE MIDLIFE PERIOD

Have you wondered what it would be like to be 20 or 30 years older than you are now? What would you be doing, feeling, and thinking if you were the age of your parents? What, in fact, are your parents thinking about and trying to accomplish as they move through their midlife years?

One thought that probably recurs all too often is the reality of their own eventual death. Their awareness that they will not live forever is a subtle but profoundly influential force that can cause them to be restless, to renew their religious faith, and to be more highly motivated to master the developmental tasks of midlife. This motivation and the awareness of the inevitability of death combine to produce the dynamic concept of being at "the prime of life"—a time when there seems to be a great deal to accomplish and relatively little time in which to accomplish it.

Achieving Generativity

In a very real sense, midlife persons are asked to do something they have not been expected to do previously. As a part of their development as unique persons, they are expected to "pay back" society for the support it has given them. Most persons in midlife begin to realize that the collective society, through its institutions (families, schools, churches), has been generous in its support of their own growth and development and that it is time to replenish these resources. Younger and older persons may have needs that middle-age persons can best meet. By meeting the needs of others, midlife persons can fulfill their own needs to grow and develop. *Generativity* reflects this process of contributing to the collective good.[15] Generativity benefits both midlife persons and society.

The process of repaying society for its support is structured around familiar types of activities. Developmentally speaking, midlife persons are able to select the activities that best utilize their abilities to contribute to the good of society.[16]

The most traditional way in which midlife persons express their generativity is through parenting. Children, with their potential for becoming valuable members of the next generation, need the support of persons who recognize the contribution they can make. By supporting children, either directly through quality parenting or through institutions that function on behalf of children, middle-age persons repay society for the support they have themselves received. As they extend themselves outward on behalf of the next generation, they ensure their own growth and development. In similar fashion, their support of aging parents and institutions that serve the elderly provides another means to express generativity.

For the relatively few persons who possess artistic talent, generativity may be accomplished through the pleasure brought to others. Artists, craftsmen, and musicians have unique opportunities to speak directly to others through their respective talents. Volunteer work serves as another avenue for generativity. Most midlife persons also express generativity through their occupations, by providing quality products or services and thus contributing to the well-being of those who desire or need these goods and services.

A sense of intent is important to midlife persons in their quest for generativity. They need to feel that their efforts are recognized. This reinforces their intention to return something of real value to society. Thus generativity exists only when it is recognized in relationship to midlife growth and development. The fact that midlife adults work or have children does not ensure that their developmental obligations are being met. Without this sense of generativity, they may not feel they are continuing to grow and develop.

Reassessing the Plans of Young Adulthood

It is also essential for midlife persons to come to terms with the finality of their own deaths. Having done this, they often feel compelled to reassess the aspirations for adulthood they formulated 25 or more years previously. Their "dreams" must be revisited.[16,17] This reassessment constitutes a second developmental task of midlife adults.

By carefully reviewing the aspirations they had as young adults, middle-age persons can more clearly study their short- and long-term goals. Specifically, strengths and limitations that were unrecognizable when they were young adults are now more clearly seen. Naiveté is replaced by the insights gained through experience. A commitment to quality often replaces the desire for quantity during the second half of the life cycle. Time is valued more highly because it is now seen in a more realistic perspective. The dream for the future is more sharply delineated and the success and failures of the past are more fully understood as this developmental task of reassessing earlier plans of young adulthood is accomplished.

The Midlife Balance

What do midlife persons learn about themselves when they seek generativity and reassess their previous plans? Levinson et al.,[16] in *The Seasons of a Man's Life*, suggest that persons in midlife learn about their feelings in the areas of youthfulness, gender identification, attachment, and constructiveness. As they accomplish their developmental tasks, they find where they comfortably fit on each of four continuums suggested by Levinson.

- *Youthfulness/agedness.* How youthful should a person over 45 years of age feel? How much maturity makes a person appear too old? These questions reflect the first *polarity* that midlife persons bring into balance. If a balance is not reached, they may be too youthful and, as a consequence, appear incapable of accepting the responsibility appropriate to their position in the life cycle. By appearing to be too mature, they appear "old beyond their years." Overmaturity separates them from experiences and changes that are not only possible but also desirable.
- *Masculinity/femininity.* Before midlife, adults have carefully maintained images of their sexuality suitable for public consumption. More than likely this youthful depiction of their masculinity or femininity suppressed traits that could have been construed as being of the opposite gender identification. Men did not wish to emphasize their more feminine traits, and women did not wish to appear too masculine. In midlife the gender identification defenses are no longer necessary. A more personally satisfying expression of sexuality may emerge.

What Do You Know about Aging?

Erdman Palmore, author of the *The Facts on Aging Quiz: A Handbook,* developed the following quiz to stimulate discussions and identify misconceptions about aging. Test your knowledge about the elderly by answering yes or no to the following items.

	Yes	No
1 A person's height tends to decline in old age.	____	____
2 Older people have more acute (short-term) illnesses than people under 65.	____	____
3 The aged are more fearful of crime than are people under 65.	____	____
4 More of the aged vote than any other age group.	____	____
5 There are proportionately more older people in public office than in the total population.	____	____
6 Most old people live alone.	____	____
7 All five senses tend to decline in old age.	____	____
8 When the last child leaves home, the majority of parents have serious problems adjusting to their "empty nest."	____	____
9 Aged people have fewer accidents per driver than drivers under 65.	____	____
10 One-tenth of the aged live in long-stay institutions like nursing homes.	____	____
11 Most old people report they are seldom angry or irritated.	____	____
12 Most old people are socially isolated and lonely.	____	____
13 Most old people work or would like to have some kind of work (including housework or volunteer work).	____	____
14 Medicare pays over half of the medical expenses for the aged.	____	____
15 Social Security benefits automatically increase with inflation.	____	____

Interpretation

Odd-numbered questions are "yes", even-numbered questions are "no." Have you identified any misconceptions about the elderly that you may have had?

■ *Attachment/separation.* In the years remaining, to what extent do midlife persons need to stay actively involved in the world around them? Is it in their best interest to pull back and leave the "rat race" to younger men and women? This is the polarity of attachment versus separation. From a developmental point of view, middle-age persons are assessing their generativity. Throughout the midlife years, an overattachment to society can hinder the development of the introspective skills that will be needed in the next life cycle segment. If these persons withdraw too quickly, generativity may have been insufficiently undertaken. How much of one trait is too much?

■ *Constructiveness/destructiveness.* In what ways and to what extent have mid-life persons been of help or hindrance to the progress of others? How have they helped or hindered their own progress through life? Have they know-ingly allowed other people to do too much or too little for them? Of course, these questions are closely related to the developmental task of generativity. Midlife persons are challenged to recognize their constructiveness so that its contributive role can be continued through the lengthy midlife period. At the same time, they must recognize their history of destructiveness to others so that it can be moderated.

By searching for a balance point for each of the sets of polarized traits described above, persons in midlife take a careful look at themselves and their lives before they move toward the last segment of the life cycle.

The Midlife Crisis

midlife crisis
period of emotional up-heaval noted among some midlife persons as they struggle with the finality of death and the nature of their past and future accom-plishments.

As portrayed on television talk shows, the **midlife crisis** is a drastic and unex-plainable "throwing in the towel" on life by a few middle-age men and women. Television viewers ask, "How can they do that? Why would they leave families, jobs, and communities where they have roots to strike out into the world as if they were nothing more than adolescents? Are they middle-age crazy?"

We hope that through this discussion of midlife, we have helped you better understand why the midlife crisis can occur and why some men and women make drastic decisions during this period. We are neither condoning nor con-demning these kinds of choices. Rather, we are pointing out that midlife can be a precarious time of reflection and reassessment. For many midlife persons this reassessment coincides with a deeply personal sense of time vulnerability—life seems to be slipping by. They sense that personal growth and development should be occurring. If it is not, the alternatives appear to be limited. "Dropping out" and starting over may seem like attractive alternatives to facing the future. Have you noticed any of these characteristics in midlife adults you know?

THE JOYS OF MIDLIFE

Contrary to some stereotypic views, many midlife adults do not experience a multitude of problems that fill them with melancholy and despair. The lives of numerous midlife adults are characterized by positive elements. It is a myth that every midlife adult must have a midlife crisis. Most probably do not experience such an ordeal. Midlife adults may frequently find themselves more reflective and pensive than when they were young, but to label these behaviors detrimen-tal is to fail to appreciate the value of careful self-examination. Perhaps midlife adults just have more to think about than when they were younger.

From our perspective, much of what midlifers think about is positive. Many see themselves as being in the prime of life. Certain potentially difficult aspects of life have been completed. Many have completed a formal education, become established in an occupation, gained financial security, and raised a family. Mid-life adults can find great satisfaction with these accomplishments and can begin planning for future challenges.

By being relatively free from financial problems and no longer responsible for young children, midlife adults can pursue some of their own dreams. For exam-

Bridging the Generations

Dr. Arthur Kornhaber, president of the Foundation for Grandparenting in Jay, New York, suggests the following tips for parents to help bridge the relationship between grandparents and grandchildren:

- When possible, encourage frequent contact between your children and your parents.
- Think of yourselves as a family and not separate generations.
- Let grandparents and grandchildren have time alone together.
- Expect your parents to be less strict with your children than they were with you.
- Let your children learn different customs, ideas, and viewpoints from your parents.
- Don't cloud your children's relationships with your parents if you do not get along with them.

ple, it is not surprising to see midlife adults travel more than they did earlier in life. Many midlifers rededicate themselves to a fitness program or a hobby, such as reading or gardening. Some seem to love reliving their own college days vicariously through the lives of their college-age children. For many midlifers, joyous moments also come with being grandparents (see box above). Can you think of other ways midlife adults experience deeply satisfying feelings?

THE ELDERLY YEARS

From an organizational standpoint, we decided to separate our discussions of the midlife years and the elderly years. Most gerontologists, physicians, and other health experts see distinct developmental differences between adults in these two age groupings. These differences are reflected in the most prominent social theories of aging.

Social Theories of Aging

Becoming elderly (over 65 years of age) is perceived by many people as a terribly unattractive, undesired, and perhaps even frightening occurrence. These perceptions form a basis for the *disengagement theory* of aging. According to this theory, while society slowly withdraws (disengages) from the elderly, the elderly also withdraw from society.[5] The movement away from cooperation and interaction fosters a sense of isolation. Society no longer wants or needs the elderly and the elderly comply. Perhaps your generation, initially as younger persons and subsequently as the elderly, will largely reject this interpretation of what it means to grow old.

In contrast to a theory that depicts the elderly as being "former" members of society, proponents of the *activity theory* of aging see the elderly as being active and contributing for as long as possible. Research clearly shows that the "young

Exploring new interests after retirement.

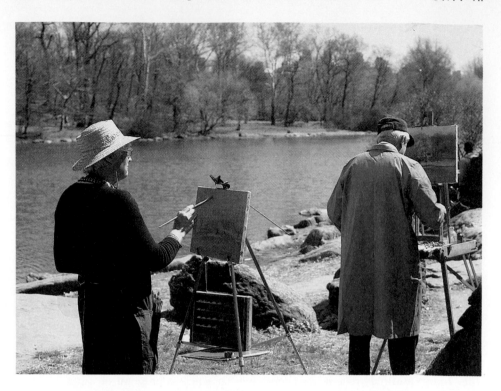

elderly" (ages 66 to 75 years) routinely describe themselves as being "middle aged." Most are active at least as long as they can do what they need to do and what they enjoy doing. Particularly for the young elderly living in urban areas and in sunbelt retirement communities, post retirement is a positive and active period of life. These elderly both contribute to the well-being of the society (through volunteer work, as foster grandparents, and as taxpayers) and work to develop or refine interests for themselves.

Quality of the Elderly Years

For the elderly, as it is for all adults, the quality of life is often judged on the basis of the status of several traits or conditions. We believe that life will be described as being "good" by older persons who have not yet shown significant declines in the majority of areas listed below.

- *Health.* As long as the person feels well, has sufficient energy, and is not limited in terms of mobility, health is not a distracting factor to a good life.
- *Social status.* As long as the elderly person continues to participate in social activities that were enjoyed before retirement or the death of the spouse, social status remains unchanged and is not a negative factor in the quality of life.
- *Economic status.* As long as income is sufficient to maintain an acceptable lifestyle, provide the basic necessities, and form a cushion against unexpected major expenses, economic status is not an erosive factor in a good life.
- *Marital status.* For the majority of men, marital status remains unchanged. For women, widowhood can prove to be a significant factor distracting from

the quality of life. If a support group can, in a sense, replace the spouse, the impact of a changed marital status can be minimized.

- *Living condition.* Only 5% of the elderly are permanently institutionalized. As long as residential arrangements are unchanged, or, if changed, undertaken with minimal disruption, living conditions are not significant factors in defining the quality of life.

- *Educational level.* Educational level in general and an active interest in learning and experimenting in particular seem to foster positive experiences during aging. Limited education may inhibit some elderly persons from learning more about the changing world around them.

- *Sexual intimacy.* Assuming the availability of a partner, sexual practices closely follow the patterns established during earlier periods of adulthood.[18] As long as both partners are satisfied, adjustment is not adversely influenced Divergent expectations can cause difficulty for one or both partners.

HEALTH CONCERNS OF ELDERLY ADULTS

In elderly persons it is frequently difficult to distinguish between changes caused by aging and those caused by disease. For virtually every body system, biomedical indexes for the old and young can overlap. In the respiratory system, for example, the oxygen uptake capacity of a man 70 years old may be no different from that of a man 55 years old who has a history of heavy cigarette smoking. Is the level in the elderly man to be considered an indicator of a disease or should it be considered a reflection of normal old age?[4] In dealing with the elderly, physicians frequently must make this kind of distinction.

In elderly persons, as in midlife persons, structural and physiological changes are routinely seen. In some cases these are closely related to disease processes, but in most cases they reflect the gradual decline that is thought to be a result of the normal aging process. The most frequently seen changes include the following.

Decrease in bone mass

Changes in the structure of bone

Decrease in muscle bulk and strength

Decrease in oxygen uptake

Loss of nonreproducing cells in the nervous system

Decrease in auditory and visual acuity

Decrease in all other sensory modalities, including the sense of body positioning (*proprioception*)

Slower reaction time

Gait and posture changes resulting from a weakening of the muscles of the trunk and legs

In addition to these changes, the most problematic change seen in the elderly is the increased sensitivity of the body's homeostatic mechanism.[4] Because of this sensitivity, a minor infection or superficial injury can be traumatic enough to disrupt markedly the body's ability to maintain its internal balance. Because of this delicate homeostatic mechanism, an illness that would be easily controlled in a younger person could even prove fatal to a seemingly healthy 75-year-old person. Health can be a precarious commodity for persons beyond the age of 65 years.

Conditions and Diseases

In many cases potentially serious health conditions diagnosed during midlife are still prevalent in persons 20 years later. Particularly, such conditions as elevated blood lipid concentrations, hypertension, osteoporosis, osteoarthritis, and depression challenge the health of the elderly more than the health of midlife persons. In addition to these conditions, the following illnesses deserve special attention.

Cardiovascular disease

As for midlife persons, cardiovascular disease remains the leading cause of death for the elderly. Atherosclerotic blockage to vessels of the heart, brain, and kidneys leads to myocardial infarction, cerebrovascular accidents (strokes), pathological hypertension, and congestive heart failure. (see Chapter 10.)

Cancer

Cancers (see Chapter 11), much like cardiovascular diseases, retain their rank as major causes of death among the elderly. Although mortality associated with specific types of cancer varies for "young" and "old" elderly persons, men continue to die of lung cancer more frequently than of any other cancer. In elderly men, prostate cancer is the second leading cause of cancer death. In elderly women lung cancer and breast cancer are replaced by colon-rectum cancer as the leading cause of cancer-related deaths.[14]

Again, because of the delicate balance of homeostasis in the elderly, the treatment of cancer may be especially incapacitating.

Exogenous depression

Whereas endogenous depression (see Chapter 11) in midlife persons is caused by subtle disturbances in brain chemistry, depression in the elderly is more often exogenous or reactive in nature. The death of a partner, growing incapacitation,

Exogenous depression can follow various life crises.

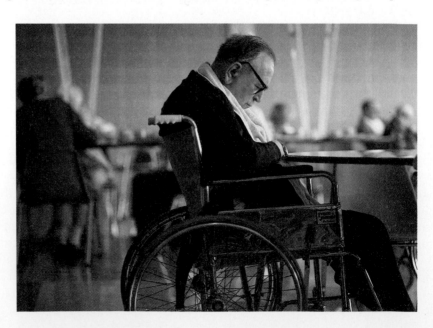

retirement, and the death of grown children drive many elderly to serious depression. Although psychotherapy would offer a measure of resolution for reactive depression, statistics indicate that relatively few of the elderly are treated for their depression in this manner. Most receive only custodial care in institutional settings or in the homes of children.

Proneness to accidents

With decline in sensory acuity, reaction time, and balance, the elderly experience a disproportionate number of accidents. More than 20% of all persons 75 years of age or older require medical treatment for injuries sustained during a fall. Most accidents of the elderly occur in the home.[5]

In light of this tendency to fall, homes should be modified to minimize accidents. Single-story residents are preferable, and homes with stairs should be equipped with handrails and nonslip surfaces. Lighting should be upgraded. Bathrooms may need to be equipped with handrails.

Simple injuries occurring to elderly people who live alone can disrupt routines and force the elderly to care for themselves. Overall health often fails quickly following relatively minor injuries.

Alzheimer's disease (organic brain syndrome)

Although it affects fewer than 1% to 2% of the elderly, organic brain syndrome, in either its acute or chronic form, is an incapacitating, heart-rending, and costly affliction. Alzheimer's disease represents the best known of the presenile dementia disorders.

The initial indication of Alzheimer's disease is often an unusual and unanticipated change in behavior—for example, a sudden inability to use a familiar applicance or a tendency to shave only one side of the face. At this stage of the disease process, the person might experience some difficulty answering questions like these:
- Where are we now?
- What month is it?
- What is today's date?
- When is your birthday?
- Who is the President?

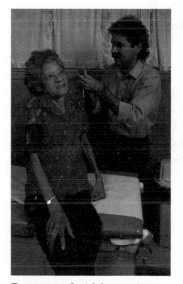

Patient with Alzheimer's disease.

During the ensuing months, victims experience greater memory loss, confusion, and dementia (or loss of reasoning). In its most advanced stage, Alzheimer's victims experience incontinence, infantile behavior, and finally total incapacitation resulting from the destruction of brain tissue. Institutionalization of persons with advanced Alzheimer's disease is certain.

The precise diagnosis of Alzheimer's disease and other similar disorders remains difficult to make before the death of the victim. At that time, the characteristic neurofibrillary tangles, neuritic plaques, and loss of neurons can be identified. Before death, all other conditions capable of leading to dementia are individually ruled out. The diagnosis of Alzheimer's disease is made based on a process of elimination.

In recent years progress in diagnosing Alzheimer's has been made. Today physicians can follow the progression of the disease using positron emission tomography (PET) and single photon emission computed tomography (SPECT).[19] Various changes in the brain can be seen occurring, and because these progress in

Strategies for Straight-Talk

When discussing sensitive topics with your aging parents (such as failing health, housing changes, and financial matters). Mark Edinberg, author of *Talking With Your Aging Parents*, suggests the following:

- Clearly explain the purpose and objectives of the conversation.
- Find out your parents' desires. Let them have a sense of control.
- Be assertive when necessary.
- Explore options; provide information that can be helpful in making decisions.
- Don't be patronizing; learn to accept the impact of potential changes in your parent(s).
- Don't make promises you cannot keep.

sequence with known behavioral changes, the diagnosis of Alzheimer's disease can be made.

Treatment of Alzheimer's disease has been attempted using a variety of drugs. The most recent treatment that appeared promising involved the use of the drug THA, or tetrahydroaminacrine. This drug has been removed from use, however, because of the development of serious side effects.

Several theories exist concerning the cause of Alzheimer's disease. The most plausible theory suggests that a genetic defect involving an extra chromosome 21, similar to that seen in Down's syndrome, may foster the development of the disease.[20] Additional theories explaining Alzheimer's disease involve abnormal proteins, infectious agents, toxins (particularly aluminum), altered blood flow, and a deficiency in acetylcholine (a neurotransmitter).

Alzheimer's-like symptoms appear in conjunction with senial dementia brought on by other conditions. Primary among these symptoms is the more sudden onset of Alzheimer's-like symptoms associated with cerebral vascular disease. When occurring in conjunction with paralysis, a stroke would be anticipated (see Chapter 10). Other causes of Alzheimer's-like symptoms include tumors, infection, and drug-related changes to cerebral function.

SPECIAL NEEDS OF AGING ADULTS

Beyond the needs applicable to all persons, aging adults have some special needs. These needs reflect the many changes associated with aging, including physical change, retirement, and the changing composition of social groups.

Housing is an area of concern to many older adults. As children leave home, income declines, and physical restrictions become more common, aging adults may need (or want) a smaller home or one with a less demanding floor plan. For some, the need for a nursing home facility becomes necessary.

We have only started to address housing needs for our aging population. The development of low-cost senior apartments, group residences, retirement communities, and life-care communities reflects some initial efforts to meet the housing needs of our aging population.

Exercise for the Elderly

In Chapter 4, physical fitness was described in terms of its components and the benefits to be derived from participation in fitness activities. Cardiovascular fitness was presented as the most beneficial component and a training program to enhance aerobic capacity was described.

With recent research indicating that life expectancy can be increased through regular physical conditioning, older adults may now be inclined more than ever before to begin or continue an endurance-based conditioning program. This can be done safely and effectively if these steps to safe exercise are considered[21]:

- Have a medical checkup and talk with your physician before beginning your program. Continue to consult with your physician during your conditioning program.

- If possible, join an exercise class for older adults. Make certain that the instructor is experienced in working with older students. Be certain your instructor is certified in CPR.

- Start your participation slowly. Keep records of your progress.

- Wear loose, comfortable clothing. Invest in good quality exercise shoes.

- Establish a schedule that allows you to exercise three to four times per week. Set aside sufficient time to warm up and cool down.

- Exercise 30 to 60 minutes per session, preferably with a friend.

- Choose a type of activity that will allow you to have fun when you are exercising. Walking is frequently the most appropriate activity for elderly persons.

- Pay attention to your body. Do not exercise if you are ill or injured. Call your doctor if you experience chest pain, breathlessness, joint discomfort, or muscle cramps.

- Become involved in your conditioning program—read books and articles. Share your experiences with other participants.

- Practice seeing yourself as a healthier, more fit person. Imagery is valuable in obtaining the maximum benefit possible from the fitness program.

Elderly persons may be better conditioned than young adults.

When cardiovascular fitness is the focus of the overall fitness program, the formula for INTENSITY presented in Chapter 4 can be used by older adults in calculating a training rate, with only a reduction in the percentage of the maximum heart rate used in the calculation. Depending on age and medical status, an intensity rate of 40% to 60% of the maximum heart rate, rather than 75%, will provide a training effect. The FREQUENCY and DURATION of training are consistent with the information presented in Chapter 4.

Transportation represents an area of need that influences the elderly more than any other group of adults. The need to shop, visit with family and friends, attend religious services, and see a physician are particularly stressful for those who are unable to drive, no longer own an automobile, or do not have access to public transportation. In some communities the inability of the elderly to get around remains a largely unmet need.

As people age, the need for health care services increases. This reflects both the greater incidence of illness as well as the prevalence of chonic problems in the elderly. For older adults the frequency and length of hospitalization increase, rehabilitation services are more likely to be become necessary, and prescription medication use increases. These services are expensive and likely to occur at the same time that earning potential is being lost to retirement and group health insurance is no longer available. Medicare offers some assistance, but many older adults are forced to use their savings to pay their health care bills.

These problems reflect the needs of aging adults and represent challenges that face society as the aging population increases.

DEVELOPMENTAL TASKS OF THE ELDERLY PERIOD

Although this textbook is primarily about young adults, their health, and their developmental tasks, in this chapter we focus on the developmental tasks confronted by midlife and elderly persons. Accepting the physical decline of aging, maintaining high levels of physical function, and establishing a sense of integrity are tasks of the elderly period.

Accepting the Decline of Aging

The general decline associated with the second half of the life cycle is particularly serious between the seventh and eighth decades. Emotionally, socially, and intellectually, elderly persons must accept at least some diminution of resources. Even a spiritual loss may be encountered at those times when life seems less ordered or less humane. Clearly, a developmental task to be accomplished by the elderly is to accept the nature and extent of these losses.[2]

To accept the losses brought about by the aging process, the elderly must first confirm them, usually in one of three ways. The elderly can verify the decline by *testing* for its presence. Depending on the area in question, the elderly can test for losses by trying to take part in activities they were previously capable of. Failure to perform in an accustomed fashion can confirm the nature and extent of the decline.

Observing others is a second way the elderly can confirm their functional, structural, and emotional losses. When a particular loss can be seen in others, elderly people are able to confirm it in themselves much more easily.

The elderly can also confirm their own decline by *consulting* experts. Physicians and experts in other dimensions of gerontology can assist the elderly in confirming the type and extent of decline that has occurred.

The process of accepting the decline brought about by aging can, we believe, be facilitated by these processes of testing, observing, and consulting. Actual acceptance of the decline, however, reflects an internalization of that which was confirmed. Of course, whether this will or will not occur in a particular elderly

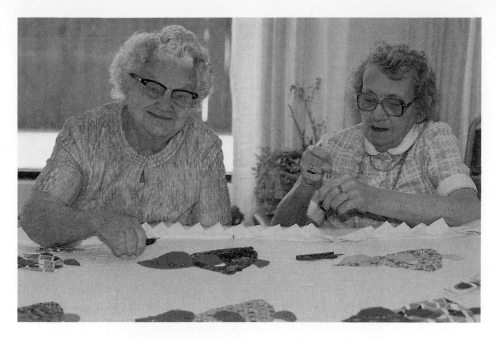

Activities enhance social contact.

person is a highly individual matter. However, we believe that this acceptance is vital for continued growth and development

Maintaining High Levels of Physical Function

Because each segment of the life cycle should be approached with the fullest level of involvement possible, the elderly also should strive to maintain the highest level of physical function possible. High-level function is not an absolute term, but rather is loosely defined as the best function possible. Two approaches to achieving this level of function are **rehabilitation** and **remediation.**

For areas of decline in which some measure of reversal is possible, the elderly are afforded an opportunity to seek rehabilitation. Whether through an individually designed program or through the aid of a skilled professional, the elderly can bring back some function to a previously high level.

The second approach, often used in combination with rehabilitation, is remediation, whereby an alternative to the area of loss is introduced. Examples of remediation include the use of hearing aids, audio cassettes, and prescription shoes. By bringing into play alternate resources, function can often be returned as well as actually improved.

rehabilitation
return of function to a previous level.

remediation
development of alternate forms of function to replace those that have been lost or were poorly developed.

Establishing a Sense of Integrity

The third major developmental task that awaits the elderly is to establish a sense of *integrity,* or a sense of wholeness, concerning the journey that may be nearly complete.[15] In a figurative sense, the elderly must look back over their lives to see the value in what they were able to accomplish. They must address the simple but critical questions, "Would I do it over again?" "Am I satisfied with what I managed to accomplish?" "Can I accept the fact that others will have experiences to which I can never return?"

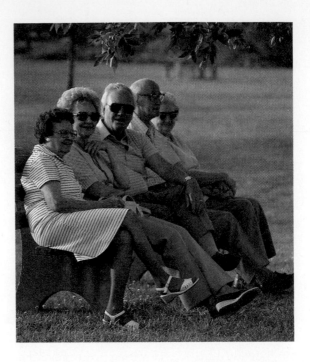

If the elderly can answer these questions positively, then they will feel a sense of wholeness, personal value, and worth. Having established this sense of integrity, they will believe that their lives have had meaning and fullness and that their resources benefitted society.

Since they have already experienced so much, many elderly people have no fear of death, even though they may fear the process of dying. Their ability to come to terms with death thus reinforces their sense of integrity.

Like all of the other developmental tasks, this critical area of growth and development is a personal experience. The elderly must assume this last developmental task with the same sense of purpose they used for earlier tasks. When elderly people can feel this sense of integrity, their reasons for having lived will be fully understood.

SUMMARY

Aging is a positive process of continued growth and development. The aging population can be categorized by a variety of demographic variables. These data provide some interesting generalizations about our older population. Aging can be viewed with respect to two general groups: midlife persons (ages 45 to 65 years) and elderly persons (over 65 years of age).

It is important for us to recognize that physical decline is inevitable. Regardless of the cause, a variety of subtle changes in the structure and function of the body occur during midlife and certain health conditions seem to be associated with these changes. Some of these conditions include adult onset obesity, hypercholesterolemia, essential hypertension, menopause, osteoporosis, osteoarthritis, type 2 (noninsulin-dependent) diabetes mellitus, and endogenous depression.

Growth and development during the midlife years also involve the mastery of two key developmental tasks: achieving generativity and reassessing the plans of young adulthood. While successfully completing these tasks, midlife persons learn about their feelings and where they fit on continuums of youthfulness, gender identification, attachment, and constructiveness. For some, this time of reflection and reassessment results in what is known as the "midlife crisis." For most, the midlife years are satisfying and productive.

The elderly years are often viewed negatively. We hope that your generation will begin to see these elderly years as meaningful ones—ones that need not be feared. The quality of life for the elderly is often judged on the basis of health, social status, economic status, marital status, living conditions, health care, educational level, and sexual intimacy.

As expected, structural and physiological changes are routinely seen in the elderly. Conditions and disease processes linked closely with the elderly include cardiovascular disease, cancer, exogenous depression, Alzheimer's disease, and accidents.

Growth and development for the elderly require mastery of three principal developmental tasks: accepting the decline of aging, maintaining high levels of physical function, and establishing a sense of integrity. We encourage you to examine your interactions with and contributions to the lives of older persons.

REVIEW QUESTIONS

1 Describe our aging population as it relates to representation in the total population, marital status, living arrangements, income, and level of education.
2 Identify the four predictable occurrences in the process of physical decline that accompanies aging.
3 Identify theories of aging that attempt to explain why body organs become dysfunctional. Which ones are most plausible?
4 Describe the following diseases or conditions and explain why each could be a health concern for persons in midlife: adult onset obesity, hypercholesterolemia, hypertriglyceridemia, essential hypertension, menopause, osteoporosis, osteoarthritis, type 2 diabetes mellitus, endogenous depression, and cancer.
5 What are the two developmental tasks midline adults must accomplish? Identify the three developmental tasks of the elderly period.
6 What is a "midlife crisis"?
7 In what seven ways do the elderly often judge the quality of their lives? Discuss each one.
8 Identify the structural and physiological changes most frequently seen in midlife and elderly adults. Are older people capable of expressing their sexuality?
9 Identify the conditions and diseases of greatest concern to the elderly population.
10 Identify and explain the three ways in which the elderly confirm the losses associated with their aging.

QUESTIONS FOR PERSONAL CONTEMPLATION

1 Think of the people you know who are between the ages of 45 and 65 years. What are the positive aspects of this age? What are the negative aspects? What can these persons do that you cannot do? What can you do that they cannot do? Now imagine yourself at age 55 years. How do you think you will look? What do you think a typical day in your life will be like?

2 Imagine yourself at age 80 years. How do you think you will look? What do you think a typical day in your life will be like at that age? How will it be different from being 55 years of age?

3 How can you change your health-related behaviors now to influence the quality of your midlife and elderly years?

4 Compare the developmental tasks of the midlife and elderly periods with those of the young adult period. How are they similar? How are they different? If you were to find out today that you only had 1 year to live, would the developmental tasks of the midlife and elderly period be important for you even though you are a young person? Explain your answer.

5 Take some time to make plans for your aging. For example, decide how you would like to look when you are older. What activities do you want to participate in? How do you want to be treated by your family and friends? How healthy do you want to be? Determine the kinds of things you must do now to help make these plans come true. What resources are available to help you?

REFERENCES

1 US Bureau of the Census: Current population report, series P-23, Pub no 153, America's centenarians, Data from the 1980 census, Washington DC, 1987, US Government Printing Office.

2 US Bureau of the Census: Statistical abstract of the United States: 1987, ed 107, Washington, DC, 1986, US Government Printing Office.

3 Cox, H: Later life: the realities of aging, ed 2, Englewood Cliffs, NJ, 1988, Prentice-Hall, Prentice Hall Press.

4 Woodruff, D, and Birren, J: Aging: scientific perspectives and social issues, New York, 1975, Van Nostrand Reinhold Co, Inc.

5 Kaluger, G, and Kaluger, M: Human development: the span of life, ed 3, St. Louis, 1984, Times Mirror/Mosby College Publishing.

6 Forbes, EJ, and Fitzsimons, VM: The older adult: a process for wellness, St. Louis, 1981, The CV Mosby Co.

7 Crooks, R, and Baur, K: Our sexuality, ed 3, Menlo Park, Calif, 1987, The Benjamin-Cummings Publishing Co.

8 Guthrie, H: Introductory nutrition, ed 7, St. Louis, 1989, Times Mirror/Mosby College Publishing.

9 American Heart Association: 1987 Heart facts, Dallas, 1987, The Association.

10 Braunwald, E, et al: Harrison's principles of internal medicine, ed 11, New York, 1987, McGraw-Hill Inc.

11 White, MK, and Rosenberg, BS: What research says about exercise and osteoporosis, Health Education 16:3-5, 1985.

12 Marble, A, et al, editors: Joslin's diabetes mellitus, ed 12, Philadelphia, 1985, Lea & Febiger.

13 Ray, O, & Kiser, C: Drugs, society, and human behavior, ed 4, St. Louis, 1987, Times Mirror/Mosby College Publishing.

14 American Cancer Society: 1987 Cancer facts and figures, New York, 1987, The Society.

15 Erikson, E: Childhood and society, New York, 1963, WW Norton & Co, Inc.

16 Levinson, D, et al: The seasons of a man's life, New York, 1978, Alfred A Knopf, Inc.

17 Sheehy, G: Passages: predictable crises of adult life, New York, 1974, Bantam Books.

18 Rienzo, BA: The impact of aging on human sexuality, Journal of School Health 55:66-68, 1985.

19 Zoler, M: Alzheimer's disease: new imaging techniques show diagnostic promise, Geriatrics 41:91-94, 1986.

20 Barnes, D: Defect in Alzheimer's is on chromosome 21, Science 235:846-847, 1987.

21 Birkel, D: Safe exercise for adults, Class handout, Muncie, Ind, 1988, School of Physical Education, Ball State University.

ANNOTATED READINGS

American Medical Association: Health and well-being after 50, New York, 1984, Random House, Inc.

> Deals with many of the problems people face as they grow older: how to cope with everyday physical problems, fatigue, and diminished vision; how to ensure continued psychological growth: myths of the midlife crisis; and how to confront the issue of personal mortality. Also presents other information to help one prepare for a satisfying future.

Brecher, EM: Love, sex, and aging, Boston, 1984, Little, Brown & Co, Inc.

> Summarizes the results of an intensive research project that involved the sampling of 4,246 men and women between the ages of 50 and 93 years. The project was undertaken by the editors of Consumer Reports Books. Ten chapters cover a variety of topics related to sexuality and aging. Responses clearly indicate that a wide range of sexual attitudes and behaviors exists among older people. Numerous quotations from the respondents are included.

Katchadourian, H: Fifty: midlife in perspective, New York, 1987, WH Freeman & Co, Publishers.

> An optimistic examination of midlife changes that encourages the reader to enjoy each stage of life for its unique qualities. The author, a Stanford psychiatrist, reminds midlifers that they are in the fastest growing segment of the population. Thus, midlifers are not alone as they journey into the future.

Mac Lean, H: Caring for your parents: a source book for options and solutions for both generations, Garden City NY, 1987, Doubleday & Co.

> A practical guide to assist people who will be taking care of their aging parents. Includes information pertaining to medical changes, medicine, insurance, home care, support groups, and future planning. Readers are reminded to encourage their parents to prepare a will.

Skinner, BF, and Vaughan, ME: Enjoy old age, New York, 1983, WW Norton & Co., Inc.

> The philosophy of this book is that old age should be a time of considerable joy and productivity. This can be accomplished with advanced planning and a positive approach. Includes thinking about old age, keeping busy, doing something about old age, having a good day, getting along with people, and how to deal with fear of death.

Stoppard, M: The best years of your life, New York, 1984, Ballantine/Del Ray/Fawcett Books.

> Discusses a variety of topics, including growing through life, personal fulfillment, fitness, diet, exercise, medical checkups, stress, depression, and loneliness. Provides information on retirement, financial and psychological issues, living with illness, adapting your environment, "age-proofing" your house to prevent accidents, and labor-saving tools for the house and garden.

Tomb, DA: Growing old: a handbook for you and your aging parent, New York, 1984, Viking Press.

> A handbook for you and your aging parents. Covers medical, social, psychological, and financial problems of taking care of elderly parents and helps the reader to distinguish normal changes from abnormal changes during the aging process. It may be used as a reference book.

CHAPTER
20

Dying and Death
The Last Transitions

Key Concepts

Personal awareness of
death encourages us to
prepare for the
inevitability of our deaths
so that we might live more
meaningful lives.

Death can be defined from
a number of perspectives.

Terminally ill people pass
through a sequence of
stages as they adjust to the
reality of their own deaths.

Hospice care uses a variety
of strategies to maximize
the quality of life for dying
persons.

Grief is a necessary process
that gradually permits
people to detach
themselves from those who
have died.

Suicide is a leading cause
of death among young
people.

Society has established a
number of rituals
associated with death.

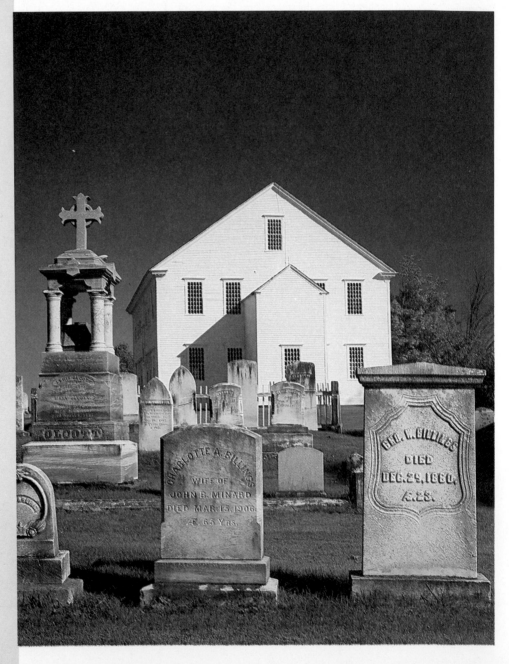

The primary goal of this chapter is to help people realize that the reality of death can serve as a focal point for a more enjoyable, productive, and contributive life.

At first this notion may seem to run counter to our emphasis on viewing life as the completion of a sequence of developmental tasks. You might argue that accepting the reality of death is a developmental task reserved for persons who have already lived full lives or for those who are in the process of dying, not for people whose best years lie ahead. In fact, in Chapter 19 we stated that the acceptance of death is an important component of an older person's establishment of a sense of integrity. We also believe that this acceptance can serve the younger adult as well. Please consider the following points. First, life has few, if any, guarantees. Each of us could die at any time. Second, most of us have older friends or relatives who may soon die. Third, the value of the present can only be judged by comparison with the past and future.

Each of these points should be viewed in its most positive light. Each day in our lives becomes especially meaningful only after we have fully accepted the reality that someday we are going to die. We can then live each day to its fullest, as if it were our last day.

Our mortality provides us with a framework from which to appreciate and conduct our lives. It should help us prioritize our activities so that we can accomplish what we want to accomplish (in our academic work, in our relationships with others, in our recreation) before we die. Quite simply, death gives us our only absolute reason for living.

PERSONAL DEATH AWARENESS

Since shortly after the turn of the century, the manner in which people experience death in this society has changed significantly. Formerly most people died in their own homes, surrounded by family and friends. Young children frequently lived in the same home with their aging grandparents and saw them grow older and eventually die. Death was seen as a natural extension of life. Children grew up with a keen sense of what death meant, both to the dying person and the grieving survivors.

Times have indeed changed. Today approximately 75% of people die in hospitals, nursing homes, and extended care facilities, not in their own homes. The extended family is seldom at the bedside of the dying person.[1] Frequently, frantic efforts are made to keep a dying person from dying. Although medical technology may have improved our lives, some persons believe that it has reduced our ability to die with dignity. Many are convinced that our way of dying has become more artificial and less civilized than it used to be. (The trend toward hospice care may be a positive response to this "high-tech" manner of dying; see pp. 591-592.)

Dying away from the home reflects one way in which we shield ourselves and our children from the reality of death. Children may grow up with distorted views of what dying and death really are. They see so many television and cartoon characters die in ridiculous, violent ways that they soon believe death is just a temporary phase. Death cannot be real.

Well-intentioned parents sometimes deny young children the opportunity to become acquainted with death. They may avoid talking about death with their children. They may refuse to let them visit a terminally ill grandparent, see a

Is this a death without dignity?

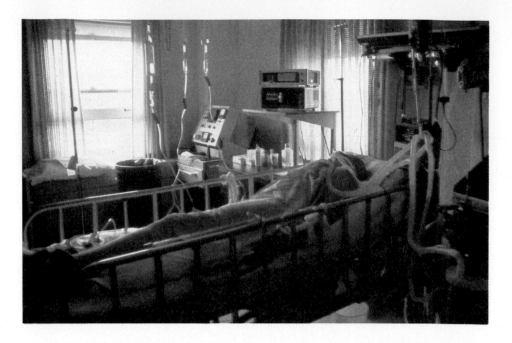

dead body, or attend a funeral. Such efforts may reinforce a child's belief that death is not real, or if it is real, that it only results from traffic accidents or gunshot blasts.

Since we have been raised in a society that shields us from death in a myriad of ways, it is natural for us to deny the reality of our own deaths. Unfortunately, by doing so we open ourselves to a variety of unpleasant situations. These situations start to present themselves when we begin to fully realize that others around us do die. We may begin to feel uneasy when a friend, grandparent, or parent dies. When we hear about disasters or terrorist bombings, we may start to believe that we, too, may die someday. Most of us persist in ignoring this thought. We continue to deny the inevitability of our own deaths.

Worden and Proctor[2] believe that the confusion or dissonance created with our death denial is unhealthy, since it breeds feelings of helplessness and vulnerability, which will eventually lead to one of the following three situations:

- *Fear and anxiety.* Unresolved fear and anxiety commonly cause neurotic behavior. Phobias, compulsions, and even hypochondriasis may result.
- *Futility and alienation.* The conflicts generated by death denial can lead to an existential type of depression in which a person can have profound doubts about the value of living. Worden and Proctor think such a depression can ultimately lead to suicide or a **willed death.**
- *Frustration and anger.* Persons who are unable to cope with the reality of death may react by becoming aggressive. Ultimately, with frustration, rage, and aggression, people can become homicidal. Perhaps they believe that by controlling the fate of another person, they have, in some manner, mastered their own fate.

Because of the pitfalls associated with the denial of death, many death educators are supporting the concept of *personal death awareness,* or the acceptance of the fact that you are going to die. Personal death awareness allows you to put your life in a clearer, more comfortable, meaningful perspective. The goal is not to make you so cognizant of your own potential death that you live in constant

willed death
A death in which a person gives up the desire to live and merely waits to die.

fear of its coming. Rather, the goal is a positive, healthy one. We can best gain personal death awareness by undertaking some of the activities that force us to deal with our own mortality. We discuss many of these activities in the section entitled "Personal Preparation for Death" on pp. 600-601.

DEFINITIONS OF DEATH

Would you be willing to stipulate in your will that your estate spend thousands of dollars a year for your body or head to be frozen in liquid nitrogen to await the development of thawing technology and a medical cure that could bring you back to life? If so, you might be interested in the pseudoscience of cryonics. Already a few hundred people have consented to be frozen in hopes of "cheating death." Scientists, however, believe that their wait will be very long.

In contrast with cryonics is the science of cryobiology, in which the effects of freezing on living tissues are studied. Already cryobiologists have contributed to our ability to preserve tissue for transplanting, such as fertilized ova. Cryobiologists doubt, however, that science will overcome the enormous problems associated with thawing a frozen human.

Neomorts are brain-dead persons kept alive artificially for purposes of perfecting surgical procedures, testing new drugs, or preserving organs for transplantation. Neomorts have been preserved for up to 10 days at a cost of about $1,000 per hour. However, the number of neomorts that have been used is very limited. The growth of neomort use could represent an intermediate level of medical research between animal studies and clinical human trials. Would you consent to have your body used in this manner?

Before many of the scientific advancements of the past 25 years, death was relatively easy to define. People were considered dead when a heartbeat could no longer be detected and when breathing ceased. Now, with the technological advancements made in medicine (especially emergency medicine), some patients and accident victims who give every indication of being dead can be resuscitated. Critically ill persons (even those in comas) can now be kept alive for years with many of their body functions maintained by medical devices, including feeding tubes and respirators.

Thus death can be a very difficult concept to define. Numerous professional associations and ad hoc interdisciplinary committees have struggled with this problem and have developed criteria by which to establish death. Some of these criteria have been adopted by state legislatures, although there certainly is no consensus definition of death that all states embrace.

Clinical determinants of death refer to measures of body functions. Often judged by a physician (who can then sign a legal document called a medical death certificate), these clinical criteria include the following:

1 Lack of heartbeat and breathing.
2 Lack of central nervous system function, including all reflex activity and environmental responsiveness. Often this can be corroborated by an **electroencephalograph** reading. If there is no brain wave activity following an initial measurement and a second measurement after 24 hours, the person is said to have undergone *brain death*.
3 The presence of **rigor mortis,** indicating that body tissues and organs are no longer functioning at the cellular level. This is sometimes referred to as *cellular death*.

electroencephalograph
instrument that measures the electrical activity of the brain.

rigor mortis
rigidity of the body that occurs after death.

Death can also be determined by a *coroner*, an elected legal official empowered to pronounce death and then sign the appropriate coroner's death certificate. Often coroners pronounce death at accident scenes, when a death results from physical violence, or when the cause of a death is suspicious. The *legal determinants* used by government officials are established by state law and often adhere closely to the clinical determinants already listed. Although a person is not legally dead until a death certificate is signed (either by a physician, coroner, or health department officer), the legal rights of a fully incapacitated comatose person may be given to a close relative by a legal procedure called *power of attorney*.

Figure 20-1
The living will is a legally binding document in many states; it allows individuals to express their wishes concerning dying with dignity. When such a document has been drawn, families and physicians are better able to deal with the wishes of persons who are near death from conditions from which there is no reasonable expectation of recovery. Individuals can construct their own living wills or use forms supplied by concerned organizations such as the form shown.

To My Family, My Physician, My Lawyer and All Others Whom It May Concern

Death is as much a reality as birth, growth, maturity and old age—it is the one certainty of life. If the time comes when I can no longer take part in decisions for my own future, let this statement stand as an expression of my wishes and directions, while I am still of sound mind.

If at such a time the situation should arise in which there is no reasonable expectation of my recovery from extreme physical or mental disability, I direct that I be allowed to die and not be kept alive by medications, artificial means or "heroic measures". I do, however, ask that medication be mercifully administered to me to alleviate suffering even though this may shorten my remaining life.

This statement is made after careful consideration and is in accordance with my strong convictions and beliefs. I want the wishes and directions here expressed carried out to the extent permitted by law. Insofar as they are not legally enforceable, I hope that those to whom this Will is addressed will regard themselves as morally bound by these provisions.

Signed_____

Date _____

Witness_____

Witness_____

Copies of this request have been given to _____

_____

_____

_____

From Concern for Dying.

Legality of the Living Will

The living will is recognized as a legally binding document in many states. Legislation pending in other states could increase even further the availability of this document. For those who use the living will, concerns about dying with dignity can be acted on in accordance with the individual's wishes. States in which living will legislation has been enacted include the following:

Alabama	Georgia	Mississippi	Tennessee
Alaska	Hawaii	Missouri	Texas
Arizona	Idaho	Montana	Utah
Arkansas	Illinois	Nevada	Vermont
California	Indiana	New	Virginia
Colorado	Iowa	Hampshire	Washington
Connecticut	Kansas	New Mexico	Wisconsin
Delaware	Louisiana	North Carolina	West Virginia
District of	Maine	Oklahoma	Wyoming
Columbia	Maryland	Oregon	
Florida		South Carolina	

Three states have upheld the living will in the courts:

Texas	Florida	Arizona

In addition to the constructs for physical and legal death described above, could it be possible that there are other forms of death? For persons who have lost contact with reality, could psychological death exist? For those who reject all contact with others, could social death exist? For persons who fail to recognize the existence of God, could spiritual death exist? If so, how many other forms of death can you identify?

EUTHANASIA

There are two types of euthanasia for desperately ill persons: they are either intentionally put to death (direct euthanasia) or allowed to die without being subjected to heroic lifesaving efforts (indirect euthanasia). **Direct (active) euthanasia** usually involves the administration of large amounts of depressant drugs, which eventually causes all central nervous system function to stop. Although direct euthanasia is commonly practiced on household pets and laboratory animals, it is illegal for humans in the United States, Canada, and most other countries.

Indirect (passive) euthanasia is increasingly occurring in a number of hospitals, nursing homes, and medical centers. Physicians who withhold heroic lifesaving techniques or drug therapy treatments or who disconnect life support systems from terminally ill patients are practicing indirect euthanasia. Although some people still consider this form of euthanasia a type of murder, indirect euthanasia seems to be gaining legal and public acceptance for victims of certain terminal illnesses—near-death cancer patients, brain-dead accident victims, and hopelessly ill newborn babies.

direct (active) euthanasia
process of inducing death, often through the injection of lethal drugs.

indirect (passive) euthanasia
process of allowing a person to die by disconnecting life support systems or withholding life saving techniques.

Figure 20-2
Opinions change on euthanasia.

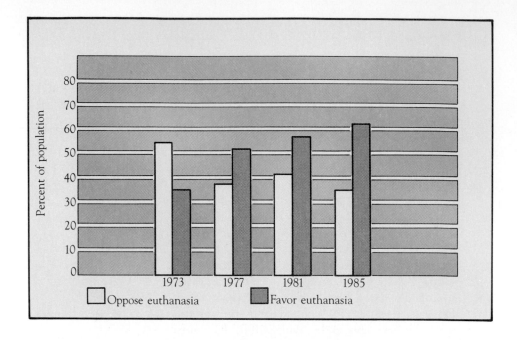

The Right to Pull
the Plug

The following figures are based on a Gallup Poll asking 995 adults how willing they would be to have their life support disconnected if each were in an irreversible coma*:

Very willing	70%
Somewhat willing	12%
Don't know	7%
Somewhat unwilling	4%
Very unwilling	6%

*Total of 99% caused by rounding of results.

Because some physicians and families find it difficult to support indirect euthanasia, many people are using a living will (See Figure 20-1). This is a document that confirms a dying person's desire to be allowed to die peacefully and with a measure of dignity if a time should arise when there is little hope for recovery from a terminal illness or major injury. As of January 1988, the living will is legally binding in 38 states and the District of Columbia (see the box on p. 585).[3] This document requires that physicians or family members carry out a person's wishes. Even in states where the living will is not legally recognized, it morally binds the surviving parties to carry out a person's desire to die with dignity while freeing them from having to make difficult decisions.

Proponents of euthanasia believe that it allows terminally ill people the opportunity to die with dignity and peace. Some people oppose euthanasia on moral grounds, claiming it is a form of murder (see Figure 20-2). Other opponents fear that our society could find it easy to accommodate increasingly active forms of euthanasia. They worry about how euthanasia decisions will be made and who will make these decisions. They fear that our society will someday find euthanasia acceptable for elderly people, terminally ill people who don't want to live, and children born with birth defects. Where will the lines be drawn? Clearly, the technology exists to support terminally ill people for extended periods of time. One wonders, however, if this technology is prolonging life or if the procedures are only prolonging death.

EMOTIONAL STAGES OF DYING

A process of self-adjustment has been observed in persons who have a terminal illness. The stages in this process have helped form the basis for the modern movement of death education. An awareness of these stages may help you understand how people adjust to other major losses in their lives.

Perhaps the most widely recognized name in the area of death education is Dr. Elizabeth Kübler-Ross. As a psychiatrist working closely with terminally ill patients at the University of Chicago's Billings Hospital, Kübler-Ross was able to observe the emotional reactions of dying persons. In her book *On Death and Dying,* Kübler-Ross summarized the psychological stages that dying people often experience[4]:

- *Denial.* This is the stage of disbelief. Patients refuse to believe that they actually will die. Denial can serve as a temporary defense mechanism and can allow patients the time to accept their prognosis on their own terms.
- *Anger.* A common emotional reaction after denial is anger. Patients can feel as if they have been cheated. By expressing anger, patients are able to vent some of their fears, jealousies, anxieties, and frustrations. Patients often direct their anger at relatives, physicians and nurses, religious symbols, and normally healthy people.
- *Bargaining.* Terminally ill persons follow the anger stage with a stage characterized by bargaining. Patients who desperately want to avoid their inevitable deaths attempt to strike bargains—often with God or a church leader. Some people undergo religious conversions. The goal is to buy time by promising to repent for past sins, to restructure and rededicate their lives, or to make a large financial contribution to a religious cause.
- *Depression.* When patients realize that at best bargaining can only postpone their fate, they may begin an unpredictable period of depression. In a sense, terminally ill people are grieving for their own anticipated death. They may become quite withdrawn and refuse to visit with close relatives and friends. Prolonged periods of silence or crying are normal components of this depression stage and should not be discouraged.
- *Acceptance.* During the acceptance stage, patients fully realize that they are going to die. Acceptance ensures a relative sense of peace for most dying persons. Anger, resentment, and depression are usually gone. Kübler-Ross describes this stage as one without much feeling. Patients feel neither happy nor sad. Many are calm and introspective and prefer to be left either alone or with a few close relatives or friends.

One or two additional points should be made about the psychological stages of dying. Just as each person's life is totally unique, so is each person's death. Unfolding deaths vary as much as do unfolding lives. Some people move through Kübler-Ross's stages of dying very predictably. Others do not. It is not uncommon for some dying people to avoid one or more of these stages entirely. Edwin S. Schneidman[5] supports this contention.

One does not find a unidirectional movement through progressive stages as much as an alternation between acceptance and denial. Denial is a most interesting psychodynamic phenomenon. For a few consecutive days a dying person is capable of shocking a listener with the breathtaking candor of his profound acceptance of imminent death and the next day shock the listener with unrealistic talk of leaving the hospital and going on a trip.

The second important point to be made about Kübler-Ross's stages of dying is that the family members or friends of dying people often pass through similar stages as they observe the dying of their loved one. When informed that a close friend or relative is dying, many people will also experience varying degrees of denial, anger, bargaining, depression, and acceptance. Because of this, as caring persons we need to recognize that the emotional needs of the living must be fulfilled in ways that do not differ appreciably from those of the dying.

Psychological Stages
of Dying

Denial
Anger
Bargaining
Depression
Acceptance

NEAR-DEATH EXPERIENCES

As Bob lay on the gymnasium floor in apparent cardiac arrest, he watched from above as the team trainer and coaches applied CPR. Turning from his observation of his own attempted resuscitation, he began walking in the direction of his uncle's voice, a voice that he had last heard a few days before his uncle's death 4 years earlier. Suddenly, his uncle instructed Bob to stop and turn back because Bob was not yet ready to join him. Over 24 hours later Bob regained consciousness in the cardiac intensive care unit of The Ohio State University Hospital.

Death brings an end to our physical existence. Perhaps this is the ultimate connection between death and our physical dimension of health. Many people believe that, in a positive sense, death brings with it a sense of relief and comfort—two qualities that may be most needed when one is dying. The work of Raymond Moody[6], who examined reports of people who had "near-death" experiences, suggests that we may have less to fear about dying than we have generally thought.

In a more recent study of over 100 persons who had near-death experiences, Kenneth Ring[7] reported these people shared a core experience. This experience was composed of some or all of the following stages:

1 An emotional component comprised of a sense of well-being and peace.
2 A body component in which the dying person floats above his or her body and is able to witness (autoscope) the activities that are occurring.
3 A period of entering into extreme blackness or darkness.
4 A shaft of intense light that generally leads upward or lies in the distance.
5 A decision to enter into the light.

Central to this experience is the need to make a decision to move toward death or to return to the body that has been temporarily vacated.

Experts are not in agreement as to whether near-death experiences are truly associated with death or more closely associated with the depersonalization that is experienced by some persons during particularly frightening situations. Regardless, for those who had near-death experiences, simply knowing that death might not be such an unpleasant experience appears to be comforting. Most seem to have formed a new orientation toward living.

INTERACTING WITH DYING PERSONS

Facing the impending death of a friend, relative, or loved one is a difficult experience. If you have yet to face this situation, be assured that, as you grow older, your opportunities will increase. This is part of the reality of living.

Most counselors, physicians, nurses, and ministers who spend time with terminally ill people suggest that you display one quality when interacting with dying people. That quality is honesty. Just the thought of talking with a dying person can make one feel uncomfortable. (Most of us have had no training in this sort of thing.) Sometimes, to make ourselves feel less anxious or depressed, we may tend to deny that the person we are with is dying. Our words and nonverbal behavior indicate that we prefer not to face the truth. Our words become stilted as we gloss over the facts and merely attempt to cheer up both our dying friend and ourselves. This behavior is rarely beneficial or supportive—for either party.

As much as possible, we should attempt to be genuine and honest. We should not try to avoid crying if we feel the need to cry. At the same time, we can provide emotional support for dying people by allowing them to express their feelings openly. We should resist the temptation of trying to "pull someone out" of the denial, anger, or depression. We should not feel obliged to talk constantly and to fill long pauses with idle talk. Sometimes, nonverbal communication, including touching, may be much more appreciated than mere talk. Since our interactions with dying persons help fulfill our needs, we too should express our emotions and concerns as openly as possible.

TALKING WITH CHILDREN ABOUT DEATH

Because most children are curious about everything, it is not surprising that they are also fascinated about death. From very young ages, children are exposed to death through mass media (cartoon shows, pictures in newspapers and magazines, and news reports), adult conversations ("Aunt Emily died today," "Uncle Bill is terminally ill"), and their discoveries (a dead bird, a crushed bug, a dead flower). The manner in which children learn about death will have an important impact on their ability to recognize and accept their own mortality and to cope with the deaths of others.

Edgar Jackson,[8] a minister and psychologist who specializes in death education, encourages parents and older friends to avoid shielding children from or misleading children about the reality of death. Young children need to realize that death is not "temporary" and it is not "like sleeping." Parents are encouraged to make certain they understand children's questions about death before they give an answer. Most children want simple, direct answers to their ques-

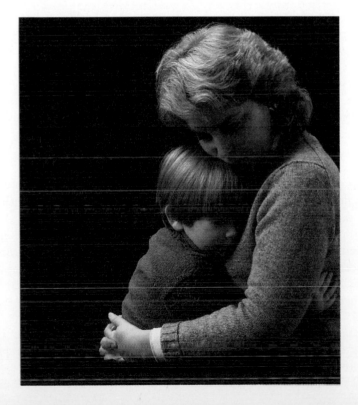

Children need support when dealing with death.

tions, not long detailed dissertations, which often confuse the issues. For example, when a 4-year-old child asks her father, "Why is Tommy's dog dead?" an appropriate answer might be, "Because he got very, very sick and his heart stopped beating." Getting involved in a lengthy discussion about "doggy heaven" or the causes of specific canine diseases may not be necessary or appropriate.

Jackson encourages parents to answer questions when they arise and always with openness and honesty. In this way young children can learn that death is a real part of life and that sad feelings are a normal part of accepting the death of a loved one.

When adults find it necessary to counsel school-age children concerning death, they should consider important guidelines. Eddy et al[9] make the following suggestions:

- Become acquainted with the manner in which children of certain ages respond to death.
- Communicate with children on their level.
- Structure explanations in a direct, simple manner.
- Answer questions truthfully.
- Avoid communicating your own anxiety and uncertainty.
- Recognize that children need to express their grief.
- Remember that children learn from even the most stressful events, such as the death of a family member or friend.

Communication structured around these guidelines should support children, both emotionally and in terms of their understanding of death.

DEATH OF A CHILD

Adults face not only the death of their parents and friends, but perhaps the death of a child. Whether because of sudden infant death syndrome (SIDS), chronic illness, accident, or suicide, children die and adults are forced to grieve the loss of someone who was "too young to die."

Coping with the death of children presents adults with a difficult period of adjustment, particularly when the death was unexpected. Experts agree the grieving adults, particularly the parents, should express their grief fully and proceed cautiously on their return to normal routines. Many pitfalls can be avoided. Adults who are grieving for dead children should:

- *Avoid coping through the use of alcohol or drugs.*
- *Make no major life changes.* Moving to a different home, relocating, or changing jobs usually doesn't help parents deal any better with the grief they are experiencing.
- *Share their feelings with others.* Grieving adults should share their feelings particularly with other adults who have experienced a similar loss. Group support is available in many communities.
- *Avoid trying to erase the death.* Giving away clothing and possessions that belonged to the child cannot erase the memories the adult may have of the child.
- *Give themselves the time and space to grieve.* On the anniversary of the child's death or on the child's birthday grievers should give themselves special time just for grieving.

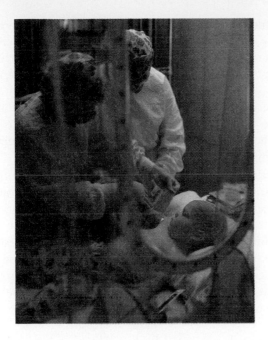

A dying child.

- *Don't attempt to replace the child.* Do not quickly have another child or use the deceased child's name for another child.

For some adults, grief over the death of a child will require an extended period of time. Eventually, however, life can return to normal.

HOSPICE CARE FOR THE TERMINALLY ILL

The thought of dying in a hospital ward, with spotless floors, pay television, and strict visiting hours, leaves many people with a cold feeling. Perhaps this thought alone has helped encourage the concept of **hospice care.** Hospice care provides an alternate approach to dying for terminally ill patients and their families. The goal of hospice care is to maximize the quality of life for dying persons and their family members. Popularized in England during the 1960s yet derived from a concept developed during the Middle Ages (where "hospitable" lodges took care of weary travelers), the hospice helps people die comfortably and with dignity by using one or more of the following strategies:

- *Pain control.* Dying persons are not usually treated for their terminal disease; they are provided with appropriate drugs to keep them free from pain, alert, and in control of their faculties. Drug dependency is of little concern and patients can receive pain medication when they feel they need it.
- *Family involvement.* Family members and friends are trained and encouraged to interact with the dying person and with each other. Family members often care for the dying person at home. If the hospice arrangement includes a hospice ward in a hospital or a separate building (also called a hospice), the family members have no restrictions on visitation.
- *Multidisciplinary approach.* The hospice concept promotes a team approach. Specially trained physicians, nurses, social workers, counselors, and volunteers work with the patient and family to fulfill important needs. The needs of the survivors receive nearly the same priority as those of the patient.

hospice care
approach to caring for terminally ill patients that maximizes the quality of life and allows death with dignity.

▪ *Patient decisions.* Contrary to most hospital approaches, hospice patients are encouraged to make their own decisions. The patient decides when to eat, sleep, go for a walk, and just be alone. By maintaining a personal schedule, the patient is more apt to feel "in control" of his or her life, even as that life is slipping away.

Another way in which the hospice approach differs from the hospital approach concerns the care given to the survivors. Even after the death of the patient, the family receives a significant amount of follow-up counseling. Helping families with their grief is an important role for the hospice team.

The number of hospices in the United States has climbed quickly to nearly 1,500.[10] People seem to be convinced that the hospice system does work effectively. Part of this approval may be the cost factor. The cost of caring for a dying person in a hospice is usually less than the cost of full (inpatient) services provided by a hospital. Although insurance companies are delighted to see the lower cost for hospice care, many are still uncertain as to how to define hospice care. Thus not all insurance companies are fully reimbursing patients for their hospice care. Before discussing the possibility of hospice care for members of your family, you should consider the extent of hospice coverage in your health insurance policy.

Kathy Charmaz,[11] in her book *The Social Reality of Death,* raises the question of whether the hospice concept can exist in the United States as it has in England and other parts of the world. She is concerned that hospices here will eventually integrate themselves into our "fee for service" medical care system.[11]

Whether the founders' commitment can survive the institutionalization of the hospice concept remains to be seen. It is even possible, that, if fully realized, it may replicate some of the worst features of nursing homes. And all kinds of knotty problems may be anticipated if attempts are made to provide hospice care to all when the existing medical care system is largely based on profit. Still, it appears that hospice workers, both here and in England, construct a context wherein the quality of life takes precedence over the quantity.

Regardless of what course the payment for hospice care takes, the value of the support that can be provided to dying persons and their families should not be denied.

GRIEF AND THE RESOLUTION OF GRIEF

The emotional feelings that persons experience after the death of a friend or relative are collectively called *grief. Mourning* is the process of experiencing these emotional feelings in a culturally defined manner.[12] See the box on p. 593 for more information on the grieving process. The expression of grief is seen as a valuable process that gradually permits people to detach themselves from the deceased. Expressing grief, then, is a sign of good health.

Although people experience grief in remarkably different ways, most people experience some of the following sensations and emotions.[13]

▪ *Physical distress.* Shortly after the death of a loved one, grieving persons display a rather similar pattern of physical discomfort. This discomfort is characterized by "sensations of somatic distress occurring in waves lasting from twenty minutes to an hour at a time, a feeling of tightness in the throat, choking with shortness of breath, need for sighing, and an empty feeling in the abdomen, lack of muscular power, and an intense subjective distress described as tension or mental pain. The patient soon learns that these waves of discomfort can be precipitated by visits, by mentioning the deceased, and by receiving sympathy."

- *Sense of unreality.* Grieving persons may feel as if they are numb or in a state of shock. They may deny the death of their loved one.
- *Feelings of detachment from others.* Grieving persons see other people as being distant from them, perhaps because the others cannot feel the loss. A person in grief can feel very lonely. This is a common response.
- *Preoccupation with image of the deceased.* The grieving person may not be able to complete daily tasks without constantly thinking about the deceased.
- *Guilt.* The survivor may be overwhelmed with guilt. Thoughts may center on how the deceased was neglected or ignored. Sensitive survivors feel guilt merely because they still are alive. Indeed, guilt is a common emotion.

The Grieving Process

The grieving process consists of four phases, each of which is variable in length and unique in form to the individual.[14] These phases are composed of the following:

1 *Internalization of the deceased person's image.* By forming an idealized mental picture of the dead person, the grieving person is freed from dealing too quickly with the reality of the death.

2 *Intellectualization of the death.* Mental processing of the death and the events leading up to its occurrence move the grieving person to a clear understanding that death has occurred.

3 *Emotional reconciliation.* During this third and often delayed phase, the grieving person allows conflicting feelings and thoughts to be expressed and eventually reconciled with the reality of the death.

4 *Behavioral reconciliation.* Finally, the grieving person is able to comfortably return to a life in which the death has been fully reconciled. Old routines are reestablished and new patterns of living are adopted where necessary. The grieving person has largely recovered.

Only time and the sequential "working through" of the death will allow earlier behaviors to be returned to in a manner that is comfortable to the persons who have suffered the loss of a spouse, friend, or child. For some the process will unfold quickly, while for others the resolution of grief may never fully occur.

If a mistake is to be made by the friends of a grieving person, it will be in terms of encouraging a return to normal behavior too quickly. When friends urge the grieving person to return to work right away, make new friends, or become involved in time consuming projects, they may be preventing necessary grieving from occurring. It is not easy or desirable to "forget" about the fact that a spouse, friend, or child has recently died.

Grief evokes feelings of profound loss.

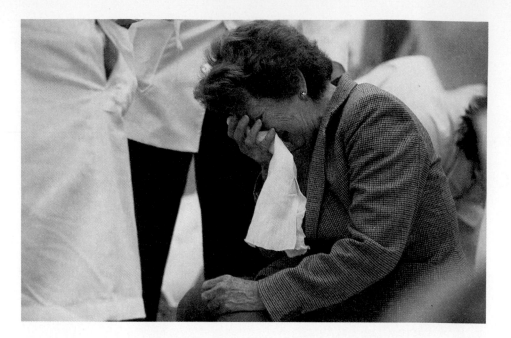

- *Hostility.* Survivors may express feelings of loss and remorse through hostility, which they direct at other family members, physicians, lawyers, and others.
- *Disruption in daily schedule.* Grieving persons often find it difficult to complete daily routines. They can suffer from an anxious type of depression. Seemingly easy tasks take a great deal of effort. Initiation of new activities and relationships can be difficult. Social interaction skills can be lost.
- *Delayed grief.* In some people, the typical pattern of grief can be delayed for weeks, months, and even years.

The grief process will continue until the bereaved person can establish new relationships, feel comfortable with others, and look back on the life of the deceased person with positive feelings. Although the duration of the grief resolution process will vary with the emotional attachments one has to a deceased person, grief usually lasts from a few months to 1 year. Professional help should be sought when grieving is characterized by unresolved guilt, extreme hostility, physical illness, significant depression, and a lack of other meaningful relationships. Trained counselors, physicians, and hospice workers can all play significant roles in helping people through grief.

SUICIDE

One of the major tragedies of our times is the high incidence of suicide. Suicide is a complex social phenomenon.[15] In the last year for which statistics are available (1983), 28,295 persons in the United States killed themselves.[16] Nearly three times as many women as men attempted suicide in 1983. With approximately 7,000 deaths annually among young people (including college students), suicides follow accidents as the second leading cause of death. Among young people, the suicide rate has nearly tripled over the last several decades.[17] In the 15 to 24 age group, the overall suicide death rate in 1983 was 11.9 deaths per

100,000 persons. Interestingly, the suicide death rate for persons age 65 and over was 19.2 per 100,000.[16]

Determining the actual incidence of suicide is somewhat difficult, since some of the deaths that appear to be accidents may actually be cases of suicide (for example, certain deaths in falls, fires, or car accidents). Furthermore, deaths related to avoiding medical care, choosing to drink excessively, or deciding not to eat might also be considered forms of suicide. It is also possible that numerous cases of suicide go unreported, perhaps to protect family and friends.

Several reasons have been proposed to explain suicides among young people, including (1) increased pressure to succeed in our society, (2) onset of depression at an early age, (3) high divorce rates, (4) unavailability of jobs, (5) use of alcohol and other drugs, and (6) inability to form meaningful relationships with friends, parents, and older role models.

It is relatively easy to become depressed when faced with some of the concerns listed above. At one time or another, most people must cope with some of these situations. In coping with problems people may at times feel somewhat depressed or "blue." What separates the potentially suicidal person from the non-suicidal person is the degree of despair and depression experienced and their inability to cope with it.

Suicidal persons tend to become overwhelmed with a range of destructive emotions, including anxiety, anger, loneliness, loss of self-esteem, and hopelessness. Suicidal persons may feel that their death is a solution to all that is afflicting them. While it is common for many people to occasionally experience periods of mild depression and thoughts of suicide, suicidal persons tend to view their own deaths as viable solutions.

What many suicidal persons fail to realize is that their death is a "permanent solution to a temporary problem." Rarely does a suicide solve a problem. In fact, suicides invariably create a multitude of additional problems for those who love

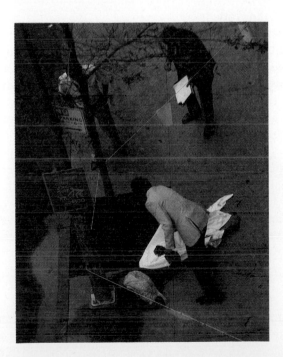

For young adults, suicide remains a leading cause of death.

the victim. Because the pressures related to higher education can make people more vulnerable to suicide, it seems clear that all persons in the college community need to be concerned with information related to suicide so that they can help other students, faculty, and family members in suicide prevention.

Eddy and Alles have stated that although each suicide case is different, demographic data concerning suicide victims permit the following generalizations[12]:

- Men commit suicide more often than women.
- Women have a greater numer of incompleted suicides than men.
- Older people commit suicide more often than younger people.
- Younger people have a greater number of incompleted suicides than older people.
- City dwellers commit suicide more often than rural residents.
- Protestants commit suicide more often than Catholics or Jews.
- Wealthy people commit suicide more often than poor people.
- Professionals commit suicide more often than nonprofessionals.
- Alcoholics commit suicide more often than social drinkers.

Additional generalizations concerning suicide indicate that men tend to select more violent means of suicide than do women, that many suicide victims give indications to others of their willingness to commit suicide, and that suicide is not a trait that is genetically passed from generation to generation.

Suicide Prevention

Warning Signs of Suicidal Behaviors

Change in appetite
Change in sleep pattern
Decreased concentration
Decreased interest in activities
    that were a source of pleasure
Sudden agitation or sudden
    slowing down in level of
    activity
Social withdrawal
Feelings of hopelessness,
    worthlessness, and self-
    reproach
Inappropriate or excessive guilt
Suicidal thoughts and/or talk
Making a suicide plan
Writing a suicide note
Giving away prized possesions
Recent humiliating life event
Lack of social supports

Many communities are recognizing the need to provide or expand suicide prevention services. Suicide prevention centers are available in many communities. Most suicide prevention centers operate 24-hour hotlines and are staffed through volunteer agencies, mental health centers, public health departments, and hospitals. Staff members in these centers have extensive training in counseling skills required to deal with suicide-prone persons. Phone numbers for these services can be found in the telephone directory.

The public is responding to the need for new approaches in suicide prevention. Specific programs are being aimed at young people and college students to teach them how to recognize and handle friends who may be depressed and suicidal. Some community programs are geared to parents, in hopes of teaching parents to communicate better with their children and to recognize when professional intervention is needed. To learn more about suicide prevention programs in your college community, you might check with the counseling center or university health center.

What signs and symptoms could indicate that a person might be considering suicide? Dr. Susan Blumenthal, chief of the behavioral medicine program at the National Institute of Mental Health, recommends that we watch for the symptoms listed in the margin. Blumenthal believes that a person needs professional help when he or she shows a clustering of these suicide warning signs for more than 2 weeks.[18]

RITUALS OF DEATH

Our society has established a number of rituals associated with death that help the survivors accept the reality of death, ease the pain associated with the grief process, and provide a safe disposal of the body. Our rituals give us the chance to formalize our "goodbyes" to a person and to receive emotional support and strength from family members and friends. In recent years more of our rituals seem to be celebrating the life of the deceased. In doing this, our rituals also reaffirm the value of our own lives.

Most of our funeral rituals take place in funeral homes, churches, and cemeteries. *Funeral homes* (or *mortuaries*) are business establishments that provide a variety of services to the families of dead people. The services are carried out by funeral directors, who are licensed by the state in which they operate. Most funeral directors are responsible for preparing the bodies for viewing, filing death certificates, preparing obituary notices, establishing calling hours, assisting in the preparation and details of the funeral, casket selection, transportation to and from the cemetery, and family counseling. Although licensing procedures vary from state to state, most new funeral directors must complete 1 year of college, 1 year of mortuary school, and 1 year of internship with a funeral home before taking a state licensing examination.[19]

Funeral Services

An ethical funeral director will attempt to follow the wishes of the deceased's family and provide only the services requested by the family. Most families want traditional, **full funeral services.** Three major components of the full funeral services are as follows.

full funeral services
all of the professional services provided by funeral directors.

Embalming Embalming is the process of using formaldehyde-based fluids to replace the blood components. Embalming helps preserve the body and return it to a natural look. Embalming permits friends and family members to view the body without being subjected to the odors associated with tissue decomposition. Embalming is often an optional procedure, except when death results from specific communicable diseases or when body *disposition* (disposal) is delayed.

Ground burial.

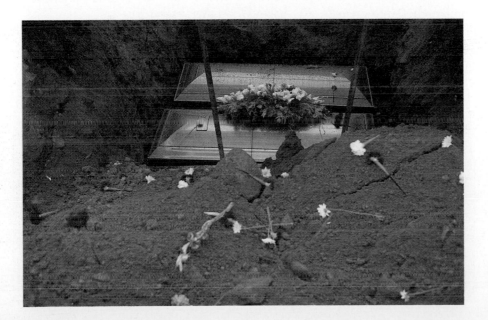

Calling hours Formerly called a *wake,* this is an established time when friends and family members can gather in a room to share their emotions and common experiences about the dead person. Generally in the same room, the body will be in a casket, whose lid may be open or closed. Open caskets assist some people to confirm that death truly did occur. Some families prefer not to have any calling hours, sometimes called visiting hours.

Funeral service Funeral services vary according to religious preference and the emotional needs of the survivors. Although some services are held in a church, most funeral services today take place in a funeral home, where a special room might serve as a chapel. Some services are held at the graveside. Families may also choose to have a simple *memorial service* within a few days after the funeral.

Disposition of the body Bodies are disposed of in one of four ways. *Ground burial* is the most common method. The casket is almost always placed in a metal or concrete vault before being buried. The vault serves to further protect the body (a need only of the survivors) and to prevent collapse of ground because of the decaying of caskets. Use of a vault is required by most cemeteries.

A second type of disposition is *entombment.* Entombment refers to nonground burial, most often in structures called **mausoleums.** A mausoleum has a series of shelves where caskets can be sealed in vaultlike areas called *niches.* Entombment can also occur in the basements of buildings, especially in old, large churches. The bodies of famous church leaders are sometimes entombed in vaultlike spaces called **crypts.**

Cremation is a third type of body disposition. In the United States, 13% to 14% of all bodies are cremated. This practice is increasing. Generally both the body and casket (or cardboard cremation box) are incinerated so that only the bone ash from the body remains. The body of an average adult produces about 5 to 7 pounds of bone ash. These ashes can then be placed in containers called *urns,* and then buried, entombed, or scattered, if permitted by state law. The cost of cremation (from $100 to $300) is much less than ground burial. Some families choose to cremate after having full funeral services.

A fourth method of body disposition is *anatomical donation.* Separate organs (corneal tissue, kidneys, heart) can be donated to a medical school, research facility, or organ donor network by using a donor card such as the one shown in Figure 20-3. Certain states permit people to indicate on their driver's licenses that they wish to donate their organs. Some people choose to donate their entire

mausoleum
above-ground structure into which caskets can be placed for disposition and which frequently resembles a small stone house.

crypts
burial locations underneath churches.

Figure 20-3
Organ donor card.

UNIFORM DONOR CARD

OF_____
Print or type name of donor
In the hope that I may help others, I hereby make this anatomical gift, if medically acceptable, to take effect upon my death. The words and marks below indicate my desires.
I give: (a) _____ any needed organs or parts
           (b) _____ only the following organs or parts

_____
Specify the organ(s) or part(s)
for the purposes of transplantation, therapy, medical research or education;
           (c) _____ my body for anatomical study if needed.
Limitations or
special wishes, if any :_____
08-21-84   100M/84

Signed by the donor and the following two witnesses in the presence of each other:

_____   _____
Signature of Donor   Date of Birth of Donor

_____   _____
Date Signed   City & State

_____   _____
Witness   Witness
This is a legal document under the Uniform Anatomical Gift Act or similar laws.
For further information consult your physician or
KF   National Kidney Foundation, Inc.
2 Park Avenue, New York, N.Y. 10016

Planning Your Funeral

In line with this chapter's positive theme of the value of personal death awareness, here is a funeral service assessment that we frequently give to our health classes. This inventory can help you assess your reactions and thoughts about the funeral arrangements you would prefer for yourself.

After answering each of the following questions, you might wish to discuss your responses with a friend or close relative.

1 Have you ever considered how you would like your body to be handled after your death?
____ Yes ____ No

2 Have you already made funeral prearrangements for yourself?
____ Yes ____ No

3 Have you considered a specific funeral home or mortuary to handle your arrangements?
____ Yes ____ No

4 If you were to die today, which of the following would you prefer?
____ Embalming ____ Ground burial
____ Cremation ____ Entombment
____ Donation to medical science

5 If you prefer to be cremated, what would you want done with your ashes?
____ Burial ____ Entombed ____ Scattered
____ Other, please specify _____

6 If your funeral plans involve a casket, which of the following ones would you prefer?
____ Plywood (cloth covered)
____ Hardwood (oak, cherry, mahogany, maple, etc.)
____ Steel (sealer or nonsealer type)
____ Stainless steel
____ Copper or bronze
____ Other, please specify _____

7 How important would a funeral service be for you?
____ Very important
____ Somewhat important
____ Somewhat unimportant
____ Very unimportant
____ No opinion

8 What kind of funeral service would you want for yourself?
____ No service at all
____ Visitation (calling hours) the day before the funeral service; funeral held at church or funeral home
____ Graveside service only (no visitation)
____ Memorial service (after body disposition)
____ Other, please specify _____

9 How many people would you want to attend your funeral service or memorial service?
____ I do not want a funeral or memorial service
____ 1-10 people
____ 11-25 people
____ 26-50 people
____ Over 51 people
____ I do not care how many people attend

10 What format would you prefer at your funeral service or memorial service? Select any of the following that you would like.

	Yes	No
Religious music	____	____
Nonreligious music	____	____
Clergy present	____	____
Flower arrangements	____	____
Family member eulogy	____	____
Eulogy by friend(s)	____	____
Open casket	____	____
Religious format	____	____
Other, please specify	_____

11 Using today's prices, how much would you expect to pay for your total funeral arrangements, including cemetary expenses (if applicable)?
____ Less than $1,500
____ Between $1,501 and $3,000
____ Between $3,001 and $4,500
____ Between $4,501 and $6,000
____ Above $6,001

body to medical science. Often this is done through prior arrangements with medical schools. Bodies still require embalming. After they are studied, the remains are often cremated and returned to the family, if requested.

Costs

The full funeral services offered by a funeral home average from $1,500 to $2,000.[19] To this price, one must add additional expenses. Casket prices vary significantly, with the average cost between $1,200 and $1,600. If the family chooses an especially fancy casket, then the costs could spiral up to $9,000 or more. Costs that extend beyond these expenses include (should one choose them) those shown in the margin. When one adds up all of the expenses associated with a typical funeral, the average cost is between $4,000 and $5,500.

With the urging of consumer activist groups, the Federal Trade Commission recently enacted a policy that stipulates that funeral homes must itemize their funeral expenses. Starting April 1984, one-price funeral package plans were no longer permitted. This policy was enacted to stop the large costs that some disreputable funeral homes were charging unwary families. The new itemized pricing policy specifies what each separate service costs. Furthermore, this information must be given over the phone, if requested.

Regardless of the rituals you select for the handling of your body (or the body of someone in your care), most educators are encouraging people to prearrange their plans. Before you die, you can save your survivors a lot of misery by putting your wishes in writing. *Funeral prearrangements* relieve the survivors of many of the details that must be handled at the time of death. You can gather much of the information for your obituary notice and your wishes for the disposition of your body. Prearrangements can be made with a funeral director, family member, or attorney. By making arrangements in advance of need, you can enhance your own peace of mind. Why leave things merely to chance?

Estimated Funeral Costs

Cemetery lot	$200-400
Opening and closing of grave	$200-400
Vault	$275+
Mausoleum space	$1000+
Honorarium for minister	$40-50+
Organist and vocalists	$25 each
Flowers over casket	$100+
Grave marker	$500+
Beautician services	$25

PERSONAL PREPARATION FOR DEATH

We hope that this chapter is helping you to discover some new perspectives about death and to develop your own personal death awareness. Remember, the ultimate goal of death education is a positive one—to help you best use and enjoy your life. Becoming aware of the reality of your own mortality is a step in the right direction. Reading about the process of dying, grief resolution, and the rituals surrounding death can also help you imagine that someday you too will die.

There are some additional ways in which you can prepare for the reality of your own death. Preparing a will, purchasing a life insurance policy, making funeral prearrangements, preparing a living will, and considering an anatomical or organ donation are measures that help you prepare for your own death. At the appropriate time, you might also wish to talk with family and friends about your own death. You may discover that an upbeat, positive discussion about death can help relieve some of your apprehensions and those of others around you.

Another suggestion to help you emotionally prepare for your own death is to prepare an *obituary notice* or **eulogy** for yourself. Include all the things you would

eulogy
composition or speech that praises someone; often delivered at a funeral or memorial service.

like to have said about you and your life. Now compare your obituary notice and eulogy with the current direction your life seems to be taking. Are you doing the kinds of activities for which you want to be known? If so, great! If not, perhaps you will want to consider why your current direction does not reflect how you would like to be remembered. Should you make some changes to restructure your life's agenda in a more personally meaningful fashion?

Another suggestion to help make you aware of your own eventual death is to write your own **epitaph.** Before doing this, you might want to visit a cemetery. (Unfortunately, most of us only visit cemeteries when we are forced to.) Reading the epitaphs of others may help you to develop your own epitaph.

epitaph
inscription on a grave marker or monument.

Further awareness of your own death might come from attempting to answer these questions (in writing, since this pushes you beyond mere thinking): (1) If I had only one day to live, how would I spend it? (2) What one accomplishment would I like to make before I die? (3) Once I am dead, what two or three things will people miss most about me? By answering these questions and accomplishing a few of the tasks suggested in this section, you will have a good start on accepting your own death and the value of life itself.

SUMMARY

The goal of this chapter is to assist you in putting dying and death into a proper framework. Our society frequently approaches death from the standpoint of death denial. Death denial tends to generate a variety of negative feelings including overwhelming fear and anxiety. To avoid this, death educators are encouraging us to develop the concept of personal death awareness. People who develop a personal death awareness learn to accept the inevitability of death and then to use this understanding as a springboard to a more meaningful life.

Death can be defined in terms of clinical and legal determinants. Euthanasia is a major controversy of the 1980s. Living wills are only one way in which people can have some control over the manner in which they die.

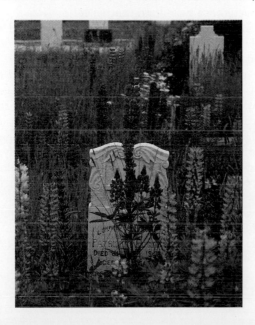

Persons for whom the dying process is protracted adjust to the reality of their death in a recognized sequence of stages. These five stages include denial, anger, bargaining, depression, and acceptance. Not everyone moves through each stage in a predictable manner. The stages can be applied to other significant losses people might experience.

Hospice care is an approach used to help terminally ill people die comfortably. It uses multidisciplinary strategies for pain control, family involvement, and personal decisions. An additional feature of hospice care is the care provided to the survivors.

Grief encompasses the emotional feelings that survivors experience after the death of a friend or relative. These sensations and emotions typically include physical distress, a sense of unreality, feelings of detachment, preoccupation with the image of the deceased, guilt, hostility, disruption in daily schedule, and delayed grief.

Suicide is a leading cause of death among young people. Although each suicide case is unique, some generalizations can be made regarding the types of people who most often commit suicide.

Death in our society is associated with a number of rituals to help the survivors cope with the death and to ensure proper disposal of the body. Activities that may help you prepare for death include preparing a will, purchasing life insurance, prearranging funeral services, and writing your own obituary or eulogy.

REVIEW QUESTIONS

1 According to Worden and Proctor, death denial leads to one of three situations. Identify and explain each one of these situations.
2 What concept do death educators support to avoid the many problems associated with the denial of death? What is the goal behind this concept?
3 Identify and explain the determinants of death and state who establishes each of them. What characterizes a near-death experience?
4 Define euthanasia. Explain the difference between direct and indirect euthanasia. What is meant by a "living will"? What is the advantage of such a document for dying persons and their survivors?
5 Identify the five psychological stages that dying people often experience. Explain each stage. What is meant by the statement, "the emotional needs of the living must be fulfilled in ways that do not differ appreciably from those of the dying"?
6 What are the recommendations for talking with children about death?
7 Identify and explain the four strategies that form the basis of hospice care. What are the advantages of hospice care for the patient and for the family?
8 Explain what is meant by the term "grief." Identify and explain the sensations and emotions most people have when they experience grief. When does the grieving process end? How can adults cope with the death of a child?
9 Identify some of the proposed explanations for suicides in young people. What generalizations can be made about suicide?
10 What purposes do the rituals of death serve? What are the major components of the full funeral service? What are the four ways in which bodies are disposed?

QUESTIONS FOR PERSONAL CONTEMPLATION

1 If you were going to die tomorrow, what would you do today? What would you say
   to those who are closest to you? Whom would you tell about your impending death?
   Whom would you not tell? Why?

2 What are your feelings about death at this point in your life? How was death handled
   in your family as you were growing up? Have any major circumstances influenced
   your attitudes about death? Do you wish your exposure or lack of exposure to death
   had been different? In what ways?

3 Examine your feelings about euthanasia. Put yourself in two hypothetical situations.
   First, consider how you would feel if you were being kept alive by machines when
   there was no chance for your recovery. What would you want to happen? Second,
   consider how you would feel if someone very close to you were being kept alive by
   machines. What would you want to happen to this person? Compare your feelings
   for both situations. Are there any differences?

4 If you could envision your own death, what would be the circumstances of your
   death? With whom would you be? Where would you be? How would you feel? Can
   thinking about your own death ever be a positive experience?

5 What are your feelings about suicide? Have you ever been close to someone who did
   commit suicide? If so, how did you feel after the suicide? Under what circumstances
   might you feel like taking your own life? What do you think you could do to stop
   someone from committing suicide?

REFERENCES

1 Ebersole, P, and Hess, P: Toward healthy aging: human needs and nursing response, ed 2, St.
   Louis, 1985, The CV Mosby Co.
2 Worden, J, and Proctor, W: PDA: personal death awareness, Englewood Cliffs, NJ, 1976,
   Prentice-Hall.
3 Concern for Dying: Personal correspondence, February, 1988, New York.
4 Kübler-Ross, E: On death and dying, New York, 1969, Macmillan Publishing Co.
5 Schneidman, ES: Death work and the stages of dying. In Death and dying: challenge and
   change, Reading, Mass, 1978, Addison-Wesley Publishing Co, Inc.
6 Moody, RA: Life after life, New York, 1975, Bantam Books.
7 Ring, K: Life at death: a scientific investigation of the near-death experience, New York, 1980,
   Coward, McCann & Geoghegan.
8 Jackson, E: When to talk about death. In Fulton, et al, editors: Death and dying: challenge
   and change, Reading, Mass, 1978, Addison-Wesley Publishing Co, Inc.
9 Eddy, JM, et al: Death counseling in school-age populations, Health Education 15:42-45, 1985.
10 Stewart, SA: Hospice care turns attention to children, USA Today October 31, 1984, p 5.
11 Charmaz, K: The social reality of death, Reading, Mass, 1980, Addison-Wesley Publishing Co,
   Inc.
12 Eddy, JM, and Alles, WF: Death education, St. Louis, 1983, The CV Mosby Co.
13 Lindemann, E: Symptomatology and management of acute grief. In Death and dying: challenge
   and change, Reading, Mass, 1978, Addison-Wesley Publishing Co, Inc.
14 Wolfelt, AD, PhD: Workshop presentation on death and grief, Muncie, Ind, 1986, Ball State
   University.
15 Kamerman, JB: Death in the midst of reality: social and cultural influences on death, grief and
   mourning, Englewood Cliffs, NJ, 1988, Prentice-Hall.
16 US Bureau of the Census: Statistical abstract of the United States: 1987, ed 107, Washington,
   DC, 1986, US Department of Commerce.
17 Simmons, K: Adolescent suicide: second leading cause of death, Journal of the American Medical Association 257:3329-3330, 1987.
18 Manning, A: We should all be on the alert for cries of help, USA Today April 18, 1984, p 4.
19 Bowman, J: Licensed funeral director, Personal interview, February 19, 1988.

ANNOTATED READINGS

Gordon, S: When living hurts, New York, 1985, Dell Publishing.

    A direct, compassionate, easy-to-read book by the famous Syracuse University professor. Focuses on how we can better confront our problems with sadness, hopelessness, anger, depression, and thoughts of suicide. Uplifting and frequently humorous, this book is a good antidote for persons going through painful life (or death) experiences.

Grollman, EA: Suicide: prevention, intervention, postvention, ed 2, 1988, Boston, Beacon Press.

    A guide for both professionals and others touched by suicide, this book is a compendium of information about suicide. Includes statistics, warning signs, prevention, intervention techniques, and help for survivor-victims. This expanded edition covers euthanasia, living wills, and provides a list of intervention centers across the country.

Kamerman, JB: Death in the midst of life, Englewood Cliffs, NJ, 1988, Prentice-Hall.

    Written by a sociologist, this brief book examines the social and cultural influences on death, grief and mourning. Kamerman indicates the many changes that have taken place in the manner in which Americans view death. The institutionalization of death is discussed, along with suicide, grief, mourning, near-death experiences, and the death of pets.

Myers, E: When parents die: a guide for adults, New York, 1986, Penguin Books.

    A valuable guide for persons who face the reality of their own parents' deaths. Contains pertinent information concerning the process of death, grief, and bereavement. Discusses funerals and the many legal procedures related to death. Myers provides an extensive appendix that outlines resources and supportive agencies.

A wide variety of children's books have been written about dying and death. Two books that we have found especially helpful in talking to our own children about death are:

Viorst, J: The tenth good thing about Barney, New York, 1975, Atheneum Publishers.

Buscaglia, L: The fall of Freddie the leaf, New York, 1982, Holt, Rinehart & Winston.

Mastering Tasks

We believe that it is to your advantage to be knowledgeable about the information in Unit VII. Although you may not be especially concerned about your own aging or the likelihood of your own death happening anytime soon, we feel that studying these topics now may help you master the developmental tasks that are meaningful for your emotional growth.

▪ **Forming an Initial Adult Self-Identity** It may be obvious that discovering your self-identity (that which makes you unique) involves first coming to grips with who you are right now—this minute or this day. However, is it also possible that your identity could be related to both your past experiences and those awaiting you in the future?

We think so. It would be hard to deny that past experiences play a major role in providing a foundation for one's developing self-identity. Clearly, we are products of our past experiences.

But we may also be products of our future experiences. How we feel about the impact of our own aging and eventual deaths is reflected in our self-identities *now*. To fear these inevitable processes may make us tentative, frightened persons during our entire lives. To ignore our aging and eventual deaths may cause us to live unfocused, less meaningful lives. To acknowledge and accept the reality of aging and dying may be the healthiest approach of all. This approach (used throughout Unit VII) allows our self-identities to emerge in an emotionally secure fashion.

▪ **Establishing a Sense of Relative Independence** Being independent is a fragile quality. Most of us will never be completely independent from other people. What comes as a surprise to many independent young and midlife adults is the probability of someday becoming the "parent" to your own parents. By understanding the needs of older adults, you will be better prepared for this reversal of dependency.

Are you prepared to alter your own independence to help your aging parents make decisions? For example, will you be able to tell your parents that they should no longer drive an automobile? Can you be truly sensitive to the loss that your parents might feel if you must finally encourage them to move into a retirement community or apartment? Can you envision comforting your parents in death as they once held and comforted you in sickness and disappointment?

▪ **Assuming Increasing Levels of Responsibility** With increasing age and maturity, you will be expected (by the collective society) to assume more and more responsibility. Although you may not consciously think about it, most young adults are probably glad to shoulder more responsibility. Indeed, by successfully assuming increasing levels of responsibility, you can improve your mental health and your overall perspective on life.

Concerning dying and death, responsibility can gradually develop in many ways. For example, you can prepare a will, make funeral prearrangements, or plan an anatomical donation. You can also learn to become more responsible to other people by helping survivors cope with the deaths of family or friends. Finally, you can help younger family members or your own children develop healthy attitudes toward death by remaining open and honest when they come to you with questions and concerns about death.

▪ **Developing the Skills for Social Interaction** The everyday references you see to the loneliness that comes with aging, death experiences, and the grieving process might lead you to believe that these experiences are solitary ones. In fact, most of the time they are not. Many persons come in contact with older people, including family members, friends, neighbors, nurses, doctors, ministers, and social service employees. Growing older and dying should not be equated with isolation from other persons.

For this reason, it is important to maintain and sharpen your communication skills over your entire lifetime. Your continued social involvement as an active, interested older person will make your life more enjoyable to you and more meaningful to others.

Commonly Used Over-the-counter Products

Cold and Cough Products		
Active Ingredient*†	**Physiological Function**	**Potential Side Effect**
Decongestant (sympathemimetic amine) Phenylephrine hydrochloride	Vasoconstriction, which decreases blood flow into nasal tissues, thus decreasing fluid loss	Nervousness, sweating
Antihistamine Chlorpheniramine maleate	Blockage of histamine's vasodilating effect on capillaries within nasal tissue, thus reducing fluid loss (runny nose)	Drowsiness, drying of the mouth
Analgesic Acetaminophen	Pain relief and fever reduction	Generally few side effects with the amounts found in cold and cough preparations—see p. A3 for additional information on side effects

Cough suppressant
  Dextromethorphan hydrobromide
  Codeine
	Suppression of sensitivity of the brain's cough control center and reduces CNS activity, thus reducing coughing and facilitating sleep	Mild sedation

Alcohol 20% to 25% per unit volume	CNS depression	Reduction in inhibitions when taken in quantity

*Popular cold and cough medications generally contain an ingredient from each of the five categories listed.
†*Expectorants*, which stimulate respiratory tract secretions, and *bronchodilators*, which increase the diameter of air passages, have also been employed in the formulations of cold and cough medications. Their roles are to some degree controversial and are currently under study.

Deodorant and Antiperspirant Products

Two avenues exist for controlling odor resulting from the action of microbes on the organic matter in the perspiration of the apocrine sweat glands.

Product/Function	Active Agents	Adverse Side Effects
Control or mask odor		
Mild deodorant soaps	Hexachlorophene (0.75% or less) Triclocarban (TCC) Tribromosalicylanilide (TBS)	Swelling Blistering on exposure to sun
Deodorant (toilet water, colognes, perfumes, deodorants)	Alcohol Essential oils Vitamin E	Allergic reactions
Reduce release of perspiration		
Antiperspirants	Aluminum chloride Aluminum chlorohydrate Aluminum sulfate	Allergic reactions Should not be used for excessive, offensive, or colored perspiration

Personal Dental Hygiene Products

Product	Recommendations for Selection or Use
Toothbrush	Round, soft bristles in four rows; use 3 to 4 minutes with a proven technique; replace brush when bristles lose their original alignment
Disclosing solution	Use periodically to familiarize yourself with the locations in which plaque accumulates and to assess the effectiveness of your brushing and flossing technique; sequence: disclose-brush-inspect-brush-redisclose
Dental floss	Waxed or unwaxed cotton fiber thread for use in removing food debris from areas not generally reached by brushing alone; pull thread through adjoining tooth surfaces, gently elevating gingival tissues
Toothpaste	Tartar-control toothpaste is recommended. Select a fluoridated product in the midrange of abrasiveness; products designed to "brighten" or "whiten" teeth are generally too abrasive for general use; dentifrice intended for use with false teeth should not be used on natural teeth

Continued.

Personal Dental Hygiene Products—cont'd

Product	Recommendations for Selection or Use
Dental irrigator	Device using a pressurized stream of water to "pick" food debris lodged between teeth; model with a self-contained pump is considered more effective than one using household water pressure
Mouthwash	Freshens the breath; capable of effecting some plaque reduction only when used in combination with regular brushing and flossing; fluoridated dental rinses can contribute to the prevention of dental caries when used in combination with brushing and flossing

Pain Relievers

Product	Physiological Function	Potential Side Effect
Aspirin (only) Aspirin (with caffeine)	Analgesic (pain relief) Antipyretic (fever reduction) Antirheumatic (inflammation reduction) Anticoagulant (slowed clotting time)	Hypersensitivity Gastrointestinal disturbance Internal bleeding Ototoxicity (toxic action on the ear) Prothrombin depression Overdose potential Reye's syndrome
Acetaminophen (only) Acetaminophen (with aspirin) Acetaminophen (with caffeine) Acetaminophen (with aspirin and caffeine)	Analgesic (pain relief) Antipyretic (fever reduction)	Liver damage Gastric erosion Kidney failure Irregular heartbeat
Ibuprofen	Analgesic (pain relief) Antirheumatic (inflammation reduction)	Gastrointestinal disturbance Headache Nervousness Vision distortion Fluid retention Rash

Acne Products

Active Ingredient	Representative Brands	Effectiveness
Benzoyl peroxide medications	PanOxyl bar Oxy-5 and Oxy-10 Clearasil cream Noxzema Acne 12	The most effective OTC active ingredient; benzoyl peroxide aids in the prevention of new lesion formation
Salicylic acid cleaners	Clearasil Medicated Cleanser Stri-Dex Maximum Strength Pads PROPA pH Cleaning Pads and Lotion	Salicylic acid aids in unseating blackheads; alcohol base helps remove surface oils; no suppression of lesion formation is associated with these products
Sulfur-based medications	Acnomel Cream Fostril Lotion	Does not prevent lesion formation; active ingredient does help dry areas associated with lesions
Alcohol-based cleansers	Sea Breeze Antiseptic for the Skin Noxzema Antiseptic Skin Cleanser	Noneffective
Scrubs	Epi-Clear Scrub Cleanser Komix Cleanser	Too abrasive
Medicated soaps	Clearasil Antibacterial Soap Fostex Medicated Cleansing Bar	No more effective than ordinary soap and water

Sun Tanning Products

Sun Protection Factors and Classifications

2 to 4	Minimal protection from sunburn; permits fullest tanning
4 to 6	Moderate protection from sunburn; permits some tanning
6 to 8	Extra protection from sunburn; permits limited tanning
8 to 15	Maximal protection from sunburn; permits little or no tanning
15+	Ultraprotection from sunburn; permits no tanning

NOTE: Protection factor 65 is available in sun tanning products.

Safe and Effective Sunscreens

Aminobenzoic acid
Cinoxate
Diethanolamine p-methoxycinnamate
Digalloyl trioleate
Dioxybenzone
Ethyl 4-bis(hydroxypropyl)aminobenzoate
2-Ethylhexyl 2-cyano-3,3-diphylacrylate
Ethylhexyl p-methoxycinnamate
2-Ethylhexyl salicylate

Adverse Reactions to Excessive Sun Tanning

Skin cancer
Skin aging
Photosensitivity
Allergies

Continued.

Sun Tanning Products—cont'd

Safe and Effective Sunscreens—cont'd

Glyceryl aminobenzoate
Homosalate
Lawsone with dihydroxyacetone
Menthyl anthranilate
Oxybenzone
Padimate A
Padimate O
2-Phenylbenzimidazole-5-sulfonic acid
Red petrolatum
Sulisobenzone
Titanium dioxide
Triethanolamine salicylate

From Cornacchia, H, and Barrett, S: Consumer health: a guide to intelligent decisions, St. Louis, 1989, Times Mirror/Mosby College Publishing.

First Aid and Personal Safety

APPENDIX

2

Accidents are the leading cause of death for people ages 1-37.* Injuries sustained in accidents can often be tragic. They are grim reminders of our need to learn first aid skills and to practice preventive safety habits.

First aid knowledge and skills allow you to help people who are in need of immediate emergency care. They also can help you save yourself if you should become injured. We recommend that our students enroll in Red Cross first aid and safety courses, which are available in local communities or through colleges or universities. In this appendix we will briefly present some information about common first aid emergencies. After this, we will offer a variety of useful recommendations that can make your personal, residential, and recreational lives safer. (Please note that our information is *not* a substitute for comprehensive Red Cross first aid institution.)

FIRST AID

General Principles

1. Keep a list of important phone numbers near your phone (your doctor, ambulance service, hospital, poison control center, police and fire departments).
2. In case of serious injury or illness, call the appropriate emergency service for immediate help (if uncertain, call "911" or "0").

SPECIFIC PROBLEM	WHAT TO DO
Mouth-to-Mouth Breathing	
Victim stops breathing and skin, lips, tongue, and fingernail beds turn bluish or gray.	Adult: Tip head back with one hand on forehead and other lifting the lower jaw near the chin.
	Look, listen, and feel for breathing.
	If not breathing, place your mouth over victim's mouth, pinch the nose, get a tight seal, and give 2 slow, full breaths.
	Recheck the breathing; if still not breathing, give breaths once every 5 seconds for an adult, once every 4 seconds for a child, once every 3 seconds for infants (do not exaggerate head tilt for babies).

*Source: Bever, DL: *Safety: a personal focus*, ed 2, St. Louis, 1988, Times Mirror/Mosby College Publishing.

A6

SPECIFIC PROBLEM	*WHAT TO DO*

Bleeding

Victim bleeding severely can quickly go into shock and die within 1 or 2 minutes.

With the palm of your hand, apply firm, direct pressure to the wound with a clean dressing or pad.

Elevate the body part if possible.

Do not remove blood-soaked dressings; add additional layers, continue to apply pressure, and elevate the site.

Choking

Accidental ingestion or inhalation of food or other objects causes suffocation that can quickly lead to death. There are over 3,000 deaths annually, mostly of infants, small children, and the elderly.

The procedure for coping with airway obstruction is easy to learn. However, the Heimlich maneuver must be learned from a qualified instructor. The procedure varies somewhat for infants, children, adults, pregnant women, and obese persons.

Hyperventilation

A situation in which a person breathes too rapidly; often the result of fear or anxiety; may cause confusion, shortness of breath, dizziness, or fainting. Intentional hyperventilation because an underwater swim is especially dangerous, since it may cause a swimmer to "pass out" in the water and drown.

Have the person relax and rest for a few minutes. Provide reassurance and a calming influence. Having the victim take a few breaths in a paper bag (not plastic) may be helpful. Do not permit swimmers to practice hyperventilation before attempting to swim.

Bee Stings

Not especially dangerous except for persons who have developed an allergic hypersensitivity to a particular venom. Those who are not hypersensitive will indicate swelling, redness, and pain. Hypersensitive persons may develop extreme swelling, chest constriction, breathing difficulties, hives, and shock signs.

For nonsensitive persons: Scrape stinger from skin and apply cool compresses or over-the-counter topical preparation for insect bites.

For sensitive persons: Get professional help immediately. Scrape the stinger from skin; position the person so that the bitten body part is below the level of the heart; help administer prescribed medication (if available); apply cold compresses.

Poisoning

Often poisoning can be prevented with adequate safety awareness. Children are frequent victims.

Dilute with 1 glass of water or milk (if victim is conscious and not in convulsions).

Call the poison control center immediately; follow the instructions provided.

Keep syrup of ipecac on hand.

Shock

A life-threatening depression of circulation, respiration, and temperature control. Recognized by a victim's cool, clammy, pale skin; weak and rapid pulse; shallow breathing; weakness; nausea; or unconsciousness.

Provide psychological reassurance.

Keep victim calm and in a comfortable, reclining position; loosen tight clothing.

Prevent loss of body heat; cover if necessary.

Elevate feet 8 to 12 inches (if no head, neck, or back injuries).

Do not give fluids (unless aid will be delayed an hour or more).

Seek further emergency assistance.

SPECIFIC PROBLEM	WHAT TO DO
Burns	
Burns can cause major tissue damage and lead to serious infection and shock.	Minor burns; immerse in cold water and then cover with sterile dressings; do not apply butter or grease to burns.
	Major burns: seek help immediately; cover affected area with large quantities of clean dressings or bandages; do not try to clean the burned area or break blisters.
	Chemical burns: flood the area with running water.
Broken Bones	
Fractures are a common result of car accidents, falls, and recreational accidents.	Do not move the victim unless absolutely necessary to prevent further injury.
	Immobilize the affected area.
	Treat for shock while waiting for further emergency assistance.

Epilepsy: Recognition and First Aid

Seizure Type	What It Looks Like	Often Mistaken For	What To Do	What Not To Do
Convulsive				
Generalized tonic-clonic (also called grand mal)	Sudden cry, fall, rigidity, followed by muscle jerks, frothy saliva on lips, shallow breathing or temporarily suspended breathing, bluish skin, possible loss of bladder or bowel control, usually lasts 2-5 minutes; normal breathing then starts again; there may be some confusion and/or fatigue, followed by return to full consciousness	Heart attack Stroke Unknown but life-threatening emergency	Look for medical identification Protect from nearby hazards Loosen ties or shirt collars Place folded jacket under head Turn on side to keep airway clear; reassure when consciousness returns If single seizure lasted less than 10 minutes, ask if hospital evaluation wanted If multiple seizures, or if one seizure lasts longer than 10 minutes, take to emergency room	Don't put any hard implement in the mouth Don't try to hold tongue. It can't be swallowed Don't try to give liquids during or just after seizure Don't use oxygen unless there are symptoms of heart attack Don't use artificial respiration unless breathing is absent after muscle jerks subside, or unless water has been inhaled Don't restrain

Continued.

Epilepsy: Recognition and First Aid—cont'd

Seizure Type	What It Looks Like	Often Mistaken For	What To Do	What Not To Do
Nonconvulsive	This category includes many different forms of seizures, ranging from temporary unawareness (petit mal) to brief, sudden, massive muscle jerks (myoclonic seizures).	Daydreaming, acting out, clumsiness, poor coordination, intoxication, random activity, mental illness, and many others.	Usually no first aid necessary other than to provide reassurance and emotional support. Any nonconvulsive seizure that becomes convulsive should be managed as a convulsive seizure. Medical evaluation is recommended.	Do not shout at, restrain, expect verbal instructions to be obeyed, or grab a person having a nonconvulsive seizure (unless danger threatens).

Modified from Epilepsy Foundation of America.

PERSONAL SAFETY

Self-protection and the prevention of sexual assault are viable health issues that can threaten each of us—male or female. As violence in our society increases, the incidence of physical injury, sexual assault, and rape correspondingly rises. (See Chapter 14 for information concerning rape and sexual assault.) The recommendations that we present are intended to encourage you to think critically about how you can prevent personal assaults from happening to you:

1 Never assume that you are an unlikely candidate for personal assault.
2 Think carefully about your patterns of movement to and from class or work. Alter your routes frequently.
3 Walk briskly with a sense of purpose. Try not to walk alone at night.
4 Dress so that the clothes you wear do not unnecessarily restrict your movement or make you more vulnerable.
5 Always be aware of your surroundings. Look over your shoulder occasionally. Know where you are so you won't get lost.
6 If you think you are being followed, look for a safe retreat. This might be a store, a fire or police station, or a group of people.
7 Be especially cautious of first dates, blind dates, or people you meet at a party or bar who push to be alone with you.
8 Let trusted friends know where you are and when you plan to return.
9 Keep your car in good working order. Think beforehand how you would handle the situation should your car break down.
10 Trust your best instincts if you are assulted. Each situation is different. Do what you can to protect your life.

RESIDENTIAL SAFETY

Many serious accidents and personal assaults occur in dorm rooms, apartments, and houses. As a responsible young adult, you should make every reasonable effort to prevent these tragedies from happening. One good idea is to discuss some of the following points with your roommates (or housemates) and see what cooperative strategies you can implement:

1 Fireproof your residence. Are all electrical appliances and heating and cooling systems in safe working order? Are flammable materials safely stored?

2 Prepare a fire escape plan. Install smoke or heat detectors.

3 Do not give personal information over the phone to a stranger.

4 Use initials for first names on mailboxes and in phone books.

5 Install a peephole and deadbolt locks on outside doors.

6 Within reason, avoid living in first floor apartments. Change locks when moving to a new apartment or home.

7 Put locks on all windows.

8 Require repairmen or deliverymen to show valid identification.

9 Do not use an elevator if it is occupied by someone who makes you feel uneasy.

10 Be cautious around garages, laundry rooms, and driveways (especially at night). Use lighting for preventive reasons.

RECREATIONAL SAFETY

The thrills we get from risk taking are an essential part of our recreational endeavors. Sometimes we can get into serious accidents because we fail to consider important recreational safety information. Do some of the following recommendations apply to you?

1 Seek appropriate instruction for your intended activity. Few skill activities are as easy as they look.

2 Always wear your automobile seat belt.

3 Make certain that your equipment is in excellent working order.

4 Involve yourself gradually in an activity before attempting more complicated, dangerous skills.

5 Enroll in a Red Cross first aid course to enable you to cope with unexpected injuries.

6 Remember that alcohol use greatly increases the likelihood that people will get hurt.

7 Protect your eyes from serious injury.

8 Learn to swim. Drowning occurs most frequently to people who never intended to be in the water.

9 Obey the laws related to your recreational pursuits. Many laws are directly related to the safety of the participants.

10 Be aware of weather conditions. Many outdoor activities turn to tragedy with sudden shifts in the weather. Always prepare yourself for the worst possible weather.

FIREARM SAFETY

Each year about 10,000 Americans are murdered with guns and another 2,000 die in gun-related accidents. Most of the murders are committed with handguns. (Shotguns and rifles tend to be more cumbersome than handguns, and, thus, are not as frequently used in murders, accidents, or suicides.) Over half of all murders result from quarrels and arguments between acquaintances or relatives. With many homeowners arming themselves with handguns for protection against intruders, it is not surprising that over half of all gun accidents occur in the home. Children are frequently involved in gun accidents, often after they discover a gun they think is unloaded. Handgun owners are reminded to adhere to the following safety reminders:

1 Make certain that you follow the gun possession laws in your state. Special permits may be required to carry a handgun.
2 Make certain that your gun is in good mechanical order.
3 If you are a novice, enroll in a gun safety course.
4 Consider every gun to be a loaded gun, even if someone tells you it is unloaded.
5 Never point a gun at an unintended target.
6 Keep your finger off the trigger until you are ready to shoot.
7 When moving with a handgun, keep the barrel pointed down.
8 Load and unload your gun carefully.
9 Store your gun and ammunition safely in a locked container. Use a trigger lock on your gun when not in use.
10 Take target practice only at approved ranges.
11 Never "play" with guns at parties. Never handle a gun when intoxicated.
12 Educate children about gun safety and the potential dangers of gun use. Children must never believe that a gun is a toy.

MOTOR VEHICLE SAFETY

The greatest number of accidental deaths in America take place on highways and streets. When you are a young person, the most likely way that you will die is from a motor vehicle accident. According to Bever, the following is a description of a prime candidate for such a death:

. . . a male, 15 to 24 years of age, driving on a two-lane, rural road between the hours of 10 PM and 2 AM on a Saturday night. If he has been drinking and is driving a subcompact car or motorcycle, the likelihood that he and his passengers will have a fatal accident is even more pronounced.

Disabling injuries also result from motor vehicle accidents. With nearly 2 million such injuries each year, concern for the prevention of motor vehicle accidents should be important for all college students, regardless of age. With this thought in mind, we offer some important safety tips for motor vehicle operators:

1 Make certain that you are familiar with the traffic laws in your state.
2 Do not operate an automobile or motorcycle unless it is in good mechanical order. Regularly inspect your brakes, lights, and exhaust system.
3 Do not exceed the speed limit. Observe all traffic signs.
4 Always wear safety belts, even on short trips. Require your passengers to buckle up. Always keep small children in child restraints.

*Source: Bever, DL: *Safety: a personal focus*, ed 2, St. Louis, 1988, Times Mirror/Mosby College Publishing.

5 Never drink and drive. Avoid horseplay inside a car.

6 Be certain that you can hear the traffic outside your car. Keep the car's music system at a reasonable decible level.

7 Give pedestrians the right-of-way.

8 Drive defensively at all times. Do not challenge other drivers. Refrain from drag racing.

9 Look carefully before changing lanes.

10 Be especially careful at intersections and railroad crossings.

11 Carry a well-maintained first aid kit that includes flares or other signal devices.

12 Alter your driving behaviors during bad weather.

HOME ACCIDENT PREVENTION FOR CHILDREN AND THE ELDERLY

Approximately one person in ten is injured each year in a home accident. Children and the elderly spend significantly more hours each day in a home setting than do young adults and midlife persons. It is especially important that accident prevention be given primary consideration for these groups. Here are some important tips to remember. Can you think of others?

For both groups:

1 Be certain that you have adequate insurance protection.

2 Install smoke detectors appropriately.

3 Keep stairways clear of toys or debris. Install railings.

4 Maintain electrical and heating equipment.

5 Make certain that inhabitants know how to get emergency help.

For children:

1 Know all the ways to protect from accidental poisoning.

2 Use toys that are appropriate for the age of the child.

3 Never leave young children unattended, especially infants.

4 Keep any hazardous items (guns, poisons, etc.) locked up.

5 Keep small children away from kitchen stoves.

For elderly:

1 Protect from falls. (Consider rugs, floors, and stairs.)

2 Install safety equipment in the bathroom (rails, slip-resistant surfaces).

3 Be certain that elderly persons have a good understanding of the medications they may be taking. Know the side effects.

4 Encourage elderly persons to seek assistance when it comes to home repairs.

5 Make certain that all door locks, lights, and safety equipment are in good working order.

Bever, DL: *Safety: a personal focus*, ed 2, St. Louis, 1988, Times Mirror/Mosby College Publishing.

A Look at
Canadian Health

Satisfaction With Life as a Whole and With the Major Life Domains

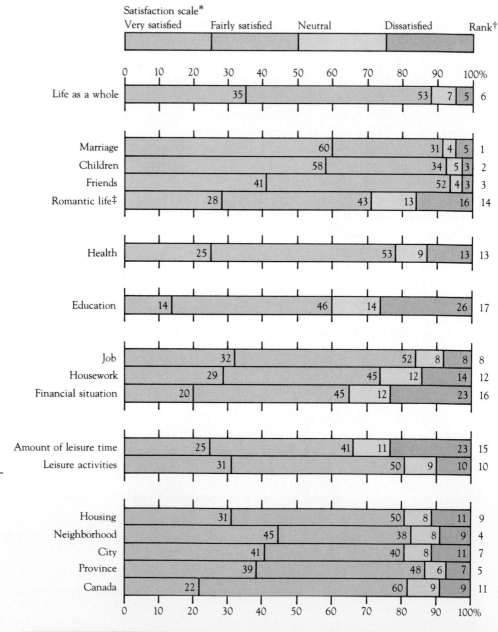

From Statistics Canada.

*Those surveyed were asked to rate their degree of satisfaction on a scale of 1 to 11. "Very Satisfied" includes those who responded 10 and 11; "Fairly Satisfied"—7, 8, and 9; "Neutral"—6; and "Dissatisfied"—1 to 5.

†Represents the ranking of the average rating for the respective domains.

‡Includes only unmarried persons.

Social Characteristics of Active Versus Sedentary Canadians, Age 15 + *

Characteristic	Persons (Thousands)	Active (%)	Moderate (%)	Sedentary (%)
Total, age 15 +	18,805	54	33	12
Education				
Elementary	2,473	41	31	25
Some secondary	5,402	53	33	12
Secondary or more	5,324	56	34	8
Certificate or diploma	2,920	58	33	7
University degree	2,193	63	31	5
Unknown	494	42	24	31
Occupation*				
Manager/professional	2,907	60	34	6
Other white collar	4,320	53	36	8
Blue collar	3,199	48	38	10
Unknown	409	49	33	15
Marital status				
Single	5,360	63	27	8
Married	11,063	49	37	12
Other	2,193	55	24	19
Unknown	189	42	26	30

From Canada Fitness Survey.
Note: The balance on each row consists of unknown activity levels, averaging about 3%.
*For those who reported employment in the 2 weeks preceding the survey.

Participation* in Sports or Exercise Activities by Age and Sex

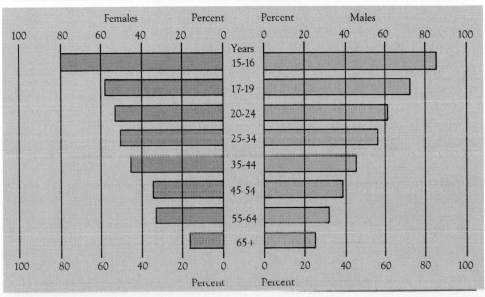

From Statistics Canada.
*Participation during the week before the survey.

Characteristics of Alcohol Consumers, 15 years of Age and Over*

	Percentage of Users		
	Females	Males	Total
Age			
15-17 years	60.1	69.0	64.7
18-19 years	90.3	84.7	87.5
20-24 years	83.3	91.5	87.4
25-29 years	90.2	91.7	91.0
30-39 years	85.1	91.7	88.0
40-49 years	81.5	90.1	85.8
50-64 years	76.2	85.6	80.8
65 years and over	48.6	71.6	58.2
Region			
British Columbia	78.9	91.7	85.2
Prairie region	77.6	85.5	81.7
Ontario	75.4	85.0	80.2
Quebec	81.8	86.4	84.1
Atlantic region	60.8	78.8	69.9
Income			
Under $5,000	60.2	78.5	67.2
$ 5,000-9,999	71.6	78.7	74.8
$10,000-14,999	75.4	81.4	78.5
$15,000-19,999	82.6	90.1	86.5
$20,000 and over	86.8	92.7	90.0
Education			
Grade B and under	63.7	81.1	72.6
Secondary	67.0	84.4	81.1
Technical institute	86.8	89.7	88.3
University	88.8	92.3	90.7
Occupation			
Professional/managerial	84.7	90.7	87.7
Sales/white collar	86.0	87.6	86.8
Skilled labor	83.0	86.5	84.8
Unskilled labor	68.6	88.3	79.8
Farmer	67.7	78.2	73.8
Unemployed	69.8	87.8	80.5
Size of community			
Under 10,000 and rural	70.8	82.7	76.9
10,000-30,000	79.6	82.9	81.0
30,000-100,000	75.4	86.5	81.1
100,000-500,000	79.0	87.4	82.8
Over 500,000	80.5	88.3	84.5
TOTAL	76.6	85.7	81.1

From Statistics Canada.
*Does not include Northwest Territories and Yukon.

Apparent Consumption of Beverage Alcohol, Canada and Provinces

Province	Thousands of Liters Consumed		
	Beer	Wine	Spirits
Newfoundland	39,213	1,827	4,094
Prince Edward Island	8,940	562	825
Nova Scotia	64,300	5,362	6,084
New Brunswick	51,090	3,202	3,446
Quebec	605,003	74,275	23,895
Ontario	803,561	85,663	62,642
Manitoba	81,632	7,570	8,369
Saskatchewan	65,209	5,458	7,817
Alberta	173,514	24,725	23,087
British Columbia	223,194	47,309	23,731
Yukon	3,143	357	269
Northwest Territory	4,154	293	539
TOTAL CANADA	2,122,953	256,603	164,798

From Statistics Canada.

Liters of Absolute Alcohol* Per Person Aged 15 Years and Over, Canada and Provinces

Province	1977-1978	1978-1979	1979-1980	1980-1981	1981-1982	1982-1983
Newfoundland	10.81	10.88	11.28	10.87	10.65	10.60
Prince Edward Island	10.76	11.14	10.61	10.43	9.36	9.57
Nova Scotia	10.37	10.40	10.37	10.26	10.06	9.85
New Brunswick	8.26	9.38	9.40	9.27	8.91	8.80
Quebec	10.37	10.42	9.80	10.03	9.78	9.19
Ontario	11.51	11.52	11.50	11.47	11.40	11.16
Manitoba	11.39	10.74	11.07	11.35	11.21	10.85
Saskatchewan	10.46	10.22	10.22	10.28	9.98	9.98
Alberta	12.71	12.79	13.29	10.44	13.58	12.94
British Columbia	13.22	12.77	13.36	13.19	13.38	12.83
Yukon	20.04	19.87	21.52	23.81	21.27	19.39
Northwest Territory	14.64	13.90	13.19	13.64	13.90	13.90
TOTAL CANADA	11.30	11.28	11.24	11.03	11.20	10.82

From Statistics Canada.
*To convert liters of beverage to liters of absolute alcohol, the following average values were employed: beer—5% alcohol by volume; wine—13%; and spirits—40%.

Proportion of Canadian Students Reporting Drug Use*

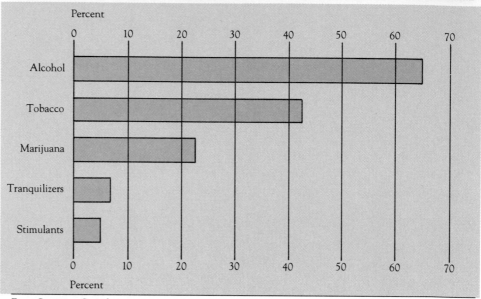

From Statistics Canada.
*The Crude Weighted Average of the proportion of drug users (used at least once in the last 6 months) in six studies.

Percentage of Regular Cigarette Smokers in the Population 15 Years of Age and Over by Sex and Age Group, Canada

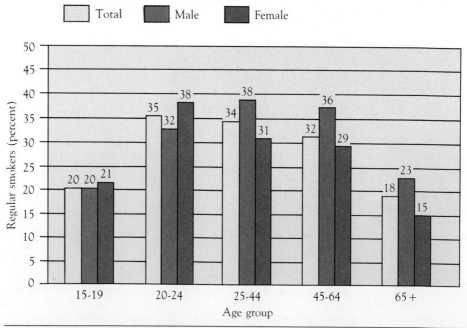

From Statistics Canada.

Death and Potential Years of Life Lost (PYLL) Attributable to Smoking to Age 70*

| | Causes of Death | | | | | | | |
| | Cancer of Trachea, Bronchus, and Lung | Cancer of Oral Cavity and Pharynx, Larynx, and Esophagus | Chronic Bronchitis and Emphysema | Ischemic Heart Disease | Cerebro-vascular Disease | Total | | |
						Male	Female	Total
Total deaths (1-70 years)	4,726	1,003	931	19,368	3,752	22,156	7,624	29,780
Percentage of deaths due to smoking	63.4	65.5	41.9	23.6	12.3	35.8	14.9	30.4
Deaths attributable to smoking	2,996	657	390	4,570	462	7,936	1,139	9,075
Total potential years of life lost (PYLL)	49,328	12,728	9,438	208,443	44,606	244,295	80,248	324,543
Percentage of PYLL due to smoking	61.4	65.8	33.2*	30.7	14.5	39.8	18.8	34.6
PYLL attributable to smoking	30,287	8,375	3,133*	63,992	6,468	97,157	15,098	112,255

From Statistics Canada.
*Includes men only; no data available for women.

Satisfaction with Romantic Relationship by Age

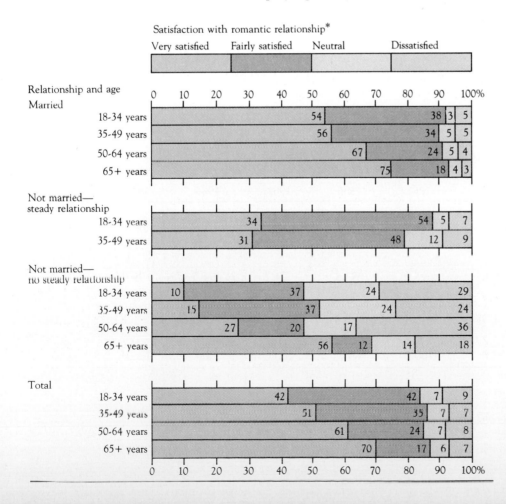

From Statistics Canada.
*See the chart on p. A-13.
†Older age groups not included because of insufficient respondents.

Divorce Rates by Province*

	1968†	1970	1974	1976	1977	1978	1980	1981	1982	1983	1984	1985
Newfoundland	3.0	27.1	55.5	76.0	81.1	75.0	95.8	100.2	109.8	123.0	101.8	96.6
Prince Edward Island	18.2	59.1	82.3	98.1	113.1	110.7	131.0	152.6	167.8	173.4	155.6	167.6
Nova Scotia	64.8	105.2	195.6	211.6	215.7	233.1	271.3	269.6	267.6	272.3	260.3	265.4
New Brunswick	22.9	61.6	114.1	138.5	140.0	165.9	187.4	191.6	237.9	274.8	200.1	189.1
Quebec	10.2	80.9	200.1	243.6	230.8	236.6	220.2	298.1	286.6	266.3	257.2	240.3
Ontario	69.3	164.9	188.7	224.9	235.7	243.2	261.7	251.4	271.3	261.7	242.1	230.0
Manitoba	47.9	125.5	177.6	190.0	202.2	211.8	221.7	233.8	231.1	252.3	247.1	216.3
Saskatchewan	40.0	92.6	114.6	131.0	157.4	150.7	189.3	199.5	185.3	201.5	197.6	189.0
Alberta	125.7	236.4	288.6	309.9	307.6	310.4	364.2	376.2	383.3	372.5	359.9	344.9
British Columbia	110.8	240.2	285.6	333.7	330.4	326.7	358.4	347.4	364.3	331.0	313.1	288.0
Yukon	200.0	241.2	237.1	Yukon/North-								
Northwest Territories	36.7	51.5	157.3	west Territories		217.1	244.6	204.7	259.5	244.7	244.4	228.0
TOTAL CANADA	54.8	139.8	200.6	235.8	237.7	243.4	259.1	278.0	285.9	275.5	259.4	244.4

From Statistics Canada.
*Rate per 100,000 persons.
†Divorce laws were liberalized in Canada in 1968.

Census Family Heads by Marital Status, 1941-1976

	1941	1951	1956	1961	1966	1971	1976
Married family heads							
Currently married*	87.8	90.1	91.4	91.6	91.8	90.7	90.3
Separated†	1.8	2.9	2.3	2.6	2.5	2.5	2.5
Spouse absent	—	—	—	—	—	0.6	0.5
Total, married‡	89.6	93.0	93.7	94.2	94.3	93.9	93.3
Widowed	8.9	6.6	5.8	5.2	5.0	4.3	4.0
Divorced	1.3§	0.3	0.3	0.4	0.5	1.1	2.0
Single, never-married	0.2	0.1	0.1	0.2	0.2	0.7	0.7
TOTAL, FAMILY HEADS	100.0	100.0	100.0	100.0	100.0	100.0	100.0

From Statistics Canada.
*This is the count of husband-wife families.
†Includes spouse absent until 1971.
‡Includes those married, spouse absent and separated.
§Includes those permanently separated.

Percentage of Population Using Nonprescription Remedies,* by Province

	Percentage Making†			
	Daily Use	Weekly Use	Monthly Use	Yearly Use
Prince Edward Island	29	60	85	96
Nova Scotia	41	56	85	96
New Brunswick	39	57	83	95
Quebec	48	65	87	95
Ontario	50	66	90	96
Manitoba	45	58	88	96
Saskatchewan	45	66	90	97
Alberta	55	70	91	98
British Columbia	53	68	88	97
Canada‡	49	65	88	96

From Statistics Canada.
*Non-prescription remedies include any drugs that may be purchased without a doctor's prescription: for example, aspirin, cough and cold remedies, laxatives, vitamins, etc.
†Usage was determined as follows: daily: reported daily use during the last month; Weekly: reported using remedy at least once a week during the last month; monthly: reported monthly use but did not indicate whether or not the remedies were used daily or weekly; yearly: reported using remedy at least once during the past year.
‡Newfoundland, Yukon and Northwest Territories not included.

Major Causes of Death, by Sex

Cause	Male	Female	Total
Diseases of the circulatory system	43,535	36,874	80,409
Neoplasms	23,640	18,724	42,364
Accidents, poisonings, and violence	10,045	4,120	14,165
Diseases of the respiratory system	7,574	4,664	12,238
Diseases of the digestive system	3,800	3,153	6,953
Endocrine, nutritional, and metabolic diseases and immunity disorders	1,826	2,288	4,114
Symptoms, signs, and ill-defined conditions	1,426	1,039	2,465
Diseases of the genitourinary system	1,247	1,082	2,329
Certain conditions originating in certain causes of perinatal period mortality	904	609	1,513
Diseases of the nervous system and sense organs	1,290	1,164	2,454
Congenital anomalies	823	646	1,469
Other causes	1,944	1,996	3,940
TOTAL ALL CAUSES	98,054	76,359	174,413

From Statistics Canada.

Suicide Death Rate by Age and Sex, Canada

Age Group	Sex	1951*	1976*	1981*	1984*	1985*
15-19	M	3.9	18.6	20.3	22.0	20.1
	F	1.8	4.5	3.8	3.5	3.5
20-24	M	8.8	33.6	32.1	33.0	31.4
	F	3.2	7.7	6.5	5.0	4.7
25-29	M	7.6	28.1	28.9	31.0	27.7
	F	3.9	8.6	7.5	7.0	6.3
30-34	M	10.4	24.3	26.6	29.0	26.5
	F	3.8	10.4	8.0	8.5	7.2
35-39	M	13.2	25.2	24.7	24.5	23.9
	F	4.6	10.9	8.6	9.0	7.5
40-44	M	19.6	27.3	26.2	28.0	25.3
	F	6.4	10.8	10.4	11.5	9.6
45-49	M	21.6	29.3	29.1	22.5	24.9
	F	7.2	14.0	12.4	11.5	9.6
50-54	M	26.4	32.7	29.7	30.0	30.2
	F	8.3	13.4	13.6	11.5	9.9
55-59	M	27.2	26.6	29.6	32.0	29.5
	F	7.3	13.7	12.3	11.0	9.8
60-64	M	30.8	24.1	27.2	29.0	25.1
	F	9.0	11.9	11.2	11.0	8.8
65-69	M	28.2	24.3	26.8	26.0	24.2
	F	9.3	9.9	10.3	11.5	8.8
70-74	M	29.5	26.3	30.1	30.5	29.2
	F	6.3	8.4	9.3	8.0	7.0
75-79	M	32.8	24.9	34.4	35.0	28.1
	F	5.9	5.8	7.1	6.0	5.8
80-84	M	25.1	21.2	41.7	36.5	32.4
	F	2.0	7.3	6.9	8.0	5.0
Standardized	M	15.7	26.5	27.5	28.1	26.3
Rate†	F	5.2	9.6	8.7	8.2	7.1

*Averages for 1950 and 1951, 1975 and 1976, 1980 and 1981, 1983 and 1984, 1984 and 1985, respectively.
†Age structure of Canada in 1976 was used as standard.
From: Statistics Canada.

Deaths From Artery Disease, Hypertension, and Ulcers

Cause	1969	1971	1973	1975	1976	1977	1982
Arteriosclerosis							
Male	1,314	1,437	1,629	1,503	1,434	1,528	1,302
Female	1,521	1,749	1,899	1,851	1,874	1,812	1,809
TOTAL	2,835	3,186	3,528	3,354	3,308	3,140	3,111
Hypertension							
Male	136	123	113	107	108	105	104
Female	151	144	148	152	125	145	163
TOTAL	287	267	261	259	233	250	267
Ulcers							
Male	687	657	577	521	445	435	444
Female	268	261	267	245	258	234	385
TOTAL	955	918	844	766	703	669	829

From Statistics Canada.

Mental Disorders

CATEGORIES OF MENTAL DISORDERS

Anxiety Disorders

Anxiety disorders are characterized by a fear that leads to overarousal of heartbeat, muscle tension, and shakiness.

  a. *Phobic disorder.* Excessive irrational fears. Examples are agoraphobia (fear of open places), claustrophobia (fear of enclosed places), and acrophobia (fear of heights).
  b. *Panic disorder.* Overwhelming fear of losing control or going crazy. Panic attacks can last from a minute to an hour or more. No clear reason why panic attacks occur.
  c. *Generalized anxiety disorder.* Continued, free-floating anxiety that lasts for at least 1 month.
  d. *Obsessive-compulsive disorder.* Obsessive behavior is characterized by recurring, irrational thoughts that remain out of control. Compulsive behavior reflects an irresistible urge to act repeatedly.

Dissociative Disorders

Dissociative disorders in which there is a sudden, temporary change in consciousness or self-identity.

  a. *Psychogenic amnesia.* Inability to recall a stressful event.
  b. *Psychogenic fugue.* Disorder in which a person loses memory of his or her past, moves to another locale, and takes on a new identity.
  c. *Multiple personality.* Disorder characterized by several distinct personalities occupying the same person.

Somatoform Disorders

Persons with somatoform disorders complain of a physical ailment, yet no physical abnormality can be found.

  a. *Conversion disorder.* Major, unexplained loss of some physical ability (such as eyesight or use of the legs).
  b. *Hypochondriasis.* The belief that one is sick, although no medical evidence can be found.

Affective Disorders

In affective disorders a disturbance exists in a person's ability to express emotions.

  a. *Dysthymic disorder.* Persistent feelings (lasting for at least 2 years) characterized by lack of energy, loss of self-esteem, pessimistic outlook, inability to enjoy other people or pleasurable activities, and thoughts about suicide. This disorder is likely the most common psychological problem in humans.
  b. *Major depressive disorder.* Depression more severe than dysthymic disorder. Evidenced by poor appetite and major weight loss, psychomotor symptoms, impaired reality testing, and recurrent thoughts of suicide.
  c. *Bipolar disorder.* Mood swings from elation to depression (formerly known as manic-depression).

Source: Rathus, SA: Psychology, New York 1987, Holt, Rinehart, & Winston.

Schizophrenic Disorders

Schizophrenic disorders are largely recognized by a person's verbal behavior. These disorders are characterized by disturbances in thought, perception, and attention. Schizophrenics may speak in a meaningless fashion, switch from topic to topic, and convey little important information. They may have delusions of grandeur or persecution, hallucinations, or excited or slowed motor activity. Usually schizophrenics do not think that their thoughts and actions are abnormal.

a. *Disorganized type.* Characterized by disorganized delusions and frequent hallucinations that may be sexual or religious in nature. Exaggerated social impairment is common.

b. *Catatonic type.* Characterized by a marked impairment in motor activity. May hold one body position for hours and not respond to the speech of others.

c. *Paranoid type.* Characterized by delusions of persecution, often ones that are complex and systemized. Paranoid schizophrenics may experience vivid hallucinations that support their delusions.

THERAPEUTIC APPROACHES TO MENTAL DISORDERS

A variety of approaches can be used to help persons who have mental disorders. These approaches involve psychotherapy or the use of biological therapies. A brief outline of the more widely known strategies follows, as a comprehensive presentation on this topic is beyond the scope of this appendix.

Insight-Oriented Therapies

Underlying this category of therapeutic approaches is the belief that the client must gain insight into the experiences that led up to his or her problem or maladaptive behavior. By being able to recognize the underlying motives for one's behavior, a client will be better able to objectively view his or her beliefs, feelings, and thinking patterns. These underlying motives often are beneath the person's level of consciousness. Insight-oriented forms of psychotherapy include cognitive therapy, psychoanalysis, person-centered therapy, transactional analysis, and gestalt therapy.

Behavior Therapy

Discussed briefly in Chapters 2 and 6, behavior therapy (also called behavior modification) attempts to produce behavior change in a client by using scientifically tested principles of classical and operant conditioning and observational learning. Techniques of behavior therapy include operant conditioning (behavior reinforcement), aversive conditioning, systematic desensitization, assertiveness training, and self-control techniques.

Group Therapy

This form of therapy involves a therapist and several clients who have similar problems. Examples might be group therapy for persons with eating disorders, smoking concerns, sexual problems, family problems, or relationship concerns.

By meeting together and working to resolve their similar concerns, clients often receive support from other group members. With multiple members, a larger volume of pertinent information exists for clients to share. In a practical sense, group therapy is usually less expensive than individual therapy and the therapist can reach more clients at once.

Biological Therapies

Psychiatrists and other physicians are qualified to approach mental disorders from a medical framework. They are able to use chemotherapy (tranquilizers, antidepressants, lithium), electroconvulsive therapy (ECT or shock therapy), and even psychosurgery (brain surgery). Often these approaches are used with clients who have especially serious psychiatric disorders or who do not respond well to psychotherapy.

Body Systems

The major organ systems of the body. The many organs that, working together, carry out the principal activities of the body are traditionally grouped together as organ systems.

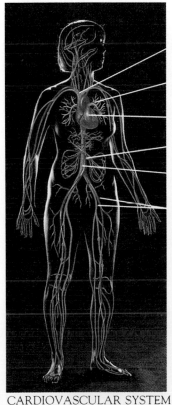

Superior
vena cava

Pulmonary
artery

Heart

Aorta

Inferior
vena cava

Femoral artery
and vein

CARDIOVASCULAR SYSTEM

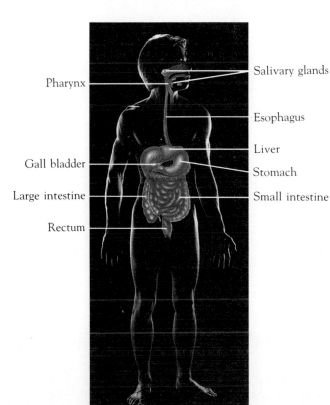

Pharynx

Gall bladder

Large intestine

Rectum

Salivary glands

Esophagus

Liver

Stomach

Small intestine

DIGESTIVE SYSTEM

Pituitary

Parathyroids
(behind thyroid)

Thyroid

Thymus

Adrenals

Pancreas

Ovaries
(in females)

Testis
(in males)

ENDOCRINE SYSTEM

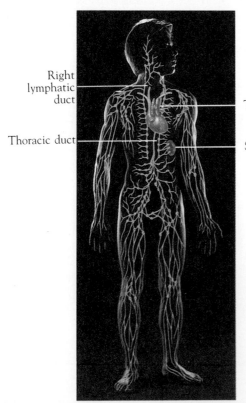

Right
lymphatic
duct

Thymus gland

Thoracic duct

Spleen

LYMPHATIC SYSTEM

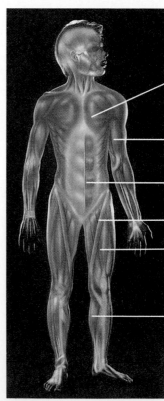

Pectoralis
Major

Biceps

Rectus
Abdominus

Sartorius

Quadriceps

Gastrocnemius

MUSCULAR SYSTEM

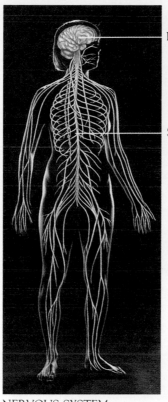

Brain

Spinal Cord

NERVOUS SYSTEM

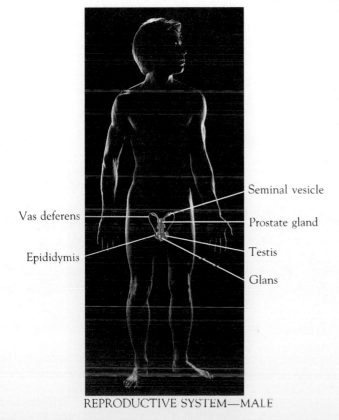

Seminal vesicle

Vas deferens

Prostate gland

Epididymis

Testis

Glans

REPRODUCTIVE SYSTEM—MALE

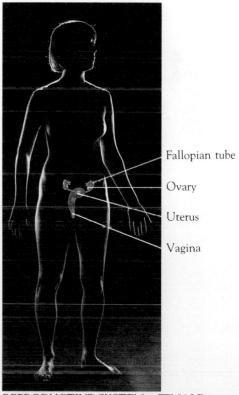

Fallopian tube

Ovary

Uterus

Vagina

REPRODUCTIVE SYSTEM—FEMALE

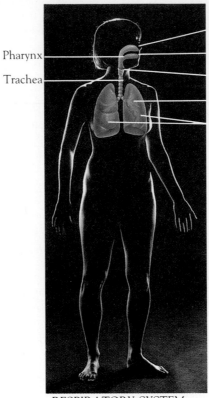
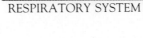

Nasal cavity

Pharynx

Oral cavity

Trachea

Larynx

Bronchus

Lungs

RESPIRATORY SYSTEM

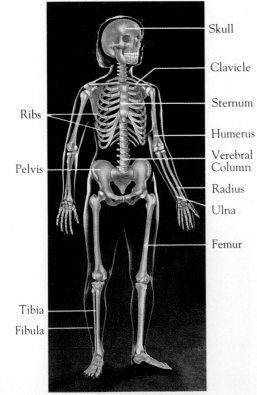

Skull

Clavicle

Sternum

Ribs

Humerus

Verebral
Column

Pelvis

Radius

Ulna

Femur

Tibia

Fibula

SKELETAL SYSTEM

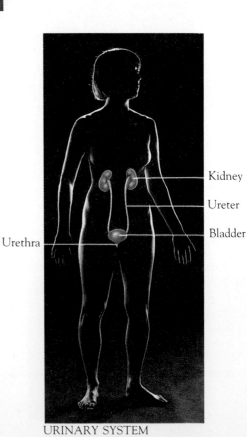

Kidney

Ureter

Bladder

Urethra

URINARY SYSTEM

A

abortion induced premature termination of a pregnancy (p. 449).

absorption passage of nutrients or alcohol through the walls of the stomach or intestinal tract into the bloodstream (p. 204).

acid-base balance acidity-alkalinity of body fluids (p. 103).

acid fog fog composed of water droplets that are more acidic (lower pH) than that normally associated with fog (p. 523).

acid rain rain that is more acidic (lower pH) than that normally associated with rain (p. 523).

acquired immunity major component of the immune system associated with the formation of antibodies and specialized blood cells that are capable of destroying pathogens (p. 334).

ACTH adrenocorticotropic hormone (p. 230).

actively acquired immunity type of acquired immunity resulting from the body's response to naturally occurring pathogens (p. 334).

activity requirement calories required for daily physical work (p. 142).

activity theory theory of aging that suggests that the elderly must (and desire to) remain in familiar and/or new areas of involvement (p. 567).

acupuncture process that attempts to alter the body's electroenergy fields to cure diseases (p. 151).

acute alcohol intoxication potentially fatal elevation of the blood alcohol concentration, often resulting from heavy, rapid consumption of alcohol (p. 206).

acute rhinitis the common cold; the sudden onset of nasal inflammation (p. 337).

adaptive thermogenesis physiological response of the body to adjust its metabolic rate to the presence of food (p. 137).

addiction term used interchangeably with physical dependency (p. 166).

addictive personality personality traits that may predispose a person to drug abuse (p. 169).

additive effect combined (but not exaggerated) effect produced by the concurrent use of two or more drugs (p. 185).

adrenal cortex outer cell layers of the adrenal glands; cells of the cortex, on stimulation by ACTH, produce corticoids (p. 50).

adrenal glands paired triangular endocrine glands situated above each kidney; site of epinephrine and corticoid production (p. 50).

adrenalin powerful stress response hormone (see epinephrine) (p. 51).

adrenocorticotropic hormone (ACTH) hormone produced in the pituitary gland and transmitted to the cortex of the adrenal glands; stimulates production and release of corticoids (p. 50).

aerobic energy production body's production of energy when the respiratory and circulatory systems are able to process and transport a sufficient amount of oxygen to muscle cells (p. 75).

affect priorities, predispositions, and values; affect influences cognition and performance (p. 32).

affective pertaining to one's beliefs, values, and predispositions (p. 377).

agent causal pathogen of a particular disease (p. 331).

agility ability of the body to move quickly with frequent changes in direction (p. 71).

AIDS Acquired Immune Deficiency Syndrome; viral-based destruction of the immune system leading to illness and death from opportunistic infections (p. 340).

alcoholism pattern of alcohol use characterized by emotional and physical dependence as well as a general loss of control over the use of alcohol (p. 216).

allergens environmental substances to which persons may be hypersensitive; allergens function as antigens (p. 314).

allopathy system of medical practice in which specific remedies are used to produce effects different from those produced by a disease (p. 494).

alveoli thin, saclike terminal ends of the airways; the sites at which gases are exchanged between the blood and inhaled air (p. 241).

Alzheimer's disease gradual development of memory loss, confusion, and loss of reasoning; can eventually lead to total intellectual incapacitation, brain degeneration, and death (p. 571).

ambivalence simultaneous holding of two incongruent ideas or aspirations: love-hate, attraction-rejection (p. 25).

amino acids chief components of protein; synthesized by the body or obtained from dietary sources (p. 102).

amotivational syndrome behavioral pattern characterized by widespread apathy toward productive activities (p. 182).

amyloid a protein-related waste found in the tissue of the elderly (p. 559).

anabolic steroids drugs that function like testosterone to produce increase in weight and strength (p. 89).

anaerobic energy production body's production of energy when needed amounts of oxygen are not readily available (p. 74).

analgesic drugs drugs that reduce the sensation of pain (p. 310).

anaphylactic shock life-threatening congestion of the airways resulting from hypersensitivity to a foreign protein (p. 314).

androgen hormones male sex hormones (p. 362).

androgyny the blending of both masculine and feminine characteristics (p. 379).

anemia condition reflecting abnormally low levels of hemoglobin (p. 322).

anesthetic drugs capable of blocking pain sensations (p. 471).

angina pectoris chest pain that results from impaired blood supply to the heart muscle (p. 269).

angiogenesis factor chemical messenger that stimulates the development of additional capillaries into the tumor (p. 293).

angioplasty surgical insertion of a balloon-tipped catheter into the coronary artery to open areas of narrowing (p. 271).

anorexia nervosa psychogenic disorder in which appetite and hunger are suppressed, and marked weight loss occurs (p. 155).

anovulatory not ovulating (p. 373).

antagonistic effect effect produced when one drug nullifies (reduces, offsets) the effects of a second drug (p. 185).

antibodies chemical compounds produced by the immune system to destroy antigens and their toxins (p. 52).

anticonvulsant drugs drugs that slow the electrical activity within the brain and thus reduce the occurrence of seizures (p. 317).

antigens disease-producing microorganisms or foreign substances that on entering the body trigger an immune response (p. 334).

antihistamines drugs that block the release of histamines (p. 315).

antiinflammatory agents drugs that reduce inflammation (p. 315).

antioncogenes genes whose function is to prevent the activation of oncogenes (p. 294).

aortic valve valve that controls the blood flow into the aorta from the left ventricle of the heart (p. 264).

ARC AIDS related complex; condition suggesting some deterioration of the immune system as a result of infection by the HIV agent (p. 343).

arrhythmias irregularities of the heart's normal rhythm or beating pattern (p. 270).

arteriosclerosis calcification of an artery's wall that makes the vessel less elastic, more brittle, and more susceptible to bursting; hardening of the arteries (p. 274).

artificial insemination depositing of sperm in the female reproductive tract in an attempt to impregnate; sperm may be those of the partner or of a donor (p. 476).

artificially acquired immunity type of acquired immunity resulting from the body's response to pathogens introduced into the body through immunizations (p. 334).

asbestos fiberous material found in insulation and many other building materials; asbestosis (p. 523).

asceticism philosophically centered denial of the importance of the body (p. 393).

asphyxiation death resulting from lack of oxygen to the brain (p. 206).

atherosclerosis a condition that produces narrowing of arteries through accumulation of fatty deposits (p. 266).

audiologists health care professionals trained to assess auditory function (p. 540).

auditory acuity clarity or sharpness at which a particular sound can be heard (p. 540).

authentic self postive self-identity that underlies the individual's more temporary mood identities; the most basic self-concept (p. 22).

autoimmune immune response against the cells of a person's own body (p. 318).

autonomic nervous system nervous system that controls the involuntary functions of the body; sympathetic and parasympathetic branches activate and deactivate body responses as conditions warrant (p. 51).

axon portion of a neuron that conducts electrical impulses to the dendrites of adjacent neurons;

neurons typically have one axon (p. 170).

AZT (azidothymidine) the first drug approved for use in the treatment of AIDS, capable of reducing symptoms and possibly extending life expectancy of the AIDS victim (p. 343).

B

balanced diet diet featuring food selections from each of the four food groups (p. 110).

bariatrician physician who specializes in the study and treatment of obesity (p. 137).

basal cells foundation cells that underlie the epithelial cells (p. 240).

basal metabolism rate (BMR) the amount of energy (in calories) your body requires to maintain basic functions (p. 137).

basement membrane thin layer of tissue that separates the basal cells of the airway tissue from the underlying connective tissue (p. 241).

behavior modification behavioral therapy designed to change the learned behavior of an individual (p. 151).

behavioralism psychological school of thought that believes that human behavior arises in response to the presentation of stimuli (p. 24).

being needs needs associated with actualization and spiritual growth (p. 27).

being values values associated with higher human potential: truth, beauty, goodness (p. 27).

benign noncancerous (p. 293).

bestiality alternate term for zoophilia (p. 411).

beta blockers drugs that prevent overactivity of the heart, which results in angina pectoris (p. 269).

binge drinking alcohol use characterized by periods of intense alcohol consumption, for example, drinking heavily on the weekend (p. 213).

bioavailability speed and extent to which a drug becomes biologically active within the body; bioavailability for a drug varies between individuals and within a given individual over the course of time (p. 511).

biochemical defenses body's immune system (p. 333).

biochemical oxygen demand index of water pollution based on the rate and extent that matter uses up dissolved oxygen from a sample of water (p. 527).

biofeedback self-monitoring of physiological processes as they occur within the body (p. 55).

biological sexuality male and female aspects of sexuality (p. 361).

biological toxins poisons produced by microorganisms during the course of an infectious disease (p. 118).

biologically available term used to describe the ability of a particular material to be used by the body (p. 124).

biologicals living materials that hold, or are believed to possess, properties usable in the treatment of disease or illness (p. 510).

birth control all of the procedures that can prevent the birth of a child (p. 421).

birthing centers nonhospital, home-like setting where pregnant women can receive prenatal care and give birth (p. 474).

birthing rooms hospital facilities that serve as both a labor and a delivery room (p. 474).

bisexual choosing members of both sexes as one's sex object preference (p. 408).

blackout temporary state of amnesia experienced by an alcoholic; an inability to remember events that occur during a period of alcohol use (p. 215).

blood alcohol concentration (BAC) proportion of alcohol in a measured quantity of blood (p. 204).

blood analysis chemical analysis of various substances in the blood; helps determine changes and possible disturbances in the body (p. 83).

body fat analysis determination of the percentage of body tissue composed of fat (p. 83). (See Chapter 6 for further elaboration.)

body image our subjective perception of how our body appears (p. 131).

bodybuilding sports activity in which the participants train their bodies to reach desired goals of muscular size, symmetry, and proportion (p. 88).

bonding important, initial sense of recognition established between the newborn and those adults on whom the newborn will be dependent (p. 472).

brain death the absence of brain wave activity after an initial measurement followed by a second measurement 24 hours later (p. 583).

brand name specific patented name assigned to a drug or product by its manufacturer (p. 511).

Braxton-Hicks contractions false labor contractions; mild and of irregular spacing (p. 467).

breakthrough bleeding midcycle uterine bleeding; spotting (p. 443).

breech position birth position in which the baby's feet or buttocks are presented first (p. 469).

brown fat cells specialized fat cells that are thought to regulate adaptive thermogenesis (p. 137).

bulimarexia binge eating followed by purging of the food (p. 156).

bulimia psychogenic disorder in which binge eating patterns are established; usually accompanied by purging (p. 156).

C

calcium channel blockers drugs that prevent arterial spasms, used in the long-term management of angina pectoris (p. 269).

calendar method form of natural family planning in which the variable lengths of a woman's menstrual cycle are used to calculate her fertile period (p. 429).

caloric balance calorie input equals caloric output; weight remains constant (p. 141).

Calories units of heat (energy); specifically, 1 Calorie equals the heat required to raise 1 gram of water 1° C (p. 99).

cannula hollow metal or plastic tube through which materials can be aspirated (p. 450).

carbohydrates chemical compounds comprising sugar or saccharide units; the body's primary source of energy (p. 99).

carbon monoxide chemical compound (CO) that can inactivate red blood cells (p. 225).

carcinogenic relates to the production of cancerous changes; property of environmental agents, including drugs, that may stimulate the development of cancerous changes within cells (p. 528).

carcinogens substances that stimulate the development of cancer (p. 225).

carcinoma in situ cancer at its site of origin (p. 242).

cardiac pertaining to the heart (p. 52).

cardiac muscle specialized, smooth muscle tissue that forms the middle (muscular) layer of the heart wall (p. 264).

cardiogram reading of heart and lung function from a cardiograph machine (p. 83).

cardiovascular pertaining to the heart (cardio) and blood vessels (vascular) (p. 261).

cardiorespiratory endurance ability of the body to process and transport oxygen required by muscle cells so that these cells can continue to contract (p. 71).

CAT scan computerized axial tomography; x-ray procedure designed to visualize structures within the body that would not normally be seen through conventional x-ray procedures (p. 277).

catabolism metabolic process of breaking down tissue for the purpose of converting it into energy (p. 147).

catastrophic health insurance health insurance designed to cover illnesses whose associated costs exceed the coverage provided by any other health insurance policies (p. 509).

cauterize to apply a small electrical current and permanently close a tube or vessel; to burn (p. 444).

celibacy the practice of being sexually abstinent (p. 387).

cellular cohesiveness tendency of normal cells to "stick togther" rather than to move independently throughout the body (p. 293).

cellular immunity form of acquired immunity that uses specialized white blood cells to destroy specific antigens that enter the body (p. 335).

cellulite term used by some clinicians to describe localized areas of fat with accompanying connective tissue strands that cause dimpling (p. 136).

cellulose chemical compound that forms the nondigestible fiber component within food (p. 109).

central nervous system the brain and spinal cord (p. 50).

cereal germ highly nutritious portions of the cereal grain, often removed during milling (p. 111).

cerebral cortex outer covering of the brain, site of intellect, memory, thought processes, and rationalization (p. 50).

cerebral hemorrhage hemorrhage from the cerebral arteries within the brain (p. 276).

cerebrovascular accident stroke; brain tissue damage resulting from impaired circulation of blood vessels in the brain (p. 238).

cerebrovascular occlusions blockages to arteries supplying blood to the cerebral cortex of the brain; strokes (p. 276).

cervical cap small, thimble-shaped device designed to fit over the cervix (p. 438).

cesarean section surgical removal of a fetus through the abdominal wall (p. 350).

chemical name name used to describe the molecular structure of a drug (p. 511).

chemoprevention cancer prevention based on the selection of foods whose nutrient composition is thought to protect the body from certain forms of cancer (p. 305).

chiropractors nonallopathic practitioners who treat illness through manipulation of the vertebral column (p. 496).

chlamydia the most prevalent sexually transmitted disease, caused by a nongonococcal bacterium (p. 346).

chlorofluorocarbons (CFCs) gaseous chemical compounds that contain chlorine and fluorine (p. 523).

cholesterol fat-related substance in alcohol form; lipid material manufactured within the body as well as derived through dietary sources (p. 102).

chorionic villi sampling (CVS) microscopic examination of the cells of the chorionic villi derived from the embryo; process for identifying genetic defects earlier than can be done with amniocentesis (p. 475).

chronic bronchitis persistant inflammation and infection of the smaller airways within the lungs (p. 241).

chronic Epstein-Barr virus (CEEV) syndrome a generalized illness thought to be the result of an infection by Epstein-Barr virus (p. 338).

cilia small, hairlike structures that extend from cells that line the air passages (p. 240).

cirrhosis condition characterized by pathological changes to the liver resulting from chronic, heavy alchol consumption; a frequent cause of death among heavy alcohol users (p. 219).

clitoris small shaft of erectile tissue located in front of the vaginal opening; the female homolog of the male penis (p. 362).

cochlea small, snail-shaped organ of the inner ear in which the energy of sound is converted into electrical energy for transmission to the brain (p. 540).

coenzyme vitamin-based organic compound that assists a particular enzyme in performing its role in regulating biochemical reactions (p. 103).

cognition information-processing skills; cognition influences *affect* and *performance* (p. 32).

cohabitation sharing of a residence by two unrelated, unmarried people; living togther (p. 405).

coitus penile-vaginal intercourse (p. 386).

coitus interruptus (withdrawal) a contraceptive practice in which the erect penis is removed from the vagina before ejaculation (p. 428).

cold turkey immediate, total discontinuation of tobacco use or of other addictive substances (p. 249).

collateral circulation growth and/or enlargement of blood vessels in the area of a myocardial infarction to restore blood supply to heart tissue (p. 265).

colostomy surgically created opening on the abdominal wall for the elimination of body wastes (p. 299).

companionate love friendly affection and deep attachment, based on extensive familiarity with another person (p. 399).

compatible needs needs of a potential mate that are the same as the needs possessed by the partner (p. 395).

complementary needs needs of a potential mate that are different from those possessed by the partner (p. 395).

complex carbohydrates carbohydrates composed of long molecular chains containing many saccharide units; starches (p. 126).

compulsion compelling emotional desire to engage in a particular behavior (p. 229).

condom latex shield designed to cover the erect penis and retain semen upon ejaculation; "rubber" (p. 434)

conflict-habituated marriage marriage characterized by unending conflict and disagreement (p. 400).

confrontation an approach to convince drug-dependent people to enter treatment (p. 188).

congestive heart failure inability of the vascular system to return blood to the heart and to provide for adequate oxygenation of the blood (p. 273).

consumer fraud marketing of unreliable and ineffective services, products, or information under the guise of curing disease or improving health; quackery (p. 512).

contact inhibition ability of a tissue, on reaching its mature size, to suppress additional growth (p. 293).

contraception any procedure that prevents fertilization (p. 421).

contraceptive sponge soft, sponge disk that is moistened and inserted over the cervical area (p. 439).

contraindications factors that make the use of a drug inappropriate or dangerous for a particular person (p. 487).

cool down stretching and walking following exercise (p. 84).

coronary arteries vessels that supply oxygenated blood to heart muscle tissues (p. 266).

coronary artery bypass surgery surgical procedure designed to improve blood flow to the heart by providing alternate routes for blood to take around points of blockage (p. 271).

corpus luteum cellular remnant of the graafian follicle after the release of an ovum (p. 375).

corticotropin-releasing factor chemical messenger produced by the hypothalamus and released into the closed circulatory pathway shared with the pituitary gland; stimulates the pituitary's production of ACTH (p. 50).

corticoids hormone generated by the adrenal cortex; corticoids influence the body's control of glucose, protein, and fat metabolism (p. 51).

CPR cardiopulmonary resuscitation; first aid procedure designed to restore breathing and heart function (p. 270).

crack a crystalline form of cocaine that is smoked; instantaneous effect and highly dependency producing (p. 178).

creativity innovative ability; insightful capacity to adopt means to ends; to move beyond analytical-logical approaches to experience (p. 28).

cross-tolerance transfer of tolerance from one drug to another within the same general category (p. 167).

crosstraining use of more than one aerobic activity to achieve cardiovascular fitness (p. 89).

crowning first appearance of the head at the vaginal opening (p. 469).

cryobiology the study of the effects of freezing on living tissue (p. 583).

cryonics pseudoscience of freezing bodies in an attempt to bring them back to life at a later date through thawing (p. 583).

crypts burial locations underneath churches (p. 598).

cueing providing clues to ensure that an individual responds to a stimulus (p. 24).

cunnilingus oral stimulation of the vulva or clitoris (p. 390).

cystitis infection of the urinary bladder (p. 353).

D

decongestants drugs to relieve nasal and chest congestion (p. 315).

deficiency needs survival requirements; needs associated with normal function as a physical being (p. 27).

dehydration abnormal depletion of fluids from the body; severe dehydration can lead to death (p. 108).

delirium tremens (DTs) uncontrollable shaking associated with withdrawal from heavy chronic alcohol use (p. 217).

demyelination destruction of myelin (p. 317).

demythologization transfer of faith from one orientation based on teachings gained outside oneself to an orientation developed within onself (p. 31).

dendrite portion of a neuron that receives electrical stimuli from adjacent neurons; neurons typically have several such branches or extensions (p. 170).

dependency development of a psychological and/or physical need for a particular drug (p. 166).

depressants the psychoactive drugs that reduce the function of the central nervous system (p. 179).

designated driver a person that abstains or carefully limits alcohol in order to drive others safely (p. 211).

designer drugs drugs that chemically resemble drugs on the FDA Schedule 1 (p. 184).

desirable weight weight range deemed appropriate for persons of a specific gender, age, and frame size (p. 131).

devitalized marriage marriage that lacks the vitality or dynamic nature it once possessed (p. 400).

diagnosis-related groups prospective billing categories established by the federal government for Medicare reimbursements to hospitals for patients' illnesses, injuries, and surgical procedures (p. 509).

diaphragm soft, rubber vaginal cup designed to cover the cervix (p. 436).

diastolic pressure blood pressure against blood vessel walls when the heart relaxes (p. 273).

dietary cholesterol cholesterol obtained through food consumed (p. 119).

diffusion movement of a substance across a cell wall membrane from an area of greater concentration to an area of lesser concentration (p. 204).

dilation gradual expansion of an opening or passageway (p. 450).

dilation and curettage (D & C) surgical procedure in which the cervical canal is dilated to allow the uterine wall to be scraped (p. 451).

dilation and evacuation (D & E) surgical procedure using cervical dilation and vacuum aspiration to remove uterine wall material and fetal parts (p. 451).

dioxin powerful and potentially harmful chemical compound found in some herbicides (p. 531).

direct (active) euthanasia process of inducing death, often through the injection of a lethal drug (p. 584).

disaccharides sugars composed of two monosaccharide units; sucrose, lactose, and maltose (p. 100).

disengagement theory theory of aging that suggests that society slowly withdraws from the elderly and they in turn slowly withdraw from society (p. 567).

dissonance feeling of uncertainty that occurs when a person believes two equally attractive but opposite ideas (p. 233)

distillation production of alcoholic beverages by the vaporization and condensation of plant material; the process that produces liquor (p. 200).

distress stress that diminishes the quality of life; commonly associated with disease, illness, and maladaptation (p. 42).

diuresis increased discharge of fluid from the body; frequent urination (p. 311).

doublings the time required for the cells of a particular tissue to undertake reproductive divisions; 30 doublings are thought to be the time required for a cancerous process to be clinically observable (p. 293).

diuretic drugs drugs that aid the body in removing excess fluid (p. 310).

dose-related drug-related response pattern that changes according to the amount of a drug within the body (p. 230).

drug synergism enhancement of a drug's effect as a result of the presence of additional drugs within the system (p. 210).

duct system collection or system of tubes within the embryo that eventually gives rise to various reproductive structures (p. 361).

duration length of time one needs to exercise at the target heart rate to produce the training effect (p. 81).

dynamic in a state of change; health is dynamic in the sense that it is influenced by factors from both within and outside the individual (p. 7).

dyspnea labored breathing (p. 82).

E

ECG electrocardiograph, an instrument to measure and record the electrical activity within the heart (p. 264).

ecosystem an ecological unit made up of both animal and plant life that interact to produce a stable system.

electrocardiography procedure that uses high-frequency sound waves to visualize the structure and function of the heart (p. 271).

ectomorph somatotype represented by the tall, thin individual; an individual who experiences little difficulty with excess weight (p. 136).

ectopic pregnancy a pregnancy wherein the fertilized ovum implants at a site other than the uterus, typically in the fallopian tube (p. 443).

EEG patterns patterns reflecting the type and extent of electrical activity occurring in the cerebral cortex of the brain (p. 235).

effacement a thinning and pulling back of the cervical opening to allow movement of the fetus from the uterus (p. 467).

effective dose dose level that produces a desired effect (p. 185).

ego the conscious egocentric contact with reality; the self-assertive and self-preserving tendencies of the individual (p. 25).

egocentric unable to take into account the views of others; self-centered (p. 23).

electroconvulsive therapy (ECT) use of electrical shock to alter the neurotransmitter activity within the brain (p. 316).

electroencephalograph instrument that measures the electrical activity of the brain (p. 94).

electrolyte balance proper concentration of various minerals within the blood and body fluids (p. 219).

embolism potentially fatal situation in which a circulating blood clot lodges itself in a smaller vessel (p. 245).

embryo developing human from the end of the second week through the end of the second month of intrauterine development (p. 361).

encephalitis inflammation of the brain (p. 339).

endocervical cultures laboratory tests in the cervix are grown in a culture medium (p. 348).

endocrine system ductless glands that secrete one or more chemical messengers (hormones) into the bloodstream (p. 50).

endogenous (primary) depression form of depression caused by the chemical makeup of an individual; a depression resulting from a genetically based abnormal production of neurotransmitter chemicals (p. 562).

endometrium innermost lining of the uterus, broken down and discharged during menstruation (p. 372).

endomorph somatotype represented by the short, round, obese individual (p. 136).

endorphins opiate-like substances within the central nervous system; endorphins are thought to create a euphoric effect 200 times greater than an equivalent dose of morphine (p. 56).

enriched process of returning to foods some of the nutritional elements (B vitamins and iron) removed during processing (p. 111).

Environmental Protection Agency (EPA) federal agency charged with the protection of natural resources and the quality of the environment (p. 528).

enzyme chemical substances that regulate physiological processes (p. 103).

epidemic rapid spread of a disease among individuals within a given area or within a given population (p. 329).

epinephrine powerful adrenal hormone whose presence in the bloodstream prepares the body for maximal energy production and skeletal muscle response (p. 51).

episiotomy a surgical procedure to enlarge the vaginal opening before giving birth (p. 471).

epitaph inscription on a grave marker or monument (p. 601).

erection the engorgement of erectile tissue with blood; characteristic of the penis, clitoris, nipple, labia minora, and scrotum (p. 386).

eros unconscious urge toward life and love; in freudian tenets, the powerful life force (p. 24).

erotic dreams dreams whose content elicits a sexual response (p. 389).

essential amino acids nine amino acids that can be obtained only from dietary sources (p. 102).

essential hypertension hypertension (high blood pressure) resulting from chronic widespread constriction of arterioles (p. 274).

estrogen ovarian hormone that initiates the development of the uterine wall (p. 312).

estrogen replacement therapy medically administered estrogen to replace estrogen lost as the result of menopause (p. 314).

eulogy composition or speech that praises someone; often delivered at a funeral or memorial service (p. 600).

eustress stress that adds a positive, enhancing dimension to the quality of life (p. 42).

eutrophication enrichment of a body of water with nutrients, which allows for overabundant growth of plants (p. 527).

exchange diet diet constructed around the interchanging of foods; important aspect in the management of diabetes mellitus (p. 115).

excitement stage initial arousal stage of the sexual response pattern (p. 383).

exhibitionism exposure of one's genitals for the purpose of shocking other persons (p. 412).

exogenous depression form of depression that results from factors outside the individual; secondary depression (p. 570).

expectorants drugs that help bring mucus and phlegm up from the respiratory system (p. 336).

expressionistic sexuality complete expression of one's personally defined concept of sexuality (p. 377).

extended care facility institution designed to provide long-term medical or custodial care for persons who do not require hospitalization (p. 554).

externality tendency of obese individuals to be highly sensitive to food-related stimuli (p. 138).

F

faith predisposition to apply one's concept of an ultimate environment to life's experiences; the purpose and meaning that underlie the individual's hopes and strivings (p. 30).

fallopian tubes paired tubes that allow passage of ova from the ovaries to the uterus: the oviducts (p. 372).

false labor conditions that tend to resemble the start of true labor; may include irregular uterine contractions, pressure, and discomfort in the lower abdomen (p. 467).

false negative test result that indicates that a condition does not exist when in fact the condition does exist (p. 462).

false positive test result that indicates that a condition exists when in fact the condition does not exist (p. 462).

fast foods convenience foods; foods featured in a variety of restaurants, including hamburgers, pizza, and tacos (p. 120).

fast-twitch (FT) fibers type of muscle cells especially suited for anerobic activity (p. 72).

fatty acid acid component that in combination with glycerol forms the dietary fat molecule (p. 102).

FDA Schedule 1 list comprising drugs that hold a high potential for abuse but have no medical use (p. 184).

fecundity the ability to produce offspring (p. 180).

fellatio oral stimulation of the penis (p. 390).

femininity behavioral expressions traditionally observed in females (p. 361).

fermentation chemical process whereby plant products are converted into alcohol by the action of yeast cells on carbohydrates (p. 199).

fertility ability to reproduce (p. 421).

fertility awareness technique combined use of three rhythm techniques of contraception (p. 428).

fertilization the union of ovum and sperm resulting in a fertilized egg; conception (p. 463).

fetal alcohol syndrome characteristic birth defects noted in the children of some women who consume alcohol during their pregnancies (p. 208).

fetal monitoring electronic monitoring of uterine contractions, fetal respiration, and heart rate (p. 475).

fetal stage stage of human development from the end of the eighth week of gestation until the time of birth (p. 463).

fetishism choice of a body part or inanimate object as a source of sexual excitement (p. 411).

fiber cellulose-based plant material that cannot be digested; found in cereal, fruits, and vegetables (p. 109).

fight-or-flight response physiological changes in response to a stressor (p. 40).

five dimensions of health major areas of health in which specific strengths or limitations will be found: physical, emotional, social, intellectual, and spiritual (p. 8).

flaccid nonerect; the state of erectile tissue when vasocongestion is not occurring (p. 370).

flashbacks unpredictable return of a psychedelic trip (p. 180).

flexibility ability of joints to function through intended range of motion (p. 70).

folacin folic acid; a vitamin of the B-complex group used in the treatment of nutritional anemia (p. 125).

follicle-stimulating hormone (FSH) gonadotrophic hormone required for initial development of ova (in

the female) and sperm (in the male) (p. 369).

fomite nonliving carrier of a disease (p. 331).

food additives chemical compounds that are intentionally or unintentionally added to our food supply (p. 118).

food supplements nutrients taken in addition to those obtained through the diet: powdered protein, vitamins, mineral extracts, and so on (p. 121).

foreplay activities, often involving touching and caressing, that prepare individuals for sexual intercourse (p. 389).

formaldehyde chemical found in many common building materials and home furnishings (p. 523).

fraternal twins (dizygotic) twins resulting when two separate ova are fertilized by different sperm (p. 465).

freebase altered form of cocaine that can be smoked (p. 178).

frequency (1) number of times per week one should exercise to achieve a training effect (p. 82). (2) rate at which a sound source vibrates, measured in cycles per second (p. 540).

G

gamete intrafallopian transfer (GIFT) retrieved ovum and partner's sperm are positioned in the fallopian tube for fertilization and subsequent movement into the uterus for implantation (p. 476).

gaseous phase portion of tobacco smoke containing carbon monoxide and many other physiologically active gaseous compounds (p. 233).

gastric bubble bubble surgically positioned and inflated within the stomach to stimulate satiety (p. 150).

gender general term reflecting a biological basis of sexuality; the male gender or the female gender (p. 365).

gender adoption lengthy process of learning the behaviors that are traditional for one's gender (p. 366).

gender identification achievement of a personally satisfying interpretation of one's masculinity or femininity (p. 368).

gender identity recognition of one's gender (p. 365).

gender preference emotional and intellectual acceptance of the gender that one is (p. 365).

gender schema mental image of the cognitive, affective, and performance characteristics appropriate to a particular gender; a mental picture of being a man or being a woman (p. 367).

general adaptation syndrome sequenced physiological response to the presence of a stressor; the alarm, resistance, and exhaustion stages of the stress response (p. 39).

generativity midlife developmental task; repaying society for its support through contributions associated with parenting, creativity, and occupation (p. 563).

generic name common or nonproprietary name of a drug (p. 511).

genetic counseling medical counseling regarding the transmission and management of inherited conditions (p. 322).

genetic marker a gene known to lie in close proximity to a disease-producing gene (p. 280).

genetic predisposition inherited tendency to develop a disease process if necessary environmental factors exist (p. 311).

genital sexuality sexuality that is centered in the recreational use of reproductive structures; the sexuality that encompasses sexual performance and eroticism (p. 377).

genital tubercle undifferentiated tissue within the embryo from which the penis (in the male) or

the clitoris (in the female) develops (p. 362).

glucose blood sugar; the body's primary source of energy (p. 51).

glycerol alcohol component that is a common constituent in dietary fats (p. 102).

glycogen storage form of the body's energy supplies; composed of a network of glucose molecules (p. 74).

goblet cells cells within the epithelial lining of the airways that produce the mucus required for cleaning the airways (p. 240).

gonadotrophic hormones hormones that influence the functioning of the testes and ovaries (p. 363).

greenhouse effect warming of the Earth's surface that is produced when solar heat becomes trapped by layers of carbon dioxide and other gases (p. 522).

grief the emotional feelings associated with death (p. 592).

guided imagery process of visualizing oneself responding in a positive and controlled fashion to a stressor (p. 58).

Guillain-Barré syndrome uncommon, often temporary paralysis that results from exposure to certain influenza viruses or vaccinations (p. 338).

H

habituation term used interchangeably with psychological dependency (p. 166).

hallucinogens psychoactive drugs capable of producing hallucinations (distortions of reality) (p. 180).

hashish resins collected from the flower tops of marijuana plants (p. 181).

health maintenance organizations (HMO) groups that supply prepaid comprehensive health care with an emphasis on prevention (p. 506).

health promotion movement in which knowledge, practices, and value stances are transmitted to

people for their use in lengthening their lives, reducing the incidence of illness, and feeling better (p. 2).

heart catheterization procedure wherein a thin catheter is introduced through an arm or leg vein into the coronary circulation to visualize areas of blockage (p. 271).

heart-lung machine device that oxygenates and circulates blood during bypass surgery (p. 271).

hemorrhaging bleeding; often implies profuse bleeding (p. 470).

herbicide chemical compound used to kill vegetation (p. 531).

herniated disk protrusion of an intervertebral disk from its normal position between adjoining vertebra (p. 319).

heterosexual having a preference for a member of the opposite sex as one's sexual partner (p. 408).

high nicotine–low tar cigarette cigarette whose high nicotine content could satisfy the user's dependency on nicotine while reducing the risks associated with exposure to high levels of tar (p. 230).

HIV human immune deficiency virus (p. 341).

holistic health encompassing view of the nature of health; views health in terms of its physical, emotional, social, intellectual, and spiritual makeup (p. 2).

homeostasis the body's preferred state of dynamic balance among body systems (p. 47).

homeostatic mechanism complex biological mechanism that attempts to moderate processes within the body so that a balance or equilibrium is maintained (p. 316).

homogamy existence of similar or shared traits among members of a group (p. 395).

homosexual choosing a member of one's own sex as one's sex object preference (p. 408).

hospice care approach to caring for terminally ill patients that maximizes the quality of life and allows death with dignity (p. 591).

hot flashes temporary feelings of warmth experienced by women during and following menopause, caused by blood vessel dilation (p. 561).

human chorionic gonadotropin (HCG) gonadotropic hormone that maintains the ovaries' production of progesterone (p. 462).

humoral immunity form of acquired immunity that uses antibodies to counter specific antigens that enter the body (p. 335).

hurry sickness excessive time dependency; seen in persons whose lives are geared to rigid schedules and high achievement aspirations (p. 57).

hydrogen bonding chemical bonds within compounds occurring at the points at which hydrogen atoms are found (p. 102).

hydrostatic weighing weighing the body while submerged in water (p. 133).

hydrotherapy form of physical therapy in which water is used as the therapeutic agent (p. 561).

hyperactivity above-normal physical movement; often accompanied by an inability to concentrate well on a specified task; also called hyperkinesis (p. 177).

hypercellular obesity form of obesity seen in individuals who possess an abnormally large number of fat cells (p. 137).

hypercholesterolemia excessively elevated levels of cholesterol (p. 559).

hyperglycemia elevated blood glucose levels; an important indicator of diabetes mellitus (p. 311).

hyperparathyroidism condition reflecting the overactive production of parathyroid hormone by the parathyroid glands (p. 313).

hyperplasia abnormal cell growth leading to an excessive accumulation of tissue (p. 241).

hyperthermia excess production of body heat; abnormally elevated core body temperature (p. 51).

hypertonic saline solution salt solution with a concentration higher than that found in human fluids (p. 452).

hypertriglyceridemia excessively elevated levels of triglycerides (p. 559).

hypertrophic obesity form of obesity in which fat cells are enlarged (p. 138).

hypervitaminosis excessive accumulation of vitamins within the body; associated with the fat-soluble vitamins (p. 103).

hypochondriasis neurotic conviction that one is ill or afflicted with a particular disease (p. 559).

hypoglycemia condition in which too little glucose circulates in the bloodstream (p. 562).

hypothalamus portion of the midbrain that provides a connection between the cerebral cortex and pituitary gland (p. 50).

hypothyroidism condition in which the thyroid gland produces an insufficient amount of its hormone, thyroxin (p. 139).

hysterectomy surgical removal of the uterus (p. 446).

I

id the unconscious pleasure drive (p. 25).

identical twins (monozygotic) twins resulting when only one ovum is fertilized but divides into two zygotes early in its development (p. 465).

immune system system of biochemical and cellular elements that protect the body from invading pathogens and foreign materials (p. 333).

immunizations laboratory-prepared pathogens that are introduced into the body for the purpose of stimulating the body's immune system (p. 334).

immunoassay pregnancy test pregnancy test that uses an antigen-antibody response to determine the presence of HCG in a urine sample (p. 462).

in vivo fertilization and embryo transfer (IVF-ET) fertilization in the laboratory of an ovum taken from the woman with subsequent return of the developing embryo into the woman's uterus (p. 476).

incest marriage or coitus (sexual intercourse) between closely related individuals (p. 412).

incomplete protein food food that lacks one or more of the essential amino acids (p. 103).

incubation stage time required for a pathogen to multiply significantly enough for signs and symptoms to appear (p. 331).

independent practice association (IPA) a modified HMO in which a group of physicians provide prepaid health care, but not from a central location within an HMO (p. 507).

indirect (passive) euthanasia process of allowing a person to die by disconnecting life support systems or withholding lifesaving techniques (p. 584).

individuative-reflective stage state of faith development generally associated with the young adult; stage in which one translates symbols into personally meaningful concepts; living within one's own structure of faith (p. 31).

inducer substance chemical substance produced by the male embryo that helps support the development of the male internal reproductive structures (p. 362).

indulgence strong emotional desire to engage in a particular behavior solely for one's own enjoyment or benefit (p. 229).

infatuation an often shallow, intense attraction to another person (p. 397).

inferior vena cava large vein that returns blood from lower body regions to the right atrium of the heart (p. 263).

infertility inability of a male to impregnate, or of a female to become pregnant (p. 476).

inhalants psychoactive drugs that enter the body through inhalation (p. 183).

inhibitions inner controls that prevent a person's engaging in certain types of behavior (p. 197).

insulin pancreatic hormone required by the body for the effective metabolism of carbohydrates (p. 310).

intensity (1) level of effort one puts into an activity (p. 80). (2) strength or loudness of a particular sound, measured in decibels (p. 540).

interstitial cell stimulating hormone (ICSH) a gonadotropic hormone of the male required for the production of testosterone (p. 368).

interstitial cells specialized cells within the testicles that on stimulation by ICSH produce the male sex hormone testosterone (p. 368).

intimacy any close, mutual verbal or nonverbal behavior within a relationship (p. 393).

intrauterine device (IUD) small, plastic, medicated or unmedicated device that when inserted in the uterus prevents continued pregnancy (p. 440).

ionizing radiation form of radiation capable of releasing electrons from atoms (p. 533).

isokinetic exercises muscular strength training exercises that use machines to provide variable resistances throughout the full range of motion (p. 68).

isometric exercises muscular strength training exercises that use a resistance so great that the resistance object cannot be moved (p. 67).

J

jaundice yellowing of the skin as a result of the abnormal accumulation of bile pigment within the body (p. 323).

K

kwashiorkor protein deficiency disease, associated with early weaning of children and a diet lacking complete protein (p. 103).

L

labia majora larger, more external skin folds that surround the vaginal opening (p. 362).

labia minora small, liplike folds of skin immediately adjacent to the vaginal opening (p. 362).

labioscrotal swelling undifferentiated tissue within the embryo which becomes either the scrotum (in the male) or the labia majora (in the female) (p. 362).

lactating breastfeeding; nursing (p. 121).

lactator female who is producing breast milk (p. 134).

lactic acid chemical by-product of anaerobic energy (p. 74).

laminaria plugs made of seaweed that on exposure to moisture expand and dilate the canal into which they have been placed (p. 452).

lay midwives persons who have received specialized training in midwifery but who do not possess the academic credentials of the registered nurse midwife (p. 171).

legumes peas and beans; plant sources high in the essential amino acids (p. 103).

lesbianism female homosexuality (p. 408).

lethal dose dose level capable of causing death (p. 185).

life cycle artificial segmenting of the life span; each segment represents a developmental period (p. 1).

lightening movement of fetus deeper into the pelvic cavity before the onset of the birth process (p. 467).

lipofuscin pigment found in the tissues of the elderly; "age spots" (p. 557).

lipogenesis process whereby the body develops (and fills) adipose cells (p. 137).

lipoprotein protein-like structure in the bloodstream to which circulating fatty materials attach; associated with cardiovascular disease (p. 238).

lipoprotein profile analysis of the relative amounts of HDLs to LDLs in the blood (p. 286).

liposuction surgical aspiration of localized pockets of fat (p. 150).

living will document confirming a person's desire to be allowed to die peacefully and with a measure of dignity in case of terminal illness or major injury (p. 586).

longitudinal studies research studies in which a group of subjects is studied over the course of many years; long-term studies (p. 282).

lordotic curvature characteristic curve in the lower portion of the spinal column (p. 318).

low back pain chronic discomfort (pain) in the lower back and hips (p. 70).

low tar and nicotine brands cigarettes containing 15 mg of tar or less (p. 227).

luteinizing hormone (LH) female gonadotropic hormone required for fullest development and release of ova; ovulating hormone (p. 375).

M

macrobiotic diet vegetarian diet composed almost entirely of brown rice (p. 123).

macrocytic anemia form of anemia in which large red blood cells predominate, but in which total red blood cell count is depressed (p. 125).

mammogram x-ray examination of the breast (p. 297).

masculinity behavioral expressions traditionally observed in males (p. 361).

masochism sexual excitement while being injured or humiliated (p. 412).

mastery when applied to growth within the young adult segment of the life cycle, mastery implies becoming more self-aware, independent, responsible, and socially interactive (p. 7).

maternal supportive tissues general term referring to the development of the placenta and other tissues specifically associated with pregnancy (p. 139).

mausoleum above-ground structure into which caskets can be placed for disposition; it frequently resembles a small stone house (p. 598).

maximum heart rate maximum number of times the heart can beat per minute (p. 81).

mechanical defenses the body's initial defensive line against pathogenic agents, skin, mucous membranes, hairs, cilia, etc. (p. 333).

Medicaid noncontributory governmental health insurance for persons receiving other types of public assistance (p. 508).

Medicare contributory governmental health insurance, primarily for persons 65 years of age or older (p. 508).

meltdown the overheating and eventual melting of the uranium fuel rods in the core of a nuclear reactor (p. 537).

memorial service form of funeral service in which the body or casket often is not present (p. 598).

menarche time of a female's first menstrual period (cycle) (p. 362).

menopause decline and eventual cessation of hormone production by the reproductive system (p. 364).

menstrual extraction procedure using vacuum aspiration to remove uterine wall material within 2 weeks following a missed menstrual period (p. 449).

menstrual phase phase of the menstrual cycle during which the broken-down lining of the uterus (endometrium) is discharged from the body (p. 373).

menstruate to undergo cyclic buildup and destruction of the uterine wall (p. 373).

mentor person who functions as a teacher, counselor, and role model for a younger person (p. 50).

mesomorph somatotype represented by the broad-shouldered, well-muscled individual (p. 136).

mesonephric duct system within the male embryo that gives rise to several internal reproductive structures (p. 362).

metabolic rate rate or intensity at which the body produces energy (p. 51).

metabolites any substance the body uses to promote cell growth and maintenance (p. 557).

metaneeds needs beyond the normal survival needs; the higher transcending human needs (p. 27).

metastasis spread of cancerous cells from their site of origin to other areas of the body (p. 293).

midlife period between 45 and 65 years of age (p. 553).

midlife crisis period of emotional upheaval noted among some midlife persons as they struggle with the finality of death and the nature of their past and future accomplishments (p. 566).

migraine headaches severe, recurrent headaches, usually affecting one side of the head (p. 443).

minerals chemical elements that serve as structural elements within body tissue or participate in physiological processes (p. 106).

minipills low-dose progesterone oral contraceptive (p. 443).

mitral (bicuspid) valve two-cusp valve that regulates blood flow between the left atrium and the left ventricle of the heart (p. 264).

monogamous paired relationship with one partner (p. 405).

monoclonal antibodies antibodies produced by clones from one original antigen-antibody complex (p. 304).

mononuclear leukocytes large white blood cells that have only one nucleus (p. 338).

mononucleosis ("mono") viral infection characterized by weakness, fatigue, swollen glands, and low-grade fever (p. 338).

monosaccharides simple sugars; carbohydrate compounds of one saccharide unit (p. 99).

monounsaturated fats fats made of compounds in which one hydrogen-bonding position remains to be filled; semisolid at room temperature; derived primarily from peanut and olive oils (p. 102).

moral realism literal interpretation of rules; real values as opposed to idealistic assumptions (p. 23).

morning-after pill high-dose progesterone-based oral contraceptives used to terminate a suspected pregnancy (p. 444).

mourning culturally defined manner of expressing grief (p. 592).

mucus clear, sticky material produced by specialized cells within the mucous membranes of the body; mucus traps much of the suspended particulate matter from tobacco smoke (p. 240).

multiorgasmic capacity potential to have several orgasms within a single period of sexual arousal (p. 386).

murmur atypical heart sound that suggests a backwashing of blood into a chamber of the heart from which it has just left (p. 279).

muscular endurance ability of a muscle or muscle group to continue functioning; depends on well-developed respiratory and circulatory systems (p. 69).

muscular strength ability to contract skeletal muscles to engage in work (p. 67).

mutagenic capable of promoting genetic alterations in cells (p. 528).

mutation spontaneous alteration of genetic material (p. 293).

myelin white, fatty, insulating material that surrounds the axons of many nerve cells (p. 317).

myocardial infarction heart attack; the death of heart muscle as a result of a blockage in one of the coronary arteries (p. 268).

myotonia buildup of neuromuscular tonus within a particular tissue (p. 387).

N

narcolepsy sleep-related disorder in which a person has a recurrent, overwhelming, and uncontrollable desire to sleep (p. 177).

narcotics psychoactive drugs derived from the oriental poppy plant; narcotics serve to relieve pain and induce sleep (p. 182).

national health coverage comprehensive health insurance coverage provided by a federal government for all of its citizens (p. 509).

natural family planning combined use of all three rhythm techniques of contraception (p. 429).

natural immunity component of the immune system that uses chemicals produced by the body to destroy pathogens (p. 333).

naturopaths a largely unregulated group of practitioners who treat/ prevent illness through the use of an array of "natural" factors, including food, sunshine, water, and exercise (p. 496).

needle biopsy procedure minor surgical procedure in which a needle is injected into an anesthetized portion of a muscle tissue and a sample of that tissue is removed for microscopic examination (p. 92).

negative dependency behavior behavior that can not only create psychological dependence but can also harm structure and function (p. 53).

neomorts brain-dead person kept alive for purposes of medical research (p. 583).

nerve blockers drugs that can stop the flow of electrical impulses through the nerves into which they have been injected (p. 318).

neuritic plaques characteristic changes to brain tissue found in association with Alzheimer's disease (p. 571).

neurofibrillary tangles characteristic changes to brain tissue found in association with Alzheimer's disease (p. 571).

neuromuscular tonus level of nervous tension within the muscle (p. 387).

neuron nerve cell; the structural unit of the nervous system (p. 176).

neurophysiological nervous system function; processes through which the body senses and responds to its internal and external environments (p. 136).

neuroscientist scientist who studies the anatomical and physiological relationships of the nervous system (p. 170).

neurotransmitters chemical messengers released by neurons that permit electrical impulses to be transferred from one nerve cell to another (p. 170).

nicotine physiologically active, dependency-producing drug found in tobacco (p. 225).

nocturnal emission ejaculation that occurs during sleep; "wet dream" (p. 363).

nonoxynol-9 a commonly used spermicide in contraceptive devices (p. 439).

nontraditional students administrative term used by colleges and universities for students who, for whatever reason, are pursuing undergraduate work at an age other than that associated with traditional college years (18-22) (p. 3).

norepinephrine adrenalin-like chemical produced within the nervous system (p. 235).

normative standards statements of societal expectations concerning behavioral conduct (p. 393).

nostrums ineffective medications or products sold by quacks (p. 513).

nuclear autumn a less devastating scenario than that of nuclear winter; less severe lowering of the temperature and fewer deaths from starvation caused by failed crop production (p. 535).

nuclear fallout radioactive debris that reaches the Earth's surface after a nuclear explosion (p. 533).

nuclear winter the lowering of atmospheric temperature caused by the loss of solar heat resulting from dust covering produced during nuclear war (p. 535).

nurse practitioners registered nurses who have taken specialized training in one or more clinical areas and are able to engage in limited diagnosis and treatment of illnesses (p. 499).

nutrient density quantity of selected nutrients in 1,000 Calories of food (p. 126).

nutrients elements in foods that are required for the growth, repair, and regulation of body processes (p. 99).

O

obesity condition in which body weight exceeds desirable weight by over 15% (p. 131).

obituary notice biographical sketch that appears in a newspaper shortly after a person's death (p. 600).

oncogenes genes that are believed to activate the development of cancer (p. 298).

oncologist physician who specializes in the treatment of malignancies (p. 294).

oogenesis production of ova in biological mature female (p. 373).

oral contraceptive pill pill taken orally, composed of synthetic female hormones that prevent ovulation or implantation; "the pill" (p. 441).

orgasmic platform expanded outer third of the vagina that during the plateau phase of the sexual response grips the penis (p. 372).

orgasmic stage third stage of the sexual response pattern; the stage during which neuromuscular tension is released (p. 383).

orthodontics dental specialty that focuses on the proper alignment of the teeth (p. 497).

osteoarthritis arthritis that develops with age (p. 322).

osteopathy a form of allopathic medicine whose historical beginnings were centered in the manipulation of the musculoskeletal system (p. 496).

osteoporosis resorption of calcium from the bone caused by the inability of the body to use dietary calcium, seen primarily in postmenopausal women (p. 124).

outercourse sexual behaviors that do not involve intercourse (p. 421).

ovary female reproductive structure that produces ova and the female gonadal sex hormones estrogen and progesterone (p. 372).

overload principle principle (often used in training programs to increase muscular strength) whereby a person gradually increases the resistance load that must be moved or lifted (p. 67).

overweight condition in which body weight exceeds desirable weight by 1% to 15% (p. 131).

ovolactovegeterianism diet that excludes the use of all meat but does allow the consumption of eggs and dairy products (p. 120).

ovulation the release of a mature egg from the ovary (p. 375).

oxidation chemical conversion (detoxification) of alcohol by the liver into water, carbon dioxide, and calories (p. 205).

oxygen debt physical state that occurs when the body can no longer process and transport sufficient amounts of oxygen for continued muscle contraction (p. 74).

ozone layer layer of triatomic oxygen that surrounds the Earth and filters much of the sun's radiation before it can reach the Earth's surface (p. 523).

P

pacemaker sinoatrial of SA node; an area of cells within the heart that contol its electrical activity (p. 264).

palliative measure taken to reduce pain and discomfort but not to cure a disease (p. 304).

pandemic spread of a disease process over a wide geographical area (p. 329).

Pap smear cancer screening procedure in which cells removed from the cervix are examined (p. 350).

paracervical anesthetic anesthetic injected into tissues surrounding the cervical opening (p. 450).

paramesonephric duct system within the female embryo that gives rise to several internal reproductive structures (p. 362).

parental image characteristics of a potential mate that remind a person of traits of his or her parent of the opposite sex (p. 395).

particulate phase portion of tobacco smoke composed of small suspended particles (p. 233).

particulate pollutants class of air pollutants composed of small solid particles and liquid droplets (p. 524).

parturition childbirth (p. 467).

passionate love state of extreme absorption in another; tenderness, elation, anxiety, sexual desire, and ecstacy (p. 399).

passive smoking inhalation of air that is heavily contaminated with tobacco smoke (p. 249).

passive-congenial marriage marriage that primarily supports the outside interests of the partners (p. 400).

passively acquired immunity temporary immunity achieved by providing antibodies to a person exposed to a particular pathogen (p. 334).

pathogen disease-causing agent (p. 230).

patient education health education delivered in a hospital or health care setting (p. 489).

peak stage stage of an infectious disease at which symptoms are most fully expressed; acute stage (p. 332).

pedophilia sexual contact with children as a source of sexual excitement (p. 412).

pelvic inflammatory disease (PID) acute or chronic infections of the peritoneum or lining of the abdominopelvic cavity; associated with a variety of symptoms and a potential cause of sterility; generalized infection of the pelvic cavity that results from the spread of an infection through a woman's reproductive structure (p. 346).

performance psychomotor skills or behaviors in which an individual is engaged; performance influences cognition and affect (p. 32).

periodontal disease destruction of soft tissue and bone that surround the teeth (p. 246).

peritonitis inflammation of the peritoneum or lining of the abdominopelvic cavity (p. 246).

pesticide agent used to destroy pests (p. 528).

phenol chemical found in tobacco smoke thought to inactivate the cilia lining air passages (p. 240).

phenylpropanolamine (PPA) active chemical compound found in most over-the-counter diet products (p. 148).

physical dependency need to continue using a drug to maintain normal body function and to avoid withdrawal illness; also called addiction (p. 166).

physical proximity physical closeness of individuals in terms of their places of residence, employment, and recreation (p. 395).

pituitary gland "master gland" of the endocrine system; the wide variety of hormones produced by the pituitary are sent to structures throughout the body (p. 50).

placebo effect improved status of one's health attributable only to the belief that one is being helped (p. 496).

placebo pills pills that contain no active ingredients (p. 441).

placenta structure through which nutrients, metabolic wastes, and drugs (including alcohol) pass from the bloodstream of the mother into the bloodstream of the developing fetus (p. 208).

plateau stage second stage of the sexual response pattern; a leveling off of arousal immediately before orgasm (p. 283).

platelet adhesiveness tendency of platelets to clump together, thus enhancing speed at which the blood clots (p. 238).

platonic close association between two people that does not include a sexual relationship (p. 405).

pleurisy inflammation of the lining of the chest cavity and outer surface of the lung (p. 322).

podiatrists specialists who treat a variety of ailments of the feet (p. 498).

polychlorinated biphenyls (PCBs) class of chlorinated organic compounds similar to the herbicide DDT (p. 528).

polyneuropathy gradual destruction of nervous system functioning resulting from influence of alcohol on nerve cells (p. 219).

polysaccharide complex carbohydrate; a compound of a long chain of glucose units; found primarily in vegetables, fruits, and grains (p. 100).

polyunsaturated fats fats composed of compounds in which multiple hydrogen-bonding positions remain open; these fats are liquids at room temperature; derived from a variety of vegetable sources (p. 102).

positive caloric balance state in which the body takes in more calories than it expends (p. 132).

positron emmission tomography (PET) diagnostic procedure used in the identification of Alzheimer's disease (p. 571).

postpartum period of time after the birth of a baby during which the uterus returns to its prepregnancy size (p. 471).

potentiated effect phenomenon whereby the use of one drug intensifies the effect of a second drug (p. 185).

preferred provider organization a group of physicians who market their professional services to an insurance company at predetermined fees (p. 507).

private hospitals profit-making hospitals; proprietary hospitals (p. 502).

problem drinking alcohol use pattern in which a drinker's behavior creates personal difficulties or difficulties for other persons (p. 212).

procreation reproduction (p. 392).

prodromal stage stage of an infectious disease process in which only general symptoms appear (p. 332).

professional nurses registered nurses who hold bachelors degrees in nursing from colleges and universities (p. 499).

progesterone ovarian hormone that continues the development of uterine wall that was initiated by estrogen (p. 375).

progressive resistance exercises muscular strength training exercises that use traditional barbells and dumbbells with fixed resistances (p. 68).

proliferative phase first half of the menstrual cycle (p. 375).

proof twice the percentage of alcohol by concentration; 100 proof alcohol is 50 percent alcohol (p. 201).

prospective pricing system system of establishing in advance the reimbursement rates for health services (p. 509).

prostaglandin inhibitors drugs that block the production of prostaglandins, thus eliminating the hormonal stimulation of smooth muscles (p. 310).

prostaglandin intrauterine injection introduction of hormonelike chemicals that on injection into the amniotic sac cause uterine muscles to contract and expel fetal contents (p. 452).

prostaglandins chemical substances that stimulate smooth muscle contractions (p. 452).

prosthodontics dental speciality that focuses on the construction and fitting of artificial appliances to replace missing teeth (p. 497).

proteins compounds composed of chains of amino acids; primary components of muscle and connective tissue (p. 102).

protooncogenes normal genes that hold the potential of becoming cancer-causing oncogenes (p. 293).

psychoactive drug any substance capable of altering one's feelings, moods, or perceptions (p. 165).

psychological dependency need to consume a drug for emotional reasons; also called habituation (p. 166).

psychosocial sexuality masculine and feminine aspects of sexuality (p. 365).

puberty achievement of reproductive ability (p. 362).

public hospitals hospitals operated by governmental agencies and supported by tax dollars (p. 502).

pulmonary pertaining to the lungs and breathing (p. 52).

pulmonary emphysema irreversible disease process in which the alveoli are destroyed (p. 241).

pulmonary valve valve that controls the flow of blood into the pulmonary arteries from the right ventricle of the heart (p. 263).

purge use of vomiting or laxatives to remove undigested food from the body (p. 156).

Q

quackery marketing of unreliable and ineffective services, products, or information under the guise of curing disease or improving health (p. 512).

R

radiation sickness illness characterized by fatigue, nausea, weight loss, fever, bleeding from mouth and gums, hair loss, and immune deficiencies, resulting from overexposure to ionizing radiation (p. 533).

radioreceptor assay test pregnancy test that uses a radioactive substance to determine the presence of HCG in a serum sample (p. 462).

radon gas a naturally occurring radioactive gas produced by the decay of uranium (p. 539).

range of motion distance through which a joint can be moved; measured in degrees (p. 68).

rape an act of violence against another person wherein that person is forced to engage in sexual activities (p. 412).

rapid eye movement (REM) sleep dream stage of sleep characterized by twitching movements of the eyes beneath the eyelids (p. 94).

rebound effect excessive congestion that results from the overuse of nosedrops and sprays (p. 336).

recovery stage stage of an infectious disease at which the body's immune system has overcome the infectious agent and recovery is underway; convalescence stage (p. 332).

refractory phase that portion of the male's resolution stage during which sexual arousal cannot occur (p. 386).

refractory errors incorrect patterns of light wave transmission through the structures of the eye (p. 498).

registered nurse midwives registered nurses (RNs) who have completed postgraduate education in prenatal care and childbirthing and are licensed or certified to practice midwifery (p. 474).

rehabilitation return of function to a previous level (p. 575).

reinforcement schedule sequencing of rewards so that desired responses continue (p. 24).

relaxation response physiological state of opposition to the fight-or-flight response of the general adaptation syndrome (p. 55).

relaxation training the use of various techniques to produce a state of relaxation (p. 55).

reliability consistent performance (p. 485).

remediation development of alternate forms of function to replace those which had been lost or were poorly developed (p. 575).

reproductive sexuality sexuality that is centered in the structural, functional, and behavioral aspects of reproduction (p. 377).

resorption withdrawal of a chemical substance from a site in which it had been initially deposited (p. 312).

resolution stage fourth stage of the sexual response pattern; the return of the body to a preexcitement state (p. 383).

rheumatic heart disease chronic damage to the heart (especially heart valves) resulting from a streptococcal infection within the heart; a complication associated with rheumatic fever (p. 278).

rheumatoid arthritis the result of autoimmune deterioration of the joints (p. 322).

rigor mortis rigidity of the body that occurs after death (p. 583).

role of health mission of health within a persons' life cycle (p. 7).

rubella German (or 3-day) measles; a viral infection which, when contracted by the pregnant mother, is capable of causing congenital heart defects in the infant (p. 339).

rubeola red or common measles (p. 339).

S

sadism sexual excitement achieved while inflicting injury or humiliation on another person (p. 412).

sadomasochism combination of sadism and masochism into one sexual activity (p. 412).

salt sensitive descriptive of people who overreact to the presence of sodium by retaining fluid and thus increasing blood pressure (p. 275).

satiety value food's ability to satisfy feelings of hunger (p. 101).

saturated fats fats made up of compounds in which no further hydrogen bonding can occur; these are fats in solid form at room temperature; primarily animal fats (p. 102).

sclerotic changes thickening or hardening of tissues (p. 294).

screenings relatively superficial evaluations designed to identify deviations from normal (p. 302).

secondary bacterial infection bacterial infection that develops as a consequence of a primary infection (p. 337).

secondary hypertension high blood pressure that results from a specific cause or pathological event; pathological hypertension (p. 560).

secretory cells specialized cells within the breast that will, on stimulation, produce milk (p. 315).

secretory phase second half of the menstrual cycle (p. 307).

sediments fine particles of soil that are washed into a body of water, become suspended, and eventually settle to the bottom (p. 529).

self-accepted moral principles moral behavior selected by the individual as opposed to socially imposed ethical standards (p. 24).

self-actualization highest level of personality development; self-actualized persons recognize their roles in life and use personal strengths to the fullest (p. 28).

self-care movement trend toward individuals taking increased responsibility for prevention or management of certain health conditions (p. 499).

self-limiting capable of not progressing beyond a specific point; self-correcting (p. 499).

semen secretion containing sperm and other nutrients discharged from the urethra at ejaculation (p. 370).

sense of well-being subjective, positive feeling resulting from an assessment of the progress being made in controlling the course that life is taking (p. 2).

sensitized lymphocytes specialized white blood cells that produce lymphokine, a chemical that inactivates fungi, viruses, and cancer cells (p. 334).

sensory modalities vision, hearing, taste, touch, and smell; pathways for stimuli to register with the body (p. 50).

sensory receptors receiving sites at which stimuli for vision, hearing, taste, touch, and smell enter the body (p. 170).

serum lipid analysis analysis of fat substance in the bloodstream; includes cholesterol and triglyceride measurements (p. 83).

set point genetically programmed range of body weight (p. 137).

sex flush reddish skin response that results from increasing sexual arousal (p. 386).

sex reassignment operation surgical procedure designed to remove the external genitalia and replace them with genitalia appropriate to the opposite sex (p. 410).

sexual fantasies fantasies with sexual themes; sexual daydreams or imaginary events (p. 389).

sexual harassment unwanted attention of a sexual nature that creates embarrassment or stress (p. 415).

sexual object preference one's preference concerning the nature of a sexual partner (p. 408).

sexual victimization sexual abuse of children, family members, or subordinates by a person in a position of power (p. 412).

sexuality the quality of being sexual; can be viewed from many biological and psychosocial perspectives (p. 361).

sexually transmitted diseases (STDs) infectious diseases that are spread primarily through intimate sexual contact (p. 345).

shaft body of the penis (p. 370).

shingles viral infection affecting the nerve endings of the skin (p. 348).

shock profound collapse of many vital body functions; evident during acute alcohol intoxication and other serious health emergencies (p. 206).

simple carbohydrates carbohydrates composed of short molecular chains containing few saccharide units; simple sugars (p. 126).

single photon emission computed tomography (SPECT) diagnostic procedure used in the identification of Alzheimer's disease (p. 571).

singlehood the state of not being married (p. 404).

sinus cavities hollow air cavities within the skull and facial bones that connect with the nasal cavities through a shared mucous membrane (p. 336).

skinfold measurement measurement to determine the thickness of the fat layer that lies immediately below the skin (p. 138).

sliding scale method of payment by which patient fees are scaled according to income levels (p. 190).

slow wave (SW) sleep stage of sleep characterized by minimal dream activity (p. 94).

slow-twitch (ST) fibers type of muscle cell especially suited for aerobic activities (p. 92).

smegma cellular discharge that can accumulate beneath the clitoral hood and the foreskin of an uncircumcised penis (p. 372).

smog air pollution composed of a combination of smoke, photochemical compounds, and fog (p. 523).

smokeless tobacco tobacco products (chewing tobacco and snuff) that are chewed or sucked rather than smoked (p. 227).

snuff finely shredded smokeless tobacco; used for dipping (p. 246).

sodomy penile-anal intercourse (p. 392).

specificity training concept that fitness components can be increased for very specific tasks or functions (p. 69).

spermatogenesis process of sperm production (p. 364).

spermicides chemicals capable of killing sperm (p. 433).

spontaneous abortion miscarriage; the expulsion of a fetus before it is sufficiently capable of survival; naturally occurring termination of a pregnancy (p. 441).

sputum mucus-based material that can be expectorated from the lungs and airways (p. 242).

starch complex carbohydrate; a polysaccharide; a compound of long-chain glucose units (p. 100).

sterilization generally permanent birth control techniques that surgically disrupt the normal passage of ova or sperm (p. 444).

stewardship acceptance of responsibility for the wise use and protection of the Earth's natural resources (p. 546).

stillborn baby that is dead at the time of birth (p. 244).

stimulants psychoactive drugs that stimulate the function of the central nervous system (p. 171).

stimulus (pl. stimuli) changing condition within the environment to which the individual will respond (p. 24).

stress physiological and psychological state of imbalance caused by the body's response to an unanticipated, disruptive, or stimulating event (p. 39).

stress test examination and analysis of heart-lung function while the body is undergoing physical exercise; generally accomplished when the client walks or runs on a treadmill device while being monitored by cardiograph (p. 83).

stressors factors or events, real or imagined, that elicit a state of stress (p. 39).

subcutaneous fat fat layer immediately below the skin (p. 133).

sudden cardiac death immediate death resulting from a sudden change in the rhythm of the heart (p. 237).

superego the higher social mores and values; the moral conscience and self-critical nature of the individual (p. 25).

superfund 10 billion dollar fund to be used in cleaning-up selected toxic waste sites; EPA controlled (p. 531).

superior vena cava body's largest vein; the vessel that brings blood from the upper body regions back to the right atrium of the heart (p. 263).

surrogate parenting one of several arrangements in which a woman becomes pregnant and gives birth for an infertile couple (p. 477).

sustainable environment an environment capable of supporting habitation; made possible by the efforts of individuals, organizations, and all levels of government (p. 546).

synaptic junction (synapse) location at which an electrical impulse from one neuron is transmitted to an adjacent neuron (p. 170).

synergistic drug effect heightened, exaggerated effect produced by the concurrent use of two or more drugs (p. 185).

synesthesia perceptual process in which a stimulus produces a response from a different sensory modality (p. 180).

synovial cells cells that produce the lubricating fluid required for smooth function of the joints (p. 323).

synthetic narcotics opiate-like drugs that are not by-products of the oriental poppy plant; laboratory-manufactured narcotics (p. 183).

synthetic conventional stage stage of faith development generally associated with adolescence in which one lives within the constructs formulated for the individual by others (p. 30).

systolic pressure blood pressure against blood vessel walls when the heart contracts (p. 273).

T

target heart rate (THR) number of times per minute that the heart must contract to produce a training effect (p. 80).

teaching hospital hospital in which preprofessional students and graduates receive clinical experience (p. 502).

teratogenic capable of producing birth defects (p. 528).

testes male reproductive structures that produce sperm and the gonadal hormone testosterone (p. 368).

thanatos unconscious urge toward death and hate; in freudian tenets, the powerful and destructive death force (p. 25).

thermal inversion weather condition in which a layer of warm, stable air forms above a cooler, polluted layer, inhibiting dispersal of pollutants (p. 525).

thorax the chest; portion of the torso above the diaphragm and within the rib cage (p. 263).

titration determining a particular level of a drug within the body (p. 229).

T-lymphocytes small circulating white blood cells, that, in the presence of specific antigens, form small sensitized lymphocytes, the basic components of the body's cellular immunity (p. 335).

T-type personality person who intentionally pursues risk-taking behavior (p. 58).

tar particulate phase of tobacco smoke with nicotine and water removed (p. 236).

technical nurses registered nurses (RNs) who hold diplomas or associate degrees from schools of nursing or university nursing programs (p. 499).

testosterone male sex hormone that stimulates tissue development (p. 89).

tolerance increasing loss of sensitivity to the effects of a particular quantity of a given drug. Acquired reaction to drugs that necessitates an increase in dosage to maintain a given reaction or effect (p. 149).

total marriage marriage in which the needs and goals of each partner are assigned a lower priority for the good of the partnership (p. 401).

total person holistic view of the person, incorporating the dynamic interplay of physical, emotional, social, intellectual, and spiritual factors (p. 2).

toxic dose dose level that produces a poisonous effect (p. 185).

toxic shock syndrome potentially fatal condition resulting from the proliferation of certain bacteria in the vagina that enter the general blood circulation (p. 340).

TPA tissue plasminogen activator; drug given immediately following a heart attack in an attempt to minimize damage by restoring blood supply to heart muscle (p. 270).

trace elements minerals that are present in the body in very small amounts; micronutrient elements (p. 108).

training effect significant positive effect that exercise has on the heart, lungs, and blood vessels (p. 80).

transcenders self-actualized people who have achieved a quality of being ordinarily associated with higher levels of spiritual growth (p. 28).

transient ischemic attack (TIA) temporary spasm of a cerebral artery that produces symptoms similar to those of a minor stroke; often a forewarning of a true cerebrovascular accident (p. 276).

transition the third and last phase of the first stage of labor; full dilation of the cervix (p. 469).

transsexualism the profound rejection of the gender to which the individual has been born (p. 412).

transvestism recurrent, persistent cross-dressing as a source of sexual excitement (p. 411).

tricuspid valve three-cusp (leaves) valve that regulates blood flow between the right atrium and the right ventricle of the heart (p. 263).

triglycerides fats made up of glycerol units, each having three fatty acid molecules (p. 102).

trimester three-month period of time; human pregnancies encompass three trimesters (p. 467).

tubal ligation sterilization procedure in which the fallopian tubes are cut and the ends tied back (p. 445).

tumescence state of being swollen or enlarged (p. 386).

type I alcoholism inherited predisposition supported by environmental factors favoring alcoholism (p. 218).

type II alcoholism male-limited alcohlism; an inherited form of alcoholism passed from father to son (p. 218).

type 1 (insulin-dependent) diabetes mellitus form of diabetes generally seen for the first time in childhood or adolescence; juvenile onset diabetes (p. 310).

type 2 (noninsulin-dependent) diabetes mellitus form of diabetes generally seen for the first time in persons 35 years of age and older; adult onset diabetes (p. 310).

U

ultimate environment abstract concept referring to a set of conditions in which one individual comfortably understands himself, others, and the material world (p. 30).

ultralow tar and nicotine brands cigarettes containing less than 4 mg of tar (p. 227).

ultrasound (1) high-intensity sound waves used to create an image of internal body structures (p. 271). (2) high-intensity sound waves used to elevate the internal temperature of cancer cells, thus killing the cells (p. 305).

unbalanced diet diet lacking adequate representation from each of the four food groups (p. 123).

underweight condition in which body weight is below desirable weight (p. 131).

uniquenesses and competencies those functional traits that make a particular person recognizably different from others (p. 4).

urethra passageway through which urine leaves the urinary bladder (p. 346)

urethritis infection of the urethra (p. 353).

urogenital folds undifferentiated tissue within the embryo from which the penile urethra (in the male) or the labia minora (in the female) develop (p. 362).

uterine perforation penetration of a foreign object through the uterine wall (p. 440).

V

vaccination medical procedure through which specially prepared antigens are introduced into the body for the purpose of activating the immune system (p. 334).

vacuum aspiration abortion procedure in which the cervix is dilated and vacuum pressure is used to remove the uterine contents (p. 450).

vaginal contraceptive film (VCF) spermicide-impregnated film that clings to the cervical opening (p. 432).

validity (1) the acuracy and soundness of one's perceptions. (2) scientific accuracy (p. 485).

variant different from the statistical average (p. 411).

vas deferens (pl. vasa deferentia) passageway through which sperm move from the epididymis to the ejaculatory duct (p. 369).

vascular system body's blood vessels; arteries, arterioles, capillaries, venules, and veins (p. 262).

vasectomy surgical procedure in which the vasa deferentia are cut to prevent the passage of sperm from the testicles; the most common form of male sterilization (p. 320).

vasocongestion retention of blood within a particular tissue (p. 387).

vegan vegetarian diet vegetarian diet that excludes the use of all animal products, including eggs and dairy products (p. 121).

vicariously formed stimuli erotic stimuli that originate in one's imagination (p. 386).

vital marriage marriage in which the needs and goals of the individual, as well as the needs of the marital union, are given top priority (p. 402).

vitamins organic compounds that facilitate the action of enzymes (p. 103).

voluntary hospitals nonprofit hospitals operated by a variety of organizations, including religious orders and fraternal groups (p. 502).

voyeurism watching others undressing or engaging in sexual activities (p. 412).

vulval tissues tissues surrounding the vaginal opening (p. 346).

W

warm-up physical and mental preparation for exercise (p. 84).

wellness a broadly based term used to describe a highly developed level of health (p. 3).

wellness centers units within hospitals or clinics that provide a wide range of rehabilitation, disease prevention, and health enhancement programs (p. 502).

whole-grain flour flour made from grain that has received only minimal processing (milling); flour containing many nutrients lost to more highly processed flour (p. 111).

will legal document that describes how a person wishes his or her estate to be disposed of after death (p. 600).

withdrawal illness uncomfortable, perhaps toxic process whereby the body attempts to maintain homeostasis in the absence of a drug on which it has been physically dependent; also called abstinence syndrome (p. 166).

work movement of mass over distance (p. 67).

Y

yeast single-cell plant responsible for the fermentation of plant products (p. 199).

young adult years segment of the life cycle from ages 18 to 22; a transitional period between adolescence and adulthood (p. 3).

Z

zoophilia sexual contact with animals as a preferred source of sexual excitement (p. 411).

Credits

Chapter 1 pp 1 and 3, FourByFive, Inc; p 5, Rob Nelson, Stock Boston; p 6, Danuta Otfinowski, Archive Pictures, Inc; p 8 *top*, Wilbert Blaine, Taurus Photos; p 8 *bottom*, BI Ullman, Taurus Photos; p 9, Joseph Nettis, Photo Researchers, Inc.

Chapter 2 p 20, FourByFive, Inc; p 22, Lenore Weber, Taurus Photos; p 25, Modified from The Life Cycle Completed, A Review, by Erik H Erikson, by permission of WW Norton & Company, Inc, © 1982 by Rikan Enterprises; p 27, "Hierarchy of needs" from Motivation and personality, by Abraham H Maslow, © 1954, 1970 by Abraham H Maslow, reprinted by permission of Harper & Row, Publishers, Inc; p 28, Constantine Manos, Magnum Photos; p 30, RC Paulson, H Armstrong Roberts, Inc; p 32, Erika Stone, Peter Arnold, Inc; p 33, Peter Menzel, Stock Boston; p 35, N Clevenger, H Armstrong Roberts, Inc.

Chapter 3 p 38, R Mayer, H Armstrong Roberts, Inc; p 40, Michael Hayman, Stock Boston; p 41, Reprinted with permission from Journal of Psychosomatic Research, 2, TH Holmes and RH Rahe: The social adjustment rating scale, © 1967, Pergamon Press, Ltd; p 43, from Lyle H Miller and Alma Dell Smith, Boston University Medical Center; p 45, Alex Von Koschembahr, Photo Researchers, Inc; p 46, JD Sloan, The Picture Cube; p 54, FourByFive, Inc; p 57 *top*, Owen Franken, Stock Boston; p 57 *right*, modified from Friedman, M, and Rosenman, R: Type A behavior and your heart; p 59, D Degnam, H Armstrong Roberts, Inc.

Chapter 4 p 65, Michael Douglas, The Image Works; p 67, Gregg Mancuso, Stock Boston; p 69, J Myers, H Armstrong Roberts, Inc; p 70, Zefa, H Armstrong Roberts, Inc; p 71, From Prentice, WE and Bucher, CA: Fitness for college and life, ed 2, Times Mirror/Mosby College Publishing, 1988; p 74, Krebs/Zefa, H Armstrong Roberts, Inc; p 76, data from the National Fitness Foundation; pp 76-77, Photos by Diana Linsley; p 79, A Hubicu, H Armstrong Roberts, Inc; p 80, Dan Sindelar; p 83, Ellis Herwig, Stock Boston; p 85, Suzanne Wu, Jerobaum, Inc; p 86-87, Copyright 1986, USA Today, excerpted with permission; p 87, art by Donald O'Connor; pp 88 and 94, FourByFive, Inc; p 90, Copyright 1987, USA Today, excerpted with permission; p 91, art by Donald O'Connor; p 95, Taurus Photos.

Chapter 5 p 98, Diana Linsley; p 100 *top*, R Krubner, H Armstrong Roberts, Inc; p 101, Composition of foods, Agriculture Handbook No. 8-4, Washington DC, US Department of Agriculture, 1979, Procter and Gamble; p 102, art by Donald O'Connor; p 103, Stacy Pick, Stock Boston; p 106, Copyright 1986, USA Today, excerpted with permission, art by Donald O'Connor; p 107-109, Federal Register 41-46172 October 19, 1976; p 110, Frank Siteman, The Picture Cube; p 112, Modified from Guthrie, H: Introductory nutrition, ed 7, 1989, Times Mirror/Mosby College Publishing; p 113, adapted from Food and Nutrition Board, National Research Council: Recommended Dietary Allowances, ed 9, Washington, DC, 1980, National Academy of Sciences; p 114, Modified from Hegarty: Decisions in nutrition, 1988, Times Mirror/Mosby College Publishing; p 116-117, © 1987, USA Today, reprinted with permission; p 120, Gardon/Reflexion, H Armstrong Roberts, Inc; p 121, Nancy Dudley, Stock Boston; p 122, data on four food groups from Guthrie, H: Introductory nutrition, ed 7, 1987, Times Mirror/Mosby College Publishing; p 124, Ethan Hoffman, Archive Pictures, Inc; p 125, American Dietetic Association, art by Donald O'Connor.

Chapter 6 p 130, Phillippe Gontier, The Image Works; p 132, Ellis Herwig, The Picture Cube; p 133, Diana Linsley; p 134, Prentice, WE, and Bucher, CA: Fitness for college and life, ed 2, 1988, Times Mirror/Mosby College Publishing; p 135, Metropolitan Life Insurance Company; p 138, Bob Daemmrich, The Image Works; pp 139 H Armstrong Roberts, Inc; p 141, Gary Goodman, The Picture Cube; p 142 and 153, art by Donald O'Connor; p 145, data from Bannister, EW and Brown, SR: The relative energy requirements of physical activity. In HB Falls, editor: Exercise physiology, New York, 1968, Academic Press; Howley, ET and Glover, ME: The caloric costs of running and walking one mile for men and women, Medicine and Science in Sports 6:235, 1974; Passmore, R, and Durnin, JVGA: Human energy expenditure, Physiological Reviews 35:801, 1955; p 146, Philip Jon Bailey, The Picture Cube; p 149, © 1987, USA Today, excerpted with permission, art by Donald O'Connor; p 150 and 151 *top*, From Hegarty, V: Decisions in nutrition, Times Mirror/Mosby Publishing, 1988; p 151 *center*, Andrew Brilliant, The Picture

Cube; p 151 *bottom*, H Armstrong Roberts, Inc; p 152 *bottom*, Frederic Lewis, Inc; p 155, Williams, SR: Nutrition and diet therapy, ed 6, Times Mirror/Mosby Publishing, 1989; p 157, FourByFive, Inc; p 163, Mark Dobson.

Chapter 7 p 164, Adam Hart-Davis, Science Photo Library, Photo Researchers, Inc; pp. 166, 179, 181, and 185, FourByFive, Inc; p 167, Ray Ellis, Photo Researchers, Inc; p 171, art by Donald O'Connor; pp 172-175, © 1987, the Muncie Star, reprinted with permission; p 176, Sources: C Lecos, The latest caffeine scoreboard, FDA Consumer March 1984, p 14, Measuring your life with coffee spoons, Tufs University Diet and Nutrition Letter, April 1984; pp 3-6, Expert Panel on Food Safety and Nutrition, Institute of Food Technologists: Evaluation of caffeine safety, from the Institute of Food Technologists, 221 N LaSalle Street, Chicago, IL 60601, 1986; p 178, Stanley Rowin, The Picture Cube; p. 180, S Ekstrand, H Armstrong Roberts, Inc; p 183, L Lorusso, The Picture Cube; p 187 and 188, Bob Daemmrich, Stock Boston; p 192, Charles Gatewood, The Image Works.

Chapter 8 p 196, Julie Houck, Stock Boston; p 198 *top*, W Keith McManus, Archive Pictures, Inc; p 198 *bottom*, Alen MacWeeney, Archive Pictures, Inc; p 199, from G Heileman Brewing Company, Inc; Lacrosse, WI; p 200, US Department of Health and Human Services: Alcohol and health: fourth special report to the US Congress, Washington, DC 1981, DHHS Pub No ADM 81-1080; p 201, US Department of Transportation, National Highway Safety Administration: Adapted from Alcohol and the impaired driver, (AMA); p 208, From Guthrie, H: Introductory nutrition, ed 7, Times Mirror/Mosby College Publishing, 1989; p 210, Rob Nelson, Stock Boston; p 213 *top*, American Demographics and National Center for Health Statistics; pp 213 *bottom* and 216, H Armstrong Roberts, Inc.; p 217, Copyright 1987, the Muncie Star, reprinted with permission; p 218, GL, French, H Armstrong Roberts, Inc; p 219, Bohdan Hrynewych, Stock Boston; p 221, Nik Kleinberg, Stock Boston.

Chapter 9 p 224, Goersch/Bavaria, H Armstrong Roberts, Inc; p 225, RJ Bennett, H Armstrong Roberts, Inc; p 227, RP Kingston, The Picture Cube; p

228, Martin Rogers, Stock Boston; p 229, Adapted from Statistical Supplement to Federal Trade Commission Report to Congress, 1984, and Smoking and Health Reporter, 2: 4, July 1986; pp 231 and 248, American Cancer Society, Inc; p 232, M Uselmann, H Armstrong Roberts, Inc; p 240, Taurus Photos; p 243, Elizabeth Crews, The Image Works; p 245, Michael O'Brien, Archive Pictures, Inc; p 247, American Health, January/February 1988 and the Muncie Star, 1987, adapted with permission; p 251, National Interagency Council on Smoking and Health; p 252, H Armstrong Roberts, Inc; p 253, Susan Van Etten, The Picture Cube.

Chapter 10 p 260, Zefa, H Armstrong Roberts, Inc; p 264, Peter Saloutos, Photographic Resources; p 265, Billy Barnes, Stock Boston; p 266 and 286, American Heart Association; p 268, Reproduced with permisison, © 1988, American Heart Association: Heart Facts; p 269, FourByFive, Inc; p 270, Ethan Hoffman, Archive Pictures, Inc; p 272, Martin Dohrn, Photo Researchers, Inc; p 274, H Armstrong Roberts, Inc; p 278, Stacy Pick, Stock Boston; pp 280-281, Reproduced with permission, © 1988, American Heart Association: Heart Facts; p 283, Frederic Lewis, Inc, pp 284-285, Michigan Heart Association, reproduced with permission American Heart Association.

Chapter 11 p 290, Keith McManus, Archive Pictures, Inc; p 292, Photo Researchers, Inc; p 294, Burt Glinn, Magnum Photos; pp 295, 296, 297 *top*, 298, 302, 303, and 305, American Cancer Society, Inc; p 297 American Cancer Society, Inc; p 297, Photo Researchers, Inc; pp 299 and 300, American Academy of Dermatology; p 304, Martin Dohrn, Photo Researchers, Inc; pp 308-309, Modified from American Cancer Society, Inc: Cancer: assessing your risks, New York; p 312, K Benser/Zefa, H Armstrong Roberts, Inc; p 313, © 1984, USA Today, Excerpted with permission; 313, Howard Dratch, The Image Works; p 316, Yvonne Freund, Photo Researchers, Inc; p 319, Bill Longcore, Photo Researchers, Inc; p 320, Diana Linsley; p 321, A Teufen, H Armstrong Roberts, Inc; p 322, courtesy of the Arthritis Foundation; p 324, The Picture Cube.

Chapter 12 p 328, Joel Gordon; p 330, Art by Donald O'Connor; p 332, Howard Dratch, The Image Works; p 334, JE

Pasquier-Rapho, Photo Researchers, Inc; p 335 *top*, Artwork by Allen Carroll and Dale Glasgow, © National Geographic Society; p 335 *bottom*, Alex Webb, Magnum Photos, Inc; p 337, FourByFive, Inc; p 341, Jeff Albertson, Stock Boston; p 343, Ellis Herwig, Taurus Photos; p 344, Tom McHugh, Photo Researchers, Inc; pp 347, 348, and 349 *bottom*, Centers for Disease Control, Atlanta; p 349 *top*, Modified from Haas, K and Haas, A: Understanding sexuality, Times Mirror/Mosby College Publishing, 1987; p 351, Centers for Disease Control, Atlanta; p 354, Sam C Pierson, Jr, Photo Researchers, Inc.

Chapter 13 p 360, Elizabeth Crews, The Image Works; p 363, Nancy Sheehan, The Picture Cube; p 366, S Feld, H Armstrong Roberts, Inc; p 367, J Myers, H Armstrong Roberts, Inc; p 378 *left*, Elizabeth Crews, The Image Works; p 378 *right*, Kindra Clineff, The Picture Cube.

Chapter 14 pp 382 and 403, FourByFive, Inc; p 389 and 394, Willie Hill, Jr, The Image Works; p 394, Mikki Ansin, Taurus Photos; p 396, Modified from USA Today; p 397, Lenore Weber, Taurus Photos; p 398, Nancy Ferguson, Photographic Resources; p 401, Suzanne Szasz, Photo Researchers, Inc; p 402, H Armstrong Roberts, Inc; p 404, Haas, K, and Haas, A: Understanding sexuality, Times Mirror/Mosby College Publishing, 1987; p 406, Gerald L French, Frederic Lewis, Inc; p 407, quiz from the joy of being single, by Joyce Harayda, © 1986 by Joyce Harayda, reprinted by permission of Doubleday, Dell Publishing Group, Inc; p 409, Paul Fusco, Magnum Photos; p 410, Owen Franken, Stock Boston; p 416, Tony Schanuel, Photographic Resources.

Chapter 15 pp. 420, 432, 433, 435, 438, 439 *center and bottom*, 400 *top*, 441, and 442, Joel Gordon Photography; p 422, Mike Mazzasche, Stock Boston; p 423, H Armstrong Roberts, Inc; pp 424-425, Lisken, L, et al: Youth in the 1980s: social and health concerns, Population Reports, Series M, No 9, Population Information Program, Johns Hopkins University, November-December, 1985; p 427, Modified from Hatcher, RA, et al: Contraceptive technology: 1986-1987, ed 13, New York, 1986, Irvington Publishers, Inc; pp 434, 437, 439 *top*, and 451, Modified from Denney, N, and Quadagno, D, Human sexuality, Times Mirror/Mosby College Publishing, 1988; pp 440 *bottom* and 447, From Haas, K and Haas, A, Understanding sexuality, Times Mirror/Mosby College Publishing, 1987; p 448, Vernon Doucette, Stock Boston; p 449, Tomas Sennett, Magnum Photos; p 450, Erika Stone, Photo Researchers, Inc.

Chapter 16 pp 456 and 471, H Armstrong Roberts, Inc; p 461, Francis Leroy, Photo Researchers, Inc; p 462, Petite Format/Nestle/Science Source, Photo Researchers, Inc; p 464, courtesy of Washington University Medical School; p 465, Rob Nelson, Picture Group; p 472, Erika Stone, Photo Researchers, Inc; p 473, David Madison; p 475, From Denney, N, and Quadagno, D, Human sexuality, Times Mirror/Mosby College Publishing, 1988; p 476, John Griffin, The Image Works; p 479, Howard Dratch, The Image Works.

Chapter 17 p 484, Dan Sindelar; p 486, data from Health care practices and perceptions: highlights of a consumer survey of self medication, Washington, DC, 1984, Proprietary Association; p 487, from Marion Laboratories, Inc; Pharmaceutical Division, Kansas City, MO; p 488, from Cornacchia, HJ, and Barrett, S: Consumer health: a guide to intelligent decision making; ed 4, St Louis, Times Mirror/Mosby College Publishing; pp 490 and 515, FourByFive, Inc; p 492 and 493 *right*, Mark Antman, The Image Works; p 494, Grace Moore, Medichrome/Stock Shop; p 497, James Holland, Stock Boston; p 498, John Griffin, The Image Works; pp 500-501, From Fuerst, ML: Home diagnostic tests: self-help health? Generics, 2:42-44; July, 1986; p 502, Modified from Farley, D: Do-it-yourself medical testing, FDA Consumer, 20:22-28, February, 1986; p 510 *top*, Martin Rotker, Taurus Photos; p. 513 from Subak-Sharpe, GJ (editor): The physicians manual for patients, by the Biomedical Information Corporation, © 1984, reprinted by permission of Random House, Inc; p 514, The Image Works.

Chapter 18 p 520, S Feld, H Armstrong Roberts, Inc; p 522, Shostal Associates; p 523, Michael O'Brien, Archive Pictures, Inc; p 524, © 1987 Time Inc, all rights reserved, reprinted by permission from TIME; p 529, H Armstrong Roberts, Inc; p 530, Photo Media, H Armstrong Roberts, Inc; p 531 *top*, Carlin, The Picture Cube; p 531 *bottom*, Ellis Herwig, The Picture Cube; p 532, art by Donald O'Connor; p 534, F Siteman, Photographic Resources; p 536, P Degginger, H Armstrong Roberts, Inc; p 537, art by Donald O'Connor; pp 538 and 544, modified from Miller, G, © 1988,

Living in the environment, ed 5, Belmont, CA, Wadsworth Publishing Co; p 539 adapted by permission of Practical Homeowner magazine, formerly New Shelter, © Rodale Press, Inc, all rights reserved; p 540, John Running, Stock Boston; p 541, modified from American Academy of Otolaryngology, Head and Neck Surgery: Noise, ears, and hearing, 1985, Washington, DC; p 543 *top*, David Burnett, Contact Press Images; p 543 *bottom*, Ken Regan, Camera 5; p 545 *left*, from National Wildlife Federation, 1985, conservation directory ed 30, Washington, DC; p 546, logos courtesy of The Wilderness Society, USDA, Forest Service, and Sierra Club; Greenpeace logo courtesy of Greenpeace USA, a nonprofit, environmental organization, 1436 U Street, NW, Washington, DC 20009; Cousteau Society logo used with permission of the Cousteau Society, a nonprofit, membership-supported organization, dedicated to the improvement of the quality of life.

Chapter 19 p 552, Frank Oberle, Photographic Resources; pp 553 and 560, FourByFive, Inc; p 554, US Census Bureau; p 555, Lou Harris and Associates, Inc, survey conducted for The Commonwealth Fund Commission on Elderly People Living Alone; p 556, Statistical Bulletin, 1987; pp 557, 568, 573, and 575, Photographic Resources; p 558, K Benser/Zefa, H Armstrong Roberts, Inc; p 559, David Madison; p 565, From The Facts on Aging Quiz, by Erdman Palmore © 1988, Springer Publishing Company, New York, used by permission; p 570, Charles Harbutt, Archive Pictures, Inc; p 571, Bob Daemmrich, Stock Boston; p 576, Glennon Donahue, Photographic Resources.

Chapter 20 p 580, H Abernathy, H Armstrong Roberts, Inc; p 582, JL Anderson, H Armstrong Roberts, Inc; p 584 and 585, Reprinted with permission from Concern for Dying, 250 W 57th Street, New York, NY, 10107; p 586 *top*, Inside America; p 589, J Myers, H Armstrong Roberts, Inc; p 591, Burt Glinn, Magnum Photos, Inc; p 594, A Webb, Magnum Photos, Inc; p 595, Leonard Freed, Magnum Photos, Inc; p 596, From Blumenthal, SJ: Suicide: a guide to risk factors: assessment and treatment of suicidal patients, Medical Clinics of North America, 72:937-971, 1988; p 597, Harry Wilks, Stock Boston; p 598, from Nation Kidney Foundation, Inc, New York, NY; p 599, J Bowman, Meeks Mortuary, Muncie, IN; p 601, Eastcott/Momatiuk, The Image Works.

Appendix 3 p A13, Statistics Canada; p A14, *top*; Canada Fitness Survey, 1983; *bottom*: Statistics Canada, from February 1978 Survey on selected leisure time activities, Education, Science, and Culture Division, adapted from Ouellet, B: Health field indicators, Canada and provinces, 1979, Health and Welfare Canada, 1979; p A15, Statistics Canada, from MacGregor, Betty, Alcohol consumption in Canada—some preliminary findings of a national survey in November-December 1976, adapted from Ouellet B: Health field indicators, Canada and provinces, Health and Welfare Canada, 1979; p A16, *top*, Statistics Canada, The control and sale of alcohol beverages in Canada 1980 and 1981, Statistics Canada Catalogue No 63-202, 1982-1986; *bottom*, Statistics Canada, The control and sale of alcohol beverages in Canada 1980 and 1981, Statistics Canada Catalogue No 63-202, 1982 and 1983, Statistics Canada Daily Catalogue 11-001, August 2, 1984; p A17, *top*; Statistics Canada, 1976, *bottom*; Statistics Canada, Labour force survey supplement, 1985; p A18, *top*: Statistics Canada, Causes of death, Catalogue 84-203, 1977, adapted from Ouellet, B, Romeder, JM, and Lance, JM: Premature mortality attributable to smoking and hazardous drinking in Canada, volume 1: summary, volume 2: detailed calculations, Health and Welfare Canada, 1977; *bottom*: Statistics Canada; p A19, *top*, Statistics Canada, Vital statistics: marriages and divorces, Catalogue 84-205; *bottom*, Statistics Canada, 1941 Census of Canada, vol I, 1951 Census of Canada, vol 3, 1956 Census of Canada, vol 1, 1961 Census of Canada, Catalogue 93-516, 1966 Census of Canada, Catalogue 93-608, 1971 Census of Canada, Catalogue 93-718, 1976 Census of Canada, Catalogue 93-809; p A20, *top*, Statistics Canada, Courtney, Heeler, Hustad, and Zarry: Investigation of use and reasons for use of non-prescription drugs, report D: National purchase diary, for CH & Z Ltd, 1974, adapted from McWhinnie, JR, Ouellet, B, and Lance, JM: Health field indicators, Canada and provinces, 1976; *bottom*, Statistics Canada, Mortality, Catalogue 84-206, 1982; A21, Statistics Canada, Causes of death, Catalogue No 84-203; A22, Statistics Canada, Mortality, Catalogue 84-206, 1982 issue, March 1984.

Appendix 5 Terry Cockerham, Synapse Media Productions, Dallas, Tx, illustrations by Cynthia Turner, Alexander & Turner, Santa Rosa Beach, Fla.